# Tissue Engineering and Regeneration in Dentistry

# Tissue Engineering and Regeneration in Dentistry

Editor: Lawrence Davis

AMERICAN
MEDICAL PUBLISHERS
www.americanmedicalpublishers.com

AMERICAN
MEDICAL PUBLISHERS
www.americanmedicalpublishers.com

**Cataloging-in-Publication Data**

Tissue engineering and regeneration in dentistry / edited by Lawrence Davis.
p. cm.
Includes bibliographical references and index.
ISBN 978-1-63927-062-0
1. Dental materials. 2. Tissue engineering. 3. Dentistry--Methodology.
4. Periodontium--Regeneration. 5. Regenerative medicine. I. Davis, Lawrence.
RK320.T47 T57 2022
617.634 059 2--dc23



American Medical Publishers,
41 Flatbush Avenue,
1st Floor, New York,
NY 11217, USA

ISBN 978-1-63927-062-0 (Hardback)

# Contents

# Preface

This book aims to highlight the current researches and provides a platform to further the scope of innovations in this area. This book is a product of the combined efforts of many researchers and scientists, after going through thorough studies and analysis from different parts of the world. The objective of this book is to provide the readers with the latest information of the field.

The specialty within biomedical engineering which makes use of engineering, cells and materials methods as well as physicochemical factors is termed as tissue engineering. It seeks to restore, improve, maintain or replace diverse types of biological tissues. Regenerative medicine is a branch of medicine which focuses on regenerating, replacing or engineering human cells and tissues to restore normal function. Tissue engineering and regenerative medicine are used to design dental therapies to repair, restore and regenerate dental tissues. Research is being conducted in this field to regenerate single dental tissues such as the pulp or dentine. This book traces the progress of this field and highlights some of the key concepts and applications of tissue engineering and regenerative medicine in dentistry. It strives to provide a fair idea about this discipline and to help develop a better understanding of the latest advances within this field. As this field is emerging at a rapid pace, the contents of this book will help the readers understand the modern concepts and applications of the subject.

I would like to express my sincere thanks to the authors for their dedicated efforts in the completion of this book. I acknowledge the efforts of the publisher for providing constant support. Lastly, I would like to thank my family for their support in all academic endeavors.

**Editor**

1

# Dental pulp stem cells as a multifaceted tool for bioengineering and the regeneration of craniomaxillofacial tissues

**Edited by:**
Thimios Mitsiadis,
University of Zurich, Switzerland

***Correspondence:**
Fernando Unda
fernando.unda@ehu.eus;
Gaskon Ibarretxe
gaskon.ibarretxe@ehu.eus

† These authors have contributed equally to this work.

*Maitane Aurrekoetxea †, Patricia Garcia-Gallastegui †, Igor Irastorza, Jon Luzuriaga, Verónica Uribe-Etxebarria, Fernando Unda * and Gaskon Ibarretxe **

*Department of Cell Biology and Histology, Faculty of Medicine and Dentistry, University of the Basque Country, Leioa, Spain*

Dental pulp stem cells, or DPSC, are neural crest-derived cells with an outstanding capacity to differentiate along multiple cell lineages of interest for cell therapy. In particular, highly efficient osteo/dentinogenic differentiation of DPSC can be achieved using simple *in vitro* protocols, making these cells a very attractive and promising tool for the future treatment of dental and periodontal diseases. Among craniomaxillofacial organs, the tooth and salivary gland are two such cases in which complete regeneration by tissue engineering using DPSC appears to be possible, as research over the last decade has made substantial progress in experimental models of partial or total regeneration of both organs, by cell recombination technology. Moreover, DPSC seem to be a particularly good choice for the regeneration of nerve tissues, including injured or transected cranial nerves. In this context, the oral cavity appears to be an excellent testing ground for new regenerative therapies using DPSC. However, many issues and challenges need yet to be addressed before these cells can be employed in clinical therapy. In this review, we point out some important aspects on the biology of DPSC with regard to their use for the reconstruction of different craniomaxillofacial tissues and organs, with special emphasis on cranial bones, nerves, teeth, and salivary glands. We suggest new ideas and strategies to fully exploit the capacities of DPSC for bioengineering of the aforementioned tissues.

**Keywords: DPSC, differentiation, tooth, bone, salivary gland, nerve, cell therapy**

## INTRODUCTION: DPSC AND TISSUE ENGINEERING OF THE ORAL CAVITY

The oral cavity is a complex multi-organic structure. Because oral tissues and organs are functionally connected at many levels, irreversible damage to any of them is likely to eventually affect the others, causing extensive malfunction. Tooth decay, periodontal disease, alveolar bone resorption, orthodontic problems, orofacial neuropathic pain, and impaired salivary gland function are conditions that seriously affect oral health of a large part of the world population. Owing to their functional connectivity, once damage is diagnosed to one organ of the oral cavity it is important to intervene rapidly and efficiently, to repair or replace the injured or lost tissues, to avoid severe degradation of oral health.

Synthetic replacement materials and prostheses (fillings, bridges, implants, etc.) have traditionally been the treatment of choice to treat dental decay. However, all functions of the original biological tooth are not fully restored by this kind of replacement therapies. Other organs of the oral cavity (e.g., nerves, salivary glands) are simply not amenable to mechanical substitution approaches. Thus, tissue engineering represents a new collection of treatment options for the complete biological regeneration of craniomaxillofacial tissues and organs. The development of this field requires three essential components: (i) stem cells, (ii) biomaterial scaffolds, and (iii) stimulating factors or inductive signals. Tissue engineering is now fully considered as an alternative to the conventional treatments for dental injury and disease, offering substantial advantages over traditional dental restoration techniques (Nör, 2006; Wang et al., 2012).

Stem cells are the cornerstone of regenerative cell therapy. An enormous variety of multipotent stem cells have been isolated and studied from different human tissues, such as the bone marrow (Ding and Morrison, 2013), adipose tissue (Kapur et al., 2015), skin (Blanpain and Fuchs, 2009), and the umbilical cord (Yan et al., 2013; Kalaszczynska and Ferdin, 2015). Among them, mesenchymal stem cells (MSC) are the most promising for clinical purposes (Rastegar et al., 2010; Ménard and Tarte, 2013). In the oral cavity, adult tooth tissues also contain different active populations of stem cells with mesenchymal phenotype (Huang et al., 2009). Unlike other types of MSC, dental stem cells originate from the neural crest (Janebodin et al., 2011) and are lineage-related with peripheral nerve glial progenitor cells (Kaukua et al., 2014), which places them in a privileged position to mediate regeneration of both connective and nerve tissues (Ibarretxe et al., 2012; Martens et al., 2013). Several types of human dental stem cells have been identified. Among them; DFPC, Dental Follicle progenitor cells; PDLSC, Periodontal ligament stem cell; SCAP, Stem cells from apical papilla; SHED, Stem cells from primary exfoliated deciduous teeth; DPSC, Dental pulp stem cells, which are without a doubt the most used for research purposes (**Figure 1**). Although it still remains a considerable challenge to obtain all the different types of neuronal and glial cells from DPSC, their differentiation to specialized connective tissue cells has proven to be relatively simple. Efficient protocols for obtaining adipocytes, chondroblasts and osteo/odontoblasts are firmly established in the literature (Gronthos et al., 2002; Huang et al., 2009; Kawashima, 2012).

In this review, we summarize the current understanding of DPSC and their capacity to regenerate injured orofacial tissues, with special focus on the teeth and associated periodontal tissues, peripheral cranial nerves, and the salivary glands. We present the different strategies used in experimental restorative models with potential applications in dentistry and oral medicine, together with the different scaffold biomaterials and stimulating factor combinations employed to elicit an optimal cellular response required to regenerate damaged tissues. We critically comment on some crucial aspects to be considered for bioengineering and the regeneration of each of these tissues, based on our own research experience.

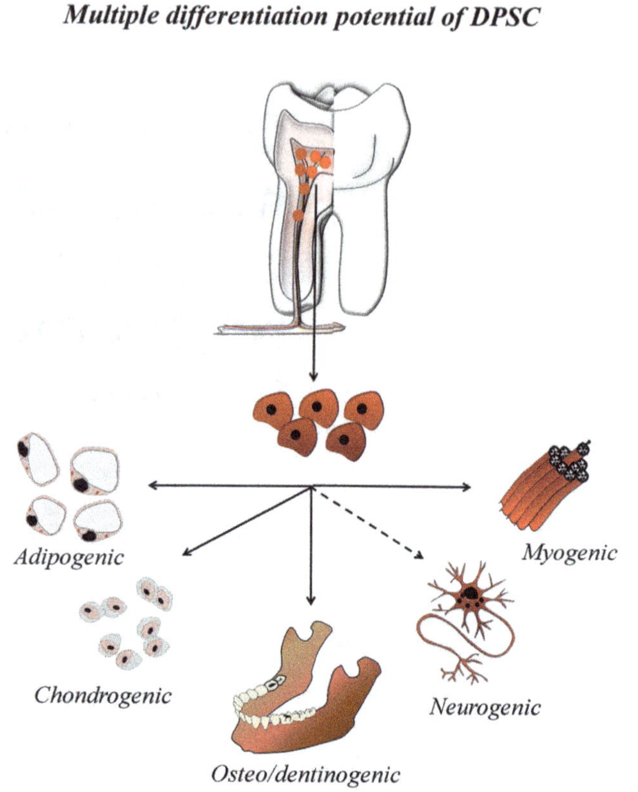


**FIGURE 1 | Multiple differentiation potential of DPSC.** DPSC are isolated from the adult dental pulp and can be *in vitro* expanded and differentiated to multiple cell lineages, including all connective tissue-lineages and some neural cell lineages.

## DPSC FOR BONE REGENERATION

Regeneration of maxillary and mandibular bone is fundamental in the field of implantology (Lee et al., 2014). Osteogenic differentiation of DPSC is easily induced *in vitro* by adding ascorbic acid (Asc), dexamethasone (Dexa), and β-glycerophosphate (β-gly) to the culture medium, along with fetal bovine serum (Laino et al., 2005; Langenbach and Handschel, 2013). Asc is an essential enzyme cofactor to generate pro-collagen (Vater et al., 2011), which is necessary for the correct synthesis of Collagen type I, the main organic component of the bone matrix. Dexa is required for osteoblast differentiation, working as Runx2 inductor by activating WNT/β-catenin signaling in MSC (Hamidouche et al., 2008). Runx2 transcription factor expression is fundamental in driving cellular commitment to osteogenic lineages. Finally, β-gly is a donor of inorganic phosphate, which is essential for creating hydroxyapatite mineral, and as a signaling molecule to induce DPSC osteo-differentiation (Foster et al., 2006; Fatherazi et al., 2009; Tada et al., 2011).

The application of this differentiation cocktail is highly effective in inducing DPSC to generate a mineralized bone-like extracellular matrix *in vitro*. When DPSC are exposed to this differentiation cocktail for 7–21 days, they start to strongly express different osteoblast differentiation markers, such as Osterix, Runx2, osteocalcin, and bone sialoprotein. Alkaline phosphatase (ALP), and Alizarin red staining are positive under these conditions, and are used to demonstrate effective differentiation of DPSC to functional osteoblasts, and the generation of a calcified hydroxyapatite (HA)-containing extracellular matrix (Mangano et al., 2010; Yu et al., 2010; Li et al., 2011). DPSC-derived osteoblasts are phenotypically and functionally similar to normal primary osteoblasts, although some differences remain in terms of their gene expression profiles (Carinci et al., 2008). Naïve undifferentiated DPSC are negative for the adult osteo/odontoblast differentiation marker Osterix, but nevertheless exhibit detectable levels of Runx2, suggesting they are primed or pre-committed to differentiate to osteo/odontoblasts (Yu et al., 2010). When the osteogenic differentiation cocktail is added to DPSC, Runx2, and Osterix expression increase and these cells generate extracellular calcified bone-like matrix nodules, that stain distinctively and positively with Alizarin red (Laino et al., 2005; **Figure 2**).

In the last few years the use of DPSC for *in vivo* bone regeneration by tissue engineering has been extensively studied by relying on these protocols and using different experimental models and types of scaffolds with different results (Morad et al., 2013). Woven bone chips obtained by human DPSC (hDPSC) osteoinduction are able to induce the generation of adult bone tissue with an integral blood supply, when they are heterotopically transplanted in immune-compromised (IC) animals (d'Aquino et al., 2007). However, the use of scaffolding materials is often necessary to optimize the 3D structure of the formed bone tissue and enhance the osteoblastic differentiation of hDPSC. To this end, different materials have been successfully employed as a vehicle of hDPSC, including 3D gelatin scaffolds (Li et al., 2011), self-assembling biodegradable peptide nanofiber hydrogels (Chan et al., 2011), CaP/PLGA (calcium phosphate/polylactic-co-glycolic acid) scaffolds (Graziano et al., 2008a,b), particulate hydroxyapatite/tricalcium phosphate (HA/TCP) ceramic scaffolds (Zhang et al., 2008), and natural scaffolds like biocoral (Mangano et al., 2011) and chitosan/collagen (Yang et al., 2011). Finally, alginate and PuraMatrix™ hydrogels also provide a three dimensional (3D) biodegradable carrier of stem cells for bone tissue engineering purposes, with the additional large advantage that these formulations are injectable, forming 3D hydrogels upon contact with the physiological environment and thus completely filling the tissue lesion, with minimally invasive dental and orthopedic surgeries. Dental stem cells encapsulated in either alginate or PuraMatrix™ exhibited high capacities for osteo-differentiation both *in vitro* and *in vivo* (Misawa et al., 2006; Cavalcanti et al., 2013; Moshaverinia et al., 2013).

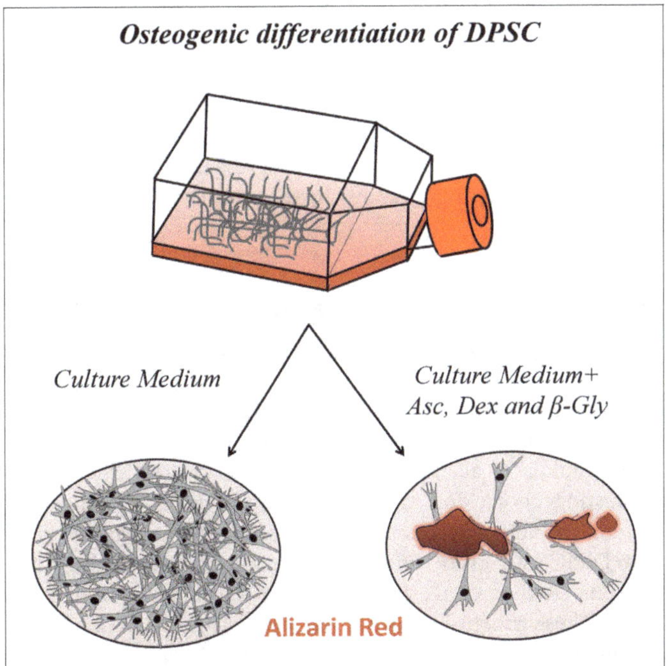


**FIGURE 2 | Osteogenic differentiation of DPSC.** In the presence of a three-ingredient cocktail containing dexamethasone, β-glycerophosphate and ascorbate added to the culture medium for 7 days, DPSC differentiate to osteoblast-like cells that generate a mineralized bone tissue matrix that stains positively for Alizarin red.

Inductive signals also play a critical role to stimulate development of new bone tissue. The development of a well-defined, safe, and controlled technique to obtain and locally deliver growth factors derived from autologous plasma has provided a powerful tool to enhance bone tissue regeneration, which has been successfully implemented in the clinical practice (Anitua et al., 2008, 2012). Formulations such as Platelet-rich plasma (PRP), Platelet-rich fibrin (PRF), and Plasma rich in growth factors (PRGF) provide a biologically enriched culture medium for the stimulation and functional differentiation of primary cells with latent regenerative potential. Several studies have shown that PRGF in particular provides additional benefits for bone regeneration (Paknejad et al., 2012; Rivera et al., 2013). It has been reported that PRP and PRGF induce proliferation and enhance osteogenic differentiation in SHEDs, DPSCs, and PDLSCs (Lee et al., 2011). Other studies have used recombinant human Bone morphogenetic protein 2 (rhBMP-2) to enhance osteogenic differentiation of DPSC in animal models of alveolar bone reconstruction (Liu et al., 2011). The use of rhBMP-2 is approved and widely extended to perform maxillary sinus floor augmentation in dental practice (Nazirkar et al., 2014; Freitas et al., 2015).

Despite a large body of preclinical evidence, very few clinical trials have still been performed to evaluate new advanced therapeutic medicinal products (ATMP) for bone regeneration based on DPSC (La Noce et al., 2014). A notable exception is one clinical trial performed with seven patients to repair mandibular bone defects by transplant of DPSC in a collagen scaffold (d'Aquino et al., 2009). After 3 years of follow-up, the clinical outcomes were positive (Giuliani et al., 2013). However, several obstacles remain, including a changing regulatory framework, a shortage of technology for automation of cell production by Good manufacturing practice (GMP) standards, a non-alignment between academic and industrial research, and a need for long-term product follow-up (La Noce et al., 2014; Leijten et al., 2015).

These limitations have hampered the emergence of DPSC as a tool to enhance bone regeneration at clinical level.

## DPSC FOR DENTAL PULP REGENERATION

Caries and root fracture are the cause of approximately fifty percent of all tooth extractions. Tooth injuries such as pulp exposure, deep caries and irreversible pulpitis are currently treated by endodontics and dental refilling/reconstruction. This procedure usually entails the amputation or entire removal of the dental pulp and replacement of the tissue with an inert material. Root fracture and tooth loss are closely related to this loss of pulp vitality because innervation and vasculature affect pulp homeostasis and root dentin regeneration. The regeneration of pulp injuries has become a goal for functional tooth restoration in dentistry (Nakashima and Akamine, 2005; Nakashima et al., 2009).

The first research reports on DPSC showed that these cells present optimal characteristics to attain functional regeneration of the dental-pulp chamber. Xenogenic transplant of HA/TCP scaffolds with hDPSC into the dermis of IC mice resulted in the formation of pulp-like tissue and polarized odontoblasts that produced tubular dentin, showing that dentinogenic differentiation was one of the prime or default programs established in the DPSC phenotype (Gronthos et al., 2000, 2002). Recently, more refined studies combining SHED with injectable scaffolds (Puramatrix™ and rhCollagen type I) have demonstrated that dental stem cells are not only kept alive when injected into human premolar root canals *in vivo*, but are also able to fully reconstruct vascularized pulp tissue throughout the root canal, and to differentiate to DSPP and DMP-expressing odontoblasts that generate new dentin (Rosa et al., 2013). In a similar experimental design, other authors employed combinations of DPSC and umbilical vein endothelial cells embedded in Puramatrix™ scaffold, to improve vascularization and angiogenesis of *de novo* formed dental pulp-like tissue (Dissanayaka et al., 2015).

Other studies have focused on the regenerative potential of different cytokines and growth factors, with the goal to improve cellular chemotaxis and cell homing into the emptied dental pulp space *in vivo*. Different combinations of cytokines and growth factors which included basic Fibroblast growth factor (bFGF), Platelet derived growth factor (PDGF), or Vascular endothelial growth factor (VEGF) in the presence of basal levels of Nerve growth factor (NGF) and BMP-7 were effective in regenerating a revascularized and recellularized dental pulp-like tissue integrated into endodontically-treated root canal dentinal walls *in vivo* (Kim et al., 2010). In addition, it has been shown that bFGF and Stromal-derived factor (SDF1) also exert a potent chemotactic recruitment on DPSC, while BMP-7 induces their differentiation (Suzuki et al., 2011). In a recent study, SDF1 loaded onto silk-fibroin scaffolds promoted the complete regeneration and revascularization of the dental pulp of mature dog teeth that had been subjected to endodontic treatment *in situ* (Yang et al., 2015), suggesting a promising future for the functional reconstruction of dental pulp tissue in next generation dentistry.

## DPSC FOR COMPLETE DENTAL REGENERATION

In 2009, a ground-breaking report was published by the group of T. Tsuji on the generation of complete and fully functional teeth by combining isolated mouse dental epithelial and MSC (Ikeda et al., 2009). More recently, in 2011, the same research group developed a complete tooth unit consisting of a mature tooth, periodontal ligament and alveolar bone, using a similar recombination technique (Oshima et al., 2011). These tooth units were transplanted into toothless mouse jaw regions *in vivo*, and erupted correctly and in occlusion. They also presented an adequate dental structure, an adequate hardness of enamel and dentin, a proper function of the periodontal ligament, a positive alveolar bone remodeling response to orthodontic forces, and a positive response to noxious stimuli such as mechanical stress and pain.

Although precise replication of these results has not yet been reported on the literature, the aforementioned work represents a substantial advance in stem cell combination technology, with the potential to develop completely new bioengineered replacement organs for next generation regenerative therapy. One of the main limitations to date is probably the lack of consistent sources of epithelial cells that can be combined with dental mesenchymal cells (DPSC or others) to generate a complete bioengineered tooth germ. The team of T. Tsuji employed embryonic mouse tooth germ epithelia as precursors of the enamel organ, a structure that fully disappears in adult teeth. In the search for dental-competent sources of epithelial stem cells, some authors have reported success using adult gingival epithelial cells, which upon recombination with mesenchymal cells generate mature teeth and form enamel and dentin (Angelova Volponi et al., 2013). Other authors have employed iPS-derived cells to generate mature bioengineered teeth by similar recombination methods (Wen et al., 2012; Cai et al., 2013; Otsu et al., 2014). The substantial progress made in the field of dental bioengineering warrants further research on this line for the next years.

## DPSC FOR REGENERATION OF NERVE TISSUE AND DAMAGED CRANIAL NERVES

DSPC originate from the neural crest (Janebodin et al., 2011) and share a common origin with peripheral nerve glial progenitor cells (Kaukua et al., 2014). These features make DPSC a very interesting choice for regeneration of the peripheral nervous system, including nerves of the oral cavity. Some reports claim that DPSC can even differentiate to functionally active adult neurons (Arthur et al., 2008; Kiraly et al., 2009; Gervois et al., 2015). These conclusions are based on the acquisition of neuron-specific gene and protein markers by DPSC, and also on their capacity to generate neuronal-like voltage-dependent sodium and calcium currents, and action potential-like membrane voltage oscillations. However, it should be noted that to date there has been no definite proof of differentiation of DPSC to genuine neurons that can exhibit repetitive firing of action potentials upon electrical stimulation, and establish synapses showing functional plasticity as identified by transmission electron microscopy (TEM).

However, it is undeniable that DPSC present some striking similarities with neural stem cells. When DPSC are grown in culture conditions lacking fetal serum, they reorganize morphologically and switch from a uniform cell monolayer to a more quiescent state characterized by the appearance of prominent spheroid structures that resemble CNS-derived neurospheres which stain positively for the neural stem cell marker Nestin (Ibarretxe et al., 2012; Bonnamain et al., 2013; Xiao and Tsutsui, 2013; Gervois et al., 2015; **Figure 3**). Migratory cells are occasionally observed to leave the DPSC spheroids and virtually all these cells express the neuron-lineage marker β3-tubulin. Moreover, their morphology is in some cases surprisingly similar to migratory neuroblasts, with a long and thin leading process terminated by a prominent growth cone, and a trailing cell body displaying a few short cytoplasmic processes (Marín et al., 2006). However, a note of caution should be added: another cell type of the dental pulp, the odontoblast, is also characterized by the expression of Nestin, the generation of voltage-dependent Na+ currents, and a similar morphology (Fujita et al., 2006; Ichikawa et al., 2012). The DPSC population grown in these conditions is fairly heterogeneous, both morphologically and physiologically, with a range of different morphologies from fibroblast-like to neuroblast-like cells, and also a variable rate of response to stimulation with neurotransmitter receptor agonists.

Regardless of the debate on the true capacity of DPSC to differentiate to neurons and other neural cell lineages, there is little doubt that these cells could be a very interesting choice to repair injured nerve tissues as a result of their active secretion of neurotrophic and immune-modulatory factors (Nosrat et al., 2004; Pierdomenico et al., 2005). The high expression of certain neural markers and neurotransmitter receptors by DPSC also suggests that these cells may actively respond to signals of the neural environment and effectively integrate into injured nerve tissues, promoting the reestablishment of functional nerve connectivity (Arthur et al., 2009; Kadar et al., 2009; Kiraly et al., 2009). For instance, some recent reports show that transplanted DPSC are able to differentiate *in vivo* to myelinating cells in the spinal cord, replacing lost cells and promoting regeneration of transected axons in acute models of spinal cord injury (Sakai et al., 2012).

In the case of the peripheral nerve system, treatment of nerve injuries represents a clinical challenge because of the difficulties of regenerating transected nerves. Though numerous surgical successes have been reported with a short nerve gap, there is still no satisfactory technique for long nerve defects, which often require a complex clinical reconstruction. Autologous nerve grafting has been considered the gold standard for repairing peripheral nerve gaps caused by traffic accidents or tumor resectioning (Kumar and Hassan, 2002; Hayashi and Maruyama, 2005; Bae et al., 2006). However, this technique has inevitable disadvantages, such as a limited supply of available nerve grafts and permanent loss of the sacrificed donor nerve function. Brain-derived neural progenitor cells also promote regeneration of

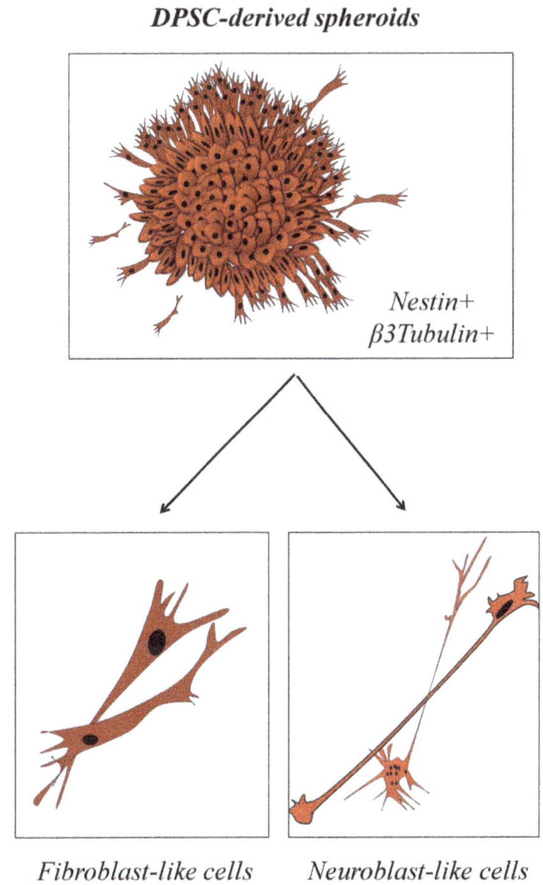


**FIGURE 3 | Neurosphere-like properties of DPSC-derived spheroids. (Top)** DPSC grown in serum-devoid conditions rearrange to form characteristic spheroids that stain positive for neural stem cell markers. **(Bottom)** Migratory cells outside of the spheroids express some neuronal markers and present a variable morphology, with either fibroblast-like or neuroblast-like features.

transected nerves (Murakami et al., 2003). However, the use of cells from other neural tissues involves potentially serious clinical complications along with ethical considerations.

Taking all these arguments into account, there is an active search for new sources of cells to be used in craniofacial nerve bridging and regeneration. Considerable advances have been made in this field using DPSC for the treatment of facial nerve injuries. Particularly, patients with facial paralysis, especially younger ones, may experience tremendous psychosocial distress about their condition (Chan and Byrne, 2011). Recent studies have used DPSC transplanted in PLGA tube scaffolds to achieve a complete functional regeneration of the facial nerve in rats to recovery levels comparable to those obtained with peripheral nerve autografts (Sasaki et al., 2011, 2014). Interestingly, recent research also indicates that hDPSC can be differentiated to Schwann-like cells that efficiently myelinate DRG neuron axons *in vitro*, a finding confirmed by ultrastructural TEM analysis (Martens et al., 2014). Considering the important role that Schwann cells play in axonal protection and regeneration of peripheral nerves (Walsh and Midha, 2009), and the difficulty of their harvesting and maintenance, the generation of DPSC-derived autologous Schwann cells may represent a milestone in the design of new treatments for conditions of peripheral nerve injury, including facial paralysis.

Finally, another important property of DPSC is their active secretion of neurotrophic factors (Nosrat et al., 2004; Bray et al., 2014), which may be exploited to treat neuropathic pain states associated with peripheral nerve injury. In the case of orofacial pain, some of the most distressing and painful conditions that can be experienced by a human being are neuralgias affecting the trigeminal nerve, or CN V. These are characterized by intense stabbing pain and spasms, usually associated with a mechanical injury, compression, demyelination and inflammation of trigeminal sensory fibers (Love and Coakham, 2001; Sabalys et al., 2013). It is known that local application of Glial derived neurotrophic factor (GDNF) exerts a potent analgesic effect and reverses the symptoms associated with neuropathic pain (Boucher et al., 2000). Because DPSC secrete important amounts of GDNF, it is conceivable that autologous DPSC transplantation to the injured trigeminal nerve may also potentially provide important benefits to treat severe orofacial pain disorders, alone or in combination with pharmacological enhancers of GDNF signaling (Hedstrom et al., 2014), some of which are even formulated to permit topical application.

## DPSC FOR SALIVARY GLAND REGENERATION

Salivary gland regeneration is an area of intense research because the most common treatment for head and neck cancer (i.e., radiotherapy) irreversibly affects salivary gland function, causing hyposalivation and xerostomia. In consequence, difficulty in mastication, swallowing, taste, speech, rampant dental caries and mucosa infections appear, leading to high discomfort in patients and a reduced quality of life (Vissink et al., 2010). Palliative treatments such as mechanical stimulation of salivary gland activity (chewing gum), or pharmacological agents such as pilocarpine (Salagen™), as well as saliva substitutes, show a limited efficacy in relieving the symptoms (Taylor, 2003).

Tissue engineering of a salivary gland replacement organ would be a conclusive way to treat these patients. To accomplish this complex task, there are some issues that must be taken into account: (i) optimization of the 3D scaffold material properties (including non-toxicity, permeability and biodegradability, among others), (ii) identification of an epithelial stem cell population capable of appropriate salivary differentiation (iii) definition of ideal culture conditions and extracellular matrix components (ECM) with laminin, integrins, MMPs to mimic the microenvironment of the gland, and (iv) selection of a population of MSC to be combined with salivary epithelial cells to generate a full bioengineered salivary gland germ. Finally, in comparison with dental bioengineering, salivary gland bioengineering presents an important additional requirement: apart from the communication between the epithelium and the mesenchyme, epithelial-axonal interactions are also required from the very beginning of salivary gland morphogenesis, because innervation plays an important role in regulating the activity of epithelial progenitor cells (Knox et al., 2010) and salivary gland branching and tubulogenesis (Nedvetsky et al., 2014). Therefore, salivary gland bioengineering strategies must also take into account that this is an organ that heavily relies on the establishment of a functional innervation to properly complete its development (Lombaert et al., 2011; Knosp et al., 2012).

Some studies indicate that isolated mouse salivary gland stem cells (cKit+, CK14+, Msi-1+, and Sca-1+) can grow and form salispheres that produce amylase (Lombaert et al., 2008). Moreover, injection of a liquid suspension containing only 300–400 cKit+ cells into the mouse SMG was shown to partially rescue the loss of morphology and function induced by irradiation insults (Lombaert et al., 2008; Coppes and Stokman, 2011; Nanduri et al., 2013). In recent years, the technology to generate salivary gland organoids *in vitro* has progressed remarkably. Recent major advances in the field include the advent of bioengineered glands constructed from dissociated cells from adult and fetal salivary glands (Ogawa et al., 2013; Nanduri et al., 2014). An important study by the group of T. Tsuji showed that the bioengineered salivary glands generated by a cell recombination protocol contained epithelium, mesenchyme, endothelium, and nerve cells. Most importantly, the entire organ could be transplanted into adult mice, reconnect with the existing ductal system and function properly (Ogawa et al., 2013; Ogawa and Tsuji, 2015). Thus, the salivary gland joins the tooth in the list of organs that can be fully generated *ex vivo* by tissue engineering. As in the case of the tooth, the main challenge to translate these findings to clinical practice is still the need for sources of stem cells that are sufficiently abundant and competent for salivary epithelial differentiation, and that do not involve destruction of donor salivary gland tissue.

In the search for stem cell sources to be employed in salivary gland bioengineering, some progress has been recently made using DPSC. It has been shown that DPSC contribute to the generation of salisphere-like structures when combined with Human salivary gland (HSG) cell lines in either Matrigel™ or hyaluronic acid hydrogel scaffolds (Janebodin and Reyes, 2012). These salispheres expressed markers of terminally differentiated acinar cells, and generated a well-irrigated salivary gland-like tissue after subcutaneous transplantation in IC mice. The principal role of DPSC in salivary gland bioengineering is to generate the salivary stroma or mesenchymal-derived compartment, and these cells are in theory one of the best choices for that purpose because the tooth mesenchyme and the salivary gland mesenchyme share a common embryonic origin (i.e., neural crest).

HSG are stable cell lines derived from neoplastic tissues (Shirasuna et al., 1981) and definitely not the best choice to bioengineer a physiologically functional salivary gland. In order to evaluate whether trophic support provided by DPSC sustains proliferation and ramification of primary salivary gland epithelia in developmental stages, *in vitro* recombination experiments between isolated embryonic mouse salivary epithelia and dissociated hDPSC may be performed in 3D laminin or other extracellular matrix scaffolds (Sequeira et al., 2013). In

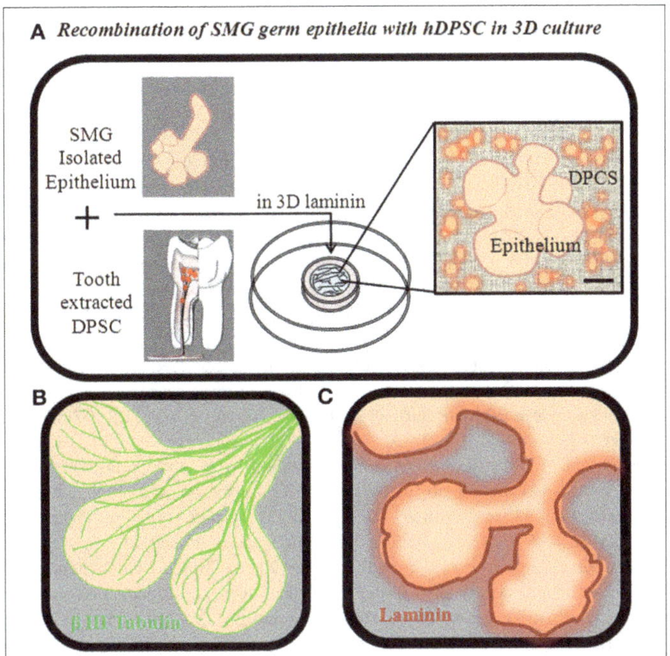


**FIGURE 4 | Recombination of salivary gland germ epithelia with DPSC in 3D culture. (A)** SMG epithelia can be mechanically and enzymatically isolated from SMG mesenchyme, and recombined with hDPSC in 3D laminin scaffolds to generate a bioengineered salivary gland germ **(B)** SMG acini from E14.5 mouse, showing the extensive natural innervation of the SMG by β3-tubulin+ nerve fibers at this developmental stage. **(C)** SMG acini from E14.5 mouse, showing the natural localization of Laminin in the basal lamina that separates the salivary epithelium and mesenchyme.

these conditions, DPSC bind and interact with isolated salivary epithelia, improving the *in vitro* viability of the tissue (**Figure 4**). However, recombination with DPSC alone is clearly insufficient to promote long-term growth and ramification of developing salivary epithelia. One missing but important potential factor is that this system cannot reproduce the extensive innervation that occurs within normal salivary gland tissues and plays a crucial role in salivary gland growth and morphogenesis (Knox et al., 2010; Knosp et al., 2012). Next steps in this direction should involve the addition of specific growth factors that sustain epithelial cell growth and commitment to salivary gland cell differentiation, as well as the use of coculture systems between bioengineered salivary glands and nerve cells to attempt to mimic the growth stimulatory effect of natural salivary innervation.

## CONCLUDING REMARKS

DPSC have emerged as a very promising tool with a great potential to be used in tissue engineering models aimed at the functional reconstruction of different craniomaxillofacial organs. Some of the main advantages of these cells are their multifaceted differentiation capacity, along with their non-tumorigenic phenotype, a high proliferation rate, a relative simplicity of extraction and culture, and their possibility of cryopreservation, which ultimately make possible to obtain patient-specific cell lines for their use in autologous cell therapy. However, many issues and challenges still need to be addressed before these cells can be employed in clinical practice. The full control of differentiation of DPSC to specific fates is still one important issue, and although DPSC derivation to certain connective tissue-lineage cells appears to be relatively simple, their differentiation into nerve-tissue lineages still poses important unanswered questions. Moreover, the development of the cell recombination technology required to create next generation bioengineered replacement organs will necessitate extensive research for the coming years. In this case, DPSC may be an ideal choice to be used in experimental models of tissue-engineered reconstruction of organs of the oral cavity, and the paradigmatic cases of the tooth and the salivary gland may constitute the leading edge of a massive research effort on next generation organ replacement therapies.

## FUNDING

This work was financed with project grants from the University of the Basque Country UPV/EHU (UFI11/44) and the Basque Government (IT831-13). MA, PG, and JL were sponsored by the University of the Basque Country (UPV/EHU) and VU by Jesus Gangoiti Barrera Foundation.

## REFERENCES

Angelova Volponi, A., Kawasaki, M., and Sharpe, P. T. (2013). Adult Human Gingival Epithelial Cells as a Source for Whole-tooth Bioengineering. *J. Dent. Res.* 92, 329–334. doi: 10.1177/0022034513481041

Anitua, E., Alkhraisat, M. H., and Orive, G. (2012). Perspectives and challenges in regenerative medicine using plasma rich in growth factors. *J. Control. Release* 157, 29–38. doi: 10.1016/j.jconrel.2011.07.004

Anitua, E., Sánchez, M., Orive, G., and Andia, I. (2008). Delivering growth factors for therapeutics. *Trends Pharmacol. Sci.* 29, 37–41. doi: 10.1016/j.tips.2007.10.010

Arthur, A., Rychkov, G., Shi, S., Koblar, S. A., and Gronthos, S. (2008). Adult human dental pulp stem cells differentiate toward functionally active neurons under appropriate environmental cues. *Stem Cells* 26, 1787–1795. doi: 10.1634/stemcells.2007-0979

Arthur, A., Shi, S., Zannettino, A. C., Fujii, N., Gronthos, S., and Koblar, S. A. (2009). Implanted adult human dental pulp stem cells induce endogenous axon guidance. *Stem Cells* 27, 2229–2237. doi: 10.1002/stem.138

Bae, Y. C., Zuker, R. M., Manktelow, R. T., and Wade, S. (2006). A comparison of commissure excursion following gracilis muscle transplantation for facial paralysis using a cross-face nerve graft versus the motor nerve to the masseter nerve. *Plast. Reconstr. Surg.* 117, 2407–2413. doi: 10.1097/01.prs.0000218798.95027.21

Blanpain, C., and Fuchs, E. (2009). Epidermal homeostasis: a balancing act of stem cells in the skin. *Nat. Rev. Mol. Cell Biol.* 10, 207–217. doi: 10.1038/nrm2636

Bonnamain, V., Thinard, R., Sergent-Tanguy, S., Huet, P., Bienvenu, G., Naveilhan, P., et al. (2013). Human dental pulp stem cells cultured in serum-free supplemented medium. *Front. Physiol.* 4:357. doi: 10.3389/fphys.2013.00357

Boucher, T. J., Okuse, K., Bennett, D. L., Munson, J. B., Wood, J. N., and McMahon, S. B. (2000). Potent analgesic effects of GDNF in neuropathic pain states. *Science* 290, 124–127. doi: 10.1126/science.290.5489.124

Bray, A. F., Cevallos, R. R., Gazarian, K., and Lamas, M. (2014). Human dental pulp stem cells respond to cues from the rat retina and differentiate to express the retinal neuronal marker rhodopsin. *Neuroscience* 280, 142–155. doi: 10.1016/j.neuroscience.2014.09.023

Cai, J., Zhang, Y., Liu, P., Chen, S., Wu, X., Sun, Y., et al. (2013). Generation of tooth-like structures from integration-free human urine induced pluripotent stem cells. *Cell Regen.* 2:6. doi: 10.1186/2045-9769-2-6

Carinci, F., Papaccio, G., Laino, G., Palmieri, A., Brunelli, G., D'Aquino, R., et al. (2008). Comparison between genetic portraits of osteoblasts derived from primary cultures and osteoblasts obtained from human pulpar stem cells. *J. Craniofac. Surg.* 19, 616–625. doi: 10.1097/SCS.0b013e31816aabc8

Cavalcanti, B. N., Zeitlin, B. D., and Nör, J. E. (2013). A hydrogel scaffold that maintains viability and supports differentiation of dental pulp stem cells. *Dent. Mater.* 29, 97–102. doi: 10.1016/j.dental.2012.08.002

Chan, B., Wong, R. W., and Rabie, B. (2011). *In vivo* production of mineralised tissue pieces for clinical use: a qualitative pilot study using human dental pulp cell. *Int. J. Oral Maxillofac. Surg.* 40, 612–620. doi: 10.1016/j.ijom.2011.01.008

Chan, J. Y., and Byrne, P. J. (2011). Management of facial paralysis in the 21st century. *Facial Plast. Surg.* 27, 346–357. doi: 10.1055/s-0031-1283053

Coppes, R. P., and Stokman, M. A. (2011). Stem cells and the repair of radiation-induced salivary gland damage. *Oral Dis.* 17, 143–153. doi: 10.1111/j.1601-0825.2010.01723.x

d'Aquino, R., De Rosa, A., Lanza, V., Tirino, V., Laino, L., Graziano, A., et al. (2009). Human mandible bone defect repair by the grafting of dental pulp stem/progenitor cells and collagen sponge biocomplexes. *Eur. Cell. Mater.* 18, 75–83.

d'Aquino, R., Graziano, A., Sampaolesi, M., Laino, G., Pirozzi, G., De Rosa, A., et al. (2007). Human postnatal dental pulp cells co-differentiate into osteoblasts and endotheliocytes: a pivotal synergy leading to adult bone tissue formation. *Cell Death Differ.* 14, 1162–1171. doi: 10.1038/sj.cdd.4402121

Ding, L., and Morrison, S. J. (2013). Haematopoietic stem cells and early lymphoid progenitors occupy distinct bone marrow niches. *Nature* 495, 231–235. doi: 10.1038/nature11885

Dissanayaka, W. L., Hargreaves, K. M., Jin, L., Samaranayake, L. P., and Zhang, C. (2015). The interplay of dental pulp stem cells and endothelial cells in an injectable peptide hydrogel on angiogenesis and pulp regeneration *in vivo*. *Tissue Eng. Part A.* 21, 550–563. doi: 10.1089/ten.tea.2014.0154

Fatherazi, S., Matsa-Dunn, D., Foster, B. L., Rutherford, R. B., Somerman, M. J., and Presland, R. B. (2009). Phosphate regulates osteopontin gene transcription. *J. Dent. Res.* 88, 39–44. doi: 10.1177/0022034508328072

Foster, B. L., Nociti, F. H. Jr., Swanson, E. C., Matsa-Dunn, D., Berry, J. E., Cupp, C. J., et al. (2006). Regulation of cementoblast gene expression by inorganic phosphate *in vitro*. *Calcif. Tissue Int.* 78, 103–112. doi: 10.1007/s00223-005-0184-7

Freitas, R. M., Spin-Neto, R., Marcantonio Junior, E., Pereira, L. A., Wikesjö, U. M., and Susin, C. (2015). Alveolar ridge and maxillary sinus augmentation using rhBMP-2: a systematic review. *Clin. Implant Dent. Relat. Res.* 17, e192–e201. doi: 10.1111/cid.12156

Fujita, S., Hideshima, K., and Ikeda, T. (2006). Nestin expression in odontoblasts and odontogenic ectomesenchymal tissue of odontogenic tumours. *J. Clin. Pathol.* 59, 240–245. doi: 10.1136/jcp.2004.025403

Gervois, P., Struys, T., Hilkens, P., Bronckaers, A., Ratajczak, J., Politis, C., et al. (2015). Neurogenic maturation of human dental pulp stem cells following neurosphere generation induces morphological and electrophysiological characteristics of functional neurons. *Stem Cells Dev.* 24, 296–311. doi: 10.1089/scd.2014.0117

Giuliani, A., Manescu, A., Langer, M., Rustichelli, F., Desiderio, V., Paino, F., et al. (2013). Three years after transplants in human mandibles, histological and in-line holotomography revealed that stem cells regenerated a compact rather than a spongy bone: biological and clinical implications. *Stem Cells Transl. Med.* 2, 316–324. doi: 10.5966/sctm.2012-0136

Graziano, A., d'Aquino, R., Laino, G., and Papaccio, G. (2008a). Dental pulp stem cells: a promising tool for bone regeneration. *Stem Cell Rev.* 4, 21–26. doi: 10.1007/s12015-008-9015-3

Graziano, A., d'Aquino, R., Laino, G., Proto, A., Giuliano, M. T., Pirozzi, G., et al. (2008b). Human CD34+ stem cells produce bone nodules *in vivo*. *Cell Prolif.* 41, 1–11. doi: 10.1111/j.1365-2184.2007.00497.x

Gronthos, S., Brahim, J., Li, W., Fisher, L. W., Cherman, N., Boyde, A., et al. (2002). Stem cell properties of human dental pulp stem cells. *J. Dent. Res.* 81, 531–535. doi: 10.1177/154405910208100806

Gronthos, S., Mankani, M., Brahim, J., Robey, P. G., and Shi, S. (2000). Postnatal human dental pulp stem cells (DPSCs) *in vitro* and *in vivo*. *Proc. Natl. Acad. Sci. U.S.A.* 97, 13625–13630. doi: 10.1073/pnas.240309797

Hamidouche, Z., Haÿ, E., Vaudin, P., Charbord, P., Schüle, R., Marie, P. J., et al. (2008). FHL2 mediates dexamethasone-induced mesenchymal cell differentiation into osteoblasts by activating Wnt/beta-catenin signaling-dependent Runx2 expression. *FASEB J.* 22, 3813–3822. doi: 10.1096/fj.08-106302

Hayashi, A., and Maruyama, Y. (2005). Neurovascularized free short head of the biceps femoris muscle transfer for one-stage reanimation of facial paralysis. *Plast. Reconstr. Surg.* 115, 394–405. doi: 10.1097/01.PRS.0000149405.89201.9E

Hedstrom, K. L., Murtie, J. C., Albers, K., Calcutt, N. A., and Corfas, G. (2014). Treating small fiber neuropathy by topical application of a small molecule modulator of ligand-induced GFRalpha/RET receptor signaling. *Proc. Natl. Acad. Sci. U.S.A.* 111, 2325–2330. doi: 10.1073/pnas.1308889111

Huang, G. T., Gronthos, S., and Shi, S. (2009). Mesenchymal stem cells derived from dental tissues vs. those from other sources: their biology and role in regenerative medicine. *J. Dent. Res.* 88, 792–806. doi: 10.1177/0022034509340867

Ibarretxe, G., Crende, O., Aurrekoetxea, M., García-Murga, V., Etxaniz, J., and Unda, F. (2012). Neural crest stem cells from dental tissues: a new hope for dental and neural regeneration. *Stem Cells Int.* 2012:103503. doi: 10.1155/2012/103503

Ichikawa, H., Kim, H. J., Shuprisha, A., Shikano, T., Tsumura, M., Shibukawa, Y., et al. (2012). Voltage-dependent sodium channels and calcium-activated potassium channels in human odontoblasts *in vitro*. *J. Endod.* 38, 1355–1362. doi: 10.1016/j.joen.2012.06.015

Ikeda, R., Morita, K., Nakao, K., Ishida, K., Nakamura, T., Takano-Yamamoto, T., et al. (2009). Fully functional bioengineered tooth replacement as an organ replacement therapy. *Proc. Natl. Acad. Sci. U.S.A.* 106, 13475–13480. doi: 10.1073/pnas.0902944106

Janebodin, K., Horst, O. V., Ieronimakis, N., Balasundaram, G., Reesukumal, K., Pratumvinit, B., et al. (2011). Isolation and characterization of neural crest-derived stem cells from dental pulp of neonatal mice. *PLoS ONE* 6:e27526. doi: 10.1371/journal.pone.0027526

Janebodin, K., and Reyes, M. (2012). Neural crest-derived dental pulp stem cells function as ectomesenchyme to support salivary gland tissue formation. *Dentistry* S13:001. doi: 10.4172/2161-1122S13-001

Kadar, K., Kiraly, M., Porcsalmy, B., Molnar, B., Racz, G. Z., Blazsek, J., et al. (2009). Differentiation potential of stem cells from human dental origin - promise for tissue engineering. *J. Physiol. Pharmacol.* 60, 167–175.

Kalaszczynska, I., and Ferdin, K. (2015). Wharton's jelly derived mesenchymalstem cells: future of regenerative medicine? recent findings and clinical significance. *Biomed. Res. Int.* 2015:430847. doi: 10.1155/2015/430847

Kapur, S. K., Dos-Anjos Vilaboa, S., Llull, R., and Katz, A. J. (2015). Adipose tissue and stem/progenitor cells: discovery and development. *Clin. Plast. Surg.* 42, 155–167. doi: 10.1016/j.cps.2014.12.010

Kaukua, N., Shahidi, M. K., Konstantinidou, C., Dyachuk, V., Kaucka, M., Furlan, A., et al. (2014). Glial origin of mesenchymal stem cells in a tooth model system. *Nature* 513, 551–554. doi: 10.1038/nature13536

Kawashima, N. (2012). Characterisation of dental pulp stem cells: a new horizon for tissue regeneration? *Arch. Oral Biol.* 57, 1439–1458. doi: 10.1016/j.archoralbio.2012.08.010

Kim, J. Y., Xin, X., Moioli, E. K., Chung, J., Lee, C. H., Chen, M., et al. (2010). Regeneration of dental-pulp-like tissue by chemotaxis-induced cell homing. *Tissue Eng. Part A* 16, 3023–3031. doi: 10.1089/ten.tea.2010.0181

Kiraly, M., Porcsalmy, B., Pataki, A., Kadar, K., Jelitai, M., Molnar, B., et al. (2009). Simultaneous PKC and cAMP activation induces differentiation of human dental pulp stem cells into functionally active neurons. *Neurochem. Int.* 55, 323–332. doi: 10.1016/j.neuint.2009.03.017

Knosp, W. M., Knox, S. M., and Hoffman, M. P. (2012). Salivary gland organogenesis. Wiley interdisciplinary reviews. *Dev. Biol.* 1, 69–82. doi: 10.1002/wdev.4

Knox, S. M., Lombaert, I. M., Reed, X., Vitale-Cross, L., Gutkind, J. S., and Hoffman, M. P. (2010). Parasympathetic innervation maintains epithelial progenitor cells during salivary organogenesis. *Science* 329, 1645–1647. doi: 10.1126/science.1192046

Kumar, P. A., and Hassan, K. M. (2002). Cross-face nerve graft with free-muscle transfer for reanimation of the paralyzed face: a comparative study of the single-stage and two-stage procedures. *Plast. Reconstr. Surg.* 109, 451–462. doi: 10.1097/00006534-200202000-00006

La Noce, M., Paino, F., Spina, A., Naddeo, P., Montella, R., Desiderio, V., et al. (2014). Dental pulp stem cells: state of the art and suggestions for a true translation of research into therapy. *J. Dent.* 42, 761–768. doi: 10.1016/j.jdent.2014.02.018

Laino, G., d'Aquino, R., Graziano, A., Lanza, V., Carinci, F., Naro, F., et al. (2005). A new population of human adult dental pulp stem cells: a useful source of living autologous fibrous bone tissue (LAB). *J. Bone Miner. Res.* 20, 1394–1402. doi: 10.1359/JBMR.050325

Langenbach, F., and Handschel, J. (2013). Effects of dexamethasone, ascorbic acid and β-glycerophosphate on the osteogenic differentiation of stem cells *in vitro*. *Stem Cell Res. Ther.* 4, 117. doi: 10.1186/scrt328

Lee, J. E., Jin, S. H., Ko, Y., and Park, J. B. (2014). Evaluation of anatomical considerations in the posterior maxillae for sinus augmentation. *World J. Clin. Cases* 2, 683–688. doi: 10.12998/wjcc.v2.i11.683

Lee, J. Y., Nam, H., Park, Y. J., Lee, S. J., Chung, C. P., Han, S. B., et al. (2011). The effects of platelet-rich plasma derived from human umbilical cord blood on the osteogenic differentiation of human dental stem cells. *In vitro Cell. Dev. Biol.* 47, 157–164. doi: 10.1007/s11626-010-9364-5

Leijten, J., Chai, Y. C., Papantoniou, I., Geris, L., Schrooten, J., and Luyten, F. P. (2015). Cell based advanced therapeutic medicinal products for bone repair: keep it simple? *Adv. Drug Deliv. Rev.* 84, 30–44. doi: 10.1016/j.addr.2014.10.025

Li, J. H., Liu, D. Y., Zhang, F. M., Wang, F., Zhang, W. K., and Zhang, Z. T. (2011). Human dental pulp stem cell is a promising autologous seed cell for bone tissue engineering. *Chin. Med. J.* 124, 4022–4028.

Liu, H. C., E, L. L., Wang, D. S., Su, F., Wu, X., Shi, Z. P., et al. (2011). Reconstruction of alveolar bone defects using bone morphogenetic protein 2 mediated rabbit dental pulp stem cells seeded on nano-hydroxyapatite/collagen/poly(L-lactide). *Tissue Eng. Part A* 17, 2417–2433. doi: 10.1089/ten.tea.2010.0620

Lombaert, I. M., Brunsting, J. F., Wierenga, P. K., Faber, H., Stokman, M. A., Kok, T., et al. (2008). Rescue of salivary gland function after stem cell transplantation in irradiated glands. *PLoS ONE* 3:e2063. doi: 10.1371/journal.pone.0002063

Lombaert, I. M., Knox, S. M., and Hoffman, M. P. (2011). Salivary gland progenitor cell biology provides a rationale for therapeutic salivary gland regeneration. *Oral Dis.* 17, 445–449. doi: 10.1111/j.1601-0825.2010.01783.x

Love, S., and Coakham, H. B. (2001). Trigeminal neuralgia: pathology and pathogenesis. *Brain* 124, 2347–2360. doi: 10.1093/brain/124.12.2347

Mangano, C., De Rosa, A., Desiderio, V., d'Aquino, R., Piattelli, A., De Francesco, F., et al. (2010). The osteoblastic differentiation of dental pulp stem cells and bone formation on different titanium surface textures. *Biomaterials* 31, 3543–3551. doi: 10.1016/j.biomaterials.2010.01.056

Mangano, C., Paino, F., d'Aquino, R., De Rosa, A., Iezzi, G., Piattelli, A., et al. (2011). Human dental pulp stem cells hook into biocoral scaffold forming an engineered biocomplex. *PLoS ONE* 6:e18721. doi: 10.1371/journal.pone.0018721

Marín, O., Valdeolmillos, M., and Moya, F. (2006). Neurons in motion: same principles for different shapes? *Trends Neurosci.* 29, 655–661. doi: 10.1016/j.tins.2006.10.001

Martens, W., Bronckaers, A., Politis, C., Jacobs, R., and Lambrichts, I. (2013). Dental stem cells and their promising role in neural regeneration: an update. *Clin. Oral Invest.* 17, 1969–1983. doi: 10.1007/s00784-013-1030-3

Martens, W., Sanen, K., Georgiou, M., Struys, T., Bronckaers, A., Ameloot, M., et al. (2014). Human dental pulp stem cells can differentiate into Schwann cells and promote and guide neurite outgrowth in an aligned tissue-engineered collagen construct *in vitro*. *FASEB J.* 28, 1634–1643. doi: 10.1096/fj.13-243980

Ménard, C., and Tarte, K. (2013). Immunoregulatory properties of clinical grade mesenchymal stromal cells: evidence, uncertainties, and clinical application. *Stem Cell Res. Ther.* 4, 64. doi: 10.1186/scrt214

Misawa, H., Kobayashi, N., Soto-Gutierrez, A., Chen, Y., Yoshida, A., Rivas-Carrillo, J. D., et al. (2006). PuraMatrix facilitates bone regeneration in bone defects of calvaria in mice. *Cell Transplant.* 15, 903–910. doi: 10.3727/000000006783981369

Morad, G., Kheiri, L., and Khojasteh, A. (2013). Dental pulp stem cells for *in vivo* bone regeneration: a systematic review of literature. *Arch. Oral Biol.* 58, 1818–1827. doi: 10.1016/j.archoralbio.2013.08.011

Moshaverinia, A., Chen, C., Akiyama, K., Xu, X., Chee, W. W., Schricker, S. R., et al. (2013). Encapsulated dental-derived mesenchymal stem cells in an injectable and biodegradable scaffold for applications in bone tissue engineering. *J. Biomed. Mater. Res. Part A* 101, 3285–3294. doi: 10.1002/jbm.a.34546

Murakami, T., Fujimoto, Y., Yasunaga, Y., Ishida, O., Tanaka, N., Ikuta, Y., et al. (2003). Transplanted neuronal progenitor cells in a peripheral nerve gap promote nerve repair. *Brain Res.* 974, 17–24. doi: 10.1016/s0006-8993(03)02539-3

Nakashima, M., and Akamine, A. (2005). The application of tissue engineering to regeneration of pulp and dentin in endodontics. *J. Endod.* 31, 711–718. doi: 10.1097/01.don.0000164138.49923.e5

Nakashima, M., Iohara, K., and Sugiyama, M. (2009). Human dental pulp stem cells with highly angiogenic and neurogenic potential for possible use in pulp regeneration. *Cytokine Growth Factor Rev.* 20, 435–440. doi: 10.1016/j.cytogfr.2009.10.012

Nanduri, L. S., Baanstra, M., Faber, H., Rocchi, C., Zwart, E., de Haan, G., et al. (2014). Purification and *ex vivo* expansion of fully functional salivary gland stem cells. *Stem Cell Rep.* 3, 957–964. doi: 10.1016/j.stemcr.2014.09.015

Nanduri, L. S., Lombaert, I. M., van der Zwaag, M., Faber, H., Brunsting, J. F., van Os, R. P., et al. (2013). Salisphere derived c-Kit+ cell transplantation restores tissue homeostasis in irradiated salivary gland. *Radiother. Oncol.* 108, 458–463. doi: 10.1016/j.radonc.2013.05.020

Nazirkar, G., Singh, S., Dole, V., and Nikam, A. (2014). Effortless effort in bone regeneration: a review. *J. Int. Oral Health* 6, 120–124.

Nedvetsky, P. I., Emmerson, E., Finley, J. K., Ettinger, A., Cruz-Pacheco, N., Prochazka, J., et al. (2014). Parasympathetic innervation regulates tubulogenesis in the developing salivary gland. *Dev. Cell* 30, 449–462. doi: 10.1016/j.devcel.2014.06.012

Nör, J. E. (2006). Tooth regeneration in operative dentistry. *Oper. Dent.* 31, 633–642. doi: 10.2341/06-000

Nosrat, I. V., Smith, C. A., Mullally, P., Olson, L., and Nosrat, C. A. (2004). Dental pulp cells provide neurotrophic support for dopaminergic neurons and differentiate into neurons *in vitro*; implications for tissue engineering and repair in the nervous system. *Eur. J. Neurosci.* 19, 2388–2398. doi: 10.1111/j.0953-816x.2004.03314.x

Ogawa, M., Oshima, M., Imamura, A., Sekine, Y., Ishida, K., Yamashita, K., et al. (2013). Functional salivary gland regeneration by transplantation of a bioengineered organ germ. *Nat. Commun.* 4, 2498. doi: 10.1038/ncomms3498

Ogawa, M., and Tsuji, T. (2015). Reconstitution of a bioengineered salivary gland using a three-dimensional cell manipulation method. *Curr. Protoc. Cell Biol.* 66, 19.17.1–19.17.13. doi: 10.1002/0471143030.cb1917s66

Oshima, M., Mizuno, M., Imamura, A., Ogawa, M., Yasukawa, M., Yamazaki, H., et al. (2011). Functional tooth regeneration using a bioengineered tooth unit as a mature organ replacement regenerative therapy. *PLoS ONE* 6:e21531. doi: 10.1371/journal.pone.0021531

Otsu, K., Kumakami-Sakano, M., Fujiwara, N., Kikuchi, K., Keller, L., Lesot, H., et al. (2014). Stem cell sources for tooth regeneration: current status and future prospects. *Front. Physiol.* 5:36. doi: 10.3389/fphys.2014.00036

Paknejad, M., Shayesteh, Y. S., Yaghobee, S., Shariat, S., Dehghan, M., and Motahari, P. (2012). Evaluation of the effect of plasma rich in growth factors (PRGF) on bone regeneration. *J. Dent.* 9, 59–67.

Pierdomenico, L., Bonsi, L., Calvitti, M., Rondelli, D., Arpinati, M., Chirumbolo, G., et al. (2005). Multipotent mesenchymal stem cells with immunosuppressive activity can be easily isolated from dental pulp. *Transplantation* 80, 836–842. doi: 10.1097/01.tp.0000173794.72151.88

Rastegar, F., Shenaq, D., Huang, J., Zhang, W., Zhang, B. Q., He, B. C., et al. (2010). Mesenchymal stem cells: molecular characteristics and clinical applications. *World J. Stem Cells* 2, 67–80. doi: 10.4252/wjsc.v2.i4.67

Rivera, C., Monsalve, F., Salas, J., Morán, A., and Suazo, I. (2013). Platelet-rich plasma, plasma rich in growth factors and simvastatin in the regeneration and repair of alveolar bone. *Exp. Ther. Med.* 6, 1543–1549. doi: 10.3892/etm.2013.1327

Rosa, V., Zhang, Z., Grande, R. H., and Nör, J. E. (2013). Dental pulp tissue engineering in full-length human root canals. *J. Dent. Res.* 92, 970–975. doi: 10.1177/0022034513505772

Sabalys, G., Juodzbalys, G., and Wang, H. L. (2013). Aetiology and pathogenesis of trigeminal neuralgia: a comprehensive review. *J. Oral Maxillofac. Res.* 3, e2. doi: 10.5037/jomr.2012.3402

Sakai, K., Yamamoto, A., Matsubara, K., Nakamura, S., Naruse, M., Yamagata, M., et al. (2012). Human dental pulp-derived stem cells promote locomotor recovery after complete transection of the rat spinal cord by multiple neuro-regenerative mechanisms. *J. Clin. Invest.* 122, 80–90. doi: 10.1172/JCI 59251

Sasaki, R., Aoki, S., Yamato, M., Uchiyama, H., Wada, K., Ogiuchi, H., et al. (2011). PLGA artificial nerve conduits with dental pulp cells promote facial nerve regeneration. *J. Tissue Eng. Regen. Med.* 5, 823–830. doi: 10.1002/term.387

Sasaki, R., Matsumine, H., Watanabe, Y., Takeuchi, Y., Yamato, M., Okano, T., et al. (2014). Electrophysiologic and functional evaluations of regenerated facial nerve defects with a tube containing dental pulp cells in rats. *Plast. Reconstr. Surg.* 134, 970–978. doi: 10.1097/PRS.0000000000000602

Sequeira, S. J., Gervais, E. M., Ray, S., and Larsen, M. (2013). Genetic modification and recombination of salivary gland organ cultures. *J. Vis. Exp.* 28:e50060. doi: 10.3791/50060

Shirasuna, K., Sato, M., and Miyazaki, T. (1981). A neoplastic epithelial duct cell line established from an irradiated human salivary gland. *Cancer* 48, 745–752.

Suzuki, T., Lee, C. H., Chen, M., Zhao, W., Fu, S. Y., Qi, J. J., et al. (2011). Induced migration of dental pulp stem cells for *in vivo* pulp regeneration. *J. Dent. Res.* 90, 1013–1018. doi: 10.1177/0022034511408426

Tada, H., Nemoto, E., Foster, B. L., Somerman, M. J., and Shimauchi, H. (2011). Phosphate increases bone morphogenetic protein-2 expression through cAMP-dependent protein kinase and ERK1/2 pathways in human dental pulp cells. *Bone* 48, 1409–1416. doi: 10.1016/j.bone.2011.03.675

Taylor, S. E. (2003). Efficacy and economic evaluation of pilocarpine in treating radiation-induced xerostomia. *Expert Opin. Pharmacother.* 4, 1489–1497. doi: 10.1517/14656566.4.9.1489

Vissink, A., Mitchell, J. B., Baum, B. J., Limesand, K. H., Jensen, S. B., Fox, P. C., et al. (2010). Clinical management of salivary gland hypofunction and xerostomia in head-and-neck cancer patients: successes and barriers. *Int. J. Radiat. Oncol. Biol. Phys.* 78, 983–991. doi: 10.1016/j.ijrobp.2010.06.052

Walsh, S., and Midha, R. (2009). Practical considerations concerning the use of stem cells for peripheral nerve repair. *Neurosurg. Focus* 26:E2. doi: 10.3171/FOC.2009.26.2.E2

Wang, Y., Preston, B., and Guan, G. (2012). Tooth bioengineering leads the next generation of dentistry. *Int. J. Paediatr. Dent.* 22, 406–418. doi: 10.1111/j.1365-263X.2011.01206.x

Wen, Y., Wang, F., Zhang, W., Li, Y., Yu, M., Nan, X., et al. (2012). Application of induced pluripotent stem cells in generation of a tissue-engineered tooth-like structure. *Tissue Eng. Part A* 18, 1677–1685. doi: 10.1089/ten.tea. 2011.0220

Xiao, L., and Tsutsui, T. (2013). Characterization of human dental pulp cells-derived spheroids in serum-free medium: stem cells in the core. *J. Cell. Biochem.* 114, 2624–2636. doi: 10.1002/jcb.24610

Yan, M., Sun, M., Zhou, Y., Wang, W., He, Z., Tang, D., et al. (2013). Conversion of human umbilical cord mesenchymal stem cells in Wharton's jelly to dopamine neurons mediated by the Lmx1a and neurturin *in vitro*: potential therapeutic application for Parkinson's disease in a rhesus monkey model. *PLoS ONE* 8:e64000. doi: 10.1371/journal.pone.0064000

Yang, J. W., Zhang, Y. F., Wan, C. Y., Sun, Z. Y., Nie, S., Jian, S. J., et al. (2015). Autophagy in SDF-1α-mediated DPSC migration and pulp regeneration. *Biomaterials* 44, 11–23. doi: 10.1016/j.biomaterials.2014.12.006

Yang, X., Han, G., Pang, X., and Fan, M. (2011). Chitosan/collagen scaffold containing bone morphogenetic protein-7 DNA supports dental pulp stem cell differentiation in vitro and *in vivo*. *J. Biomed. Mater. Res. Part A 2011*. doi: 10.1002/jbm.a.34064. [Epub ahead of print].

Yu, J., He, H., Tang, C., Zhang, G., Li, Y., Wang, R., et al. (2010). Differentiation potential of STRO-1+ dental pulp stem cells changes during cell passaging. *BMC Cell Biol.* 11:32. doi: 10.1186/1471-2121-11-32

Zhang, W., Walboomers, X. F., van Osch, G. J., van den Dolder, J., and Jansen, J. A. (2008). Hard tissue formation in a porous HA/TCP ceramic scaffold loaded with stromal cells derived from dental pulp and bone marrow. *Tissue Eng. Part A* 14, 285–294. doi: 10.1089/tea.2007.0146

# 2

# Use of Rat Mature Adipocyte-Derived Dedifferentiated Fat Cells as a Cell Source for Periodontal Tissue Regeneration

**Edited by:**
Thimios Mitsiadis,
University of Zurich, Switzerland

***Correspondence:**
Masaki Honda
honda-m@dpc.agu.ac.jp

*Daisuke Akita [1], Koichiro Kano [2], Yoko Saito-Tamura [3], Takayuki Mashimo [4], Momoko Sato-Shionome [5], Niina Tsurumachi [3], Katsuyuki Yamanaka [6], Tadashi Kaneko [6], Taku Toriumi [7], Yoshinori Arai [8], Naoki Tsukimura [1], Taro Matsumoto [9], Tomohiko Ishigami [1], Keitaro Isokawa [7] and Masaki Honda [10]**

[1] *Department of Partial Denture Prosthodontics, School of Dentistry, Nihon University, Tokyo, Japan,* [2] *Laboratory of Cell and Tissue Biology, College of Bioresource Science, Nihon University, Fujisawa, Japan,* [3] *Department of Orthodontics, School of Dentistry, Nihon University, Tokyo, Japan,* [4] *Department of Oral and Maxillofacial Surgery, Faculty of Medicine, Juntendo University, Tokyo, Japan,* [5] *Department of Pediatric Dentistry, School of Dentistry, Nihon University, Tokyo, Japan,* [6] *GC Corp. R&D, Tokyo, Japan,* [7] *Department of Anatomy, School of Dentistry, Nihon University, Tokyo, Japan,* [8] *School of Dentistry, Nihon University, Tokyo, Japan,* [9] *Division of Cell Regeneration and Transplantation, Department of Functional Morphology, School of Medicine, Nihon University, Tokyo, Japan,* [10] *Department of Oral Anatomy, School of Dentistry, Aichi-Gakuin University, Nagoya, Japan*

Lipid-free fibroblast-like cells, known as dedifferentiated fat (DFAT) cells, can be generated from mature adipocytes with a large single lipid droplet. DFAT cells can re-establish their active proliferation ability and can transdifferentiate into various cell types under appropriate culture conditions. The first objective of this study was to compare the multilineage differentiation potential of DFAT cells with that of adipose-derived stem cells (ASCs) on mesenchymal stem cells. We obtained DFAT cells and ASCs from inbred rats and found that rat DFAT cells possess higher osteogenic differentiation potential than rat ASCs. On the other hand, DFAT cells show similar adipogenic differentiation, and chondrogenic differentiation potential in comparison with ASCs. The second objective of this study was to assess the regenerative potential of DFAT cells combined with novel solid scaffolds composed of PLGA (Poly *d, l*-lactic-co-glycolic acid) on periodontal tissue, and to compare this with the regenerative potential of ASCs combined with PLGA scaffolds. Cultured DFAT cells and ASCs were seeded onto PLGA scaffolds (DFAT/PLGA and ASCs/PLGA) and transplanted into periodontal fenestration defects in rat mandible. Micro computed tomography analysis revealed a significantly higher amount of bone regeneration in the DFAT/PLGA group compared with that of ASCs/PLGA and PLGA-alone groups at 2, 3, and 5 weeks after transplantation. Similarly, histomorphometric analysis showed that DFAT/PLGA groups had significantly greater width of cementum, periodontal ligament and alveolar bone than ASCs/PLGA and PLGA-alone groups. In addition, transplanted fluorescent-labeled DFAT cells were observed in the periodontal ligament beside the newly formed bone and cementum. These findings suggest that DFAT cells have a greater potential for enhancing periodontal tissue regeneration than ASCs. Therefore, DFAT cells are a promising cell source for periodontium regeneration.

**Keywords: periodontal tissue regeneration, dedifferentiated fat cells (DFAT cells), PLGA scaffold, cell transplantation, periodontal fenestration defect**

## INTRODUCTION

The use of adult mesenchymal stem cells (MSCs) seems to be ideal for practical periodontal regenerative medicine, because they are not subject to the restrictions such as embryonic stem cells (ESCs) or induced pluripotent stem cells (Prockop, 1997; Pittenger et al., 1999; Zuk et al., 2001; Reyes et al., 2002; Safford et al., 2002; Akita et al., 2014). ASCs may be a promising cell source for periodontal-tissue regeneration (Tobita et al., 2008; Tobita and Mizuno, 2013; Akita et al., 2014). The use of ASCs has several advantages over bone marrow-derived or dental tissue-derived MSCs such as dental follicle (Honda et al., 2007, 2010, 2011), dental pulp (Aurrekoetxea et al., 2015; Sato et al., 2015), and periodontal ligament (Saito et al., 2013). Adipose tissue contains large numbers of stromal cells and is available in larger quantities than bone marrow and dental tissue (Fraser et al., 2006). Furthermore, the method for obtaining adipose tissue is relatively easy and is less invasive than that for bone marrow, and adipose tissue can be obtained from patients without teeth. The utility of ASCs for periodontal tissue regeneration has been demonstrated in rat and canine models in several studies, but successful use of human ASCs for such purpose has not been described yet (Tobita et al., 2008; Tobita and Mizuno, 2013; Akita et al., 2014).

Adipose tissue is connective tissue composed mostly of adipocytes surrounded by fibroblasts. Mature adipocytes with a large single lipid droplet are generally considered to be terminally differentiated cells which have lost their proliferative ability. However, by using a ceiling culture methods based on buoyancy, lipid-free fibroblast-like cells, known as dedifferentiated fat (DFAT) cells, can be separated from mature adipocytes in our previous studies (Yagi et al., 2004; Nobusue et al., 2008; Nobusue and Kano, 2010). DFAT cells can re-establish their active proliferation ability and can differentiate into various cell types under appropriate culture conditions (Matsumoto et al., 2008; Kono et al., 2014). DFAT cells may have the potential to contribute to dental tissue regeneration (Kaku et al., 2015).

A three-dimensional (3D) biodegradable scaffold is likely to be necessary for the delivery of stem cells or progenitor cells to periodontal defect, both to preserve space for the formation of new periodontal tissue and to provide initial support for the growing transplanted cells (Wang et al., 2005). Since the most extensively used synthetic polymers in tissue engineering studies are poly(glycolic acid), poly(lactic acid), and their copolymers (e.g., Poly *d, l*-lactic-co-glycolic acid; PLGA), we previously examined the *in vivo* performance of solid PLGA scaffolds seeded with ASCs (Akita et al., 2014). Solid PLGA scaffolds have large fully interconnected pores and substantially higher compressive strength than sponge-like PLGA-based scaffolds. Recently, the possibility of using DFAT cells to promote periodontal tissue regeneration was raised by researchers who seeded an atelocollagen sponge-like scaffold with DFAT cells (Sugawara and Sato, 2014). An advantage of the higher compressive strength of solid PLGA scaffolds is that they typically offers higher primary stability than natural scaffolds such as those composed of atelocollagen. Our results showed that the PLGA scaffolds maintained their structural integrity for 5 weeks when used for *in vivo* transplants (Akita et al., 2014). We concluded that these solid PLGA scaffolds are useful for regeneration of periodontium.

To date, no studies evaluating DFAT cells combined with solid PLGA scaffolds for periodontal tissue regeneration have been published. We first compared the characteristics of rat DFAT cells with those of rat ASCs—including proliferative and multipotent differentiation potential. We then evaluated the *in vivo* potential for periodontal tissue regeneration of rat DFAT cells combined with solid PLGA scaffolds in periodontal fenestration defects created in mandibular alveolar bone, and compared the performance of rat DFAT cells in this context with that of ASCs.

## MATERIALS AND METHODS

All animal experiments were reviewed and approved by the Animal Research and Care Committee at the Nihon University School of Dentistry (AP10D014 and AP15D006).

### Isolation of Rat DFAT Cells and ASCs

To isolate DFAT cells and ASCs, 9-week-old male F344 rats ($n = 5$, body weight $190 \pm 10$ g) were purchased from CLEA Japan, Inc. (Tokyo, Japan). Isolation of DFAT cells from mature adipocytes was done with a modified version of a method that has been described previously (Matsumoto et al., 2008). Briefly, ~1 g of inguinal subcutaneous fat tissue was washed extensively with phosphate-buffered saline (PBS; Wako, Osaka, Japan) and minced and digested in 0.1% (w/v) collagenase solution (C6885; Sigma-Aldrich, St. Louis, MO) at 37°C for 60 min with gentle agitation. After filtration and centrifugation at 135 g for 3 min, the floating primary mature adipocytes in the top layer were collected. After three washes with PBS, cells ($5 \times 10^4$) were placed in 12.5 cm$^2$ culture flasks (BD Falcon, England) filled completely with Dulbecco's modified Eagle's medium (DMEM; Sigma-Aldrich, UK) and supplemented with 20% fetal bovine serum (FBS; Nichirei Bioscience Inc., Tokyo, Japan), and were incubated at 37°C in 5% $CO_2$. Mature adipocytes floated up and adhered to the top inner surface (ceiling surface) of the flasks. After about a week, the medium was removed and changed into DMEM supplemented with 20% FBS, and the flasks were inverted so that the cells were on the bottom (**Figure 1**). The medium was changed every 4 days until the cells reached confluence.

Cultured ASCs were prepared as described previously (Tobita et al., 2008; Tobita and Mizuno, 2013; Akita et al., 2014). Briefly, the stromal vascular fraction (SVF) was isolated as the pellet fraction from collagenase-digested adipose tissue by centrifugation at 180 g for 5 min after collecting of the floating uppermost layer as described above. The remaining cells were plated in DMEM supplemented with 20% FBS and 1% antibiotics as a growth medium. The cells were referred to as SVF cells, and were cultured at 37°C in a humidified atmosphere containing 5% $CO_2$ (**Figure 1**). In the comparison experiments, second and third passage ASCs and DFAT cells from the same samples were used. All animal experiments were reviewed and approved by the Animal Research and Care Committee at the Nihon University School of Dentistry (AP10D014 and AP15D006).

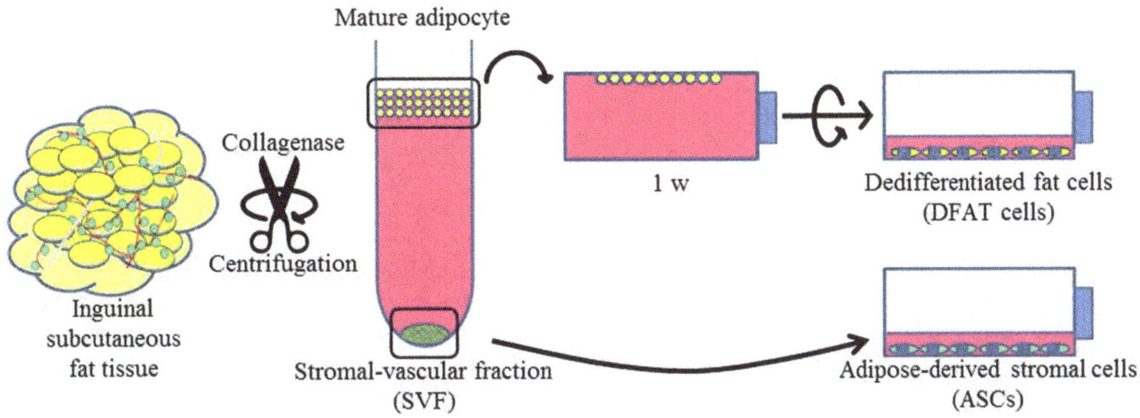


**FIGURE 1 | Isolation of DFAT cells and ASCs.** The upper section shows the method used to isolate DFAT cells from floating unilocular adipocytes. The floating cells were attached to the upper surface of the flasks and then DFAT cells emerged by asymmetrical division of floating cells for 1 week. The lower section shows the method used to isolate ASCs. After centrifugation, the SVF fraction was separated by sedimentation from floating cells and the SVF fraction was cultured for isolation of ASCs.

## Adipogenic, Osteoblastic, and Chondrocytic Differentiation *In vitro*

Differentiation assays for adipocytes, osteoblasts, and chondrocytes were performed as previously described (Matsumoto et al., 2008; Mikami et al., 2011; Saito et al., 2013; Akita et al., 2014; Sato et al., 2015). The three cell lines obtained from three rats were used in those studies.

For adipogenic differentiation, the cells were plated in 6-well plates at a density of 5 × $10^4$ cells and grown to confluency with growth medium. The cells were then incubated for 21 days in DMEM containing 10% FBS, 1 mM dexamethasone (Sigma-Aldrich), 0.5 mM isobutylmethylxanthine (Sigma-Aldrich), and 1× insulin-transferrin-selenium-A (ITS; GIBCO, Grand Island, NY) as an adipogenic induction medium, and lipid vacuole formation was examined by Oil red O staining (Wako Pure Chemical Industries, Osaka, Japan). To evaluate the adipogenic differentiation ability, Oil red O-positive cells were count under the phase contrast microscope.

For osteogenic differentiation, cells were plated in 6-well plates at a density of 5 × $10^4$ cells and grown to confluency with growth medium. The growth medium was replaced with osteogenic induction medium including DMEM containing 10% FBS, 100 nM dexamethasone, 10 mM glycerol 2-phosphate disodium salt hydrate (Sigma-Aldrich), and 50 mM L-ascorbic acid phosphate magnesium salt *n*-hydrate (Wako Pure Chemical Industries). The cells were cultured with the osteogenic induction medium for 21 days and stained with alkaline phosphatase (ALP) activity using nitro-blue tetrazolium plus 5-bromo-4-chloro-3′-indolyphosphate (NBT/BCIP) ready-to-use tablets, pH 9.5 (Roche Diagnostics, Pentzberg, Germany). To detect calcium deposition, cells were incubated in 1% Alizarin red S (Sigma-Aldrich). $Ca^{2+}$ evaluated was also determined by measuring $Ca^{2+}$ uptake using the Calcium *E*-test (Wako Pure Chemical Industries).

For chondrogenic differentiation, cell pellets were collected in centrifuge tube (2.5 × $10^4$ cells/tube) with growth medium. After 2 days in culture, the growth medium was replaced with chondrogenic induction medium including DMEM containing 1% FBS, 50 μM L-ascorbic acid phosphate magnesium salt n-hydrate, 40 μg/mL proline (Sigma-Aldrich), 100 μg/mL pyruvate (Sigma-Aldrich), 10 ng/mL recombinant human TGF-β3 (R&D Systems, Inc., Minneapolis, MN, USA), and 1 × ITS for 21 days. The microscopic structure of cells was examined after cell pellets were fixed for 10 min with 10% neutral buffered paraformaldehyde, dehydrated in a graded series of ethanol solutions, embedded in paraffin, and cut into 7 μm sections. After deparaffinization, sections were stained with Alcian blue (0.1 N, pH 1.0). Each test was conducted three times and results are presented as the mean ± standard deviation.

## Preparation of Cell-Scaffold Complex

The PLGA-based solid scaffolds (LA:GA = 75:25, Mw. 25 kDa; PLGA scaffold, GC Dental Product Co. Ltd.), with a porosity of 80%, were prepared as previously described (Akita et al., 2014; Yamanaka et al., 2015). Briefly, PLGA scaffolds were resized to ~2 × 3 × 1 $mm^3$ and soaked in 70% ethanol for 30 min to improve wetting, and then a vacuum pump was used to remove air bubbles. The scaffolds were then washed three times (30 min each) in PBS to remove residual ethanol, and 100 μL aliquots of the cell suspension (1 × $10^7$ cells/mL, 1 × $10^6$ cells/scaffold) were seeded onto the tops of prewetted PLGA scaffolds and left undisturbed in an incubator for 1 h. As a negative control, empty PLGA scaffolds were prepared.

## Cell Transplantation

Fifteen healthy male F344 rats (10-weeks-old; 200 ± 10 g) were used for *in vivo* experiment. Under inhalational device of Isoflurane (KN-1071 Marcobit-E; Natsume Seisakusho Co. Ltd., Tokyo, Japan), the rat periodontal fenestration defect model was prepared as previously described (King et al., 1997; Yang et al., 2010; Han et al., 2013; Akita et al., 2014). A skin incision was made along the inferior border of the left mandible, then the masseter muscle and the periosteum covering the buccal surface of the mandible were elevated as a flap. The alveolar bone overlying the mandibular first and second molar roots was removed with a dental inverted bur. The size of the periodontal defect was $\sim 2 \times 3 \times 1$ mm in height, width, and depth, respectively, with the anterior margin mesial to the distal root of the first molar and the posterior margin just distal to the second molar. The coronal margin was ~1.5 mm apical to the crest of the alveolar bone and the inferior margin was ~2.5 mm apical to the alveolar crest (**Figures 2A,B**). The exposed roots of the first and second molars were denuded and cementum was completely removed together with the supporting bone, which occasionally resulted in penetration into the root dentin (**Figures 2C,D**). PLGA scaffolds with DFAT (DFAT/PLGA) or ASCs (ASCs/PLGA) were placed in the defects and covered with membrane (GC membrane; GC Dental Product Co. Ltd.). The unilateral mandibular first molar in each of the 15 rats were selected for analysis and the defects were randomly assigned to the following three treatment groups: (1) PLGA scaffolds covered with GC membrane (GC membrane; GC Dental Product Co. Ltd.) without cells (PLGA-alone group) ($n = 5$), (2) ASCs-loaded PLGA scaffolds covered with membrane (ASCs/PLGA group) ($n = 5$), and (3) DFAT cells-loaded PLGA scaffolds covered with membrane (DFAT/PLGA group) ($n = 5$). The right side of the mandibular was not operated to maintain oral function. After the masseter muscle was repositioned, the skin incision was closed to ensure healing by primary intention.

## *In vivo* Micro Computed Tomography (CT) Imaging and Analysis

*In vivo* x-ray micro computed tomography (R_mCT; Rigaku Corporation, Tokyo, Japan) was used as previously described (Akita et al., 2014). The exposure parameters were 17 s, 90 kV, and 100 μA. The isotropic voxel size was 30 μm.

Briefly, hard tissue regeneration images were obtained from each rats immediately after surgery and each week until 5 weeks after surgery. The images were constructed into 3D images using i-View (J. Morita Co., Kyoto, Japan). Bone volume was measured in the regions of interest (ROIs) from voxel images using bone volume-measuring software 3 by 4 viewer 2011 (Kitasenjyu Radist Dental Clinic I-View Image Center, Tokyo, Japan). The ROI size was $4 \times 3 \times 1.5$ mm, which covered the surgically created periodontal tissue defect. The bone volume in the ROI was measured immediately after surgery and each week until 5 weeks after surgery. The increase in bone volume in individual rats was then calculated by subtracting the bone volume on day 0 from each of the subsequent values. The increase in bone was considered to be defect re-ossification.

## Histological and Histometric Analysis

Five weeks after surgery, the harvested specimens were fixed in 10% neutral buffered paraformaldehyde for 24 h, decalcified in 10% ethylenediaminetetraacetic acid (EDTA) for 5 weeks, dehydrated through a graded series of ethanol solutions, and then embedded in paraffin. For the rat specimens, frontal plane sections (7 μm thick) were prepared with a microtome (Leica RM2165, Nussloch, Germany) and the paraffin sections of the first molar central and distal roots were stained with hematoxylin and eosin (H&E). To observe the periodontal ligament fibers and Sharpey's fibers, the paraffin sections were stained with Azan and Picrosirius-red.

For the quantitative analysis, five H&E-stained sections per specimen were selected and the thickness of newly formed cementum and periodontal ligament in the first molar central and distal roots were measured by light microscopy (ECLIPSE LV100POL, Nikon, Tokyo, Japan).

After decalcification, the sections were stained as follows: dewaxing and rehydration; immersion in 0.1% Picrosirius-red

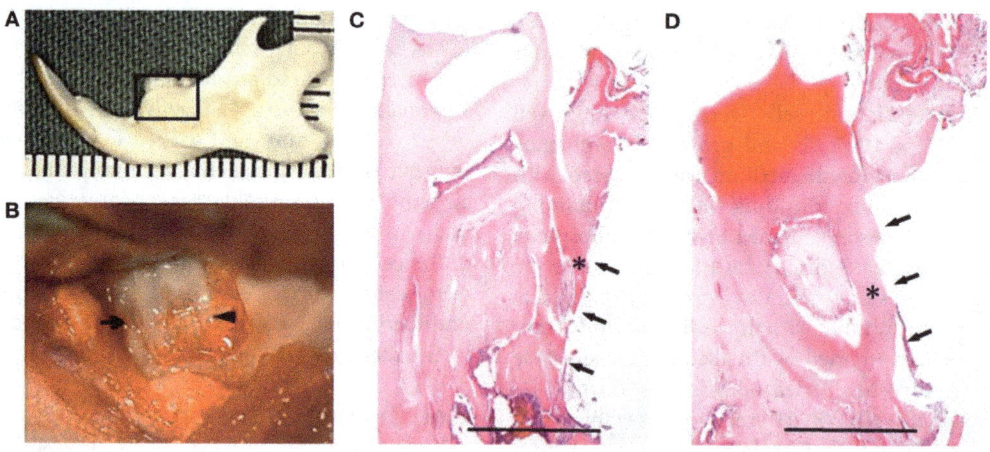


**FIGURE 2 | Creation of the periodontal fenestration defect. (A)** Rat mandibular frame specimen. The black flame indicates the site of the surgically created periodontal fenestration defect site. **(B)** Macroscopic view of a surgically created periodontal defect on the buccal surface of the mandibular first molar. The arrow indicates the first molar mesial root and the arrowhead indicates the first molar distal root. **(C)** H&E staining showing the surgically exposed central root of the first mandibular molar. The defect includes alveolar bone, periodontal ligament, and cementum. The arrows indicate the defect site and the asterisk indicates the central root of the first molar on the buccal side. Scale bar = 1000 μm. **(D)** H&E staining showing surgically exposed distal root of the first mandibular molar. The arrows indicate the defect site and the asterisk indicates the distal root of the first molar on the buccal side. Scale bar = 1000 μm.

solution (Sirius red 0.1 g dissolved into 100 mL of saturated picric acid solution) for 1 h of staining; rinsing with water for 5 min; re-staining with Harris hematoxylin for 5 min, dehydration with a gradient series of ethanol solutions; treatment with a xylene solution; and sealing with a rubber mount. The amount, distribution, and morphology of each different type of collagen were assessed by polarized light microscopy.

## Localization of Fluorescent-Labeled DFAT Cells

Four healthy male F344 rats (10-weeks-old; 200 ± 10 g) were used for this experiment. Cells harvested with 0.25% trypsin-EDTA, resuspended at 1 × $10^6$ cells/ml in DMEM, and labeled with a fluorescent dye—chloromethylbenzamido 1,1′ -dioctadecyl-3,3,3′,3′ tetramethylindocarbocyanine (DiI; Vybrant®, V22885, Life Technologies, Eugene, OR, USA). Fluorescent lipophilic tracer was added at 5 μL/mL in DMEM. After incubation for 20 min at 37°C with 5% humidified $CO_2$, the cells were centrifuged at 180 g for 5 min and washed twice with PBS. To prepare cryosections, fixed, and dehydrated specimens after 5 weeks fluorescent-labeled cell transplantation were embedded immediately in OCT compound (Sakura Finetechnical Co. Ltd., Tokyo) and frozen in liquid nitrogen. After cryosections were incubated for 30 min with a fluorescent 4′,6-diamidino-2-phenylindole solution (DAPI; Sigma-Aldrich), fluorescence microscopy (Biozero BZ-8000, Keyence, Osaka, Japan) was used to investigate the survival and localization of transplanted cells.

## Statistical Analysis

Data was expressed as the mean and standard deviation (SD) for each group. Statistical analysis was performed using ExcelStatistical File software (ystat2008.xls; Igakutosyosyuppan, Tokyo, Japan). The Mann–Whitney $U$-test was used for intergroup comparisons. $P < 0.05$ was considered statistically significant.

# RESULTS

## Characterization of Rat DFAT Cells

After ceiling culture, the adhered mature adipocytes divided asymmetrically and generated cuboidal cells with scanty cytoplasm as described previously (Matsumoto et al., 2008). The cuboidal cells formed colonies on day 7 (**Figure 3A**). We also successfully prepared ASCs from SVF fractions; these cells also expanded and formed colonies on day 7 as described in our previous reports (**Figure 3B**) (Akita et al., 2014). The morphology of the ASCs was slightly different from that of the cells derived from mature adipocytes. The ASCs have more cytoplasm than the DFAT cells.

Next, differentiation potential was analyzed. Patterns of increase in ALP activity were detected in both cell populations with or without differentiation-inducing medium. Since the extent of the formation of Alizarin Red-positive mineralized nodules in DFAT cells was slightly higher than that observed in ASCs on day 14 (**Figure 4A**), calcium accumulation was measured. Calcium accumulation in osteogenic induction medium was significantly higher in DFAT cells than in ASCs at day 14 and 21 (**Figure 4B**). Newly synthesized glycosaminoglycan, as determined by Alcian-blue positive staining, was observed in both cell populations when subjected to conditions that favor chondrogenic differentiation (**Figure 4C**). DFAT cells showed Alcian-blue positive areas in the cell pellets in chondrogenic induction medium compared with that of ASCs. The accumulation of lipid vacuoles as determined by positive Oil red O staining was observed in the cytoplasm in both cell populations when subjected to conditions that favor adipogenic differentiation (**Figure 4D**). The number of Oil red O-positive cells in the DFAT cell population was similar to that in the ASC population (**Figure 4E**).

## Hard Tissue Formation

Furcation periodontal tissue defects were artificially prepared and transplanted with PLGA-alone, ASCs/PLGA, or DFAT/PLGA scaffolds. No severe inflammation or swelling was observed in any examined sites throughout the experimental period. To evaluate hard tissue formation in the alveolar bone areas, reconstituted micro computed tomography (micro-CT) images and horizontal sections were prepared by micro-CT until week 5 because the artificially created defect area was almost filled with newly formed hard tissue by week 5 in the DFAT/PLGA scaffold group (**Figure 5**).

Newly formed hard tissue was clearly visible at the alveolar bone defect sites in all groups at week 2. Interestingly, cortical bone-like tissue was observed at the outer layer of the defect sites at 4 weeks in the DFAT/PLGA scaffold, but not the ASCs/PLGA and PLGA-alone scaffolds by the horizontal images. At 5 weeks, the newly formed hard tissue was completely connected with the native cortical bone at both mesial and distal side in the DFAT/PLGA group. The translucent image between dental root and the newly formed hard tissue was clearly visible in all the samples by week 5. Since the DFAT/PLGA scaffolds showed large amounts of newly formed hard tissue compared with the ASCs/PLGA scaffolds, we calculated the quantity of new hard tissue formation. The hard tissue volume in DFAT/PLGA scaffolds was significantly higher than that in ASCs/PLGA scaffolds at 2, 3, and 5 weeks (**Figure 6**) ($P < 0.05$).

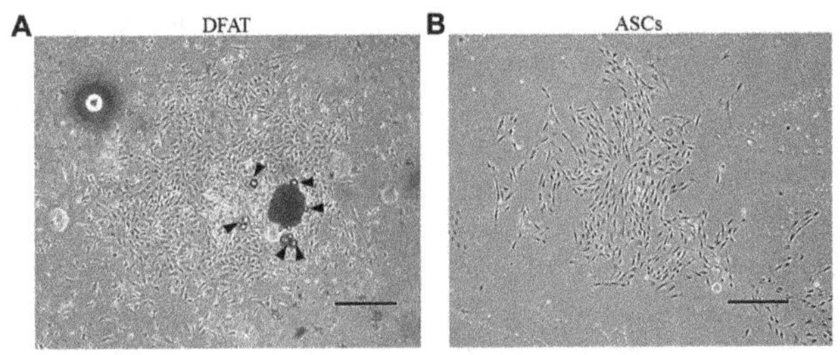


**FIGURE 3 | Morphology of primary cultured DFAT cells and ASCs. (A)** When the flasks had been inverted for 7 days, DFAT cells grew to form a colony. Some DFAT cells in the colony still have a lipid droplet (arrowheads). Scale bar = 500 μm. **(B)** Cultured ASCs are more spindle-shaped than DFAT cells. Scale bar = 500 μm.

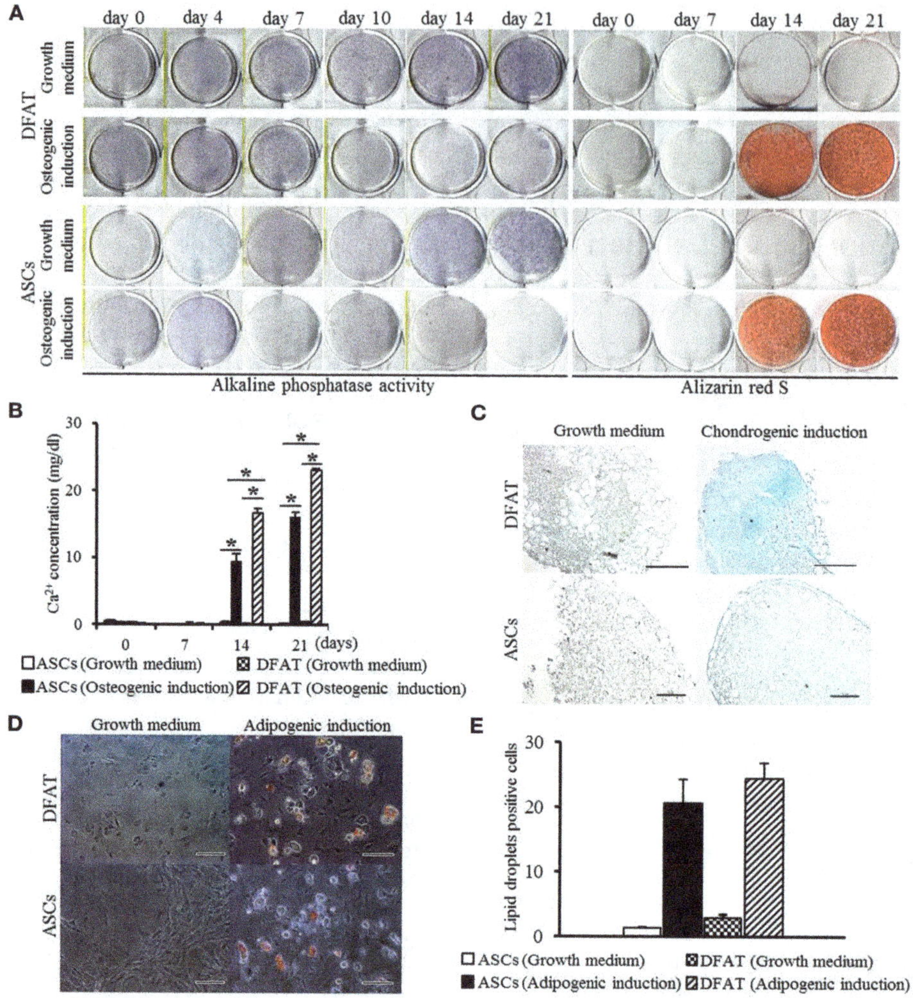


**FIGURE 4 | Multilineage potential of DFAT cells and ASCs. (A)** ALP activity and Alizarin red staining, examined to detect osteogenic potential of DFAT cells, and ASCs. **(B)** Calcium concentration determined by quantitative colorimetric assay. Each bar represents the mean ± SD ($n = 12$); $^*P < 0.05$. **(C)** Cells stained for Alcian blue to determine chondrogenic differentiation. Scale bar = 100 μm. **(D)** Adipogenic differentiation evaluated by staining with Oil red O. **(E)** Oil red O-positive lipid droplets were measured in DFAT cells and ASCs under growth and adipogenic induction media. There was no significant difference between DFAT cells and ASCs on the cell number stained by Oil red O.

## Transplantation of DFAT/PLGA Enhanced Periodontal Tissue Regeneration

By week 5, the created defect sites were easily identifiable by H&E in the PLGA-alone group because the remnant of the PLGA scaffold was clearly visible (**Figures 7A,D, 8A,D**). At low magnification, formation of mineralized tissues such as bone and cementum was evident in the DFAT/PLGA and ASCs/DFAT groups at 5 weeks (**Figures 7B,C**), but not in the PLGA-alone group (**Figure 7A**). The newly formed bone structures within the defect were coalesced with surrounding native alveolar bone (**Figures 7B,C, 8A–C**). The presence of osteoblasts lining the organic matrix and osteocytes trapped in the lacunae of newly formed bone structures was detected in the DFAT/PLGA and ASCs/PLGA groups (**Figures 7E,F, 8E,F**). Vascularization was observed in all samples (**Figures 7G–I, 8G–I**).

Periodontal ligament organization was recognized in the cementum-ligament-alveolar bone complex in the DFAT/PLGA and ASCs/PLGA groups (**Figures 7H,I, 8G–I**). The orientation of the ligament fibers, visualized by Picrosirius-red staining, resembled the oblique fibers in the functional native periodontal ligament tissue (**Figures 7K,L, 8K,L**). In the PLGA-alone group, sparse, and disorganized fibers were observed between dentin and scaffold because there was no cementum or nearby bone formation in the alveolar bone defect (**Figures 7J, 8J**).

The results of the histometric analysis are summarized in **Figure 9**. The newly formed cementum on the central root in the DFAT/PLGA group was significantly thicker than that in the ASCs/PLGA and PLGA-alone groups ($P < 0.05$) (**Figure 9A**). Furthermore, the thickness of periodontal ligament regenerated in the tissue defects at the part of the central root in the DFAT/PLGA group was also significantly larger than in the

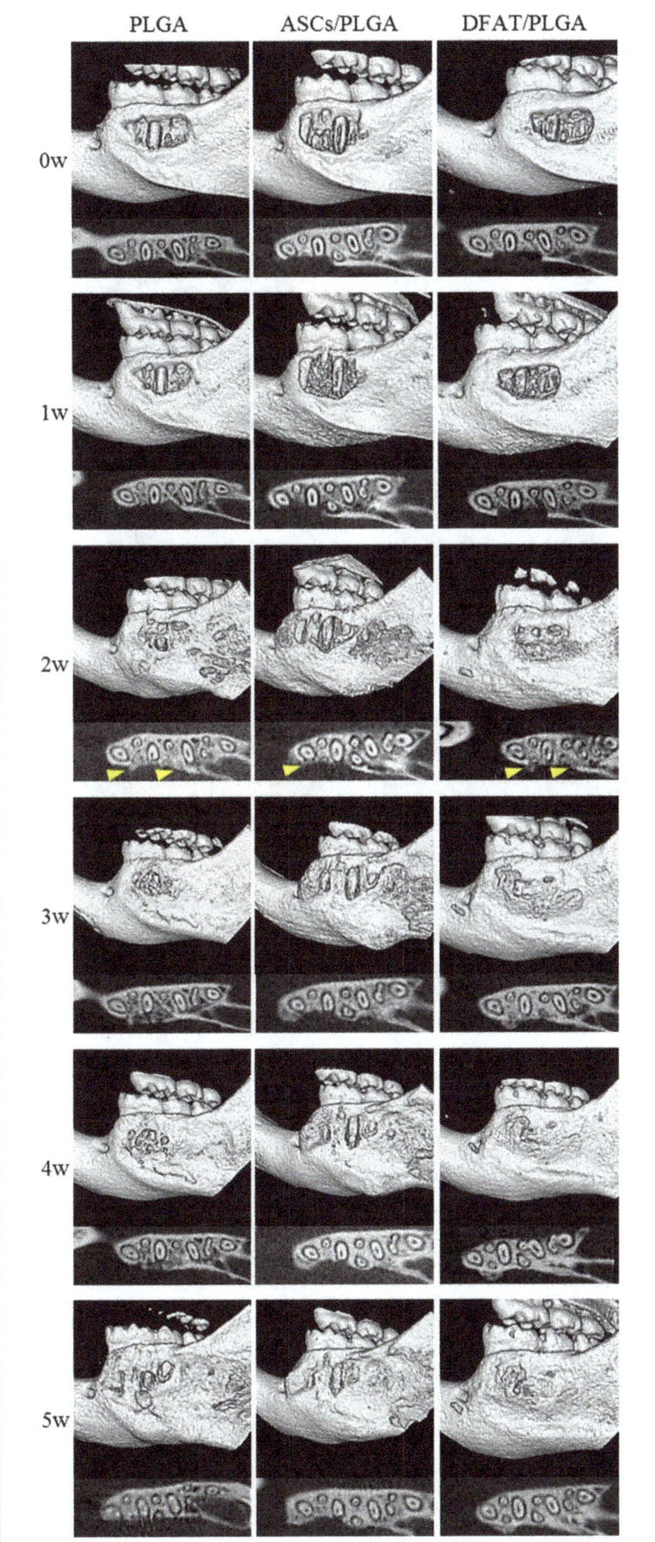


**FIGURE 5 | Micro-CT images of regenerative process in the periodontal fenestration defect.** Micro-CT images were obtained from the identical rats immediately after transplantation until 5 weeks after transplantation. The upper section of each image shows reconstructed micro-CT images. The lower section shows the horizontal plane section of the mandible. Hard tissue is visible (distinct from native bone structure) at 2 weeks (arrowheads).

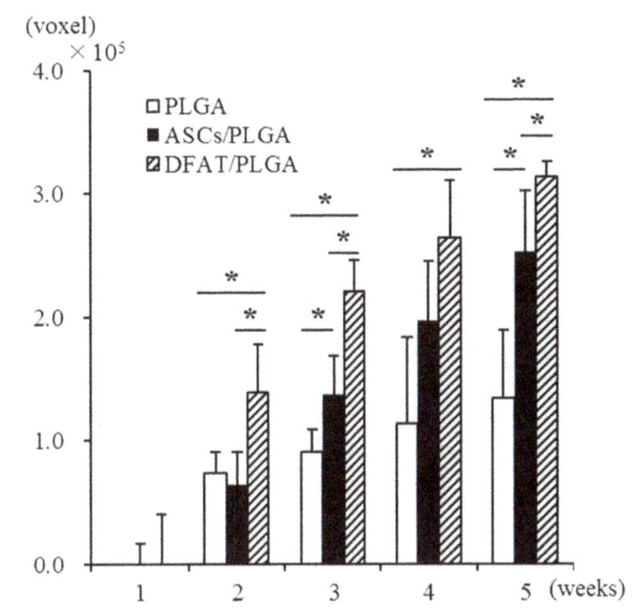


**FIGURE 6 | Quantification of newly formed hard tissue regeneration using bone volume measuring software and the data from micro-CT analysis.** A significant difference was observed between the DFAT/PLGA and ASCs/PLGA groups at weeks 2, 3, and 5 ($n = 12$, * $P < 0.05$).

ASCs/PLGA and PLGA-alone groups ($P < 0.05$) (**Figure 9B**). Finally, the newly formed alveolar bone at the part of central root in the DFAT/PLGA group was significantly thicker than that in the ASCs/PLGA and PLGA-alone groups.

## Localization of Transplanted DFAT Cells in the Periodontal Tissue Defects

Fluorescent-labeled DFAT cells and ASCs were visualized in the newly formed alveolar bone and cementum, as well as in the newly formed periodontal tissues (**Figures 10A–H**).

## DISCUSSION

The aim of this study was to assess the periodontal regenerative potential of DFAT cells derived from rat mature adipocytes in combination with solid PLGA scaffolds transplanted into surgically created periodontal tissue defects (King et al., 1997; Akita et al., 2014). In addition, we compared the proliferation and differentiation potential *in vitro* and periodontal tissue-forming capability *in vivo* of DFAT cells and ASCs.

A successful periodontal tissue-engineering strategy requires a suitable scaffold that maintains space for cell growth and differentiation. A suitable scaffold for periodontal tissue regeneration should be biodegradable, so that it can eventually be replaced by regenerated tissue (Rungsiyanont et al., 2012). We previously demonstrated the *in vivo* performance of a PLGA scaffold seeded with ASCs (Akita et al., 2014). When a PLAG-alone scaffold was transplanted into a periodontal defect in the present study, the defect space was occupied by connective tissue. In addition, newly formed connective tissue was observed

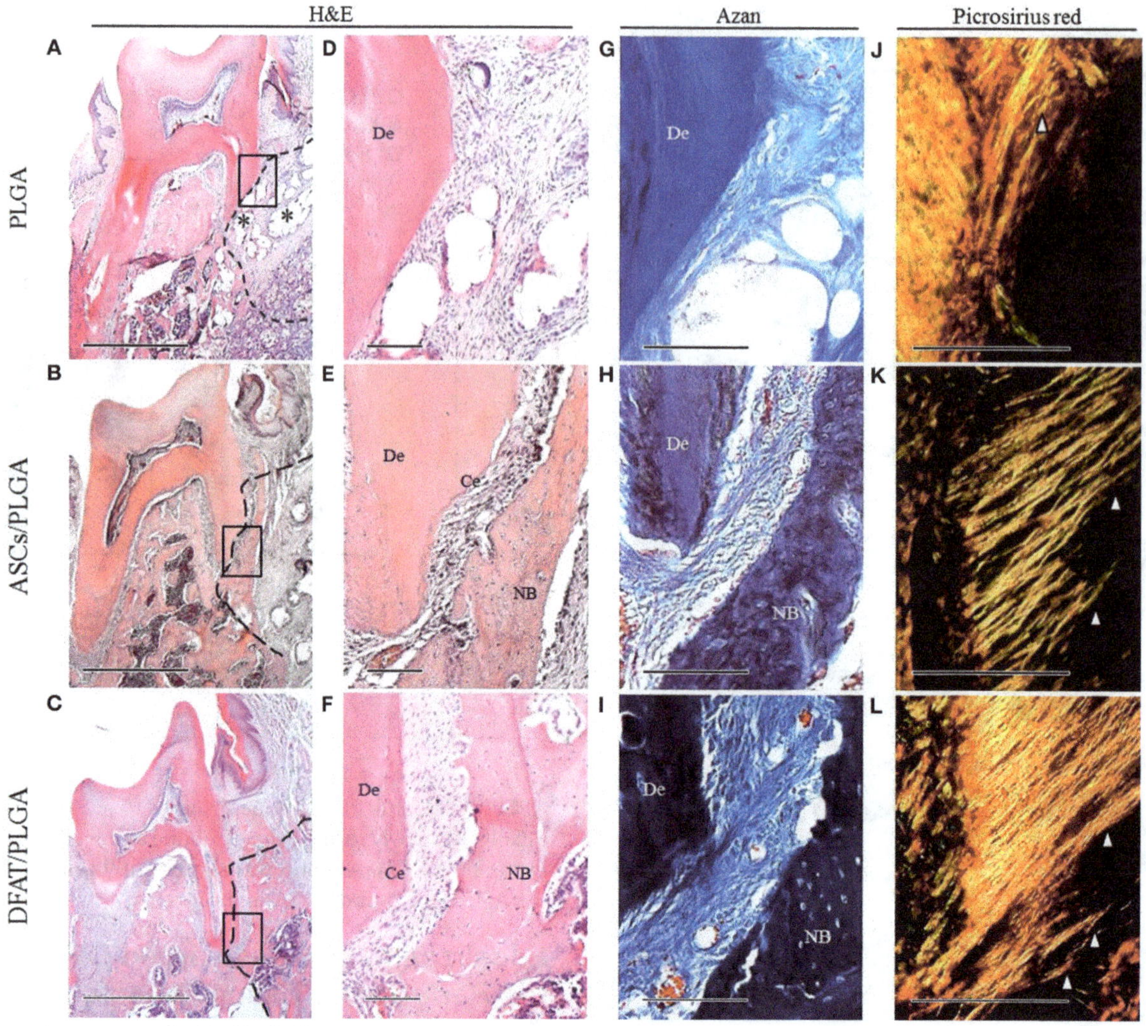


**FIGURE 7 | Representative histological observation of frontal plane section in central root of first molar. (A–C)** Overview of H&E staining. No alveolar bone formation was observed in the PLGA-alone group. Asterisk indicate scaffold remnant. Alveolar bone formation was observed in the ASCs/PLGA and DFAT/PLGA groups. The dotted line indicates defect site. Scale bar = 1000 μm. **(D–F)** Higher magnification of the framed areas in **(A–C)**, respectively. No cementum formation was observed in the PLGA-alone group and newly formed cementum was observed in the ASCs/PLGA and DFAT/PLGA groups. Scale bar = 100 μm. **(G–I)** Higher magnification of the framed area in **(A–C)**, respectively, with Azan staining to observe the periodontal ligament fibers. Scale bar = 100 μm. **(J–L)** Enlarged images of the area equivalent to **(G–I)**, stained with Picrosirius-red to show Sharpey's fibers. Arrowheads indicate newly formed collagen fibers. Scale bar = 100 μm. NB, newly formed bone; Ce, newly formed cementum; De, root dentin.

around the remaining scaffold 5 weeks after transplantation and no inflammation was observed during the 5-week experimental period. These results suggest that the PLGA scaffold contribute to maintaining space for tissue regeneration in the periodontal defect because the structural integrity of the PLGA scaffold is higher than that of soft scaffolds such as those made from hydro gels and collagen sponge, which have been used in many other studies (Doğan et al., 2003; Kawaguchi et al., 2004; Zhao et al., 2004; Tobita et al., 2008; Li et al., 2009; Nuñez et al., 2012).

Interestingly, based on ALP activity and mineralization activity *in vitro*, DFAT cells showed higher osteoblastic differentiation capacity than ASCs. Furthermore, DFAT cells showed greater potential for hard tissue formation *in vivo* than ASCs by micro-CT analysis. These results indicate that the osteogenic potential of DFAT cells is higher than that of ASCs, which is consistent with previous findings (Kishimoto et al., 2013). In addition, based on Oil red O and Alcian blue analysis, DFAT cells and ASCs had similar adipogenic and chondrogenic differentiation potential. Our group has studied DFAT cells in term of tissue-specific functions and genes that regulate of differentiation, such as those encoding SFRP2, PRRX1, HEY2, AEBP1, PEG10, PRRX2, RUNX1, FZD7, and IGFBP5. The results indicate DFAT cells have a multilineage differentiation capacity and a feature of progenitor cells committed to various cell lineages rather than the stem cell fate (Ono et al., 2011). Furthermore, our previous study showed that when a single cell-derived clonal population of DFAT cells expressed the specific genes of various cell lineages, it was capable of

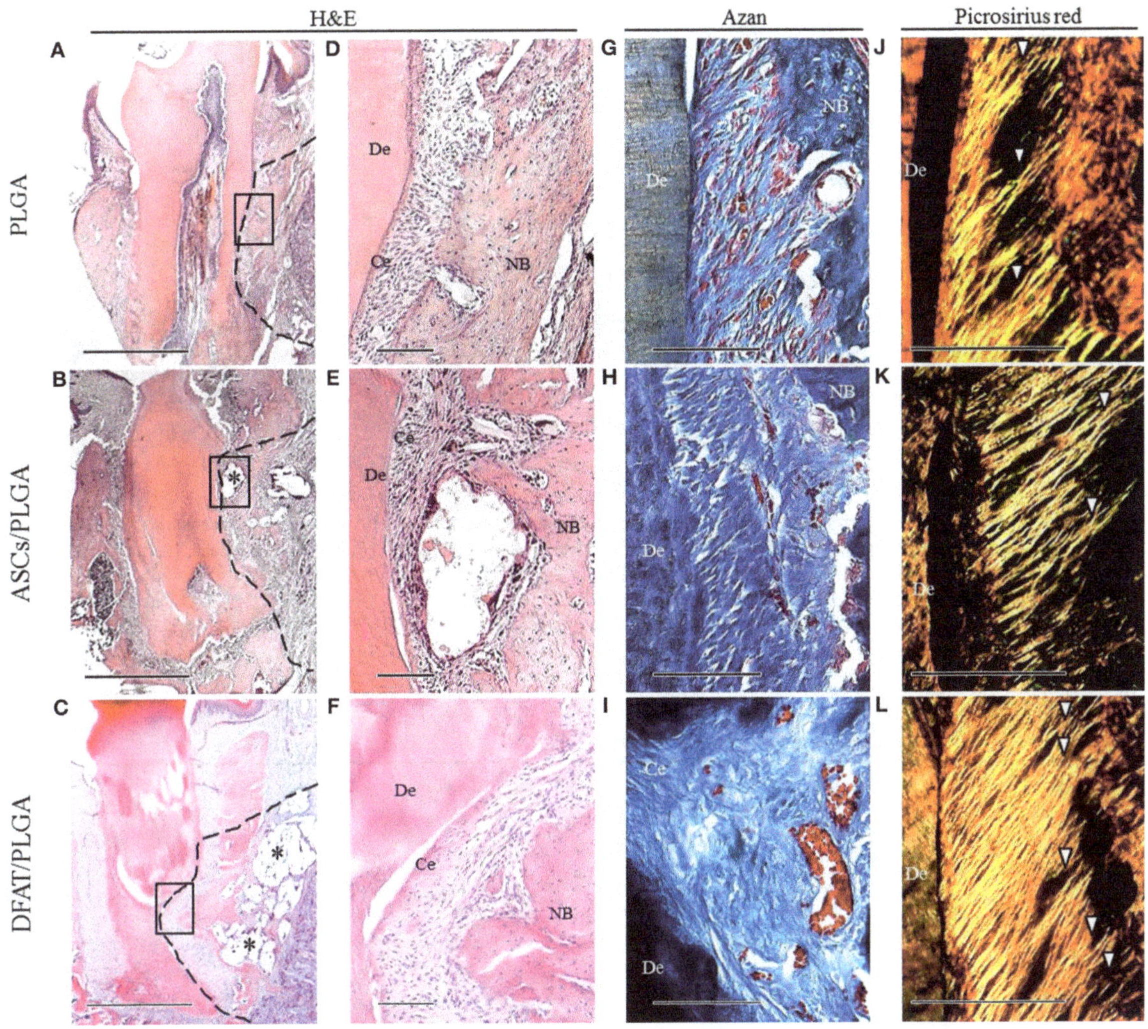


**FIGURE 8 | Representative histological observation of frontal plane section in distal root of first molar. (A–C)** Overview of H&E staining showing significant bone formation in DFAT/PLGA and ASCs/PLGA groups. Asterisks indicate scaffold remnants. The dotted line indicates defect sites. Scale bar = 1000 μm. **(D–F)** Higher magnification of the framed area in **(A–C)**, respectively. Newly formed abundant cementum was observed in the DFAT/PLGA group. Scale bar = 100 μm. **(G–I)** Azan staining at higher magnification showed collagen bundles in the PLGA-alone group. Collagen bundles of more than 100 μm width were observed in the ASCs/PLGA and DFAT/PLGA groups. Scale bar = 100 μm. **(J–L)** Enlarged images of the area equivalent to **(G–I)**, stained with Picrosirius-red staining to show periodontal ligament fibers. Arrowheads indicate newly formed collagen fibers. Scale bar = 100 μm. NB, newly formed bone; Ce, newly formed cementum; De, root dentin.

differentiating into multiple lineages (Kazama et al., 2008; Matsumoto et al., 2008). Taken together, these findings suggest that DFAT cells could have the ability to differentiate into cementoblasts, fibroblasts, and osteoblasts.

In our study, we observed *in vivo* periodontal tissue regeneration including cementum, periodontal ligament, and alveolar bone following both transplantation of DFAT cells and transplantation of ASCs. For the functional repair of the cementum-ligament-bone complex, fibrous connective tissues must insert into the cementum, and bone to achieve optimal biomechanical integration. In our study, the PLGA-alone group showed no cementum or alveolar bone formation, This is because the damaged tissue does not naturally repair owing to the lack of MSCs in periodontal tissues. In contrast, when DFAT cells or ASCs were transplanted into the periodontal tissue defect, newly formed cementum, and alveolar bone formation was observed in the periodontal fenestration defect. Interestingly, the regenerated cementum and bone volume in the DFAT/PLGA group was significant higher than in the ASCs/PLGA group. This is the first comparative study on periodontal tissue regeneration to show that rat DFAT cells have highly potential for cementum and alveolar bone formation than ASCs. However, the rat is not a reliable animal model because rats have a very high capability of regenerating bone. Therefore, we need to examine the periodontal tissue regeneration potential of DFAT cells in a large animal model before clinical use is attempted.

In contrast to our methods, Sugawara, and Sato used DFAT cells that were cultured in an osteogenic differentiation induction

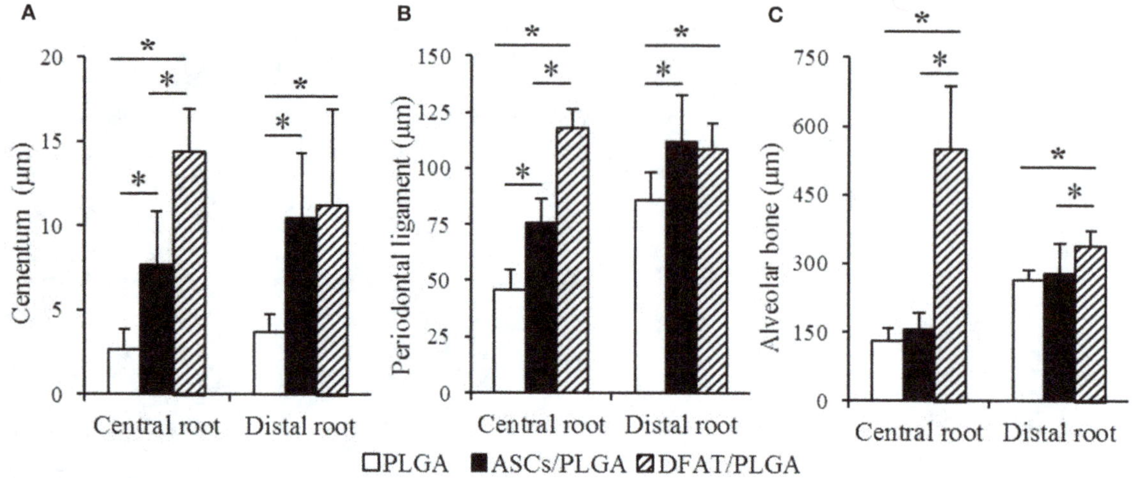


**FIGURE 9 | Histometric analysis of newly formed cementum thickness, periodontal ligament width, and alveolar bone width. (A)** In the central root of the first molar, the cementum in the DFAT/PLGA group was significantly thicker than that in the ASCs/PLGA and PLGA-alone groups. In the distal root of the first molar, there were no significant differences between DFAT/PLGA and ASCs/PLGA. **(B)** In the central root of first molar, the periodontal ligament of the DFAT/PLGA group was significantly wider than that of the ASCs/PLGA and PLGA-alone groups. In the distal root of first molar, there were no significant differences between DFAT/PLGA and ASCs/PLGA groups. **(C)** In the central root and distal root of the first molar, the alveolar bone in the DFAT/PLGA group was significantly thicker than in the ASCs/PLGA and PLGA-alone groups ($n = 12$, $^*P < 0.05$).

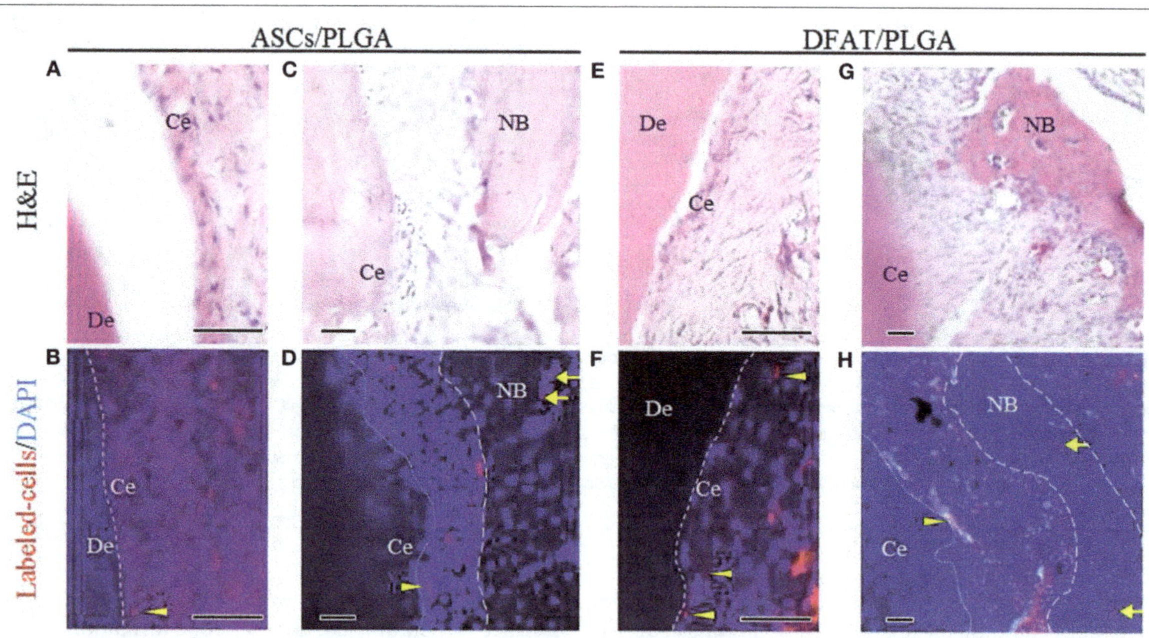


**FIGURE 10 | Localization of fluorescent-labeled ASCs and DFAT cells analyzed via fluorescence microscopy 5 weeks after transplantation. (A,C,E,G)** Highly magnified fluorescence images of the fenestration defect in the distal root of the first molar. (H&E staining; scale bar: 50 μm). **(B,D,F,H)** The dotted line indicates newly formed periodontal ligament tissue between cementum and bone. Fluorescent-labeled ASCs and DFAT cells were observed in periodontal ligament beside the bone (arrows) and cementum (arrowheads). (Blue color: DAPI; Scale bar: 50 μm.). NB, newly formed bone; Ce, newly formed cementum; De, root dentin.

medium before transplantation. They observed a small amount of a cementum on the exposed root surface (Sugawara and Sato, 2014). In our study, we found thicker cementum and alveolar bone formation. The discrepancy could be because of difference in the number of transplanted cells, the scaffold, and the treatment before transplantation. We seeded $1 \times 10^6$ DFAT cells in the PLGA scaffold. In addition, DFAT cells in our study had not been induced to undergo differentiation into specialized cells *in vitro*. Further research is needed to clarify suitable cell number and suitable pre-transplantation treatment.

We specifically observed fibrous connective tissue in the newly formed cementum and alveolar bone in the DFAT cell group and the ASC group by using Picrosirius-red staining and Azan staining. Interestingly, the periodontal ligament space in the DFAT/PLGA was wider than that in the ASCs/PLGA. The results suggest that the transplanted DFAT cells participated in the repair of periodontal tissue via secretion of trophic factors or that they could directly participate into the various cell types constituting the periodontium (Chen et al., 2008; Gnecchi et al., 2008; Mooney and Vandenburgh, 2008; Chen and Jin, 2010). Our group has reported that DFAT cells secrete several cytokines associated with bone formation and angiogenesis (Kikuta et al., 2013). In addition, some GFP-positive DFAT cells clearly remained in the regenerated periodontal tissue area, as also reported in a previous study on periodontal tissue regeneration (Sugawara and Sato, 2014). Our analysis also revealed that the transplanted DFAT cells were detected at the injection site 5 weeks after transplantation. Both of these results suggest that at least some of the DFAT cells engrafted onto injected periodontal tissue and contributed to local periodontal tissue regeneration. Further research is required to determine specifically whether the labeled DFAT cells generated the differentiated cementoblasts, osteoblasts, and periodontal ligament fibroblasts. Previous studies have demonstrated that MSCs, at least in part, can differentiated into cementoblasts, osteoblasts, and fibroblasts in regenerated periodontal tissue (Hasegawa et al., 2006; Tobita et al., 2008).

In conclusion, we found a significantly greater increase in crucial tissues, cementum, and alveolar bone in the DFAT/PLGA group compared with the ASCs/PLGA group. The regenerated periodontium restored the architecture to an arrangement that was similar to the original architecture, collagen fibers inserted into the cementum, and alveolar bone layers. DFAT cells could be a promising cell source for periodontal tissue regeneration. However, the impact of the local differentiation microenvironment on DFAT cells and the mechanisms controlling the differentiation into cementoblasts, periodontal ligament fibroblasts, and osteoblasts remain to be examined further.

## AUTHOR CONTRIBUTIONS

DA: Performed most of work, in particular *in-vivo* study. KK: Developed the technique to isolate DFAT cells. YS: Supported the experiment performed by DA. T. Mashimo: Performed *in vivo* experiments. N. Tsurumachi: Isolated DFAT cells from rat. KY: Developed the scaffolds in our study. TK: Developed the scaffold. TT: Performed Cell culture and differentiation assay. N. Tsukimura: Made the experimental design. T. Matsumoto: Established the differentiation assay and cell culture technique. TI: Prepared the manuscript. KI: Managed the overall experimental design. MH: Controlled the overall paper until completion.

## FUNDING

This work was supported in part by Grant-in-Aid for Scientific Research (B and Houga) (21390528, 15H05037, and 15K15724 to MH, and 15H04607 to KK), research grants from the Promotion Project of Medical Clustering of Okinawa Prefecture (KK), Grants from the Dental Research Center, the Nihon University School of Dentistry (MH), Nihon University Multidisciplinary Research Grant for 2012 and 2013 (MH), and the Nihon University Graduate School of Dentistry research fund (10010105 to DA). This work was also supported by the MEXT-Supported Program for the Strategic Research Foundation at Private Universities (S1411018).

## REFERENCES

Akita, D., Morokuma, M., Saito, Y., Yamanaka, K., Akiyama, Y., Sato, M., et al. (2014). Periodontal tissue regeneration by transplantation of rat adipose-derived stromal cells in combination with PLGA-based solid scaffolds. *Biomed. Res.* 35, 91–103. doi: 10.2220/biomedres.35.91

Aurrekoetxea, M., Garcia-Gallastegui, P., Irastorza, I., Luzuriaga, J., Uribe-Etxebarria, V., Unda, F., et al. (2015). Dental pulp stem cells as a multifaceted tool for bioengineering and the regeneration of craniomaxillofacial tissues. *Front. Physiol.* 6:289. doi: 10.3389/fphys.2015.00289

Chen, F. M., and Jin, Y. (2010). Periodontal tissue engineering and regeneration: current approaches and expanding opportunities. *Tissue Eng. Part B Rev.* 16, 219–255. doi: 10.1089/ten.teb.2009.0562

Chen, L., Tredget, E. E., Wu, P. Y., and Wu, Y. (2008). Paracrine factors of mesenchymal stem cells recruit macrophages and endothelial lineage cells and enhance wound healing. *PLoS ONE* 3:e1886. doi: 10.1371/journal.pone.0001886

Doğan, A., Ozdemir, A., Kubar, A., and Oygür, T. (2003). Healing of artificial fenestration defects by seeding of fibroblast-like cells derived from regenerated periodontal ligament in a dog: a preliminary study. *Tissue Eng.* 9, 1189–1196. doi: 10.1089/10763270360728099

Fraser, J. K., Wulur, I., Alfonso, Z., and Hedrick, M. H. (2006). Fat tissue: an underappreciated source of stem cells for biotechnology. *Trends Biotechnol.* 24, 150–154. doi: 10.1016/j.tibtech.2006.01.010

Gnecchi, M., Zhang, Z., Ni, A., and Dzau, V. J. (2008). Paracrine mechanisms in adult stem cell signaling and therapy. *Circ. Res.* 103, 1204–1219. doi: 10.1161/CIRCRESAHA.108.176826

Han, J., Menicanin, D., Marino, V., Ge, S., Mrozik, K., Gronthos, S., et al. (2013). Assessment of the regenerative potential of allogeneic periodontal ligament stem cells in a rodent periodontal defect model. *J. Periodont. Res.* 49, 333–345. doi: 10.1111/jre.12111

Hasegawa, N., Kawaguchi, H., Hirachi, A., Takeda, K., Mizuno, N., Nishimura, M., et al. (2006). Behavior of transplanted bone marrow-derived mesenchymal stem cells in periodontal defects. *J. Periodontol.* 77, 1003–1007. doi: 10.1902/jop.2006.050341

Honda, M. J., Imaizumi, M., Suzuki, H., Ohshima, S., Tsuchiya, S., and Satomura, K. (2011). Stem cells isolated from human dental follicles have osteogenic potential. *Oral Surg. Oral Med. Oral Pathol. Oral Radiol. Endod.* 111, 700–708. doi: 10.1016/j.tripleo.2010.08.004

Honda, M. J., Imaizumi, M., Tsuchiya, S., and Morsczeck, C. (2010). Dental follicle stem cells and tissue engineering. *J. Oral Sci.* 52, 541–552. doi: 10.2334/josnusd.52.541

Honda, M. J., Nakashima, F., Satomura, K., Shinohara, Y., Tsuchiya, S., Watanabe, N., et al. (2007). Side population cells expressing ABCG2 in human adult dental pulp tissue. *Int. Endod. J.* 40, 949–958. doi: 10.1111/j.1365-2591.2007.01301.x

Kaku, M., Akiba, Y., Akiyama, K., Akita, D., and Nishimura, M. (2015). Cell-based bone regeneration for alveolar ridge augmentation - cell source, endogenous cell recruitment and immunomodulatory function. *J. Prosthodont. Res.* 59, 96–112. doi: 10.1016/j.jpor.2015.02.001

Kawaguchi, H., Hirachi, A., Hasegawa, N., Iwata, T., Hamaguchi, H., Shiba, H., et al. (2004). Enhancement of periodontal tissue regeneration by transplantation of bone marrow mesenchymal stem cells. *J. Periodontol.* 75, 1281–1287. doi: 10.1902/jop.2004.75.9.1281

Kazama, T., Fujie, M., Endo, T., and Kano, K. (2008). Mature adipocyte-derived dedifferentiated fat cells can transdifferentiate into skeletal myocytes *in vitro*. *Biochem. Biophys. Res. Commun.* 377, 780–785. doi: 10.1016/j.bbrc.2008.10.046

Kikuta, S., Tanaka, N., Kazama, T., Kazama, M., Kano, K., Ryu, J., et al. (2013). Osteogenic effects of dedifferentiated fat cell transplantation in rabbit models of bone defect and ovariectomy-induced osteoporosis. *Tissue Eng. Part A* 19, 1792–1802. doi: 10.1089/ten.tea.2012.0380

King, G. N., King, N., Cruchley, A. T., Wozney, J. M., and Hughes, F. J. (1997). Recombinant human bone morphogenetic protein-2 promotes wound healing in rat periodontal fenestration defects. *J. Dent. Res.* 76, 1460–1470. doi: 10.1177/00220345970760080801

Kishimoto, N., Momota, Y., Hashimoto, Y., Tatsumi, S., Ando, K., Omasa, T., et al. (2013). The osteoblastic differentiation ability of human dedifferentiated fat cells is higher than that of adipose stem cells from the buccal fat pad. *Clin. Oral Investig.* 18, 1893–1901. doi: 10.1007/s00784-013-1166-1

Kono, S., Kazama, T., Kano, K., Harada, K., Uechi, M., and Matsumoto, T. (2014). Phenotypic and functional properties of feline dedifferentiated fat cells and adipose-derived stem cells. *Vet. J.* 199, 88–96. doi: 10.1016/j.tvjl.2013.10.033

Li, H., Yan, F., Lei, L., Li, Y., and Xiao, Y. (2009). Application of autologous cryopreserved bone marrow mesenchymal stem cells for periodontal regeneration in dogs. *Cells Tissues Organs* 190, 94–101. doi: 10.1159/000166547

Matsumoto, T., Kano, K., Kondo, D., Fukuda, N., Iribe, Y., Tanaka, N., et al. (2008). Mature adipocyte-derived dedifferentiated fat cells exhibit multilineage potential. *J. Cell. Physiol.* 215, 210–222. doi: 10.1002/jcp.21304

Mikami, Y., Ishii, Y., Watanabe, N., Shirakawa, T., Suzuki, S., Irie, S., et al. (2011). CD271/p75(NTR) inhibits the differentiation of mesenchymal stem cells into osteogenic, adipogenic, chondrogenic, and myogenic lineages. *Stem Cells Dev.* 20, 901–913. doi: 10.1089/scd.2010.0299

Mooney, D. J., and Vandenburgh, H. (2008). Cell delivery mechanisms for tissue repair. *Cell Stem Cell* 2, 205–213. doi: 10.1016/j.stem.2008.02.005

Nobusue, H., Endo, T., and Kano, K. (2008). Establishment of a preadipocyte cell line derived from mature adipocytes of GFP transgenic mice and formation of adipose tissue. *Cell Tissue Res.* 332, 435–446. doi: 10.1007/s00441-008-0593-9

Nobusue, H., and Kano, K. (2010). Establishment and characteristics of porcine preadipocyte cell lines derived from mature adipocytes. *J. Cell. Biochem.* 109, 542–552. doi: 10.1002/jcb.22431

Nuñez, J., Sanz-Blasco, S., Vignoletti, F., Muñoz, F., Arzate, H., Villalobos, C., et al. (2012). Periodontal regeneration following implantation of cementum and periodontal ligament-derived cells. *J. Periodont. Res.* 47, 33–44. doi: 10.1111/j.1600-0765.2011.01402.x

Ono, H., Oki, Y., Bono, H., and Kano, K. (2011). Gene expression profiling in multipotent DFAT cells derived from mature adipocytes. *Biochem. Biophys. Res. Commun.* 407, 562–567. doi: 10.1016/j.bbrc.2011.03.063

Prockop, D. J. (1997). Marrow stromal cells as stem cells for nonhematopoietic tissues. *Science* 276, 71–74. doi: 10.1126/science.276.5309.71

Reyes, M., Dudek, A., Jahagirdar, B., Koodie, L., Marker, P. H., and Verfaillie, C. M. (2002). Origin of endothelial progenitors in human postnatal bone marrow. *J. Clin. Invest.* 109, 337–346. doi: 10.1172/JCI0214327

Rungsiyanont, S., Dhanesuan, N., Swasdison, S., and Kasugai, S. (2012). Evaluation of biomimetic scaffold of gelatin-hydroxyapatite crosslink as a novel scaffold for tissue engineering: biocompatibility evaluation with human PDL fibroblasts, human mesenchymal stromal cells, and primary bone cells. *J. Biomater. Appl.* 27, 47–54. doi: 10.1177/0885328210391920

Safford, K. M., Hicok, K. C., Safford, S. D., Halvorsen, Y. D., Wilkison, W. O., Gimble, J. M., et al. (2002). Neurogenic differentiation of murine and human adipose-derived stromal cells. *Biochem. Biophys. Res. Commun.* 294, 371–379. doi: 10.1016/S0006-291X(02)00469-2

Saito, Y., Watanabe, E., Mayahara, K., Watanabe, N., Morokuma, M., Isokawa, K., et al. (2013). CD146/MCAM surface marker for identifying human periodontal ligament- derived mesenchymal stem cells. *J. Hard Tissue Biol.* 22, 115–128. doi: 10.2485/jhtb.22.115

Sato, M., Toriumi, T., Watanabe, N., Watanabe, E., Akita, D., Mashimo, T., et al. (2015). Characterization of mesenchymal progenitor cells in crown and root pulp from human mesiodentes. *Oral Dis.* 21, e86–e97. doi: 10.1111/odi.12234

Sugawara, A., and Sato, S. (2014). Application of dedifferentiated fat cells for periodontal tissue regeneration. *Hum. Cell* 27, 12–21. doi: 10.1007/s13577-013-0075-6

Tobita, M., and Mizuno, H. (2013). Adipose-derived stem cells and periodontal tissue engineering. *Int. J. Oral Maxillofac. Implants* 28, e487–e493. doi: 10.11607/jomi.te29

Tobita, M., Uysal, A. C., Ogawa, R., Hyakusoku, H., and Mizuno, H. (2008). Periodontal tissue regeneration with adipose-derived stem cells. *Tissue Eng. Part A* 14, 945–953. doi: 10.1089/ten.tea.2007.0048

Wang, H. L., Greenwell, H., Fiorellini, J., Giannobile, W., Offenbacher, S., Salkin, L., et al. (2005). Periodontal regeneration. *J. Periodontol.* 76, 1601–1622. doi: 10.1902/jop.2005.76.9.1601

Yagi, K., Kondo, D., Okazaki, Y., and Kano, K. (2004). A novel preadipocyte cell line established from mouse adult mature adipocytes. *Biochem. Biophys. Res. Commun.* 321, 967–974. doi: 10.1016/j.bbrc.2004.07.055

Yamanaka, K., Yamamoto, K., Sakai, Y., Suda, Y., Shigemitsu, Y., Kaneko, T., et al. (2015). Seeding of mesenchymal stem cells into inner part of interconnected porous biodegradable scaffold by a new method with a filter paper. *Dent Mate J.* 34, 78–85. doi: 10.4012/dmj.2013-330

Yang, Y., Rossi, F. M., and Putnins, E. E. (2010). Periodontal regeneration using engineered bone marrow mesenchymal stromal cells. *Biomaterials* 31, 8574–8582. doi: 10.1016/j.biomaterials.2010.06.026

Zhao, M., Jin, Q., Berry, J. E., Nociti, F. H. Jr., Giannobile, W. V., and Somerman, M. J. (2004). Cementoblast delivery for periodontal tissue engineering. *J. Periodontol.* 75, 154–161. doi: 10.1902/jop.2004.75.1.154

Zuk, P. A., Zhu, M., Mizuno, H., Huang, J., Futrell, J. W., Katz, A. J., et al. (2001). Multilineage cells from human adipose tissue: implications for cell-based therapies. *Tissue Eng.* 7, 211–228. doi: 10.1089/107632701300062859

3

# Manufacturing of dental pulp cell-based products from human third molars: current strategies and future investigations

**Edited by:**
*Thimios Mitsiadis, University of Zurich, Switzerland*

***Correspondence:**
*Jean-Christophe Farges, Laboratoire de Biologie Tissulaire et Ingénierie thérapeutique, Institut de Biologie et Chimie des Protéines, UMR5305 Centre National de la Recherche Scientifique/Université Claude Bernard Lyon 1, 7 passage du Vercors, 69367 Lyon, France jean-christophe.farges@univ-lyon1.fr*

*Maxime Ducret[1,2,3], Hugo Fabre[1], Olivier Degoul[4], Gianluigi Atzeni[4], Colin McGuckin[4], Nico Forraz[4], Brigitte Alliot-Licht[5], Frédéric Mallein-Gerin[1], Emeline Perrier-Groult[1] and Jean-Christophe Farges[1,2,3*]*

[1] Laboratoire de Biologie Tissulaire et Ingénierie thérapeutique, UMR5305 Centre National de la Recherche Scientifique/Université Claude Bernard Lyon 1, Lyon, France, [2] Faculté d'Odontologie, Université de Lyon, Université Claude Bernard Lyon 1, Lyon, France, [3] Hospices Civils de Lyon, Service de Consultations et Traitements Dentaires, Lyon, France, [4] CTI-BIOTECH, Cell Therapy Research Institute, Meyzieu, France, [5] Faculté d'Odontologie, Institut National de la Santé et de la Recherche Médicale UMR1064, Centre de Recherche en Transplantation et Immunologie, Université de Nantes, Nantes, France

In recent years, mesenchymal cell-based products have been developed to improve surgical therapies aimed at repairing human tissues. In this context, the tooth has recently emerged as a valuable source of stem/progenitor cells for regenerating orofacial tissues, with easy access to pulp tissue and high differentiation potential of dental pulp mesenchymal cells. International guidelines now recommend the use of standardized procedures for cell isolation, storage and expansion in culture to ensure optimal reproducibility, efficacy and safety when cells are used for clinical application. However, most dental pulp cell-based medicinal products manufacturing procedures may not be fully satisfactory since they could alter the cells biological properties and the quality of derived products. Cell isolation, enrichment and cryopreservation procedures combined to long-term expansion in culture media containing xeno- and allogeneic components are known to affect cell phenotype, viability, proliferation and differentiation capacities. This article focuses on current manufacturing strategies of dental pulp cell-based medicinal products and proposes a new protocol to improve efficiency, reproducibility and safety of these strategies.

**Keywords: human dental pulp, stem cells, tissue engineering, immunophenotyping, expansion, cryopreservation, good manufacturing practices, cell-based medicinal products**

## Introduction

Over the two last decades, mesenchymal stromal cells (MSC) have been intensely studied due to their potential clinical applicability to treat tissue and organ defects resulting from diseases, trauma or aging (Caplan, 1991). Their use has been proposed to repair and regenerate human mesenchymal tissues, alone or combined to scaffolds and/or morphogenic molecules (Langer and Vacanti, 1993). Bone marrow and adipose tissue are conventional sources of MSC, but invasive cell collection protocols, frequent use of general anesthesia and risk of morbidity at the collection site have stimulated the search for alternative tissues (Huang et al., 2009; Zuk, 2010;

Davies et al., 2015). Third molars are frequently removed for therapeutic reasons and the connective tissue it contains, the dental pulp, can be easily recovered. They are now considered a valuable source of MSC for tissue repair and regeneration (Mayo et al., 2014). In this context, numerous investigators have attempted to obtain clinical-grade dental pulp stem/progenitor cells (DPSC) from these teeth. However, most manufacturing procedures reported so far may not be totally satisfactory, since they may alter the biological properties of the cells and the quality of the derived cell-based products (Ménard and Tarte, 2013). If such procedures are currently permitted by European and American regulation authorities, further studies are necessary to develop more efficient, reproducible, safe and standardized manufacturing processes of dental pulp cell-based medicinal products (Tirino and Papaccio, 2012; Albuquerque et al., 2014; Eubanks et al., 2014; Huang and Garcia-Godoy, 2014; La Noce et al., 2014; Nakashima and Iohara, 2014).

Dental pulp mesenchymal cells have been successfully used to regenerate human craniofacial bone (d'Aquino et al., 2009; Giuliani et al., 2013). However, these studies were performed in the absence of defined, universally accepted protocols for large-scale, clinical-grade production of DPSC (Fekete et al., 2012). This point is important in the light of recent reports indicating moderate, irreproducible and non-suitable benefits of therapies performed with various sources of MSC (Allison, 2009; Tyndall, 2011; Daley, 2012). These results were explained in part by the fact that cell performances are affected by cell isolation and expansion conditions and indicate the need for optimized and standardized procedures for MSC-based products' manufacturing (Allison, 2009; Pacini, 2014). The European Union (EU) and United States (US) have established classifications and recommended guidelines for manufacturing MSC-based products. In Europe, MSC are defined as "cell therapy products" and referred to as Advanced Therapy Medicinal Products (ATMP) (European Regulation 1394/2007). ATMP are considered Cell-Based Medicinal Products (CBMP) when containing living cells or tissues. CBMP are "medicinal products presented as having properties for, or used in or administered to, human beings with a view to treating, preventing or diagnosing a disease in which the pharmacological, immunological or metabolic actions are carried out by cells or tissues" (Schneider et al., 2010; Pacini, 2014). DPSC belong to this category and can be referred to as Dental Pulp (DP)-CBMP. In the US, DPSC are considered as Human Cells, Tissues or cellular and tissue-based Products (HCT/Ps) (Code of Federal Regulation (CFR) Title 21 CFR 1271). They are classified in two categories: (1) products that are "minimally manipulated" and used clinically in a homologous manner, and (2) products that are either "more than minimally manipulated" or used in a non-homologous manner. A cell-based product is considered as being "more than minimally manipulated" when the inherent biological characteristics of the cells have been significantly altered (Pacini, 2014).

Production and delivery of MSCs should be made in accordance with European Good Manufacturing Practices (GMP), whereas, in the US, it must comply with Current Good Tissue Practice requirements (GTP) (Fekete et al., 2012; Kellathur and Lou, 2012; Sensebé et al., 2013). GMP/GTP require many quality controls regarding donor eligibility, sample recovery, label, transport and receipt, process and storage, laboratory equipment, supplies and reagents, cell-based product distribution to recipient patients and documentation that must be maintained by the handler (Alici and Blomberg, 2010; Abou-El-Enein et al., 2013; Sensebé et al., 2013; Wuchter et al., 2015). These controls make GMP/GTP procedures long and costly, and further studies are encouraged to develop shorter, less expensive and more standardized procedures for DP-CBMP manufacturing (Albuquerque et al., 2014; Eubanks et al., 2014; Huang and Garcia-Godoy, 2014; La Noce et al., 2014; Nakashima and Iohara, 2014; Hilkens et al., 2015). In the present paper, we will firstly review current international guidelines regarding the five manufacturing steps of DP-CBMP (**Figure 1**), and then we will highlight the drawbacks and potential risks of actual strategies. Finally we will propose modifications of the protocols intended to increase the efficiency, reproducibility and safety of these strategies, from tooth extraction to the harvest of clinical-grade DP-CMBP.

## Teeth Collection and Pulp Tissue Recovery

Since the discovery of DPSC by Gronthos et al. (2000), numerous papers have reported the isolation of stem/progenitor cells from the dental pulp of human third molars. However, since there are no rules specifying the best tooth development stages for pulp cell collection, teeth were collected in patients of various ages and therefore at various developmental stages. It also greatly impairs the interpretation and comparison of the experimental results.

Transport from the operating block to the laboratory notably requires a medium that does not affect cell viability. It was previously shown that DPSC remain viable up for 5 days when extracted teeth are maintained in phosphate-buffered saline (PBS) (Perry et al., 2008; Woods et al., 2009) and this time is more than enough for the transport of samples to the laboratory and pulp recovery.

## Dental Pulp Cell Isolation and Enrichment

After dental pulp recovery, two options are possible for isolating dental pulp cells: enzymatic dissociation and explant culture. Enzymatic dissociation consists of digesting the pulp tissue with collagenase and dispase enzymes to liberate the cells that are then plated on culture dishes. However, a growing number of authors consider that enzymatic dissociation is not adapted to medicinal manufacturing, owing to its putative consequences on cell phenotype and properties (Shah et al., 2013; Busser et al., 2014; Ohnuma et al., 2014). In addition, tissues and cells exposed to collagenase are considered "more than minimally manipulated" by FDA [Code of Federal Regulation (CFR) Title 21 CFR 1271] and potentially require the use of pharmaceutical grade manufactured enzymes, which significantly increases the scale-up costs. By contrast, cell isolation by explant culture increasingly appears easier, faster, safer, less expensive and more in line with GMP guidelines to obtain clinical-grade amounts of MSC (Hilkens et al., 2013). It is based on the growth of cells out of tissue fragments (explants) that are plated on culture dishes. It recently allowed for efficient recovery of human adipose or Wharton jelly stem/progenitor cells in serum-free,

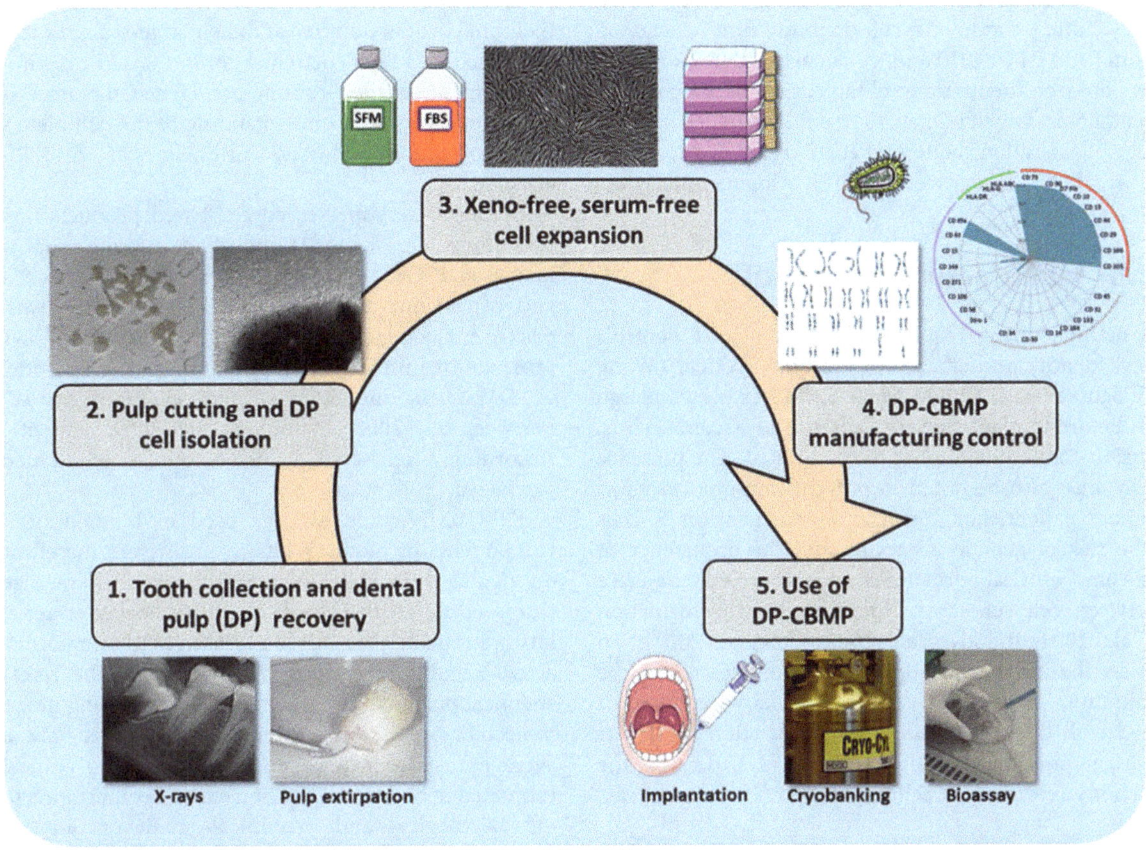


**FIGURE 1 | Standardization of the DP-CBMP manufacturing process.** It requires five major steps: tooth selection and use of the easiest technique for pulp recovery (Step 1), HDPC isolation with fast, safe and less expensive procedures (Step 2), cell expansion in defined, serum-free culture conditions with xeno-free reagents (Step 3), advanced monitoring and control of DP-CBMP manufacturing (Step 4), use of clinical-grade DP-CMBP, for immediate implantation, cryobanking or development of a bioassay (Step 5).

xeno-free medium conditions (Busser et al., 2014; Swamynathan et al., 2014). Additionally, explant-derived DPSC display similar or enhanced differentiation abilities compared with cells from dissociated tissue (Spath et al., 2010; Hilkens et al., 2013).

Cell selection by sorting methods has been proposed to enrich the cultured cell population in stem/progenitor cells based on their expression of specific surface markers such as CD34, CD184, Stro-1, CD146, CD271, and MSCA-1 (Shi and Gronthos, 2003; d'Aquino et al., 2009; Waddington et al., 2009; Yu et al., 2010; Jiang et al., 2012; Tomlinson et al., 2015). However, the use of such a procedure is today limited by the complexity of the technique and the prohibitive cost (Kawashima, 2012; Nakashima and Iohara, 2014). Besides, multiplying steps and using additional reagents increase the risk of microbial contamination and the difficulty to obtain CBMP in GMP conditions. The same reservation can be made regarding the use of biophysical markers that have been found relevant to isolate MSC in an easier and more predictable way than biochemical markers (Lee et al., 2014).

## Dental Pulp Cell Culture and Expansion

Among other factors, the composition of the culture medium and the presence of a coating material on the culture dish may influence the nature and the quality of the final CBMP and therefore the clinical results (Lopez-Cazaux et al., 2006; Majd et al., 2009; Jung et al., 2012; Pisciotta et al., 2012; Pacini, 2014). Currently, CBMP manufacturing under GMP procedures recommends the use of xeno-free materials and reagents to prevent the risk of viral, bacterial, fungal and prion contamination, and the possible induction of immunizing effects in the final recipient. Additionally, industrial production is responsible for frequent batch-to-batch serum variability and the serum itself can promote early cell differentiation (Mannello and Tonti, 2007; Jung et al., 2012). For these reasons, the supplementation of the cell culture medium with xeno- or allogeneic products should be limited to "cases for which a valid alternative cannot be found" (European Regulation 1394/2007). Today, the development of xeno-free, serum-free, defined media, able to rapidly expand stem/progenitor cells without impairing their differentiation capabilities, represents a major objective for the standardization of DP-CBMP production (Tekkatte et al., 2011; Jung et al., 2012; Bonnamain et al., 2013; Carvalho et al., 2013). Multiple passages are often necessary to obtain a clinical-scale amount of cells, but they may lead to a slow-down of the proliferation rate, progressive cell senescence and loss of multipotentiality that prevent future cell differentiation (Baxter et al., 2004; Bork et al., 2010; Yu et al., 2010; Sensebé et al., 2013). In our culture conditions, cell doubling times remained constant from P1 to P4 (≈40 h) and we calculated that more than $25.10^7$ cells could be theoretically obtained after four passages with one dental pulp, which is likely to be a sufficient cell number for one pulp regeneration, bone socket filling, or for localized periodontal treatment (Kaigler et al., 2013; Albuquerque et al., 2014).

## DP-CBMP Manufacturing Control

DP-CBMP manufacturing requires advanced quality controls of the safety, identity and efficacy of the final product (Wang et al., 2005; Sensebé et al., 2013). Since CBMP cannot undergo sterilization before implantation, the absence of bacteria, virus, fungi and prion contamination has to be checked. The presence of endotoxin must also be tested to prevent immune reactions in the recipient patient. Long-term *ex vivo* expansion of cells increases the risk of genetic instability and the occurrence of potential chromosomal abnormalities, since there exists a close relation between cell senescence and risk of transformation (Baxter et al., 2004; Rubio et al., 2005; Campisi, 2007). To limit this risk, the number of population doublings should be kept to a minimum. In addition, conventional karyotyping must be combined with fluorescence *in situ* hybridization (FISH) or comparative genomic hybridization (CGH array) to assess the genomic stability of scaled-up cell populations (Barkholt et al., 2013).

The control of the population identity into expanding cell cultures is generally realized by flow cytometry analysis of surface antigens. During the past decade, most of these controls have been realized in compliance with the recommendations of the International Society of Cellular Therapy (ISCT) (Dominici et al., 2006). However, it is today acknowledged that several markers initially proposed by ISCT for the positive characterization of MSC (for instance CD73, CD90, and CD105) are shared by several populations of cells including progenitor cells, mature fibroblasts or perivascular cells (Russell et al., 2010; Alt et al., 2011; Halfon et al., 2011; Al-Nbaheen et al., 2013; Lv et al., 2014).

## DP-CBMP Uses

Over recent years, DP-CBMP were clinically tested with the aim to regenerate human craniofacial bone. DP-CBMP were implanted, in association with a collagen I-based sponge scaffold, in mandibular bone sockets in a phase I clinical trial (d'Aquino et al., 2009). Three years after DP-CBMP grafting, the tissue regenerated in the graft site was compact bone (Giuliani et al., 2013). Case reports of osteoradionecrosis treatment using DP-CBMP were also reported (Manimaran et al., 2014). The angiogenic, neurogenic and odontogenic potential of DP-CBMP was also successfully tested in preclinical studies (Gandia et al., 2008; Iohara et al., 2009; Sakai et al., 2012; Ishizaka et al., 2013). In addition, a phase I clinical trial is currently under progress to evaluate the DP-CBMP potential to regenerate the human dental pulp (Nakashima and Iohara, 2014). Despite these successes, potential applicability of DP-CBMP will be closely dependent on their final production cost and their large-scale clinical outcomes. In particular, a high cost-efficacy ratio would constitute a serious impediment for their routine use. Hence, it is necessary to have a clear overview and understanding of the complete value chain to try to reduce costs (Abou-El-Enein et al., 2013, 2014; Leijten et al., 2015).

Storage of cryopreserved cell-based products (cryobanking) over long periods of time offers unique opportunities to increase DP-CBMP applicability. However, similar to cell culture and expansion, cryopreservation is associated with infective, prion, toxicological and immunological risks owing to the presence of human or animal components and additives such as DMSO in the storage medium (Papaccio et al., 2006; Perry et al., 2008; Woods et al., 2009; Lee et al., 2012). Accordingly, xeno-free, defined cryopreservation media must be privileged.

DP-CBMP could also be used in biomedical research as components of bioassay kits to investigate the effects of drugs on dental pulp cells in a reproducible "humanized" system (Jurga et al., 2010; Leeb et al., 2011; Forraz et al., 2013). Such kits are reliable preclinical alternatives to animal models in the actual regulatory context. Assessment of the risks related to chemical products' use and screening or testing new therapeutic molecules are indeed extremely complicated and costly. The average costs to take a blockbuster drug to clinical trials are estimated to be around 1 billion euros. Furthermore, the accuracy of toxicological and preclinical studies greatly depends on the experimental animal models used for such evaluations. In particular, rodent species, widely use, are known to only partially mimic the human biological system. Development of DP-CBMP bioassay kits would offer a prime platform to successfully induce dentinogenesis, osteogenesis or neurogenesis *in vitro* (Zhang et al., 2006; Woloszyk et al., 2014; Jensen et al., 2015; Leijten et al., 2015).

## Proposals for a Protocol with a More GMP Compliant Approach (Figure 2)

We recently proposed the use of impacted third molars between Nolla's developmental stages 5 (crown almost completed) and 7 (one third root completed). The presence of large, open apices in teeth without roots or with roots partially developed allows for an easy access to the pulp tissue and its gentle, atraumatic extirpation from the enamel/dentin shell with fine tweezers. It avoids the cell stress resulting from the crown-root mechanical separation with a drill or a clamp that is necessary for recovering pulps from teeth with more developed or complete roots (Perry et al., 2008; Takeda et al., 2008; Ducret et al., in press). Additionally, human dental pulp cells (HDPC) isolated at around the crown-completed stage displayed short cell doubling times and high growth rate (Takeda et al., 2008). We found similar results in our study. We also selected impacted teeth to minimize the risk of pulp tissue contamination and disease transmission by oral microorganisms (Nolla, 1960; Ducret et al., in press). This choice may enable to skip the step of sample disinfection performed

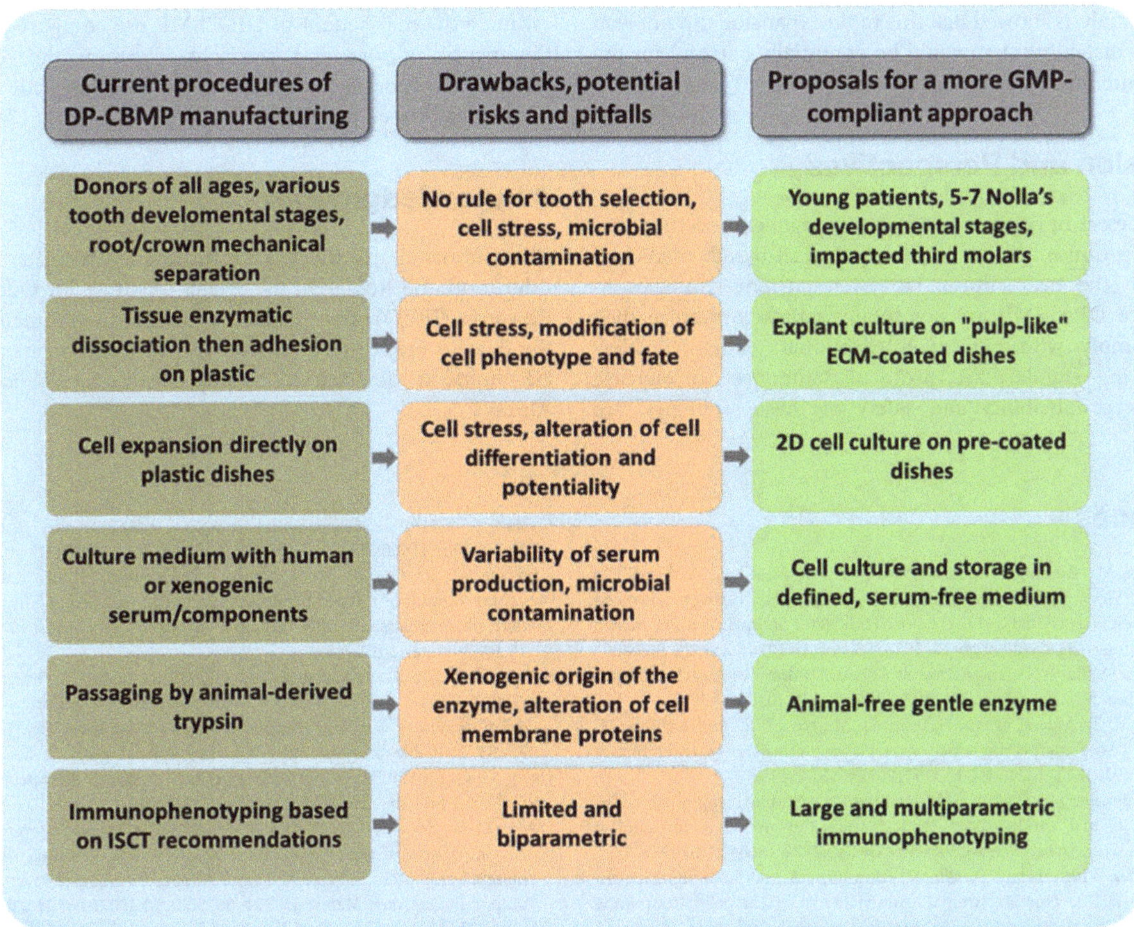


**FIGURE 2 | Important steps during DP-CBMP manufacturing that require modification.** Major drawbacks, risks and pitfalls are highlighted for each one, and proposals are made for the development of more GMP-compliant procedures.

with chemicals such as chlorhexidine or povidone-iodine/sodium thiosulfate (Perry et al., 2008; d'Aquino et al., 2009). When using PBS as a transport medium, we failed to detect any contamination in cultures of HDPC ($n > 50$ patients) during the isolation and expansion steps, contrary to others (Perry et al., 2008; Ducret et al., in press). This might be related to our selection of impacted teeth from young patients (13–17 year-old) that have never been in contact with the septic oral cavity, versus the selection of erupted ones from older patients (18–30 year-old) by those authors.

Regarding cell isolation, we used explant culture for recovering human dental pulp cells for clinical application. Each pulp sample was cut into about 20 explants that allowed for the harvest of a total of one million dental pulp cells after 14 days of culture (Ducret et al., in press). This result is in agreement with other studies reporting that, whatever the technique used (tissue dissociation or explant culture), 2 weeks of culture allow for the recovery of about $10^6$ cells from one third molar pulp (Eubanks et al., 2014).

We pre-coated the culture dish surface for cell isolation and culture with an equal mixture of human placental collagens I and III. This composition was chosen because they are the two most abundant collagens in the dental pulp extracellular matrix. Xeno-free dissociating reagents (such as TrypLe® or Accutase®) and xeno-free defined culture medium (such as SPE-IV® [ABCell-Bio, France], containing clinical grade human albumin, α-MEM, rhIGF-1 and rhFGF-2) are recommended for cell culture and passaging instead of the products commonly used (Carvalho et al., 2013; Ducret et al., in press). Moreover, cryopreservation of dental pulp cells in serum-free medium had no negative impact on cell doubling times and cumulative cell numbers (Ducret et al., in press). Although the viability of cells cryopreserved in serum-free medium was decreased compared to fresh cells, it is similar to that previously reported (Lee et al., 2012).

Future investigations are required for identifying more specific membrane markers for these cells. In our study, immunophenotypic analysis of 17 surface markers revealed that our dental pulp cell expanding population was made of mesenchymal cells, a percentage of whom expressed the mesenchymal stem cell/progenitor markers CD146 and MSCA-1. The number of cells expressing these markers remained similar from P1 to P4, suggesting that the cell fate was not significantly affected by our culture conditions. In addition, cell karyotyping by G-band analysis showed that this rapid expansion did not lead to genomic instability that would be potentially harmful for the recipient patient (Ducret et al., in press).

## Conclusion and Perspectives

Recent successes in bone and dental pulp regeneration therapies carry the promise to use dental pulp-cell-based medicinal products in the near future. However, current strategies to manufacture DP-CBMP are not totally satisfactory since they do not comply with current international guidelines. New manufacturing standardized protocols, intended to increase efficiency, reproducibility and safety of these strategies, are urgently needed. Further investigations are also warranted to estimate the real benefit of DP-CBMP use compared to current therapeutic options and precisely determine the cost-efficacy ratio that risks being a major block for the large-scale clinical use of these cell-based products.

## Acknowledgments

The authors thank the CNRS, the French Ministry of Higher Education and Research, the French Institute for Odontological Research (IFRO), the Société Française de Rhumatologie and the Société Française d'Endodontie for their financial support. HF holds a doctoral fellowship from the Région Rhône-Alpes.

## References

Abou-El-Enein, M., Römhild, A., Kaiser, D., Beier, C., Bauer, G., Volk, H. D., et al. (2013). Good Manufacturing Practices (GMP) manufacturing of advanced therapy medicinal products: a novel tailored model for optimizing performance and estimating costs. *Cytotherapy* 15, 362–383. doi: 10.1016/j.jcyt.2012.09.006

Abou-El-Enein, M., Bauer, G., and Reinke, P. (2014). The business case for cell and gene therapies. *Nat. Biotechnol.* 32, 1192–1193. doi: 10.1038/nbt.3084

Albuquerque, M. T., Valera, M. C., Nakashima, M., Nör, J. E., and Bottino, M. C. (2014). Tissue-engineering-based strategies for regenerative endodontics. *J. Dent. Res.* 93, 1222–1231. doi: 10.1177/0022034514549809

Alici, E., and Blomberg, P. (2010). GMP facilities for manufacturing of advanced therapy medicinal products for clinical trials: an overview for clinical researchers. *Curr. Gene Ther.* 10, 508–515. doi: 10.2174/156652310793797757

Al-Nbaheen, M., Vishnubalaji, R., Ali, D., Bouslimi, A., Al-Jassir, F., Megges, M., et al. (2013). Human stromal (mesenchymal) stem cells from bone marrow, adipose tissue and skin exhibit differences in molecular phenotype and differentiation potential. *Stem Cell Rev.* 9, 32–43. doi: 10.1007/s12015-012-9365-8

Allison, M. (2009). Genzyme backs Osiris, despite Prochymal flop. *Nat. Biotechnol.* 27, 966–967. doi: 10.1038/nbt1109-966

Alt, E., Yan, Y., Gehmert, S., Song, Y. H., Altman, A., Vykoukal, D., et al. (2011). Fibroblasts share mesenchymal phenotypes with stem cells, but lack their differentiation and colony-forming potential. *Biol. Cell* 103, 197–208. doi: 10.1042/BC20100117

Barkholt, L., Flory, E., Jekerle, V., Lucas-Samuel, S., Ahnert, P., Bisset, L., et al. (2013). Risk of tumorigenicity in mesenchymal stromal cell-based therapies–bridging scientific observations and regulatory viewpoints. *Cytotherapy* 15, 753–759. doi: 10.1016/j.jcyt.2013.03.005

Baxter, M. A., Wynn, R. F., Jowitt, S. N., Wraith, J. E., Fairbairn, L. J., and Bellantuono, I. (2004). Study of telomere length reveals rapid aging of human marrow stromal cells following *in vitro* expansion. *Stem Cells* 22, 675–682. doi: 10.1634/stemcells.22-5-675

Bonnamain, V., Thinard, R., Sergent-Tanguy, S., Huet, P., Bienvenu, G., Naveilhan, P., et al. (2013). Human dental pulp stem cells cultured in serum-free supplemented medium. *Front. Physiol.* 4:357. doi: 10.3389/fphys.2013.00357

Bork, S., Pfister, S., Witt, H., Horn, P., Korn, B., Ho, A. D., et al. (2010). DNA methylation pattern changes upon long-term culture and aging of human mesenchymal stromal cells. *Aging Cell* 9, 54–63. doi: 10.1111/j.1474-9726.2009.00535.x

Busser, H., De Bruyn, C., Urbain, F., Najar, M., Pieters, K., Raicevic, G., et al. (2014). Isolation of adipose derived stromal cells without enzymatic treatment: expansion, phenotypical and functional characterization. *Stem Cells Dev.* 23, 2390–2400. doi: 10.1089/scd.2014.0071

Campisi, J. (2007). Aging and cancer cell biology. *Aging Cell* 6, 261–263. doi: 10.1111/j.1474-9726.2007.00292.x

Caplan, A. I. (1991). Mesenchymal stem cells. *J. Orthop. Res.* 9, 641–650. doi: 10.1002/jor.1100090504

Carvalho, P. P., Gimble, J. M., Dias, I. R., Gomes, M. E., and Reis, R. L. (2013). Xenofree enzymatic products for the isolation of human adipose-derived stromal/stem cells. *Tissue Eng. Part C Methods* 19, 473–478. doi: 10.1089/ten.tec.2012.0465

d'Aquino, R., De Rosa, A., Lanza, V., Tirino, V., Laino, L., Graziano, A., et al. (2009). Human mandible bone defect repair by the grafting of dental pulp stem/progenitor cells and collagen sponge biocomplexes. *Eur. Cell Mater.* 18, 75–83. Available online at: http://www.ecmjournal.org/

Daley, G. Q. (2012). The promise and perils of stem cell therapeutics. *Cell Stem Cell.* 10, 740–749. doi: 10.1016/j.stem.2012.05.010

Davies, O. G., Cooper, P. R., Shelton, R. M., Smith, A. J., and Scheven, B. A. (2015). A comparison of the *in vitro* mineralisation and dentinogenic potential of mesenchymal stem cells derived from adipose tissue, bone marrow and dental pulp. *J. Bone Miner. Metab.* 33, 371–382. doi: 10.1007/s00774-014-0601-y

Dominici, M., Le Blanc, K., Mueller, I., Slaper-Cortenbach, I., Marini, F., Krause, D., et al. (2006). Minimal criteria for defining multipotent mesenchymal stromal cells. The International Society for Cellular Therapy position statement. *Cytotherapy* 8, 315–317. doi: 10.1080/14653240600855905

Ducret, M., Fabre, H., Farges, J.-C., Degoul, O., Atzeni, G., McGuckin, C., et al. (in press). Production of human dental pulp cells with a medicinal manufacturing approach. *J. Endod.* doi: 10.1016/j.joen.2015.05.017

Eubanks, E. J., Tarle, S. A., and Kaigler, D. (2014). Tooth storage, dental pulp stem cell isolation, and clinical scale expansion without animal serum. *J. Endod.* 40, 652–657. doi: 10.1016/j.joen.2014.01.005

Fekete, N., Rojewski, M. T., Fürst, D., Kreja, L., Ignatius, A., Dausend, J., et al. (2012). GMP-compliant isolation and large-scale expansion of bone marrow-derived MSC. *PLoS ONE* 7:e43255. doi: 10.1371/journal.pone.0043255

Forraz, N., Wright, K. E., Jurga, M., and McGuckin, C. P. (2013). Experimental therapies for repair of the central nervous system: stem cells and tissue engineering. *J. Tissue Eng. Regen. Med.* 7, 523–536. doi: 10.1002/term.552

Gandia, C., Armiñan, A., García-Verdugo, J. M., Lledó, E., Ruiz, A., Miñana, M. D., et al. (2008). Human dental pulp stem cells improve left ventricular function, induce angiogenesis, and reduce infarct size in rats with acute myocardial infarction. *Stem Cells* 26, 638–645. doi: 10.1634/stemcells.2007-0484

Giuliani, A., Manescu, A., Langer, M., Rustichelli, F., Desiderio, V., Paino, F., et al. (2013). Three years after transplants in human mandibles, histological and in-line holotomography revealed that stem cells regenerated a compact rather than a spongy bone: biological and clinical implications. *Stem Cells Trans. Med.* 2, 316–324. doi: 10.5966/sctm.2012-0136

Gronthos, S., Mankani, M., Brahim, J., Robey, P. G., and Shi, S. (2000). Postnatal human dental pulp stem cells (DPSCs) *in vitro* and *in vivo*. *Proc. Natl Acad. Sci. U.S.A.* 97, 13625–13630. doi: 10.1073/pnas.240309797

Halfon, S., Abramov, N., Grinblat, B., and Ginis, I. (2011). Markers distinguishing mesenchymal stem cells from fibroblasts are downregulated with passaging. *Stem Cells Dev.* 20, 53–66. doi: 10.1089/scd.2010.0040

Hilkens, P., Gervois, P., Fanton, Y., Vanormelingen, J., Martens, W., Struys, T., et al. (2013). Effect of isolation methodology on stem cell properties and multilineage differentiation potential of human dental pulp stem cells. *Cell Tissue Res.* 353, 65–78. doi: 10.1007/s00441-013-1630-x

Hilkens, P., Meschi, N., Lambrechts, P., Bronckaers, A., and Lambrichts, I. (2015). Dental stem cells in pulp regeneration: near future or long road ahead? *Stem Cells Dev.* 24, 1610–1622. doi: 10.1089/scd.2014.0510

Huang, G. T., Gronthos, S., and Shi, S. (2009). Mesenchymal stem cells derived from dental tissues vs. those from other sources: their biology and role in regenerative medicine. *J. Dent. Res.* 88, 792–806. doi: 10.1177/0022034509340867

Huang, G. T., and Garcia-Godoy, F. (2014). Missing concepts in de novo pulp regeneration. *J. Dent. Res.* 93, 717–724. doi: 10.1177/0022034514537829

Iohara, K., Zheng, L., Ito, M., Ishizaka, R., Nakamura, H., Into, T., et al. (2009). Regeneration of dental pulp after pulpotomy by transplantation of CD31 (-)/CD146(-) side population cells from a canine tooth. *Regen. Med.* 4, 377–385. doi: 10.2217/rme.09.5

Ishizaka, R., Hayashi, Y., Iohara, K., Sugiyama, M., Murakami, M., Yamamoto, T., et al. (2013). Stimulation of angiogenesis, neurogenesis and regeneration by side population cells from dental pulp. *Biomaterials* 34, 1888–1897. doi: 10.1016/j.biomaterials.2012.10.045

Jensen, J., Kraft, D. C., Lysdahl, H., Foldager, C. B., Chen, M., Kristiansen, A. A., et al. (2015). Functionalization of polycaprolactone scaffolds with hyaluronic acid and β-TCP facilitates migration and osteogenic differentiation of human dental pulp stem cells *in vitro*. *Tissue Eng. Part A* 21, 729–739. doi: 10.1089/ten.tea.2014.0177

Jiang, L., Peng, W. W., Li, L. F., Yang, Y., and Zhu, Y. Q. (2012). Isolation and identification of CXCR4-positive cells from human dental pulp cells. *J. Endod.* 38, 791–795. doi: 10.1016/j.joen.2012.02.024

Jung, S., Panchalingam, K. M., Rosenberg, L., and Behie, L. A. (2012). *Ex vivo* expansion of human mesenchymal stem cells in defined serum-free media. *Stem Cells Int.* 2012:123030. doi: 10.1155/2012/123030

Jurga, M., Forraz, N., and McGuckin, C. P. (2010). Artificial human tissues from cord and cord blood stem cells for multi-organ regenerative medicine: viable alternatives to animal *in vitro* toxicology. *Altern. Lab. Anim.* 38, 183–192. Available online at: http://www.atla.org.uk/

Kaigler, D., Pagni, G., Park, C. H., Braun, T. M., Holman, L. A., Yi, E., et al. (2013). Stem cell therapy for craniofacial bone regeneration: a randomized, controlled feasibility trial. *Cell Transplant.* 22, 767–777. doi: 10.3727/096368912X652968

Kawashima, N. (2012). Characterisation of dental pulp stem cells: a new horizon for tissue regeneration? *Arch. Oral Biol.* 57, 1439–1458. doi: 10.1016/j.archoralbio.2012.08.010

Kellathur, S. N., and Lou, H. X. (2012). Cell and tissue therapy regulation: worldwide status and harmonization. *Biologicals* 40, 222–224. doi: 10.1016/j.biologicals.2012.01.004

Langer, R., and Vacanti, J. P. (1993). Tissue engineering. *Science* 260, 920–926. doi: 10.1126/science.8493529

La Noce, M., Paino, F., Spina, A., Naddeo, P., Montella, R., Desiderio, V., et al. (2014). Dental pulp stem cells: state of the art and suggestions for a true translation of research into therapy. *J. Dent.* 42, 761–768. doi: 10.1016/j.jdent.2014.02.018

Lee, S. Y., Huang, G. W., Shiung, J. N., Huang, Y. H., Jeng, J. H., Kuo, T. F., et al. (2012). Magnetic cryopreservation for dental pulp stem cells. *Cells Tissues Organs* 196, 23–33. doi: 10.1159/000331247

Lee, W. C., Shi, H., Poon, Z., Nyan, L. M., Kaushik, T., Shivashankar, G. V., et al. (2014). Multivariate biophysical markers predictive of mesenchymal stromal cell multipotency. *Proc. Natl. Acad. Sci. U.S.A.* 111, 4409–4418. doi: 10.1073/pnas.1402306111

Leeb, C., Jurga, M., McGuckin, C., Forraz, N., Thallinger, C., Moriggl, R., et al. (2011). New perspectives in stem cell research: beyond embryonic stem cells. *Cell Prolif.* 44(Suppl. 1), 9–14. doi: 10.1111/j.1365-2184.2010.00725.x

Leijten, J., Chai, Y. C., Papantoniou, I., Geris, L., Schrooten, J., and Luyten, F. P. (2015). Cell based advanced therapeutic medicinal products for bone repair: keep it simple? *Adv. Drug Deliv. Rev.* 84, 30–44. doi: 10.1016/j.addr.2014.10.025

Lopez-Cazaux, S., Bluteau, G., Magne, D., Lieubeau, B., Guicheux, J., and Alliot-Licht, B. (2006). Culture medium modulates the behaviour of human dental pulp-derived cells: technical note. *Eur. Cell Mater.* 11, 35–42.

Lv, F. J., Tuan, R. S., Cheung, K. M., and Leung, V. Y. (2014). Concise review: the surface markers and identity of human mesenchymal stem cells. *Stem Cells* 32, 1408–1419. doi: 10.1002/stem.1681

Majd, H., Wipff, P. J., Buscemi, L., Bueno, M., Vonwil, D., Quinn, T. M., et al. (2009). A novel method of dynamic culture surface expansion improves mesenchymal stem cell proliferation and phenotype. *Stem Cells* 27, 200–209. doi: 10.1634/stemcells.2008-0674

Manimaran, K., Sankaranarayanan, S., Ravi, V. R., Elangovan, S., Chandramohan, M., and Perumal, S. M. (2014). Treatment of osteoradionecrosis of mandible with bone marrow concentrate and with dental pulp stem cells. *Ann. Maxillofac. Surg.* 4, 189–192. doi: 10.4103/2231-0746.147130

Mannello, F., and Tonti, G. A. (2007). Concise review: no breakthroughs for human mesenchymal and embryonic stem cell culture: conditioned medium, feeder layer, or feeder-free; medium with fetal calf serum, human serum, or enriched plasma; serum-free, serum replacement nonconditioned medium, or ad hoc formula? All that glitters is not gold! *Stem Cells* 25, 1603–1609. doi: 10.1634/stemcells.2007-0127

Mayo, V., Sawatari, Y., Huang, C. Y., and Garcia-Godoy, F. (2014). Neural crest-derived dental stem cells–where we are and where we are going. *J. Dent.* 42, 1043–1051. doi: 10.1016/j.jdent.2014.04.007

Ménard, C., and Tarte, K. (2013). Immunoregulatory properties of clinical grade mesenchymal stromal cells: evidence, uncertainties, and clinical application. *Stem Cell Res. Ther.* 4:64. doi: 10.1186/scrt214

Nakashima, M., and Iohara, K. (2014). Mobilized dental pulp stem cells for pulp regeneration: initiation of clinical trial. *J. Endod.* 40, 26–32. doi: 10.1016/j.joen.2014.01.020

Nolla, C. M. (1960). The development of permanent teeth. *J. Dent. Child.* 27, 254–266.

Ohnuma, K., Fujiki, A., Yanagihara, K., Tachikawa, S., Hayashi, Y., Ito, Y., et al. (2014). Enzyme-free passage of human pluripotent stem cells by controlling divalent cations. *Sci. Rep.* 4:4646. doi: 10.1038/srep04646

Pacini, S. (2014). Deterministic and stochastic approaches in the clinical application of mesenchymal stromal cells (MSCs). *Front. Cell Dev. Biol.* 2:50. doi: 10.3389/fcell.2014.00050

Papaccio, G., Graziano, A., d'Aquino, R., Graziano, M. F., Pirozzi, G., Menditti, D., et al. (2006). Long-term cryopreservation of dental pulp stem cells (SBP-DPSCs) and their differentiated osteoblasts: a cell source for tissue repair. *J. Cell Physiol.* 208, 319–325. doi: 10.1002/jcp.20667

Perry, B. C., Zhou, D., Wu, X., Yang, F. C., Byers, M. A., Chu, T. M., et al. (2008). Collection, cryopreservation, and characterization of human dental pulp-derived mesenchymal stem cells for banking and clinical use. *Tissue Eng. Part C Methods* 14, 149–156. doi: 10.1089/ten.tec.2008.0031

Pisciotta, A., Riccio, M., Carnevale, G., Beretti, F., Gibellini, L., Maraldi, T., et al. (2012). Human serum promotes osteogenic differentiation of human dental pulp stem cells *in vitro* and *in vivo*. *PLoS ONE* 7:e50542. doi: 10.1371/journal.pone.0050542

Rubio, D., Garcia-Castro, J., Martín, M. C., de la Fuente, R., Cigudosa, J. C., Lloyd, A. C., et al. (2005). Spontaneous human adult stem cell transformation. *Cancer Res.* 65, 3035–3039. doi: 10.1158/0008-5472.CAN-04-4194

Russell, K. C., Phinney, D. G., Lacey, M. R., Barrilleaux, B. L., Meyertholen, K. E., and O'Connor, K. C. (2010). *In vitro* high−capacity assay to quantify the clonal heterogeneity in trilineage potential of mesenchymal stem cells reveals a complex hierarchy of lineage commitment. *Stem Cells* 28, 788–798. doi: 10.1002/stem.312

Sakai, K., Yamamoto, A., Matsubara, K., Nakamura, S., Naruse, M., Yamagata, M., et al. (2012). Human dental pulp-derived stem cells promote locomotor recovery after complete transection of the rat spinal cord by multiple neuro-regenerative mechanisms. *J. Clin. Invest.* 122, 80–90. doi: 10.1172/JCI59251

Schneider, C. K., Salmikangas, P., Jilma, B., Flamion, B., Todorova, L. R., Paphitou, A., et al. (2010). Challenges with advanced therapy medicinal products and how to meet them. *Nat. Rev. Drug Discov.* 9, 195–201. doi: 10.1038/nrd3052

Sensebé, L., Gadelorge, M., and Fleury-Cappellesso, S. (2013). Production of mesenchymal stromal/stem cells according to good manufacturing practices: a review. *Stem Cell Res. Ther.* 4:66. doi: 10.1186/scrt217

Shah, F. S., Wu, X., Dietrich, M., Rood, J., and Gimble, J. M. (2013). A non-enzymatic method for isolating human adipose tissue-derived stromal stem cells. *Cytotherapy* 15, 979–985. doi: 10.1016/j.jcyt.2013.04.001

Shi, S., and Gronthos, S. (2003). Perivascular niche of postnatal mesenchymal stem cells in human bone marrow and dental pulp. *J. Bone Miner. Res.* 18, 696–704. doi: 10.1359/jbmr.2003.18.4.696

Spath, L., Rotilio, V., Alessandrini, M., Gambara, G., De Angelis, L., Mancini, M., et al. (2010). Explant-derived human dental pulp stem cells enhance differentiation and proliferation potentials. *J. Cell. Mol. Med.* 14, 1635–1644. doi: 10.1111/j.1582-4934.2009.00848.x

Swamynathan, P., Venugopal, P., Kannan, S., Thej, C., Kolkundar, U. K., Bhagwat, S., et al. (2014). Are serumfree and xenofree culture conditions ideal for large scale clinical grade expansion of Wharton's jelly derived mesenchymal stem cells? A comparative study. *Stem Cell Res. Ther.* 5:88. doi: 10.1186/scrt477

Takeda, T., Tezuka, Y., Horiuchi, M., Hosono, K., Iida, K., Hatakeyama, D., et al. (2008). Characterization of dental pulp stem cells of human tooth germs. *J. Dent. Res.* 87, 676–681. doi: 10.1177/154405910808700716

Tekkatte, C., Gunasingh, G. P., Cherian, K. M., and Sankaranarayanan, K. (2011). "Humanized" stem cell culture techniques: the animal serum controversy. *Stem Cells Int.* 2011:504723. doi: 10.4061/2011/504723

Tirino, V., and Papaccio, G. (2012). A new, most likely unusual approach is crucial and upcoming for the use of stem cells in regenerative medicine. *Front. Physiol.* 2:119. doi: 10.3389/fphys.2011.00119

Tomlinson, M. J., Dennis, C., Yang, X. B., and Kirkham, J. (2015). Tissue non-specific alkaline phosphatase production by human dental pulp stromal cells is enhanced by high density cell culture. *Cell Tissue Res.* doi: 10.1007/s00441-014-2106-3. [Epub ahead of print].

Tyndall, A. (2011). Successes and failures of stem cell transplantation in autoimmune diseases. *Hematol. Am. Soc. Hematol. Educ. Program.* 2011, 280–284. doi: 10.1182/asheducation-2011.1.280

Wang, Y., Huso, D. L., Harrington, J., Kellner, J., Jeong, D. K., Turney, J., et al. (2005). Outgrowth of a transformed cell population derived from normal human bone marrow mesenchymal stem cell culture. *Cytotherapy* 7, 509–519. doi: 10.1080/14653240500363216

Woloszyk, A., Holsten Dircksen, S., Bostanci, N., Müller, R., Hofmann, S., and Mitsiadis, T. A. (2014). Influence of the mechanical environment on the engineering of mineralised tissues using human dental pulp stem cells and silk fibroin scaffolds. *PLoS ONE* 9:e111010. doi: 10.1371/journal.pone.0111010

Woods, E. J., Perry, B. C., Hockema, J. J., Larson, L., Zhou, D., and Goebel, W. S. (2009). Optimized cryopreservation method for human dental pulp-derived stem cells and their tissues of origin for banking and clinical use. *Cryobiology* 59, 150–157. doi: 10.1016/j.cryobiol.2009.06.005

Wuchter, P., Bieback, K., Schrezenmeier, H., Bornhäuser, M., Müller, L. P., Bönig, H., et al. (2015). Standardization of Good Manufacturing Practice-compliant production of bone marrow-derived human mesenchymal stromal cells for immunotherapeutic applications. *Cytotherapy* 17, 128–139. doi: 10.1016/j.jcyt.2014.04.002

Yu, J., He, H., Tang, C., Zhang, G., Li, Y., Wang, R., et al. (2010). Differentiation potential of STRO1+ dental pulp stem cells changes during cell passaging. *BMC Cell Biol.* 11:32. doi: 10.1186/1471-2121-11-32

Zhang, W., Walboomers, X. F., van Kuppevelt, T. H., Daamen, W. F., Bian, Z., and Jansen, J. A. (2006). The performance of human dental pulp stem cells on different three-dimensional scaffold materials. *Biomaterials* 27, 5658–5668. doi: 10.1016/j.biomaterials.2006.07.013

Zuk, P. A. (2010). The adipose-derived stem cell: looking back and looking ahead. *Mol. Biol. Cell* 21, 1783–1787. doi: 10.1091/mbc.E09-07-0589

4

# Changing Paradigms in Craniofacial Regeneration: Current and New Strategies for the Activation of Endogenous Stem Cells

**Edited by:**
*Thimios Mitsiadis, University of Zurich, Switzerland*

***Correspondence:**
*Papaccio Gianpaolo*
*gianpaolo.papaccio@unina2.it*

*Luigi Mele [1], Pietro Paolo Vitiello [2], Virginia Tirino [1], Francesca Paino [1], Alfredo De Rosa [3], Davide Liccardo [1], Gianpaolo Papaccio [1]* and Vincenzo Desiderio [1]*

*[1] Department of Experimental Medicine, Section of Biotechnology and Medical Histology and Embryology, Second University of Naples, Naples, Italy, [2] Medical Oncology, Dipartimento Medico-Chirurgico di Internistica Clinica e Sperimentale "F. Magrassi e A. Lanzara," Second University of Naples, Naples, Italy, [3] Department of Odontology and Surgery, Second University of Naples, Naples, Italy*

Craniofacial area represent a unique district of human body characterized by a very high complexity of tissues, innervation and vascularization, and being deputed to many fundamental function such as eating, speech, expression of emotions, delivery of sensations such as taste, sight, and earing. For this reasons, tissue loss in this area following trauma or for example oncologic resection, have a tremendous impact on patients' quality of life. In the last 20 years regenerative medicine has emerged as one of the most promising approach to solve problem related to trauma, tissue loss, organ failure etc. One of the most powerful tools to be used for tissue regeneration is represented by stem cells, which have been successfully implanted in different tissue/organs with exciting results. Nevertheless, both autologous and allogeneic stem cell transplantation raise many practical and ethical concerns that make this approach very difficult to apply in clinical practice. For this reason different cell free approaches have been developed aiming to the mobilization, recruitment, and activation of endogenous stem cells into the injury site avoiding exogenous cells implant but instead stimulating patients' own stem cells to repair the lesion. To this aim many strategies have been used including functionalized bioscaffold, controlled release of stem cell chemoattractants, growth factors, BMPs, Platelet–Rich-Plasma, and other new strategies such as ultrasound wave and laser are just being proposed. Here we review all the current and new strategies used for activation and mobilization of endogenous stem cells in the regeneration of craniofacial tissue.

**Keywords: craniofacial abnormalities, regenerative medicine, stem cell transplantation, stem cells and regenerative medicine, stem cells recruitment, SDF1, bioscaffold, BMP signaling**

## INTRODUCTION

Regenerative medicine is the field of translational research that aims to replace and repair cells, tissues and organs to restore their normal functions (Mason and Dunnill, 2008). In the last 20 years, the possibility to use endogenous and exogenous stem cells for tissue repair has emerged producing enthusiasm in the scientific and medical community, but on the other side, raising a series of ethical and practical issues. The craniomaxillofacial complex is of fundamental importance for many different functions, such as breathing and eating, others non-vital but still important for social relationships, such as aesthetics and the delivery of senses such as sight, smell, and sound. For these reasons, craniomaxillofacial tissue damages have serious physiological and psychological consequences, and it is of paramount importance to seek solutions to optimize the life of people with maxillofacial trauma (Teo and Vallier, 2010). Many disciplines, such as biology, medicine, chemistry, and engineering, are involved in the study and development of techniques or products that regenerate the native conditions of such a complicated body region as the craniofacial tissues such as bone, muscle, cartilage and nervous tissue. The research moved toward two main different directions: one that involves the study of stem cell biology, including the development of novel techniques to isolate, characterize and transplant stem cells, the other related to the material science, which aims to the creation of new biomaterials and technologies suitable for the use with stem cells. As for stem cell biology, the research focused on stem and progenitor cells isolation, characterization, expansion, and transplantation for replacing damaged tissues (Giuliani et al., 2013) and on the study of growth-factors and genetic technology to control proliferation, migration and ability in tissue repair and regeneration (Alvarez et al., 2012; Han et al., 2014).

Many types of stem/progenitor cells have been described and proposed for their ability to rescue and repair injured tissue and partially restore organ function. Stem cells are undifferentiated cells capable to undergo an indefinite number of replications (self-renewal) and give rise to progenitor and finally to specialized cells. Therefore, stem cells differ from other types of cells in the body because they are capable of sustaining self-renewal, are unspecialized, and can give rise to differentiated cell types (La Noce et al., 2014a). In the field of regenerative medicine, two main types of stem cells are used: Embryonic stem cells (ESCs) and Adult stem cells (ASCs). The embryonic stem cells are isolated from the inner cell mass (ICM) of the blastocyst, they are able to differentiate in all the tissues deriving from the three definitive germ layers, and for this reason they are considered "pluripotent." Adult stem cells reside in the adult tissues and they are pivotal for the tissue homeostasis (Mohanty et al., 2015); unlike ESCs, these cells are only able to differentiate into a limited group of cells types, and they are considered "multipotent." In the recent years a new source of stem cells for regenerative and translational medicine has been created by transfecting adult cells (mainly dermal fibroblasts) with a varying number of stem-associated genes producing the so-called *induced Pluripotent Stem Cells* (iPSCs) (Takahashi et al., 2007). In this review, only Adult Stem Cells (ASCs) or cell-free approaches in regenerative medicine will be considered. Today, multiple sources for the isolation of adult stem cells have been identified, including heart tissue (Warejcka et al., 1996), umbilical cord blood (Campagnoli et al., 2001), skeletal muscle (Wada et al., 2002), and the dermis of skin (Toma et al., 2001). To identify a suitable cell population for craniofacial regeneration, many odontogenic stem cells, including dental pulp stem cells (Gronthos et al., 2000; Laino et al., 2005; d'Aquino et al., 2007, 2011), periodontal ligament stem cells (Seo et al., 2004), stem cells from human exfoliated deciduous teeth (Cordeiro et al., 2008), and stem cells from apical papilla (Sonoyama et al., 2008) and some non-odontogenic stem cells, including adipose-derived stem cells (Hung et al., 2011), bone marrow mesenchymal stem cells (Li et al., 2007), gingival stem cells (Hakkinen et al., 2014), embryonic stem cells (Ohazama et al., 2004), neural crest cells (Jiang et al., 2008), and even hair follicle stem cells (Wu et al., 2009) have been selected for screening. Studies have demonstrated that all odontogenic stem cells have a certain degree of multipotency *in vitro* and form pulp-dentin complexes combined with scaffold materials *in vivo*, except for PDLSCs, which tend to form bone-like tissues *in vivo* (Mangano et al., 2011; La Noce et al., 2014b; Naddeo et al., 2015). In contrast, non-odontogenic stem cells other than BMSCs have not yet been confirmed to have the potential for tooth regeneration. Among these cell types, postnatal DPSCs have the most potential as stem cells for endodontic tissue regeneration (Gronthos et al., 2002; Nakashima et al., 2004, 2009; Laino et al., 2005; Murray et al., 2007; Mangano et al., 2011; Paino et al., 2014; Naddeo et al., 2015). Nevertheless there is the need for craniofacial regeneration to repair tissue such as bone and soft tissue such as adipose tissue and among the different sources of stem cells bone marrow and adipose tissue seem to be the most promising. For what concerns material science, this constitutes one of the subjects most widely studied in recent years for its application in many fields of medicine, such as tissue engineering and regenerative medicine. The real paradigm shift that took place in the last years is the overlap of the material science with the biology, in an attempt to create new materials—also defined as *smart* materials or *bio*materials—that do not only exist as passive support to living cells, but that are also able to interact and respond sensitively to environmental cues derived from these cells (Mangano et al., 2011). Moreover, the increasing understanding of the natural mechanisms involved in the development of tissues and organs has led to the creation of three-dimensional *in vitro* bioreactors, including nanotechnology and microfluidics-based bioreactors that recapitulate normal and pathological tissue development, structure and function (Rajan et al., 2014; Obregon et al., 2015) and pave the way to the idea of "printed organ," a new technique used for fabrication of organ-like constructs (Choi and Kim, 2015; Ledford, 2015). These technologies have been made possible thanks to the mind-shift that has brought scientists to create synthetic matrices that recapitulate the natural properties of the extracellular matrix (ECM) of the different tissues, as a direct consequence of the evidences that the composition of the scaffold is able to influence stem cell proliferation, differentiation and angiogenesis through integrin signaling (Pittenger et al., 1999; Hynes, 2002a,b).

## GRAFTING APPROACHES

In last years scientific findings highlighted the importance of human cell therapy. In regenerative medicine stem cells can be used from donor that is a family member (allogeneic by family), donor unrelated (allogeneic cells from unrelated volunteer) or the patient's own (autologous). Stem cell commonly used in the therapy for craniofacial region are bone marrow stem cells(Yang et al., 2014), adipose stem cells (Griffin et al., 2014) hematopoietic stem cell (Vesterbacka et al., 2012) dental pulp stem cells (Giuliani et al., 2013). Both allogeneic and autologous cell therapies may be subdivided into two types: cell therapy for acute or for chronic conditions, the first to limit the natural progression of disease, the second for full regeneration (Sadan et al., 2008; Carpenter et al., 2009). Those approaches can be exploited in many clinical situations; therefore it is important that advantages and disadvantages of both therapies are made clear.

## Allogeneic Stem Cells Transplant

### Pros

Allogeneic cells represent a therapeutic technology that fits easily in pharmaceutical production. So it is more efficient to produce cells from multiple patients and introduce them into a conventional quality control (QC) system, where it is ascertained the safety of the product and its characterization from the biological point of view. As autologous cells, allogeneic cells are expandable in culture, thus allowing the production of numerous batches of material and therefore their distribution on a large scale. This represents a great potential for economic development, promoting the improvement and expansion of this therapy (Mason and Dunnill, 2008). In medical emergencies the allogeneic cells have many advantages due to the rapid availability of these cells, which guarantee a good stability during storage and already occurred characterization. It is also not necessary to perform a biopsy on a person potentially sick, avoiding additional stress to the patient and saving time.

### Cons

The most common problem in allogeneic cell transplantation is related to the host immune response that, directed against grafted cells, can lead to strong inflammatory reaction and consequent destruction of the graft (Barker and Widner, 2004). Nevertheless, some types of stem cells as MSCs have shown immunomodulatory activity in some autoimmune disorders, such as graft-versus-host disease and systemic lupus (Sui et al., 2013; Zhao et al., 2015), but this feature seem to not be sufficient or to not apply to grafted stem cells. In fact different strategies have been proposed to overcome this problem as discussed by Guha et al. (2013). Another major problem arising with allograft is the risk of generating tumors in the host. Transplanted cells can trigger a mechanism of crosstalk with the microenvironment of the receiver, which, combined with the stem cells growth capacity, brings along the risk of uncontrolled growth after transplantation. As an example Amariglio et al. described the generation of brain benign tumor after stem cells transplantation in a patient affected by ataxia telangiectasia (Amariglio et al., 2009). This problem can also be explained by the fact that *in vitro* expanded stem cells bring increased genetic abnormalities, which can favor cancer initiation (Spits et al., 2008). In fact, before use for allogeneic transplantation, stem cells are extensively cultured, and the accumulation of genomic abnormalities may represent a risk to the recipient. Another issue in derivation and culturing stem cells for allogeneic transplantation is the use of animal products in cell culture (Foetal Bovine Serum for instance), increasing risk of graft rejection and transmission of zoonosis (Chavez et al., 2008).

## Autologous Stem Cells Transplantation

### Pros

The greatest advantage in the use of autologous cells is definitely to avoid immunological responses host-versus-graft. Furthermore during therapy with autologous cells you can prevent the immunosuppressive treatment on the patient, avoiding the risk of infections and lowering by far the costs of the therapy (Chen and Palmer, 2008). In bioaesthetic treatment this approach seems to be most suitable for the less intrusive therapies and look more natural given by the patient's own cells (Tsai et al., 2000). In the autograft, the cells used are isolated from the donor-patient and when the number of cells obtained by biopsy is sufficient for transplantation it is not necessary to amplify, avoiding the anomalies due to an excessive growth *in vitro* (Baker et al., 2007). In addition, they are not exposed to products of animal origin, removing from the risk of zoonosis. Finally, the patient-derived cells do not incur ethical battles and regulation, therefore their use is much simpler than that of allografts.

### Cons

One of the major issues concerning the autograft is the limitation of material to engage in certain patients, such as children under 6 years of age or with particular diseases (Smith et al., 2011). In addition, craniofacial reconstruction may be even more difficult in the pediatric patient because the skull is not developed enough so the split-thickness bone grafting is not tolerated (Chenard et al., 2012).

Another complication is the side effects that occur in the donor site, which involves hematoma, infection, nerve damage, bone pain and fractures. All this may adversely affect the treatment and increase the length of hospital stay (Seiler et al., 2000; Smith et al., 2008). Moreover, the cells obtained by biopsy may not be sufficient for the graft, this involves an *in vitro* expansion, time consuming and often not successful. For all these reasons, this approach is not be used in emergency situations. The material used must be processed separately for each patient with customized protocols using the patient's own serum. For this reasons the use on a large scale is hardly feasible for the costs and the time required by each therapy.

# ENDOGENOUS STEM CELLS: CURRENT APPROACHES

The ultimate goal in the stem cell field is to find a way to translate our growing body of knowledge on stem cell biology into therapeutic applications for regenerative medicine. In that regard, most of our attention has focused upon stem-cell transplantation approaches, which have been considered above. On the other hand, the need to overcome the drawbacks associated with these approaches (mainly, the necessity of manipulating the cells before the graft takes place) has led to the development of new strategies to achieve tissue repair. The finding that many adult tissues contain stem cells that function to maintain and repair tissue damage (Su et al., 2009) paved the way to the idea that we could somehow recruit these endogenous stem cells in order to enhance tissue regeneration. Moreover, whereas the grafting strategies require the exogenous activation of stem cells, an endogenous re-activation can be speculated without the need of isolation, manipulation and grafting (Miller and Kaplan, 2012). However, though the concept of adult stem cells is an old one, the idea of their exploitation for regenerative purposes has gained attention only in the last few years. This is mainly due to the experimental evidence coming from studies showing that tissue stem cell behavior can be modulated differentially in physiologic and pathologic settings both in the animal model and in the human. For example, it is now well-established that regular exercise and brain injury can enhance neurogenesis, precursor proliferation and oligodendrogenesis in rodents (Ming and Song, 2011) and these results are comparable to those from recent imaging studies that show how aerobic exercise training enhances hippocampal volume in elderly humans (Erickson et al., 2011, 2012). Another reason we are currently approaching the idea of manipulating resident stem cells is that we now know that in some cases the factors that induce the stem cell response are the same that we have studied in other contexts, e.g., the growth factor BDNF is required for exercise-induced neurogenesis (Ming and Song, 2011). Moreover, a number of growth factors that were originally identified in stem cell culture studies have been shown to activate stem cells *in vivo* (Mitchell et al., 2004). We will now focus on the different approaches that have stemmed in regenerative medicine from the above considerations, with a special focus on craniofacial regeneration.

## Scaffolds in Bone Regeneration

Understanding that the three-dimensional (3D) structure of the extracellular matrix (ECM) is integral for tissue formation and regeneration has led researchers to make an effort to recreate this environment when attempting to repair tissue defects, creating biocompatible matrices known as scaffolds. A scaffold is a three-dimension biomaterial designed to allow cell-biomaterial interactions, cell survival, proliferation and differentiation. That scaffold can be designed to biodegrade at a controllable rate and is characterized by a low degree of toxicity *in vivo*. Whether produced using synthetic or biologic materials, scaffold matrices enhance tissue growth and repair by facilitating delivery and localization of progenitor cells and growth factors to a desired location (Dhandayuthapani et al., 2011). Historically, scaffolds have been used as delivery systems in cell-based applications, whereas their use in cell-free strategies for tissue regeneration is relatively new (Bueno and Glowacki, 2009).

The use of scaffolds that accurately reproduce the structure of the native ECM (the so-called *biomimetic scaffolds*) is particularly useful in cranio-facial bone defects, as they play the role of template analogous for complex anatomical form while minimizing supply constraints. These types of scaffold vary in pore size, mechanical properties and degree of biodegrability, according to their chemical structure (Teven et al., 2015; see **Table 1**).

Though a large amount of evidence correlates bioscaffold to increased tissue regeneration, it is still not clear whether this effect can be explained by the activation of endogenous stem cells (Zaky and Cancedda, 2009). For this reason, in the practice, scaffold-based approaches are generally combined with cell- and/or growth factor-based approaches. The former have already been discussed above (see section above), while the latter will be now presented.

## Growth-Factors-Mediated Activation and/or Mobilization of Stem Cells

Since several studies demonstrated the role of growth factors in stem cell biology (reviewed in Brizzi et al., 2012), it is almost impossible to ignore their potential provision to the therapeutic goal of tissue regeneration. Wagers previously reviewed how the use of growth factors in the clinic has already led to successful therapies in hematology and orthopedics (respectively, G-CSF analogs for chemotherapy-related neutropenia and parathyroid hormone analogs for osteoporosis; Wagers, 2012). In both these conditions, the support given to the stem cells is systemic, as it works in a tissue-specific fashion, with no privileged site of action. This is not the case in regenerative medicine, where the regeneration is usually desired only in a limited subset of body locations. For this reason, local delivery of growth factors to the site of lesion is a more suitable approach in regenerative medicine, and is usually pursued by binding growth factors to scaffolds (**Figure 1**). Depending on the desired release kinetic, growth factors can be either directly adsorbed to scaffolds or encapsulated in microspheres, respectively for a burst release or a sustained and delayed release. As for bone regeneration, which is the most investigated field in regenerative medicine of the craniofacial district, several growth factors have been identified with a wide range of activities *in vivo* (see **Table 2**). Bone morphogenetic proteins (BMPs) are a family of growth factors involved in embryonic development and regeneration of mesenchymal tissues (Zhao, 2003), whose roles have been investigated thoroughly in bone biology (reviewed in Luu et al., 2007). Although many isoforms of BMPs are known, only a small subset has been shown to be active in *in vivo* models of bone defects. BMP-2, among the others, is lethal in knockout mice model and was associated to orofacial clefting in case of haploinsufficiency in humans (Zhang and Bradley, 1996; Sahoo et al., 2011); for this reason, its use has been suggested for craniofacial bone reconstruction (Chenard et al., 2012). BMP-7 showed superior bone induction compared to autologous bone graft in an animal model of calvarial defect, when injected locally (Springer et al., 2005a,b). BMP-7 is also able to determine a widespread skeletal regeneration, and this led to its approval for use, along with BMP-2, in case of non-unions and open fractures of long bones (Gautschi et al., 2007). Other BMPs lack evidence of clinical relevance and their possible roles in the practice are reviewed by Bessa et al. (2008a,b). If, on one hand, BMPs support bone regeneration by activation of perilesional osteoprogenitor cells, several different growth factors can be used to stimulate mobilization of nearby or distant stem cells and their homing to the defect site (Herrmann et al., 2015).

**TABLE 1 | Most used biomimetic scaffolds for cranio-facial bone regeneration in cell-based and cell-free applications.**

| Scaffold name | Chemical structure | Features and uses | Reference(s) |
|---|---|---|---|
| **Polymer-based scaffolds** | | | |
| **NATURAL POLYMERS** | | | |
| Chitosan | Deacetylated derivative of chitin | Highly hydrophilic, osteoconductive *in vitro* and *in vivo* but not reliable for load bearing applications. | Muzzarelli et al., 1994; Seol et al., 2004 |
| Fibroin | Insoluble protein from silk | High mechanical strength and biodegradability. Highly customizable processing (gels, sponges, nets), but lower osteoconductivity. | Riccio et al., 2012; Panda et al., 2015 |
| Collagen | Fibrillar collagen | Highly biodegradable and osteoconductive. High osteoconductivity, but not reliable for load bearing applications. | Ferreira et al., 2012 |
| **SYNTHETIC POLYMERS** | | | |
| Poly(lactic-co-glycolic acid) (PLGA) | Poly(α-hydroxy esters) constituted of a combination of poly(lactic acid) (PLA) and poly(glycolic acid) (PGA) | Different combinations of the two components lead to highly customizable degradation rate, mechanical properties and osteoconductivity. | Lin et al., 2002; Gentile et al., 2014; Liu et al., 2014 |
| Poly(e-caprolactone) (PCL) | Aliphatic polyester | Long degradation time and scarce ability to mediate cellular adhesion. Useful for the production of Shape-Memory Polymers (SMPs). | Schantz et al., 2003a,b; Zhang et al., 2014 |
| **CALCIUM PHOSPHATE-BASED CERAMIC SCAFFOLDS** | | | |
| Hydroxyapatite (HA) | $Ca_{10}(PO_4)_6(OH)_2$ (Inorganic phase of native bone) | Highly biocompatible and osteoconductive. Slow rate of degradation, affected by crystallinity. Suitable for load-bearing applications. | Yoshikawa and Myoui, 2005; Bose et al., 2012 |
| β-tricalcium phosphate (β-TCP) | $Ca_3(PO_4)_2$ | Highly biocompatible and osteoconductive. Very brittle. | Rezwan et al., 2006; Kamitakahara et al., 2008 |
| Amorphous Calcium Phosphate (ACP) | $Ca_{3n}(PO_4)_{2n}$ | Highly biocompatible and osteoconductive. Degradation through a process of dissolution-precipitation to form HA. | Kobayashi et al., 2014 |
| Biphasic calcium phosphate (BCP) | Combination of HA and β-TCP | Highly biocompatible and osteoconductive. Porosity and grain size highly customizable. The addition of zinc or silicone oxide confers an increase in compressive strength and angiogenesis. | Tevlin et al., 2014 |
| **COMPOSITE SCAFFOLDS** | | | |
| Polymer-calcium phosphate composites | Addition of Ca-P nanoparticles to polymer-based scaffolds (e.g.chitosan or fibroin) | Higher biocompatibility compared to polymer-only scaffolds and improved compressive strength compared to ceramic-only scaffolds. Superior bone growth in *in vivo* calvarial defect model. | Chesnutt et al., 2009; Qi et al., 2014 |
| Poly(lactic acid)-calcium phosphate and poly(glycolic acid)-calcium phosphate | PLA, PGA or PLGA scaffolds added with HA | Increased compression modulus and tensile strength compared to PLGA scaffolds. Increased *de novo* bone formation. | Kim et al., 2006; Yoon et al., 2007 |
| Poly(e-caprolactone)- calcium phosphate composites | PCL added with TCP | Less hydrophobic than PCL alone and increased compressive strength compared to TCP alone. Suitable for load-bearing applications and osteogenic differentiation of stem cells. | Liao et al., 2013; Baykan et al., 2014 |
| Poly(1,8-octanediol-co citric acid) (POC) | Citric acid-based elastomer combined with HA and TCP | Highly biocompatible and osteoconductive. Citric acid released during polymer degradation regulates apatite nanocrystals growth, increasing stability, strength, and resistance to fracture. | Chung et al., 2011; Costello et al., 2012; Davies et al., 2014 |

Vascular Endothelial Growth Factor (VEGF) is most known for its role in angiogenesis, but has also revealed a direct involvement in supporting bone formation (Schipani et al., 2009): for this reason, numerous preclinical bone healing models involving recombinant human VEGF delivered with various biomaterials have been tested. PLGA scaffolds delivery systems showed an increase in vascular density and bone formation in cranium and calvarial defects (Murphy et al., 2004; Kaigler et al., 2006), while collagen sponge-delivered VEGF reported similar results both in calvarial and in mandibular defects (Kleinheinz et al., 2005; Behr et al., 2012; Jin and Giannobile, 2014). Sustained release of VEGF has been achieved in different ways, such as pre-encapsulation in PLGA or gelatin microspheres or co-precipitation onto BCP, in order to support angiogenesis and bone formation for a longer period of time (Patel et al., 2008; De la Riva et al., 2009, 2010; Wernike et al., 2010; Farokhi

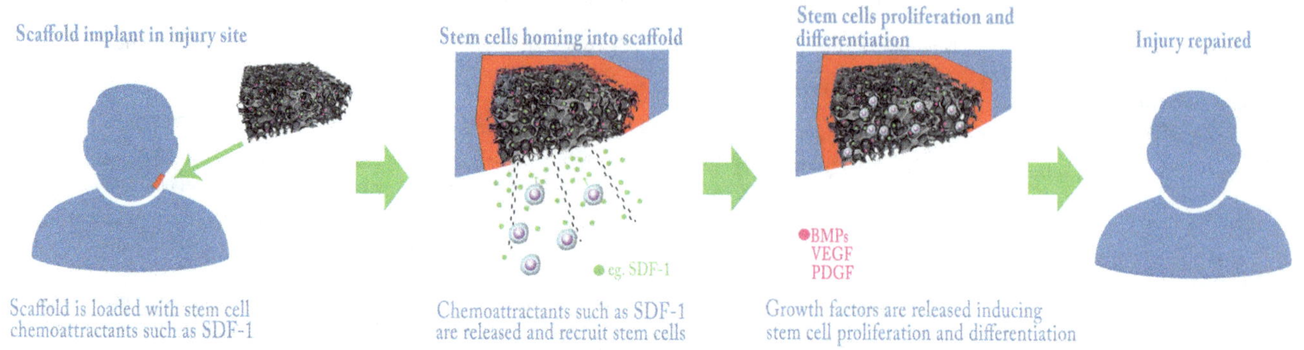


**FIGURE 1 | Example strategies for bone regeneration trough Stem Cells recruitment and activation.** A scaffold with control release of chemo-attractants and/or growth factors is grafted into the lesion, endogenous stem cells are attracted and home into the scaffold where they proliferate and differentiate repairing the tissue.

**TABLE 2 | Growth factors and other agents used for local activation and/or mobilization of stem cells in craniofacial and bone regeneration.**

| Agent | Evidence(s) | Reference(s) |
|---|---|---|
| Bone Morphogenetic Proteins (BMPs) | Activation of mesenchymal stem cells and osteogenic differentiation. Mechanisms of action and effects vary between the 15 isoforms of BMPs. The most osteoinductive are BMP-2, -6, -9, -4, -7. | Bae et al., 2001; Zhao, 2003; Luu et al., 2007 |
| BMP-2 | Knockout mice are lethal; haploinsufficiency causes orofacial clefting in humans. Use suggested for mandible, cleft, and cranial vault reconstruction. | Zhang and Bradley, 1996; Schliephake et al., 2008; Sahoo et al., 2011; Chenard et al., 2012 |
| BMP-4 | Knockout mice are lethal; heterozygous null mice exhibit skeletal defects such as craniofacial malformations and polydactyly. Enhances bone healing when co-expressed with VEGF by genetically manipulated stem cells. May be detrimental in osseointegration of oral implants coated with collagen. | Peng et al., 2002; Zhao, 2003; Stadlinger et al., 2008 |
| BMP-7 | Knockout mice are postnatal lethal and show skeletal patterning defects in skull, hindlimbs, and ribcage. Stimulates periodontal wound healing in an animal model. | Luo et al., 1995; Giannobile et al., 1998; Springer et al., 2005a |
| BMP-6 | Some evidences show this isoform to be one of the most osteogenic in animal models. | Solloway et al., 1998; Kang et al., 2004 |
| Vascular Endothelial Growth Factor (VEGF) | Delivered with PLGA or collagen scaffolds enhances bone regeneration in cranium, calvarial and mandibular defects. Sustained release (up to 5 weeks) can be obtained by pre-encapsulation of VEGF in PLGA, alginate, or gelatin microspheres or, alternatively, by VEGF co-precipitation onto BCP (Basic Calcium Phosphate). | Murphy et al., 2004; Kleinheinz et al., 2005; Patel et al., 2008; De la Riva et al., 2009, 2010; Wernike et al., 2010; Behr et al., 2012; Farokhi et al., 2013, 2014 |
| VEGF + BMP2 | A combination of these two factors showed an increased vascular density during bone regeneration but no detectable enhancement in bone formation compared to BMP2 alone in animal models of cranial and mandibular defects. This combination is also capable of facilitating bone marrow stem cells (BMSCs) homing and differentiation. | Young et al., 2009; Zhang et al., 2011; Ramazanoglu et al., 2013; Zhang et al., 2014 |
| Platelet-Derived Growth Factor (PDGF) | Local administration of PDGF in a critical-size calvarial defect has been shown to increase bone mineralization similarly to VEGF, but less than BMP-2. Use approved for periodontal repair by FDA. Chemoattractant for Mesenchymal stem cells (MSCs) | Fiedler et al., 2004; Pellegrini et al., 2009; Phipps et al., 2012; Jin and Giannobile, 2014 |
| SDF-1 | Induces extravasation and homing of mesenchymal cells through the CXCR4 receptor. SDF-1-loaded scaffolds have been studied in fracture healing models and in calvarial defects with excellent results. Capable of inducing migration, proliferation and activation of human periodontal ligament stem cells (PLSCs). | Kitaori et al., 2009; Fujio et al., 2011; Li D. et al., 2011; Du et al., 2012; Ji et al., 2013; Liu et al., 2014 |
| SDF-1 + BMP2 | The combination of SDF-1 + BMP2 increases bone volume in a calvarial defect model compared to SDF-1 alone | Jin and Giannobile, 2014 |
| Platelet-rich Plasma (PRP) | PRP is a concentrate of blood platelets that upon activation releases various growth factors, including PDGF and VEGF. It can be used to enhance tissue healing, especially in case of concomitant cell transplantation. Potential use of PRP as a stem cell activator has been suggested in the case of periodontal regeneration. | Anitua et al., 2008; Chen et al., 2010; Del Corso et al., 2012; Fekete et al., 2012 |
| Platelet-rich Fibrin (PRF) | PRF is a polymeric (fibrin-based) scaffold loaded with PRP that has shown good results in promoting craniofacial bone regeneration both in preclinical and in clinical setting | Simonpieri et al., 2012; Li et al., 2014 |

et al., 2013, 2014). Moreover, combination of VEGF and BMP-2 showed an increased vascular density during bone regeneration but no detectable enhancement in bone formation, compared to BMP-2 alone (Young et al., 2009; Zhang et al., 2011; Ramazanoglu et al., 2013). Plateled-Derived Growth Factor (PDGF) is another angiogenetic molecule, involved in maturation of newly-formed blood vessels, but after the report of its chemoattractive action on Mesenchymal Stem Cells (MSCs) it has been studied as a homing factor in bone repair (Fiedler et al., 2004; Phipps et al., 2012). Local administration of PDGF in a critical-size calvarial defect has been shown to increase bone mineralization similarly to VEGF, but less than BMP-2 (Jin and Giannobile, 2014). Notably, Chang et al. demonstrated that gene delivery of PDGF stimulates repair of oral implant extraction socket defects in a rat model (Chang et al., 2010) moreover, PDGF has been approved for periodontal repair by FDA (Pellegrini et al., 2009). One of the most investigated signaling systems for extravasation and homing of mesenchymal cells is the SDF1-CXCR4 axis (Kitaori et al., 2009). It represents the perfect target for enhancing bone regeneration, as it is involved both in MSCs and endothelial progenitor cells (EPCs) homing dynamics, thus working both as osteoinductive and pro-angiogenetic. SDF-1-loaded scaffolds have been studied in fracture healing models (Fujio et al., 2011; Li X. et al., 2011) and in cranial defects (Ji et al., 2013; Liu et al., 2014), with excellent results (**Figure 1**). There is also evidence that SDF-1 may induce migration, proliferation and activation of human periodontal ligament stem cells (PLSCs; Du et al., 2012). The association of SDF-1 with BMP-2 increases bone volume in a calvarial defect model compared to SDF-1 alone (Jin and Giannobile, 2014). Another possible approach is the use of Platelet-Rich Plasma (PRP), a concentrate of blood platelets that upon activation releases various growth factors, including PDGF and VEGF (Fekete et al., 2012), and neurotransmitters that have been shown to be fundamental for tooth repair in animal model (Baudry et al., 2015). Nevertheless, its role as activator of endogenous stem cells is still controversial, this mainly due to problems in standardize the PRP production protocol (Malhotra et al., 2013); its use seems, however, more efficient in case of soft tissue healing or in case of concomitant cell transplantation (Anitua et al., 2008). In the case of periodontal regeneration, the potential use of PRP as a stem cell activator has been suggested, but not yet demonstrated (Chen et al., 2010; Del Corso et al., 2012). On the other hand, Platelet-Rich Fibrin (PRF), a polymeric (fibrin based) scaffold loaded with PRP, has shown some very interesting results in promoting craniofacial bone regeneration both in preclinical and in clinical setting (Simonpieri et al., 2012; Li et al., 2014). The use of autologous growth factors released by platelets could overcome one of the major problems associated with growth factor-mediated recruitment/activation of stem cells: the high production costs for recombinant human growth factors-loaded scaffolds. Other strategies proposed in order to stimulate the synthesis of growth factors directly at the site of the defect, such as gene transfer by plasmids, viral vectors or by genetically modified allogeneic or autologous cells, have been reviewed by Evans CH and will not be further discussed (Evans, 2014).

## Beyond Growth Factors

### Small Molecules and Drugs

As considered in the previous section, the use of growth factors released at the site of defects to activate endogenous stem cells constitutes a valid and efficient approach for tissue regeneration, though it is encumbered by high production costs and short duration in time. If, on one hand, new preparation methods promise to decrease the costs of production, on the other hand new approaches for stem cells recruitment and activation are under investigation (Mallick and Cox, 2013). Old and new drugs are now being studied for their effects on bone and dental healing (Laurencin et al., 2014). Statins are the perfect example of drugs commonly used for hypercholesterolemia that have now shown a potential to induce bone formation (Mundy et al., 1999). The use of simvastatin-loaded scaffolds has been studied in calvarial defects in a rat model, proving an increase in bone healing; the mechanism of action seems to involve the local expression of BMP-2 and HIF-1α recruiting autogenous osteogenic and angiogenetic stem cells (Yueyi et al., 2013). AMD-3100 (octahydrochloride hydrate) is a new drug currently approved in USA (trade name: Plerixafor™) for hematopoietic stem cells mobilization in patients that do not respond well to G-CSF alone. It works as a CXCR4 antagonist (or, more accurately, as a partial agonist), interfering with the SDF-1-CXCR4 axis and disrupting stem cell homing, with a primary effect on HSCs and EPCs (Pitchford et al., 2009). Several works outlined the positive effect of AMD-3100 administration after a bone lesion in animal models (Toupadakis et al., 2013) while Kumar and Ponnazhagan evidenced MSCs mobilization from bone marrow after AMD-3100 administration, and reported a significant augmentation of bone growth when it was co-administrated with IGF-1 (Kumar and Ponnazhagan, 2012). HSCs mobilization operated by G-CSF has been investigated in a phase II clinical trial in case of tibial osteotomy: in this study, the patients who received G-CSF infusion for 3 consecutive days and 4 h before surgery manifested an improved osseointegration of the bone graft compared to controls, though no difference in the quality of the newly formed bone was seen between the two groups (Marmotti et al., 2013). Local application of G-CSF with gelatin hydrogel has shown a potential use for bone regeneration as it contributes to an ideal local environment for fracture healing (Ishida et al., 2010). FTY720 is a small-molecule analog of sphingosine-1-phosphate (S1P), that works as a selective agonist on S1P1 and S1P3-5 receptors; it has proved an angiogenetic effect of microvasculature and an increase in graft osseointegration (Petrie Aronin et al., 2010; Sefcik et al., 2011). Its local delivery with PLGA-scaffolds led to statistically significant increases in bone volumes in a rat model of critical-size calvarial defects (Huang et al., 2012). Another small compound, SVAK-12, which acts as a disruptor of the binding of the E3-ligase Smurf1 with BMP-2 pathway transducers (namely, Smads -1, -5, and -8), thus increasing downstream signaling, has been found to potentiate the transdifferentiation of myoblasts toward an osteoblastic phenotype *in vitro* (Kato et al., 2011). In another study, a single local dose of SVAK-12 enhanced bone-healing in the presence of endogenous BMPs in an animal model of femoral fracture (Wong et al., 2013).

### Physical Activation of Endogenous Stem Cells

Pharmacological means are surely a powerful way to activate and/or mobilize stem cells, but other strategies are being developed that do not need the exogenous administration of substances. Though we are still at a seminal point in this direction, the idea of pursuing stem cells activation through physical means is revolutionary. Ultrasounds are mechanical waves (sound waves) characterized by frequencies higher than the upper audible limit of the human hearing. The use of ultrasounds skyrocketed in the last decades both in diagnostics and in therapy; as for bone healing, the most used ultrasound-based technique is LIPUS (Low-Intensity Pulsed Ultrasound Stimulation), which has been tested with various successes in case of bone fractures and non-unions (Watanabe et al., 2010; Yang et al., 2010). The biology of ultrasound effects on bone tissue has been a mystery until very recently, although the role of mechanical stresses is well-known in the scientific community since a long time (Carter, 1987); therefore, today is universally accepted that mechanical forces are a major determinant of stem cells self-renewal and fate decision, as their roles have been assessed in embryonic and mesenchymal stem cells (Li D. et al., 2011). In 2013, Kusuyama et al. demonstrated how LIPUS influences the multilineage differentiation of mesenchymal stem and progenitor cells, thus finding a proof of principle for ultrasound use in bone healing (Kusuyama et al., 2014). The effects of LIPUS on mesenchymal stem cells have been also studied with regards to chondrogenic differentiation (Cui et al., 2006) and osteogenic differentiation for tooth tissue engineering (Lim et al., 2013) in two separate *in vitro* studies. Light, beside the ultrasounds, is another notable mean for endogenous stem cells recruitment. In particular, in the study by Arany et al. the use of low-power lasers (LPL) induced reactive oxygen species (ROS) in a dose-dependent manner, which in turn activated latent TGF-beta via a specific methionine residue; light-activated TGF-beta was capable of differentiating human dental stem cells *in vitro*, and the results were confirmed in an *in vivo* pulp cap model in rat teeth. Moreover, in TGF-beta-RII-null animals this response to laser was abolished, confirming a central role for TGF-beta in dental regeneration (Arany et al., 2014). The last example of physical stimulus known for its effect on gene expression and stem cell fate is heat (Fan, 2012). Heat shocks constitute natural occurring events, which can be easily reproduced under specific conditions. In a series of experiments, DPSCs have been shown to be more resistant to heat stress compared to non-stem cells (Yao et al., 2011), and this paved the way for a heat-induced activation of DPSCs (Rezai Rad et al., 2013). However, these experiments were conducted *in vitro*, and their relative importance to endogenous stem cells activation has yet to be evidenced, and thus must be considered only speculative.

## CONCLUSIONS AND FUTURE PERSPECTIVES

Regenerative medicine is today at a crucial point: we have already developed effective methods to improve tissue regeneration for some critical districts of the human body, such as the bones of the craniofacial complex, but these methods usually require the use of cells obtained from the same individual or from another individual (respectively, autologous or allogeneic graft), that need to be processed *ex vivo* before the transplant takes place. These procedures, though effective and increasingly standardized, expose the graft recipient to the risks already discussed in the previous sections. The increasing understanding of the mechanisms that regulate stem cell biology in adult tissues and their role in tissue healing in physiological and pathological conditions, along with the better comprehension of the role of the extracellular matrix in tissue dynamics, laid the foundations to newer strategies in regenerative medicine that aim to exploit the hidden potential of endogenous stem cells, such as growth factor-loaded bioscaffolds. These new approaches have been developed in order to avoid cell processing and decrease manufacturing burden, which constitute the main limitations to the spreading of the cell-based approaches. One way to reduce consistently the production costs would be the use of gene delivery strategies, in order to induce the synthesis of the growth factors directly in the host cells. However, this approach could become detrimental, as it would suffer from the same legislative and safety concerns of gene therapy (O'Reilly et al., 2015). Another critical point is that of the almost complete lack of any kind of data on human patients for growth factors-based approaches. More clinical trials are mandatory to assess the real impact of these techniques on human health, including safety assessments for the use of known mitogens. As for drug-induced stem cell activation, on the other hand, though even more molecules are under pre-clinical investigation (Kochegarov, 2009), the ones that have already proved effective in animal models should be validated for their safety and efficacy on humans. In this context, AMD-3100 could be regarded as the ideal drug to begin the clinical investigation, as it is already approved for human use, though with a different indication. Finally, concerning the physical approaches, new rigorous studies are important to understand whether these techniques can be really considered for a clinical application, as they would constitute the easiest and the less invasive way to promote tissue regeneration.

## AUTHOR CONTRIBUTIONS

ML and VP performed the literature research and wrote the manuscript. TV and PF revised the manuscript. DA proofreading. DV and PG coordinated the work, perform the proofreading, and approve the final manuscript.

## REFERENCES


Alvarez, P., Hee, C. K., Solchaga, L., Snel, L., Kestler, H. K., Lynch, S. E., et al. (2012). Growth factors and craniofacial surgery. *J. Craniofac. Surg.* 23, 20–29. doi: 10.1097/SCS.0b013e318240c6a8

Amariglio, N., Hirshberg, A., Scheithauer, B. W., Cohen, Y., Loewenthal, R., Trakhtenbrot, L., et al. (2009). Donor-derived brain tumor following neural stem cell transplantation in an ataxia telangiectasia patient. *PLoS Med.* 17:e1000029. doi: 10.1371/journal.pmed.1000029

Anitua, E., Aguirre, J. J., Algorta, J., Ayerdi, E., Cabezas, A. I., Orive, G., et al. (2008). Effectiveness of autologous preparation rich in growth factors for the treatment of chronic cutaneous ulcers. *J. Biomed. Mater. Res. B Appl. Biomater.* 84, 415–421. doi: 10.1002/jbm.b.30886

Arany, P. R., Cho, A., Hunt, T. D., Sidhu, G., Shin, K., Hahm, E., et al. (2014). Photoactivation of endogenous latent transforming growth factor-β1 directs dental stem cell differentiation for regeneration. *Sci. Trans. Med.* 6:238ra269. doi: 10.1126/scitranslmed.3008234

Bae, S. C., Lee, K. S., Zhang, Y. W., and Ito, Y. (2001). Intimate relationship between TGF-β/BMP signaling and runt domain transcription factor, PEBP2/CBF. *J. Bone Joint Surg. Am.* 83-A(Suppl. 1), S48–S55.

Baker, D. E., Harrison, N. J., Maltby, E., Smith, K., Moore, H. D., Shaw, P. J., et al. (2007). Adaptation to culture of human embryonic stem cells and oncogenesis *in vivo*. *Nat. Biotechnol.* 25, 207–215. doi: 10.1038/nbt1285

Barker, R. A., and Widner, H. (2004). Immune problems in central nervous system cell therapy. *NeuroRx* 1, 472–481. doi: 10.1602/neurorx.1.4.472

Baudry, A., Alleaume-Butaux, A., Dimitrova-Nakov, S., Goldberg, M., Schneider, B., Launay, J. M., et al. (2015). Essential roles of dopamine and serotonin in tooth repair: functional interplay between odontogenic stem cells and platelets. *Stem Cells* 33, 2586–2595. doi: 10.1002/stem.2037

Baykan, E., Koc, A., Eser Elcin, A., and Murat Elcin, Y. (2014). Evaluation of a biomimetic poly(epsilon-caprolactone)/β-tricalcium phosphate multispiral scaffold for bone tissue engineering: *in vitro* and *in vivo* studies. *Biointerphases* 9, 029011. doi: 10.1116/1.4870781

Behr, B., Sorkin, M., Lehnhardt, M., Renda, A., Longaker, M. T., and Quarto, N. (2012). A comparative analysis of the osteogenic effects of BMP-2, FGF-2, and VEGFA in a calvarial defect model. *Tissue Eng. Part A* 18, 1079–1086. doi: 10.1089/ten.TEA.2011.0537

Bessa, P. C., Casal, M., and Reis, R. L. (2008a). Bone morphogenetic proteins in tissue engineering: the road from laboratory to clinic, part II (BMP delivery). *J. Tissue Eng. Regen. Med.* 2, 81–96. doi: 10.1002/term.74

Bessa, P. C., Casal, M., and Reis, R. L. (2008b). Bone morphogenetic proteins in tissue engineering: the road from the laboratory to the clinic, part I (basic concepts). *J. Tissue Eng. Regen. Med.* 2, 1–13. doi: 10.1002/term.63

Bose, S., Roy, M., and Bandyopadhyay, A. (2012). Recent advances in bone tissue engineering scaffolds. *Trends Biotechnol.* 30, 546–554. doi: 10.1016/j.tibtech.2012.07.005

Brizzi, M. F., Tarone, G., and Defilippi, P. (2012). Extracellular matrix, integrins, and growth factors as tailors of the stem cell niche. *Curr. Opin. Cell Biol.* 24, 645–651. doi: 10.1016/j.ceb.2012.07.001

Bueno, E. M., and Glowacki, J. (2009). Cell-free and cell-based approaches for bone regeneration. *Nat. Rev. Rheumatol.* 5, 685–697. doi: 10.1038/nrrheum.2009.228

Campagnoli, C., Roberts, I. A., Kumar, S., Bennett, P. R., Bellantuono, I., and Fisk, N. M. (2001). Identification of mesenchymal stem/progenitor cells in human first-trimester fetal blood, liver, and bone marrow. *Blood* 98, 2396–2402. doi: 10.1182/blood.V98.8.2396

Carpenter, M. K., Frey-Vasconcells, J., and Rao, M. S. (2009). Developing safe therapies from human pluripotent stem cells. *Nat. Biotechnol.* 27, 606–613. doi: 10.1038/nbt0709-606

Carter, D. R. (1987). Mechanical loading history and skeletal biology. *J. Biomech.* 20, 1095–1109. doi: 10.1016/0021-9290(87)90027-3

Chang, P. C., Seol, Y. J., Cirelli, J. A., Pellegrini, G., Jin, Q., Franco, L. M., et al. (2010). PDGF-B gene therapy accelerates bone engineering and oral implant osseointegration. *Gene Ther.* 17, 95–104. doi: 10.1038/gt.2009.117

Chavez, S. L., Meneses, J. J., Nguyen, H. N., Kim, S. K., and Pera, R. A. (2008). Characterization of six new human embryonic stem cell lines (HSF7, -8, -9, -10, -12, and -13) derived under minimal-animal component conditions. *Stem Cells Dev.* 17, 535–546. doi: 10.1089/scd.2007.0216

Chen, F. M., Zhang, M., and Wu, Z. F. (2010). Toward delivery of multiple growth factors in tissue engineering. *Biomaterials* 31, 6279–6308. doi: 10.1016/j.biomaterials.2010.04.053

Chen, Z., and Palmer, T. D. (2008). Cellular repair of CNS disorders: an immunological perspective. *Hum. Mol. Genet.* 17, R84–R92. doi: 10.1093/hmg/ddn104

Chenard, K. E., Teven, C. M., He, T. C., and Reid, R. R. (2012). Bone morphogenetic proteins in craniofacial surgery: current techniques, clinical experiences, and the future of personalized stem cell therapy. *J. Biomed. Biotechnol.* 2012:601549. doi: 10.1155/2012/601549

Chesnutt, B. M., Yuan, Y., Buddington, K., Haggard, W. O., and Bumgardner, J. D. (2009). Composite chitosan/nano-hydroxyapatite scaffolds induce osteocalcin production by osteoblasts *in vitro* and support bone formation *in vivo*. *Tissue Eng. Part A* 15, 2571–2579. doi: 10.1089/ten.tea.2008.0054

Choi, J. W., and Kim, N. (2015). Clinical application of three-dimensional printing technology in craniofacial plastic surgery. *Arch. Plast. Surg.* 42, 267–277. doi: 10.5999/aps.2015.42.3.267

Chung, E. J., Sugimoto, M. J., and Ameer, G. A. (2011). The role of hydroxyapatite in citric acid-based nanocomposites: surface characteristics, degradation, and osteogenicity *in vitro*. *Acta Biomater.* 7, 4057–4063. doi: 10.1016/j.actbio.2011.07.001

Cordeiro, M. M., Dong, Z., Kaneko, T., Zhang, Z., Miyazawa, M., Shi, S., et al. (2008). Dental pulp tissue engineering with stem cells from exfoliated deciduous teeth. *J. Endod.* 34, 962–969. doi: 10.1016/j.joen.2008.04.009

Costello, L. C., Franklin, R. B., Reynolds, M. A., and Chellaiah, M. (2012). The important role of osteoblasts and citrate production in bone formation: "osteoblast citration" as a new concept for an old relationship. *Open Bone J.* 4, 27–34. doi: 10.2174/1876525401204010027

Cui, J. H., Park, K., Park, S. R., and Min, B. H. (2006). Effects of low-intensity ultrasound on chondrogenic differentiation of mesenchymal stem cells embedded in polyglycolic acid: an *in vivo* study. *Tissue Eng.* 12, 75–82. doi: 10.1089/ten.2006.12.75

d'Aquino, R., Graziano, A., Sampaolesi, M., Laino, G., Pirozzi, G., De Rosa, A., et al. (2007). Human postnatal dental pulp cells co-differentiate into osteoblasts and endotheliocytes: a pivotal synergy leading to adult bone tissue formation. *Cell Death Diff.* 14, 1162–1171. doi: 10.1038/sj.cdd.4402121

d'Aquino, R., Tirino, V., Desiderio, V., Studer, M., De Angelis, G. C., Laino, L., et al. (2011). Human neural crest-derived postnatal cells exhibit remarkable embryonic attributes either *in vitro* or *in vivo*. *Eur. Cell. Mater.* 21, 304–316.

Davies, E., Muller, K. H., Wong, W. C., Pickard, C. J., Reid, D. G., Skepper, J. N., et al. (2014). Citrate bridges between mineral platelets in bone. *Proc. Natl. Acad. Sci. U.S.A.* 111, E1354–E1363. doi: 10.1073/pnas.1315080111

De la Riva, B., Nowak, C., Sanchez, E., Hernandez, A., Schulz-Siegmund, M., Pec, M. K., et al. (2009). VEGF-controlled release within a bone defect from alginate/chitosan/PLA-H scaffolds. *Eur. J. Pharm. Biopharm.* 73, 50–58. doi: 10.1016/j.ejpb.2009.04.014

De la Riva, B., Sanchez, E., Hernandez, A., Reyes, R., Tamimi, F., Lopez-Cabarcos, E., et al. (2010). Local controlled release of VEGF and PDGF from a combined brushite-chitosan system enhances bone regeneration. *J. Control. Release* 143, 45–52. doi: 10.1016/j.jconrel.2009.11.026

Del Corso, M., Vervelle, A., Simonpieri, A., Jimbo, R., Inchingolo, F., Sammartino, G., et al. (2012). Current knowledge and perspectives for the use of platelet-rich plasma (PRP) and platelet-rich fibrin (PRF) in oral and maxillofacial surgery part 1: Periodontal and dentoalveolar surgery. *Curr. Pharm. Biotechnol.* 13, 1207–1230. doi: 10.2174/138920112800624391

Dhandayuthapani, B., Yoshida, Y., Maekawa, T., and Kumar, D. S. (2011). Polymeric scaffolds in tissue engineering application: a review. *Int. J. Polymer Sci.* 2011, 19. doi: 10.1155/2011/290602

Du, L., Yang, P., and Ge, S. (2012). Stromal cell-derived factor-1 significantly induces proliferation, migration, and collagen type I expression in a human periodontal ligament stem cell subpopulation. *J. Periodontol.* 83, 379–388. doi: 10.1902/jop.2011.110201

Erickson, K. I., Miller, D. L., and Roecklein, K. A. (2012). The aging hippocampus: interactions between exercise, depression, and BDNF. *Neuroscientist* 18, 82–97. doi: 10.1177/1073858410397054

Erickson, K. I., Voss, M. W., Prakash, R. S., Basak, C., Szabo, A., Chaddock, L., et al. (2011). Exercise training increases size of hippocampus and improves memory. *Proc. Natl. Acad. Sci. U.S.A.* 108, 3017–3022. doi: 10.1073/pnas.1015950108

Evans, C. (2014). Using genes to facilitate the endogenous repair and regeneration of orthopaedic tissues. *Int. Orthop.* 38, 1761–1769. doi: 10.1007/s00264-014-2423-x

Fan, G. C. (2012). Role of heat shock proteins in stem cell behavior. *Prog. Mol. Biol. Transl. Sci.* 111, 305–322. doi: 10.1016/B978-0-12-398459-3.00014-9

Farokhi, M., Mottaghitalab, F., Ai, J., and Shokrgozar, M. A. (2013). Sustained release of platelet-derived growth factor and vascular endothelial growth factor from silk/calcium phosphate/PLGA based nanocomposite scaffold. *Int. J. Pharm.* 454, 216–225. doi: 10.1016/j.ijpharm.2013.06.080

Farokhi, M., Mottaghitalab, F., Shokrgozar, M. A., Ai, J., Hadjati, J., and Azami, M. (2014). Bio-hybrid silk fibroin/calcium phosphate/PLGA nanocomposite scaffold to control the delivery of vascular endothelial growth factor. *Mater. Sci. Eng. C Mater. Biol. Appl.* 35, 401–410. doi: 10.1016/j.msec.2013.11.023

Fekete, N., Gadelorge, M., Furst, D., Maurer, C., Dausend, J., Fleury-Cappellesso, S., et al. (2012). Platelet lysate from whole blood-derived pooled platelet concentrates and apheresis-derived platelet concentrates for the isolation and expansion of human bone marrow mesenchymal stromal cells: production process, content and identification of active components. *Cytotherapy* 14, 540–554. doi: 10.3109/14653249.2012.655420

Ferreira, A. M., Gentile, P., Chiono, V., and Ciardelli, G. (2012). Collagen for bone tissue regeneration. *Acta Biomater.* 8, 3191–3200. doi: 10.1016/j.actbio.2012.06.014

Fiedler, J., Etzel, N., and Brenner, R. E. (2004). To go or not to go: migration of human mesenchymal progenitor cells stimulated by isoforms of PDGF. *J. Cell. Biochem.* 93, 990–998. doi: 10.1002/jcb.20219

Fujio, M., Yamamoto, A., Ando, Y., Shohara, R., Kinoshita, K., Kaneko, T., et al. (2011). Stromal cell-derived factor-1 enhances distraction osteogenesis-mediated skeletal tissue regeneration through the recruitment of endothelial precursors. *Bone* 49, 693–700. doi: 10.1016/j.bone.2011.06.024

Gautschi, O. P., Frey, S. P., and Zellweger, R. (2007). Bone morphogenetic proteins in clinical applications. *ANZ J. Surg.* 77, 626–631. doi: 10.1111/j.1445-2197.2007.04175.x

Gentile, P., Chiono, V., Carmagnola, I., and Hatton, P. V. (2014). An overview of poly(lactic-co-glycolic) acid (PLGA)-based biomaterials for bone tissue engineering. *Int. J. Mol. Sci.* 15, 3640–3659. doi: 10.3390/ijms15033640

Giannobile, W. V., Ryan, S., Shih, M. S., Su, D. L., Kaplan, P. L., and Chan, T. C. (1998). Recombinant human osteogenic protein-1 (OP-1) stimulates periodontal wound healing in class III furcation defects. *J. Periodontol.* 69, 129–137. doi: 10.1902/jop.1998.69.2.129

Giuliani, A., Manescu, A., Langer, M., Rustichelli, F., Desiderio, V., Paino, F., et al. (2013). Three years after transplants in human mandibles, histological and in-line holotomography revealed that stem cells regenerated a compact rather than a spongy bone: biological and clinical implications. *Stem Cells Trans. Med.* 2, 316–324. doi: 10.5966/sctm.2012-0136

Griffin, M., Kalaskar, D. M., Butler, P. E., and Seifalian, A. M. (2014). The use of adipose stem cells in cranial facial surgery. *Stem Cell Rev.* 10, 671–685. doi: 10.1007/s12015-014-9522-3

Gronthos, S., Brahim, J., Li, W., Fisher, L. W., Cherman, N., Boyde, A., et al. (2002). Stem cell properties of human dental pulp stem cells. *J. Dent. Res.* 81, 531–535. doi: 10.1177/154405910208100806

Gronthos, S., Mankani, M., Brahim, J., Robey, P. G., and Shi, S. (2000). Postnatal human dental pulp stem cells (DPSCs) *in vitro* and *in vivo*. *Proc. Natl. Acad. Sci. U.S.A.* 97, 13625–13630. doi: 10.1073/pnas.240309797

Guha, P., Morgan, J. W., Mostoslavsky, G., Rodrigues, N. P., and Boyd, A. S. (2013). Lack of immune response to differentiated cells derived from syngeneic induced pluripotent stem cells. *Cell Stem Cell* 12, 407–412. doi: 10.1016/j.stem.2013.01.006

Hakkinen, L., Larjava, H., and Fournier, B. P. (2014). Distinct phenotype and therapeutic potential of gingival fibroblasts. *Cytotherapy* 16, 1171–1186. doi: 10.1016/j.jcyt.2014.04.004

Han, A., Zhao, H., Li, J., Pelikan, R., and Chai, Y. (2014). *ALK5*-mediated transforming growth factor β signaling in neural crest cells controls craniofacial muscle development via tissue-tissue interactions. *Mol. Cell. Biol.* 34, 3120–3131. doi: 10.1128/MCB.00623-14

Herrmann, M., Verrier, S., and Alini, M. (2015). Strategies to stimulate mobilization and homing of endogenous stem and progenitor cells for bone tissue repair. *Front. Bioeng. Biotechnol.* 3:79. doi: 10.3389/fbioe.2015.00079

Huang, C., Das, A., Barker, D., Tholpady, S., Wang, T., Cui, Q., et al. (2012). Local delivery of FTY720 accelerates cranial allograft incorporation and bone formation. *Cell Tissue Res.* 347, 553–566. doi: 10.1007/s00441-011-1217-3

Hung, C. N., Mar, K., Chang, H. C., Chiang, Y. L., Hu, H. Y., Lai, C. C., et al. (2011). A comparison between adipose tissue and dental pulp as sources of MSCs for tooth regeneration. *Biomaterials* 32, 6995–7005. doi: 10.1016/j.biomaterials.2011.05.086

Hynes, R. O. (2002a). Integrins: bidirectional, allosteric signaling machines. *Cell* 110, 673–687. doi: 10.1016/S0092-8674(02)00971-6

Hynes, R. O. (2002b). A reevaluation of integrins as regulators of angiogenesis. *Nat. Med.* 8, 918–921. doi: 10.1038/nm0902-918

Ishida, K., Matsumoto, T., Sasaki, K., Mifune, Y., Tei, K., Kubo, S., et al. (2010). Bone regeneration properties of granulocyte colony-stimulating factor via neovascularization and osteogenesis. *Tissue Eng. Part A* 16, 3271–3284. doi: 10.1089/ten.tea.2009.0268

Ji, W., Yang, F., Ma, J., Bouma, M. J., Boerman, O. C., Chen, Z., et al. (2013). Incorporation of stromal cell-derived factor-1alpha in PCL/gelatin electrospun membranes for guided bone regeneration. *Biomaterials* 34, 735–745. doi: 10.1016/j.biomaterials.2012.10.016

Jiang, H. B., Tian, W. D., Liu, L., Tang, W., Zheng, X. H., and Chen, X. Z. (2008). [Odontoblast-like cell phenotype differentiation of cranial neural crest stem cell *in vivo*]. *Sichuan da Xue Xue Bao Yi Xue Ban* 39, 276–278.

Jin, Q., and Giannobile, W. V. (2014). SDF-1 enhances wound healing of critical-sized calvarial defects beyond self-repair capacity. *PLoS ONE* 9:e97035. doi: 10.1371/journal.pone.0097035

Kaigler, D., Wang, Z., Horger, K., Mooney, D. J., and Krebsbach, P. H. (2006). VEGF scaffolds enhance angiogenesis and bone regeneration in irradiated osseous defects. *J. Bone Miner. Res.* 21, 735–744. doi: 10.1359/jbmr.060120

Kamitakahara, M., Ohtsuki, C., and Miyazaki, T. (2008). Review paper: behavior of ceramic biomaterials derived from tricalcium phosphate in physiological condition. *J. Biomater. Appl.* 23, 197–212. doi: 10.1177/0885328208096798

Kang, Q., Sun, M. H., Cheng, H., Peng, Y., Montag, A. G., Deyrup, A. T., et al. (2004). Characterization of the distinct orthotopic bone-forming activity of 14 BMPs using recombinant adenovirus-mediated gene delivery. *Gene Ther.* 11, 1312–1320. doi: 10.1038/sj.gt.3302298

Kato, S., Sangadala, S., Tomita, K., Titus, L., and Boden, S. D. (2011). A synthetic compound that potentiates bone morphogenetic protein-2-induced transdifferentiation of myoblasts into the osteoblastic phenotype. *Molecular Cell. Biochem.* 349, 97–106. doi: 10.1007/s11010-010-0664-6

Kim, S. S., Sun Park, M., Jeon, O., Yong Choi, C., and Kim, B. S. (2006). Poly(lactide-co-glycolide)/hydroxyapatite composite scaffolds for bone tissue engineering. *Biomaterials* 27, 1399–1409. doi: 10.1016/j.biomaterials.2005.08.016

Kitaori, T., Ito, H., Schwarz, E. M., Tsutsumi, R., Yoshitomi, H., Oishi, S., et al. (2009). Stromal cell-derived factor 1/CXCR4 signaling is critical for the recruitment of mesenchymal stem cells to the fracture site during skeletal repair in a mouse model. *Arthritis Rheum.* 60, 813–823. doi: 10.1002/art.24330

Kleinheinz, J., Stratmann, U., Joos, U., and Wiesmann, H. P. (2005). VEGF-activated angiogenesis during bone regeneration. *J. Oral Maxillofac. Surg.* 63, 1310–1316. doi: 10.1016/j.joms.2005.05.303

Kobayashi, K., Anada, T., Handa, T., Kanda, N., Yoshinari, M., Takahashi, T., et al. (2014). Osteoconductive property of a mechanical mixture of octacalcium phosphate and amorphous calcium phosphate. *ACS Appl. Mater. Interfaces* 6, 22602–22611. doi: 10.1021/am5067139

Kochegarov, A. (2009). Small molecules for stem cells. *Expert Opinion Ther. Pat.* 19, 275–281. doi: 10.1517/13543770802709010

Kumar, S., and Ponnazhagan, S. (2012). Mobilization of bone marrow mesenchymal stem cells *in vivo* augments bone healing in a mouse model of segmental bone defect. *Bone* 50, 1012–1018. doi: 10.1016/j.bone.2012.01.027

Kusuyama, J., Bandow, K., Shamoto, M., Kakimoto, K., Ohnishi, T., and Matsuguchi, T. (2014). Low intensity pulsed ultrasound (LIPUS) influences the multilineage differentiation of mesenchymal stem and progenitor cell lines through ROCK-Cot/Tpl2-MEK-ERK signaling pathway. *J. Biol. Chem.* 289, 10330–10344. doi: 10.1074/jbc.M113.546382

Laino, G., d'Aquino, R., Graziano, A., Lanza, V., Carinci, F., Naro, F., et al. (2005). A new population of human adult dental pulp stem cells: a useful source of living autologous fibrous bone tissue (LAB). *J. Bone Miner. Res.* 20, 1394–1402. doi: 10.1359/JBMR.050325

La Noce, M., Mele, L., Tirino, V., Paino, F., De Rosa, A., Naddeo, P., et al. (2014a). Neural crest stem cell population in craniomaxillofacial development and tissue repair. *Eur. Cell. Mater.* 28, 348–357.

La Noce, M., Paino, F., Spina, A., Naddeo, P., Montella, R., Desiderio, V., et al. (2014b). Dental pulp stem cells: state of the art and suggestions for a true translation of research into therapy. *J. Dent.* 42, 761–768. doi: 10.1016/j.jdent.2014.02.018

Laurencin, C. T., Ashe, K. M., Henry, N., Kan, H. M., and Lo, K. W. (2014). Delivery of small molecules for bone regenerative engineering: preclinical studies and potential clinical applications. *Drug Discov. Today* 19, 794–800. doi: 10.1016/j.drudis.2014.01.012

Ledford, H. (2015). The printed organs coming to a body near you. *Nature* 520:273. doi: 10.1038/520273a

Li, D., Zhou, J., Chowdhury, F., Cheng, J., Wang, N., and Wang, F. (2011). Role of mechanical factors in fate decisions of stem cells. *Regen. Med.* 6, 229–240. doi: 10.2217/rme.11.2

Li, Q., Reed, D. A., Min, L., Gopinathan, G., Li, S., Dangaria, S. J., et al. (2014). Lyophilized platelet-rich fibrin (PRF) promotes craniofacial bone regeneration through Runx2. *Int. J. Mol. Sci.* 15, 8509–8525. doi: 10.3390/ijms150 58509

Li, X., Gao, Z., and Wang, J. (2011). Single percutaneous injection of stromal cell-derived factor-1 induces bone repair in mouse closed tibial fracture model. *Orthopedics* 34, 450. doi: 10.3928/01477447-20110427-19

Li, X., Yu, X., Lin, Q., Deng, C., Shan, Z., Yang, M., et al. (2007). Bone marrow mesenchymal stem cells differentiate into functional cardiac phenotypes by cardiac microenvironment. *J. Mol. Cell. Cardiol.* 42, 295–303. doi: 10.1016/j.yjmcc.2006.07.002

Liao, H. T., Lee, M. Y., Tsai, W. W., Wang, H. C., and Lu, W. C. (2013). Osteogenesis of adipose-derived stem cells on polycaprolactone-β-tricalcium phosphate scaffold fabricated via selective laser sintering and surface coating with collagen type I. *J. Tissue Eng. Regen. Med.* doi: 10.1002/term.1811. [Epub ahead of print].

Lim, K., Kim, J., Seonwoo, H., Park, S. H., Choung, P. H., and Chung, J. H. (2013). *In vitro* effects of low-intensity pulsed ultrasound stimulation on the osteogenic differentiation of human alveolar bone-derived mesenchymal stem cells for tooth tissue engineering. *Biomed. Res. Int.* 2013:269724. doi: 10.1155/2013/269724

Lin, H. R., Kuo, C. J., Yang, C. Y., Shaw, S. Y., and Wu, Y. J. (2002). Preparation of macroporous biodegradable PLGA scaffolds for cell attachment with the use of mixed salts as porogen additives. *J. Biomed. Mater. Res.* 63, 271–279. doi: 10.1002/jbm.10183

Liu, Y. S., Ou, M. E., Liu, H., Gu, M., Lv, L. W., Fan, C., et al. (2014). The effect of simvastatin on chemotactic capability of SDF-1alpha and the promotion of bone regeneration. *Biomaterials* 35, 4489–4498. doi: 10.1016/j.biomaterials.2014.02.025

Luo, G., Hofmann, C., Bronckers, A. L., Sohocki, M., Bradley, A., and Karsenty, G. (1995). BMP-7 is an inducer of nephrogenesis, and is also required for eye development and skeletal patterning. *Genes Dev.* 9, 2808–2820. doi: 10.1101/gad.9.22.2808

Luu, H. H., Song, W. X., Luo, X., Manning, D., Luo, J., Deng, Z. L., et al. (2007). Distinct roles of bone morphogenetic proteins in osteogenic differentiation of mesenchymal stem cells. *J. Orthop. Res.* 25, 665–677. doi: 10.1002/jor. 20359

Malhotra, A., Pelletier, M. H., Yu, Y., and Walsh, W. R. (2013). Can platelet-rich plasma (PRP) improve bone healing? A comparison between the theory and experimental outcomes. *Arch. Orthop. Trauma Surg.* 133, 153–165. doi: 10.1007/s00402-012-1641-1

Mallick, K. K., and Cox, S. C. (2013). Biomaterial scaffolds for tissue engineering. *Front. Biosci.* 5:341–360. doi: 10.2741/E620

Mangano, C., Paino, F., d'Aquino, R., De Rosa, A., Iezzi, G., Piattelli, A., et al. (2011). Human dental pulp stem cells hook into biocoral scaffold forming an engineered biocomplex. *PLoS ONE* 6:e18721. doi: 10.1371/journal.pone.0018721

Marmotti, A., Castoldi, F., Rossi, R., Marenco, S., Risso, A., Ruella, M., et al. (2013). Bone marrow-derived cell mobilization by G-CSF to enhance osseointegration of bone substitute in high tibial osteotomy. *Knee Surg. Sports Traumatol. Arthrosc* 21, 237–248. doi: 10.1007/s00167-012-2150-z

Mason, C., and Dunnill, P. (2008). A brief definition of regenerative medicine. *Regen. Med.* 3, 1–5. doi: 10.2217/17460751.3.1.1

Miller, F. D., and Kaplan, D. R. (2012). Mobilizing endogenous stem cells for repair and regeneration: are we there yet? *Cell Stem Cell* 10, 650–652. doi: 10.1016/j.stem.2012.05.004

Ming, G. L., and Song, H. (2011). Adult neurogenesis in the mammalian brain: significant answers and significant questions. *Neuron* 70, 687–702. doi: 10.1016/j.neuron.2011.05.001

Mitchell, B. D., Emsley, J. G., Magavi, S. S., Arlotta, P., and Macklis, J. D. (2004). Constitutive and induced neurogenesis in the adult mammalian brain: manipulation of endogenous precursors toward CNS repair. *Dev. Neurosci.* 26, 101–117. doi: 10.1159/000082131

Mohanty, P., Prasad, N. K., Sahoo, N., Kumar, G., Mohanty, D., and Sah, S. (2015). Reforming craniofacial orthodontics via stem cells. *J. Int. Soc. Prev. Community Dent.* 5, 13–18. doi: 10.4103/2231-0762.151966

Mundy, G., Garrett, R., Harris, S., Chan, J., Chen, D., Rossini, G., et al. (1999). Stimulation of bone formation *in vitro* and in rodents by statins. *Science* 286, 1946–1949. doi: 10.1126/science.286.5446.1946

Murphy, W. L., Simmons, C. A., Kaigler, D., and Mooney, D. J. (2004). Bone regeneration via a mineral substrate and induced angiogenesis. *J. Dent. Res.* 83, 204–210. doi: 10.1177/154405910408300304

Murray, P. E., Garcia-Godoy, F., and Hargreaves, K. M. (2007). Regenerative endodontics: a review of current status and a call for action. *J. Endodon.* 33, 377–390. doi: 10.1016/j.joen.2006.09.013

Muzzarelli, R. A., Mattioli-Belmonte, M., Tietz, C., Biagini, R., Ferioli, G., Brunelli, M. A., et al. (1994). Stimulatory effect on bone formation exerted by a modified chitosan. *Biomaterials* 15, 1075–1081. doi: 10.1016/0142-9612(94) 90093-0

Naddeo, P., Laino, L., La Noce, M., Piattelli, A., De Rosa, A., Iezzi, G., et al. (2015). Surface biocompatibility of differently textured titanium implants with mesenchymal stem cells. *Dent. Mater.* 31, 235–243. doi: 10.1016/j.dental.2014.12.015

Nakashima, M., Iohara, K., Ishikawa, M., Ito, M., Tomokiyo, A., Tanaka, T., et al. (2004). Stimulation of reparative dentin formation by *ex vivo* gene therapy using dental pulp stem cells electrotransfected with growth/differentiation factor 11 (Gdf11). *Hum. Gene Ther.* 15, 1045–1053. doi: 10.1089/hum.2004.15.1045

Nakashima, M., Iohara, K., and Sugiyama, M. (2009). Human dental pulp stem cells with highly angiogenic and neurogenic potential for possible use in pulp regeneration. *Cytokine Growth Factor Rev.* 20, 435–440. doi: 10.1016/j.cytogfr.2009.10.012

Obregon, F., Vaquette, C., Ivanovski, S., Hutmacher, D. W., and Bertassoni, L. E. (2015). Three-Dimensional Bioprinting for Regenerative Dentistry and Craniofacial Tissue Engineering. *J. Dent. Res.* 94, 143S–152S. doi: 10.1177/0022034515588885

Ohazama, A., Modino, S. A., Miletich, I., and Sharpe, P. T. (2004). Stem-cell-based tissue engineering of murine teeth. *J. Dent. Res.* 83, 518–522. doi: 10.1177/154405910408300702

O'Reilly, M., Jambou, R., Rosenthal, E., Montgomery, M., Hassani, M., Gargiulo, L., et al. (2015). The national institutes of health oversight of human gene transfer research: enhancing science and safety. *Adv. Exp. Med. Biol.* 871, 31–47. doi: 10.1007/978-3-319-18618-4_2

Paino, F., La Noce, M., Tirino, V., Naddeo, P., Desiderio, V., Pirozzi, G., et al. (2014). Histone deacetylase inhibition with valproic acid downregulates osteocalcin gene expression in human dental pulp stem cells and osteoblasts: evidence for HDAC2 involvement. *Stem Cells* 32, 279–289. doi: 10.1002/stem.1544

Panda, N. N., Biswas, A., Pramanik, K., and Jonnalagadda, S. (2015). Enhanced osteogenic potential of human mesenchymal stem cells on electrospun nanofibrous scaffolds prepared from eri-tasar silk fibroin. *J. Biomed. Mater. Res. Part B Appl. Biomater.* 103, 971–982. doi: 10.1002/jbm.b.33272

Patel, Z. S., Ueda, H., Yamamoto, M., Tabata, Y., and Mikos, A. G. (2008). *In vitro* and *in vivo* release of vascular endothelial growth factor from gelatin microparticles and biodegradable composite scaffolds. *Pharm. Res.* 25, 2370–2378. doi: 10.1007/s11095-008-9685-1

Pellegrini, G., Seol, Y. J., Gruber, R., and Giannobile, W. V. (2009). Pre-clinical models for oral and periodontal reconstructive therapies. *J. Dent. Res.* 88, 1065–1076. doi: 10.1177/0022034509349748

Peng, H., Wright, V., Usas, A., Gearhart, B., Shen, H. C., Cummins, J., et al. (2002). Synergistic enhancement of bone formation and healing by stem cell-expressed VEGF and bone morphogenetic protein-4. *J. Clin. Invest.* 110, 751–759. doi: 10.1172/JCI15153

Petrie Aronin, C. E., Shin, S. J., Naden, K. B., Rios, P. D. Jr., Sefcik, L. S., Zawodny, S. R., et al. (2010). The enhancement of bone allograft incorporation by the local delivery of the sphingosine 1-phosphate receptor targeted drug FTY720. *Biomaterials* 31, 6417–6424. doi: 10.1016/j.biomaterials.2010.04.061

Phipps, M. C., Xu, Y., and Bellis, S. L. (2012). Delivery of platelet-derived growth factor as a chemotactic factor for mesenchymal stem cells by bone-mimetic electrospun scaffolds. *PLoS ONE* 7:e40831. doi: 10.1371/journal.pone.0040831

Pitchford, S. C., Furze, R. C., Jones, C. P., Wengner, A. M., and Rankin, S. M. (2009). Differential mobilization of subsets of progenitor cells from the bone marrow. *Cell Stem Cell* 4, 62–72. doi: 10.1016/j.stem.2008.10.017

Pittenger, M. F., Mackay, A. M., Beck, S. C., Jaiswal, R. K., Douglas, R., Mosca, J. D., et al. (1999). Multilineage potential of adult human mesenchymal stem cells. *Science* 284, 143–147. doi: 10.1126/science.284.5411.143

Qi, X. N., Mou, Z. L., Zhang, J., and Zhang, Z. Q. (2014). Preparation of chitosan/silk fibroin/hydroxyapatite porous scaffold and its characteristics in comparison to bi-component scaffolds. *J. Biomed. Mater. Res. Part A* 102, 366–372. doi: 10.1002/jbm.a.34710

Rajan, A., Eubanks, E., Edwards, S., Aronovich, S., Travan, S., Rudek, I., et al. (2014). Optimized cell survival and seeding efficiency for craniofacial tissue engineering using clinical stem cell therapy. *Stem Cells Trans. Med.* 3, 1495–1503. doi: 10.5966/sctm.2014-0039

Ramazanoglu, M., Lutz, R., Rusche, P., Trabzon, L., Kose, G. T., Prechtl, C., et al. (2013). Bone response to biomimetic implants delivering BMP-2 and VEGF: an immunohistochemical study. *J. Craniomaxillofac. Surg* 41, 826–835. doi: 10.1016/j.jcms.2013.01.037

Rezai Rad, M., Wise, G. E., Brooks, H., Flanagan, M. B., and Yao, S. (2013). Activation of proliferation and differentiation of dental follicle stem cells (DFSCs) by heat stress. *Cell Prolif.* 46, 58–66. doi: 10.1111/cpr.12004

Rezwan, K., Chen, Q. Z., Blaker, J. J., and Boccaccini, A. R. (2006). Biodegradable and bioactive porous polymer/inorganic composite scaffolds for bone tissue engineering. *Biomaterials* 27, 3413–3431. doi: 10.1016/j.biomaterials.2006.01.039

Riccio, M., Maraldi, T., Pisciotta, A., La Sala, G. B., Ferrari, A., Bruzzesi, G., et al. (2012). Fibroin scaffold repairs critical-size bone defects *in vivo* supported by human amniotic fluid and dental pulp stem cells. *Tissue Eng. Part A* 18, 1006–1013. doi: 10.1089/ten.tea.2011.0542

Sadan, O., Shemesh, N., Barzilay, R., Bahat-Stromza, M., Melamed, E., Cohen, Y., et al. (2008). Migration of neurotrophic factors-secreting mesenchymal stem cells toward a quinolinic acid lesion as viewed by magnetic resonance imaging. *Stem Cells* 26, 2542–2551. doi: 10.1634/stemcells.2008-0240

Sahoo, T., Theisen, A., Sanchez-Lara, P. A., Marble, M., Schweitzer, D. N., Torchia, B. S., et al. (2011). Microdeletion 20p12.3 involving BMP2 contributes to syndromic forms of cleft palate. *A. J. Med. Genet. Part A* 155A, 1646–1653. doi: 10.1002/ajmg.a.34063

Schantz, J. T., Hutmacher, D. W., Lam, C. X., Brinkmann, M., Wong, K. M., Lim, T. C., et al. (2003a). Repair of calvarial defects with customised tissue-engineered bone grafts II. Evaluation of cellular efficiency and efficacy *in vivo*. *Tissue Eng.* 9(Suppl. 1), S127–S139. doi: 10.1089/10763270360697030

Schantz, J. T., Teoh, S. H., Lim, T. C., Endres, M., Lam, C. X., and Hutmacher, D. W. (2003b). Repair of calvarial defects with customized tissue-engineered bone grafts I. Evaluation of osteogenesis in a three-dimensional culture system. *Tissue Eng.* 9(Suppl. 1), S113–S126. doi: 10.1089/10763270360697021

Schipani, E., Maes, C., Carmeliet, G., and Semenza, G. L. (2009). Regulation of osteogenesis-angiogenesis coupling by HIFs and VEGF. *J. Bone Miner. Res.* 24, 1347–1353. doi: 10.1359/jbmr.090602

Schliephake, H., Weich, H. A., Dullin, C., Gruber, R., and Frahse, S. (2008). Mandibular bone repair by implantation of rhBMP-2 in a slow release carrier of polylactic acid–an experimental study in rats. *Biomaterials* 29, 103–110. doi: 10.1016/j.biomaterials.2007.09.019

Sefcik, L. S., Aronin, C. E., Awojoodu, A. O., Shin, S. J., Mac Gabhann, F., MacDonald, T. L., et al. (2011). Selective activation of sphingosine 1-phosphate receptors 1 and 3 promotes local microvascular network growth. *Tissue Eng. Part A* 17, 617–629. doi: 10.1089/ten.tea.2010.0404

Seiler, J. G. III, Casey, P. J., and Binford, S. H. (2000). Compartment syndromes of the upper extremity. *J. South. Orthop. Assoc.* 9, 233–247.

Seo, B. M., Miura, M., Gronthos, S., Bartold, P. M., Batouli, S., Brahim, J., et al. (2004). Investigation of multipotent postnatal stem cells from human periodontal ligament. *Lancet* 364, 149–155. doi: 10.1016/S0140-6736(04)16627-0

Seol, Y. J., Lee, J. Y., Park, Y. J., Lee, Y. M., Young, K., Rhyu, I. C., et al. (2004). Chitosan sponges as tissue engineering scaffolds for bone formation. *Biotechnol. Lett.* 26, 1037–1041. doi: 10.1023/B:BILE.0000032962.79531.fd

Simonpieri, A., Del Corso, M., Vervelle, A., Jimbo, R., Inchingolo, F., Sammartino, G., et al. (2012). Current knowledge and perspectives for the use of platelet-rich plasma (PRP) and platelet-rich fibrin (PRF) in oral and maxillofacial surgery part 2: Bone graft, implant and reconstructive surgery. *Curr. Pharm. Biotechnol.* 13, 1231–1256. doi: 10.2174/138920112800624472

Smith, D. M., Cooper, G. M., Afifi, A. M., Mooney, M. P., Cray, J., Rubin, J. P., et al. (2011). Regenerative surgery in cranioplasty revisited: the role of adipose-derived stem cells and BMP-2. *Plast. Reconst. Surg.* 128, 1053–1060. doi: 10.1097/PRS.0b013e31822b65e4

Smith, D. M., Cooper, G. M., Mooney, M. P., Marra, K. G., and Losee, J. E. (2008). Bone morphogenetic protein 2 therapy for craniofacial surgery. *J. Craniofac. Surg.* 19, 1244–1259. doi: 10.1097/SCS.0b013e3181843312

Solloway, M. J., Dudley, A. T., Bikoff, E. K., Lyons, K. M., Hogan, B. L., and Robertson, E. J. (1998). Mice lacking Bmp6 function. *Dev. Genet.* 22, 321–339. doi: 10.1002/(SICI)1520-6408(1998)22:4%3C321::AID-DVG3%3E3.0.CO;2-8

Sonoyama, W., Liu, Y., Yamaza, T., Tuan, R. S., Wang, S., Shi, S., et al. (2008). Characterization of the apical papilla and its residing stem cells from human immature permanent teeth: a pilot study. *J. Endod.* 34, 166–171. doi: 10.1016/j.joen.2007.11.021

Spits, C., Mateizel, I., Geens, M., Mertzanidou, A., Staessen, C., Vandeskelde, Y., et al. (2008). Recurrent chromosomal abnormalities in human embryonic stem cells. *Nat. Biotechnol.* 26, 1361–1363. doi: 10.1038/nbt.1510

Springer, I. N., Acil, Y., Kuchenbecker, S., Bolte, H., Warnke, P. H., Abboud, M., et al. (2005a). Bone graft versus BMP-7 in a critical size defect–cranioplasty in a growing infant model. *Bone* 37, 563–569. doi: 10.1016/j.bone.2005.05.010

Springer, I. N., Acil, Y., Spies, C., Jepsen, S., Warnke, P. H., Bolte, H., et al. (2005b). RhBMP-7 improves survival and eruption in a growing tooth avulsion trauma model. *Bone* 37, 570–577. doi: 10.1016/j.bone.2005.04.037

Stadlinger, B., Pilling, E., Huhle, M., Mai, R., Bierbaum, S., Scharnweber, D., et al. (2008). Evaluation of osseointegration of dental implants coated with collagen, chondroitin sulphate and BMP-4: an animal study. *Int. J. Oral Maxillofac. Surg.* 37, 54–59. doi: 10.1016/j.ijom.2007.05.024

Su, X., Paris, M., Gi, Y. J., Tsai, K. Y., Cho, M. S., Lin, Y. L., et al. (2009). TAp63 prevents premature aging by promoting adult stem cell maintenance. *Cell Stem Cell* 5, 64–75. doi: 10.1016/j.stem.2009.04.003

Sui, W., Hou, X., Che, W., Chen, J., Ou, M., Xue, W., et al. (2013). Hematopoietic and mesenchymal stem cell transplantation for severe and refractory systemic lupus erythematosus. *Clin. Immunol.* 148, 186–197. doi: 10.1016/j.clim.2013.05.014

Takahashi, K., Tanabe, K., Ohnuki, M., Narita, M., Ichisaka, T., Tomoda, K., et al. (2007). Induction of pluripotent stem cells from adult human fibroblasts by defined factors. *Cell* 131, 861–872. doi: 10.1016/j.cell.2007.11.019

Teo, A. K., and Vallier, L. (2010). Emerging use of stem cells in regenerative medicine. *Biochem. J.* 428, 11–23. doi: 10.1042/BJ20100102

Teven, C. M., Fisher, S., Ameer, G. A., He, T. C., and Reid, R. R. (2015). Biomimetic approaches to complex craniofacial defects. *Ann. Maxillofac. Surg.* 5, 4–13. doi: 10.4103/2231-0746.161044

Tevlin, R., McArdle, A., Atashroo, D., Walmsley, G. G., Senarath-Yapa, K., Zielins, E. R., et al. (2014). Biomaterials for craniofacial bone engineering. *J. Dent. Res.* 93, 1187–1195. doi: 10.1177/0022034514547271

Toma, J. G., Akhavan, M., Fernandes, K. J., Barnabe-Heider, F., Sadikot, A., Kaplan, D. R., et al. (2001). Isolation of multipotent adult stem cells from the dermis of mammalian skin. *Nat. Cell Biol.* 3, 778–784. doi: 10.1038/ncb0901-778

Toupadakis, C. A., Granick, J. L., Sagy, M., Wong, A., Ghassemi, E., Chung, D. J., et al. (2013). Mobilization of endogenous stem cell populations enhances fracture healing in a murine femoral fracture model. *Cytotherapy* 15, 1136–1147. doi: 10.1016/j.jcyt.2013.05.004

Tsai, R. J., Li, L. M., and Chen, J. K. (2000). Reconstruction of damaged corneas by transplantation of autologous limbal epithelial cells. *N. Engl. J. Med.* 13, 86–93. doi: 10.1056/NEJM200007133430202

Vesterbacka, M., Ringden, O., Remberger, M., Huggare, J., and Dahllof, G. (2012). Disturbances in dental development and craniofacial growth in children treated with hematopoietic stem cell transplantation. *Orthod. Craniofac. Res.* 15, 21–29. doi: 10.1111/j.1601-6343.2011.01533.x

Wada, M. R., Inagawa-Ogashiwa, M., Shimizu, S., Yasumoto, S., and Hashimoto, N. (2002). Generation of different fates from multipotent muscle stem cells. *Development* 129, 2987–2995.

Wagers, A. J. (2012). The stem cell niche in regenerative medicine. *Cell Stem Cell* 10, 362–369. doi: 10.1016/j.stem.2012.02.018

Warejcka, D. J., Harvey, R., Taylor, B. J., Young, H. E., and Lucas, P. A. (1996). A population of cells isolated from rat heart capable of differentiating into several mesodermal phenotypes. *J. Surg. Res.* 62, 233–242. doi: 10.1006/jsre.199 6.0201

Watanabe, Y., Matsushita, T., Bhandari, M., Zdero, R., and Schemitsch, E. H. (2010). Ultrasound for fracture healing: current evidence. *J. Orthop. Trauma* 24(Suppl. 1), S56–S61. doi: 10.1097/BOT.0b013e3181d2efaf

Wernike, E., Montjovent, M. O., Liu, Y., Wismeijer, D., Hunziker, E. B., Siebenrock, K. A., et al. (2010). VEGF incorporated into calcium phosphate ceramics promotes vascularisation and bone formation *in vivo*. *Eur. Cell. Mater.*19, 30–40.

Wong, E., Sangadala, S., Boden, S. D., Yoshioka, K., Hutton, W. C., Oliver, C., et al. (2013). A novel low-molecular-weight compound enhances ectopic bone formation and fracture repair. *J. Bone Joint Surg. Am.* 6, 454–461. doi: 10.2106/JBJS.L.00275

Wu, G., Deng, Z. H., Fan, X. J., Ma, Z. F., Sun, Y. J., Ma, D. D., et al. (2009). Odontogenic potential of mesenchymal cells from hair follicle dermal papilla. *Stem Cells Dev.* 18, 583–589. doi: 10.1089/scd.2008.0066

Yang, M., Zhang, H., and Gangolli, R. (2014). Advances of mesenchymal stem cells derived from bone marrow and dental tissue in craniofacial tissue engineering. *Curr. Stem Cell Res. Ther.* 9, 150–161.

Yang, M. H., Lim, K. T., Choung, P. H., Cho, C. S., and Chung, J. H. (2010). Application of ultrasound stimulation in bone tissue engineering. *Int. J. Stem Cells* 3, 74–79.

Yoon, E., Dhar, S., Chun, D. E., Gharibjanian, N. A., and Evans, G. R. (2007). *In vivo* osteogenic potential of human adipose-derived stem cells/poly lactide-co-glycolic acid constructs for bone regeneration in a rat critical-sized calvarial defect model. *Tissue Eng.* 13, 619–627. doi: 10.1089/ten.2006.0102

Yoshikawa, H., and Myoui, A. (2005). Bone tissue engineering with porous hydroxyapatite ceramics. *J. Artif. Organs* 8, 131–136. doi: 10.1007/s10047-005-0292-1

Young, S., Patel, Z. S., Kretlow, J. D., Murphy, M. B., Mountziaris, P. M., Baggett, L. S., et al. (2009). Dose effect of dual delivery of vascular endothelial growth factor and bone morphogenetic protein-2 on bone regeneration in a rat critical-size defect model. *Tissue Eng. Part A* 15, 2347–2362. doi: 10.1089/ten.tea.2008.0510

Yueyi, C., Xiaoguang, H., Jingying, W., Quansheng, S., Jie, T., Xin, F., et al. (2013). Calvarial defect healing by recruitment of autogenous osteogenic stem cells using locally applied simvastatin. *Biomaterials* 34, 9373–9380. doi: 10.1016/j.biomaterials.2013.08.060

Zaky, S. H., and Cancedda, R. (2009). Engineering craniofacial structures: facing the challenge. *J. Dent. Res.* 88, 1077–1091. doi: 10.1177/0022034509349926

Zhang, H., and Bradley, A. (1996). Mice deficient for BMP2 are nonviable and have defects in amnion/chorion and cardiac development. *Development* 122, 2977–2986.

Zhang, W., Wang, X., Wang, S., Zhao, J., Xu, L., Zhu, C., et al. (2011). The use of injectable sonication-induced silk hydrogel for VEGF(165) and BMP-2 delivery for elevation of the maxillary sinus floor. *Biomaterials* 32, 9415–9424. doi: 10.1016/j.biomaterials.2011.08.047

Zhang, W., Zhu, C., Wu, Y., Ye, D., Wang, S., Zou, D., et al. (2014). VEGF and BMP-2 promote bone regeneration by facilitating bone marrow stem cell homing and differentiation. *Eur. Cell. Mater.* 27, 1–11; discussion 11–12. doi: 10.1016/j.eurpolymj.2014.08.007

Zhao, G. Q. (2003). Consequences of knocking out BMP signaling in the mouse. *Genesis* 35, 43–56. doi: 10.1002/gene.10167

Zhao, K., Lou, R., Huang, F., Peng, Y., Jiang, Z., Huang, K et al. (2015). Immunomodulation effects of mesenchymal stromal cells on acute graft-versus-host disease after hematopoietic stem cell transplantation. *Biol. Blood Marrow Transpl.* 21, 97–104. doi: 10.1016/j.bbmt.2014.09.030

5

# Human Dental Pulp Stem Cells and Gingival Fibroblasts Seeded into Silk Fibroin Scaffolds have the Same Ability in Attracting Vessels

**Edited by:**
Gianpaolo Papaccio,
Second University of Naples, Italy

***Correspondence:**
Anna Woloszyk
anna.woloszyk@zzm.uzh.ch

[†] These authors have contributed equally to this work.

*Anna Woloszyk [1*†], Johanna Buschmann [2†], Conny Waschkies [3,4], Bernd Stadlinger [5] and Thimios A. Mitsiadis [1]*

[1] Orofacial Development and Regeneration, Center of Dental Medicine, Institute of Oral Biology, University of Zurich, Zurich, Switzerland, [2] Plastic Surgery and Hand Surgery, University Hospital Zurich, Zurich, Switzerland, [3] Institute for Biomedical Engineering, ETH and University of Zurich, Zurich, Switzerland, [4] Visceral and Transplant Surgery, University Hospital Zurich, Zurich, Switzerland, [5] Clinic of Cranio-Maxillofacial and Oral Surgery, University of Zurich, University Hospital Zurich, Zurich, Switzerland

Neovascularization is one of the most important processes during tissue repair and regeneration. Current healing approaches based on the use of biomaterials combined with stem cells in critical-size bone defects fail due to the insufficient implant vascularization and integration into the host tissues. Therefore, here we studied the attraction, ingrowth, and distribution of blood vessels from the chicken embryo chorioallantoic membrane into implanted silk fibroin scaffolds seeded with either human dental pulp stem cells or human gingival fibroblasts. Perfusion capacity was evaluated by non-invasive *in vivo* Magnetic Resonance Imaging while the number and density of blood vessels were measured by histomorphometry. Our results demonstrate that human dental pulp stem cells and gingival fibroblasts possess equal abilities in attracting vessels within silk fibroin scaffolds. Additionally, the prolonged *in vitro* pre-incubation period of these two cell populations favors the homogeneous distribution of vessels within silk fibroin scaffolds, which further improves implant survival and guarantees successful healing and regeneration.

**Keywords: regenerative medicine, vascularization, mesenchymal stem cells, human gingival fibroblasts (hGFs), human dental pulp stem cells (hDPSCs), silk fibroin scaffolds, chorioallantoic membrane (CAM)**

## INTRODUCTION

Classical bone defect treatments require the use of anatomically adapted devices that can establish tissue functionality and provide relief of symptoms to patients. However, the effectiveness and durability of treatments involving orthopedic or maxillofacial implants and transplantations of autologous bone grafts are still debatable. Indeed, the outcome of these regenerative solutions may be compromised by a variety of iatrogenic complications such as tissue morbidity and/or inflammation following implant or graft transplantation. Stem cell-based therapeutic approaches offer attractive alternatives in clinics since they can promise physiologically improved structural and functional outcomes. These therapies require a significant number of stem cell populations for implantation into specifically designed and composed scaffolds with various biological activities and compositions that can ensure their fast integration into the defect site. To avoid post-operative complications it is essential to promote rapid, constant, and complete vascularization of these implantable constructs (Giannicola et al., 2010). Different strategies have been developed in order to enhance the vascularization capabilities of the various implanted materials. Cell seeding is one of the most popular and beneficial strategies to achieve this important goal. For example, it has been demonstrated that bone marrow stem cells (BMSCs) and endothelial cells seeded together in decalcified bone scaffolds can accelerate the vascularization process during calvaria bone repair (Koob et al., 2011). Similarly, it has been shown that human amniotic fluid-derived stem cells are able to enhance and stabilize vessel attraction and formation within collagen-chondroitin sulfate scaffolds (Lloyd-Griffith et al., 2015). Cell-seeded grafts may also have immunosuppressive functions that allow an improved healing procedure, as it has been already shown for adipose-derived stem cell-seeded scaffolds (Plock et al., 2015).

The use of human dental pulp stem cells (hDPSCs; Gronthos et al., 2000; Shi et al., 2001; Huang et al., 2009) and human gingival fibroblasts (hGFs; Xu et al., 2013; Chiquet et al., 2015) for regenerative purposes has been proposed as an alternative to BMSCs, since these cell populations exhibit similar properties and have the ability to adopt a variety of alternative fates in response to extrinsic factors. Indeed, it has been shown that hGFs have distinct functional activities in the regeneration and repair of periodontal tissues (Lee et al., 2013; Chiquet et al., 2015). Similarly, numerous studies have demonstrated that hDPSCs have the potential to differentiate into different cell types such as myocytes, chondrocytes, adipocytes, neurons, and osteoblasts both *in vitro* and *in vivo* (Gronthos et al., 2000; Zhang et al., 2006; d'Aquino et al., 2007; Bluteau et al., 2008; Mitsiadis et al., 2015). In addition, *in vitro* and *in vivo* studies have shown that hDPSCs may affect endothelial cell behavior by enhancing their migration and attraction toward them (Hilkens et al., 2014). The first clinical trial using autologous hDPSCs combined with commercially available collagen scaffolds (i.e., Gingistat®) for alveolar bone reconstruction has been successfully performed several years ago (d'Aquino et al., 2009). A 3 years follow-up study has shown that the structure of the regenerated bone at the grafted site was more compact than normal spongy alveolar bone (Giuliani et al., 2013), thus indicating that the choice of the appropriate scaffold and/or stem cell population is crucial for targeted, tissue-specific, regenerative procedures.

Silk fibroin scaffolds are commonly used in the medical field for a diverse set of applications such as vascular, neuronal, skin, cartilage, and bone regeneration (Altman et al., 2003; Kundu et al., 2013). Using bioreactor devices, we have previously shown that hDPSC-seeded silk fibroin scaffolds are able to form mineralized structures *in vitro* in a very short period of time (Woloszyk et al., 2014). In another recent study using the chicken embryo chorioallantoic membrane (CAM) assay combined with magnetic resonance imaging (MRI), we have demonstrated that hDPSCs can attract vessels within silk fibroin scaffolds (Kivrak Pfiffner et al., 2015).

Here we extended our previous studies and compared the capacity of hDPSCs and human gingival fibroblasts (hGFs) to attract vessels within silk fibroin scaffolds. Vascularization of the silk fibroin scaffolds was assessed using MRI and histomorphometric measurements. The results clearly demonstrated that hDPSCs and hGFs have similar abilities in attracting vessels and thus could be equally used in clinics for generating richly vascularized tissues.

# MATERIALS AND METHODS

## Production of Silk Fibroin Scaffolds

Silk fibroin scaffolds were produced using the salt leaching technique as previously described (Sofia et al., 2001; Nazarov et al., 2004; Hofmann et al., 2007). Briefly, silkworm cocoons (Trudel Inc., Zurich, Switzerland) were boiled in 0.02 M sodium carbonate (Fluka AG, Buchs SG, Switzerland) and rinsed with ultrapure water (UPW) to extract sericin. After drying, the silk was dissolved in 9 M lithium bromide and dialyzed against UPW for 36 h followed by lyophilization (Alpha 1-2, Martin Christ GMBH, Osterode am Harz, Germany). A 17% (w/v) silk fibroin solution was prepared by dissolving lyophilized silk in 1,1,1,3,3,3-hexafluoro-2-propanol (HFIP) (abcr GmbH & Co., Karlsruhe, Germany). This solution was added to Teflon containers filled with sodium chloride (Sigma-Aldrich Chemie GmbH, Buchs SG, Switzerland) at a ratio of 1:20 (silk fibroin:NaCl). After the evaporation of HFIP, the blocks were immersed in 90% methanol for 30 min (Sofia et al., 2001). The scaffolds were dried for at least 48 h before sodium chloride was leached out in five changes of UPW in 48 h resulting in scaffolds with more than 90% porosity (Nazarov et al., 2004). Wet silk fibroin scaffolds were cut into cylinders of 5 mm diameter and 3 mm height (59 $mm^3$) and were sterilized by autoclaving at 121°C and 1 bar for 20 min.

## Cell Culture

The procedure for anonymized cell collection was approved by the Kantonale Ethikkommission of Zurich (reference number 2012-0588) and performed with written patients' consent. Human dental pulp stem cells (hDPSCs) were isolated from the dental pulp of extracted impacted wisdom teeth of healthy patients as previously described (Tirino et al., 2012). The dental pulps were enzymatically digested for 1 h at 37°C in a solution of collagenase (3 mg/mL; Life Technologies Europe B.V., Zug ZG, Switzerland) and dispase (4 mg/mL; Sigma-Aldrich Chemie GmbH, Buchs SG, Switzerland). A filtered single-cell suspension was plated in a 40 mm Petri dish with hDPSC growth medium containing DMEM/F12 (Sigma-Aldrich Chemie GmbH, Buchs SG, Switzerland) with 10% fetal bovine serum (FBS) (PAN Biotech GmbH, Aidenbach, Germany), 1% penicillin/streptomycin (P/S) (Sigma-Aldrich Chemie GmbH, Buchs SG, Switzerland), 1% L-glutamine (Sigma-Aldrich Chemie GmbH, Buchs SG, Switzerland), and 0.5 μg/ml fungizone (Life Technologies Europe B.V., Zug ZG, Switzerland) after washing away the enzyme solution. Healthy parts of gingiva were collected from biopsies. Gingival tissues were washed in phosphate buffered saline (PBS) (Life Technologies Europe B.V., Zug ZG, Switzerland), sectioned into small pieces and placed in 35 mm Petri dishes (TPP Techno Plastic Products AG, Trasadingen SH, Switzerland) for the outgrowth of human gingival fibroblasts (hGFs). The fibroblast growth medium is composed by high glucose DMEM (Life Technologies Europe B.V., Zug ZG, Switzerland), 10% FBS, 1% P/S, and 1% HEPES (Sigma-Aldrich Chemie GmbH, Buchs SG, Switzerland). hDPSCs were cultured in DMEM/F12 (Sigma-Aldrich Chemie GmbH, Buchs SG, Switzerland) supplemented with 10% fetal bovine serum (FBS) (Biochrom AG, Berlin, Germany), 1% Penicillin/Streptamycin (P/S) (Sigma-Aldrich Chemie GmbH, Buchs SG, Switzerland), and 0.5 μg/mL fungizone (Thermo Fisher Scientific AG, Reinach BL, Switzerland). hGFs were expanded in DMEM high glucose (Thermo Fisher Scientific AG, Reinach BL, Switzerland) supplemented with 10% FBS, 1% P/S, and 1% HEPES (Thermo Fisher Scientific AG, Reinach BL, Switzerland). Cells were passaged at 80–90% confluence. All experiments were performed with cells from passages 4 and 5.

## Scaffold Seeding

Sterile silk fibroin scaffolds were seeded with cells at a density of $0.5 \times 10^6$ per scaffold and then placed in a humidified incubator for 1 h at 37°C and 5% $CO_2$. The cells that were not attached to the scaffolds were washed away and then the seeded scaffolds were incubated for 1 week at 37°C before being placed on the CAM of fertilized chicken eggs. Empty scaffolds were used as controls (data not shown).

## CAM Assay

No IACUC approval is necessary when performing experiments in chicken embryos until embryonic day 14 according to Swiss animal care guidelines (TSchV, Art. 112). Fertilized Lohman white LSL chicken eggs (Animalco AG, Staufen AG, Switzerland) were pre-incubated for 3 days at 38°C at a rotation speed of 360°/4 h (Bruja 3000, Brutmaschinen-Janeschitz GmbH, Hammelburg, Germany). On embryonic day 3 (ED 3) the eggs were processed for *in ovo* cultivation, which requires the opening of the shell with a drill (Dremel§, Conrad Electronic AG, Wollerau SZ, Switzerland). 2 mL of albumen was always removed with a syringe to increase the empty space under the top of the egg shell. The eggs were stabilized in 60 mm Petri dishes (Greiner Bio-One GmbH, Frickenhausen, Germany) and the created holes of the shells were covered with another 60 mm Petri dish that was fixed with a tape before the incubation of eggs at 37°C. On ED 7, empty and cell-seeded scaffolds were placed on the CAM (1-2/egg) in the middle of silicone rings that ensure a flat surface (**Figures 1A,B**) during their incubation period of 7 days.

## *In vivo* Assessment of Perfusion Capacity Using MRI

Vascularization of the scaffolds by capillaries of the chicken embryo's CAM was studied on ED 14 using Magnetic Resonance Imaging (MRI) as previously described (Kivrak Pfiffner et al., 2015). The eggs were placed onto a custom-built sliding bed and enveloped by warm water tubing to maintain the temperature of the chicken embryo in a physiological range. To prevent motion, the chicken embryo was sedated with 5 drops of 1:100 M ketamine (Ketasol-100, Dr. E. Graeub AG, Bern BE, Switzerland) dripped onto the CAM surface. MRI was performed with a 4.7 T/16 cm Bruker PharmaScan small animal scanner (Bruker BioSpin MRI GmbH, Ettlingen, Germany) equipped with an actively decoupled two-coil system consisting of a 72 mm bird cage resonator for excitation and a 20 mm single loop surface coil for reception. Anatomical reference images were obtained in coronal, transversal, and sagittal slice orientations. T1-weighted MR images were acquired with a RARE sequence of variable TR and TE for quantitative T1 and T2 mapping. T1 maps were acquired in the samples before and after intravenous injection of 100 μL of 0.05 M Gd-DOTA MRI contrast agent (Dotarem®, Guerbet AG, Zuerich ZH, Switzerland). The time between Gd-DOTA injection and T1 mapping was kept constant at 25 min. T1 relaxation times were determined in three regions of interest: at the interface of the scaffold with the CAM (i.e., lower part), in the middle part of the scaffold, and finally at the surface of the scaffold (i.e., upper part). Perfusion capacity in these three regions was assessed through changes in the longitudinal relaxation rate $\Delta R1$ before and after injection of Gd-DOTA, as the relaxation rate changes with the amount of gadolinium present in the CAM.

## Histological Analysis

The scaffold-CAM complex was fixed in 4% paraformaldehyde (PFA) at 4°C overnight. The cell-seeded constructs were excised from the CAM, embedded in paraffin (Haslab GmbH, Ostermundigen BE, Switzerland) and sectioned vertically in 5 μm thick sections. For histological evaluation, sections from the center of the scaffolds were stained with Hematoxylin and Eosin (H&E) (Mayer's hemalum solution, Merck KGaA, Darmstadt, Germany; Eosin Y, Sigma-Aldrich Chemie GmbH, Buchs SG, Switzerland). Pictures were taken using the Axio Scan.Z1 slidescanner (Carl Zeiss AG, Oberkochen, Germany), a Hitachi HV-F202FCL camera (Hitachi, Ltd., Tokyo, Japan), and the ZEN 2012 SP2 software (Carl Zeiss AG, Oberkochen, Deutschland) provided by the Center for Microscopy and Image analysis, University of Zurich.

## Manual Vessel Analysis

The number of vessels and the percentage of vessels per scaffold area were determined by counting the number of vessels in longitudinal sections taken from the center of the scaffold (i.e., middle part). Each vessel was marked in black and ImageJ v1.48s (National Institutes of Health, USA) was used to analyze the number of marked vessels and their total area. Three sections of each sample ($3 \times$ hDPSCs, $3 \times$ hGFs) were analyzed.

## Statistics

For a comparison of the groups a one-way analysis of variance (ANOVA) was performed using GraphPad Prism v6.05 (GraphPad Software, Inc., La Jolla, CA, USA). A Bonferroni's multiple comparisons test was conducted to determine significant differences between the groups. Data were considered significant at $p < 0.05$ (*) and highly significant at $p < 0.01$ (**).

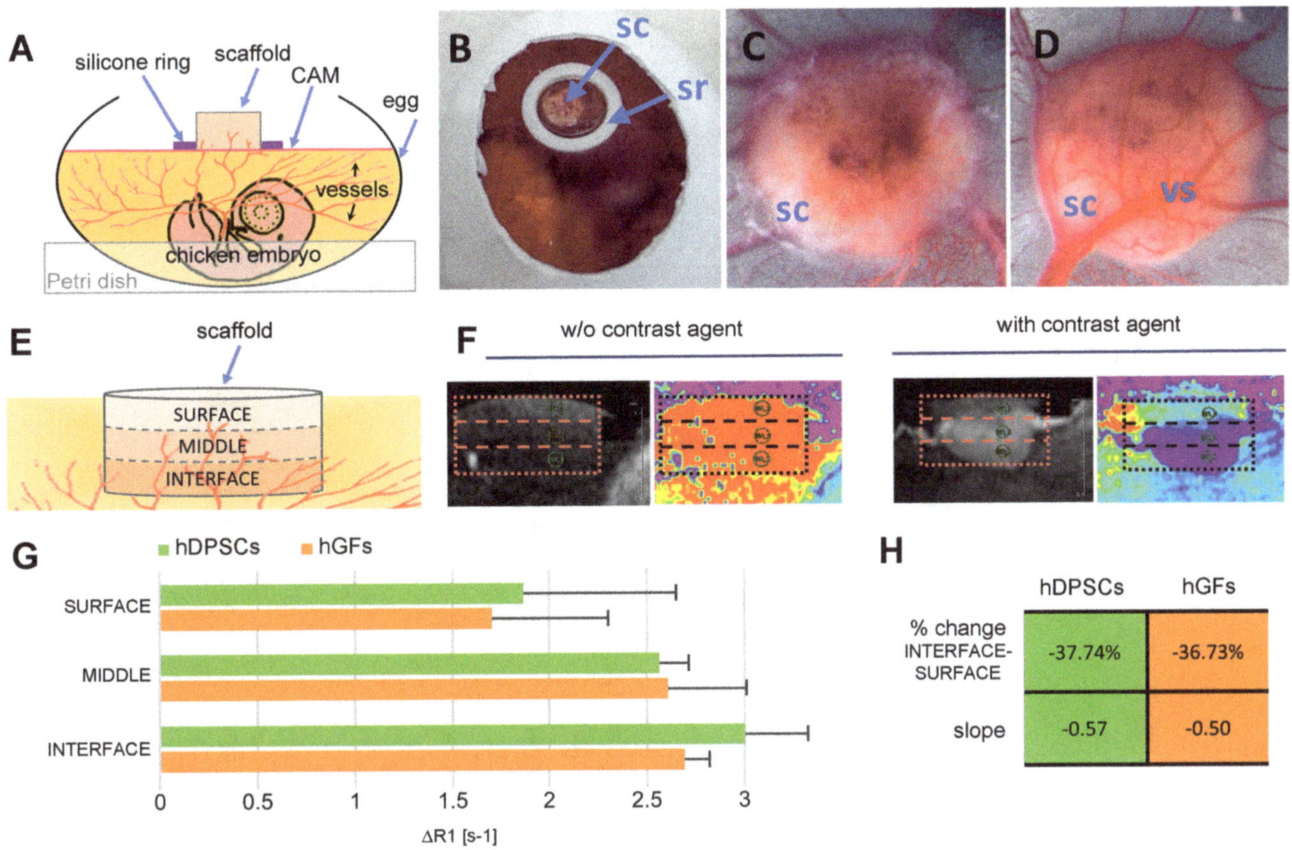


**FIGURE 1 | Experimental setup and MRI analysis. (A,B)** The scaffold is placed in the middle of a silicone ring on top of the CAM of a fertilized egg, which is stabilized in a Petri dish and incubated for 1 week. **(C)** Top and **(D)** bottom views of the scaffold after 1 week of incubation *in ovo*. **(E)** Scheme showing the analyzed parts of the samples. **(F)** Magnetic resonance image of the vascularized scaffold before and after the injection of the contrast agent Gd-DOTA. **(G)** Relaxation rate change ΔR1 in the interface, middle, and surface region of the scaffolds. Values are given as mean ± standard deviation. No statistically significant differences were found. **(H)** Percent change of the mean ΔR1 and slope of regression line between the interface and the surface layers within each group. CAM, chorioallantoic membrane; sc, scaffold; sr, silicone ring; vs, vessel; hDPSCs, human dental pulp stem cells; hGFs, human gingival fibroblasts.

# RESULTS

## Macroscopic Analysis

In growing vessels were visible on the surfaces of the hDPSC- and hGF-seeded silk fibroin scaffolds, both on the top (**Figure 1C**) and on the bottom (**Figure 1D**) of the samples after their CAM incubation for 1 week.

## MRI Analysis

For a more precise analysis of the perfusion capacity of the samples, the scaffolds were divided into three equally sized regions, specified as "interface" (i.e., bottom of the scaffold touching the CAM), "middle," and "surface" (**Figure 1E**). Thereafter, their perfusion capacity was determined by calculating the change of $R_1$ relaxation rates ($\Delta R_1$) measured by MRI before and after contrast enhancement by injected Gd-DOTA, a paramagnetic contrast agent (**Figure 1F**). The $\Delta R_1$ values within the three regions of the scaffolds showed a gradual decrease of their perfusion capacity toward the surface region (**Figure 1G**). A comparison of the perfusion capacity between the hDPSC- and hGF-seeded silk fibroin scaffolds showed no significant differences of $\Delta R_1$ within any of the three scaffold regions (**Figure 1G**). Both cell-seeded scaffolds showed only a percent change from interface to surface of approximately −37% (**Figure 1H**) resulting in much flatter slopes of −0.57 (hDPSCs) and −0.50 (hGFs) when compared to a slope of −1.33 observed in empty silk scaffolds (data not shown; Kivrak Pfiffner et al., 2015).

## Histological and Manual Vessel Analysis

Qualitative and quantitative analyses of the vascularized scaffolds were performed using sections stained with Hematoxylin and Eosin (H&E). These histological sections showed large areas of tissue expansion (depicted by the blue dashed line) into the scaffold (depicted by the red dotted line) (**Figure 2A**). While in the samples seeded with hDPSCs the growing tissue filled approximately half of the scaffold areas (**Figure 2A1**), the tissue occupied roughly two-thirds of the scaffolds seeded with hGFs (**Figure 2A2**). CAM-derived blood vessels have penetrated both hDPSC- and hGF-seeded scaffolds (**Figures 2A3–6**). A manual analysis was performed in order to determine the number and

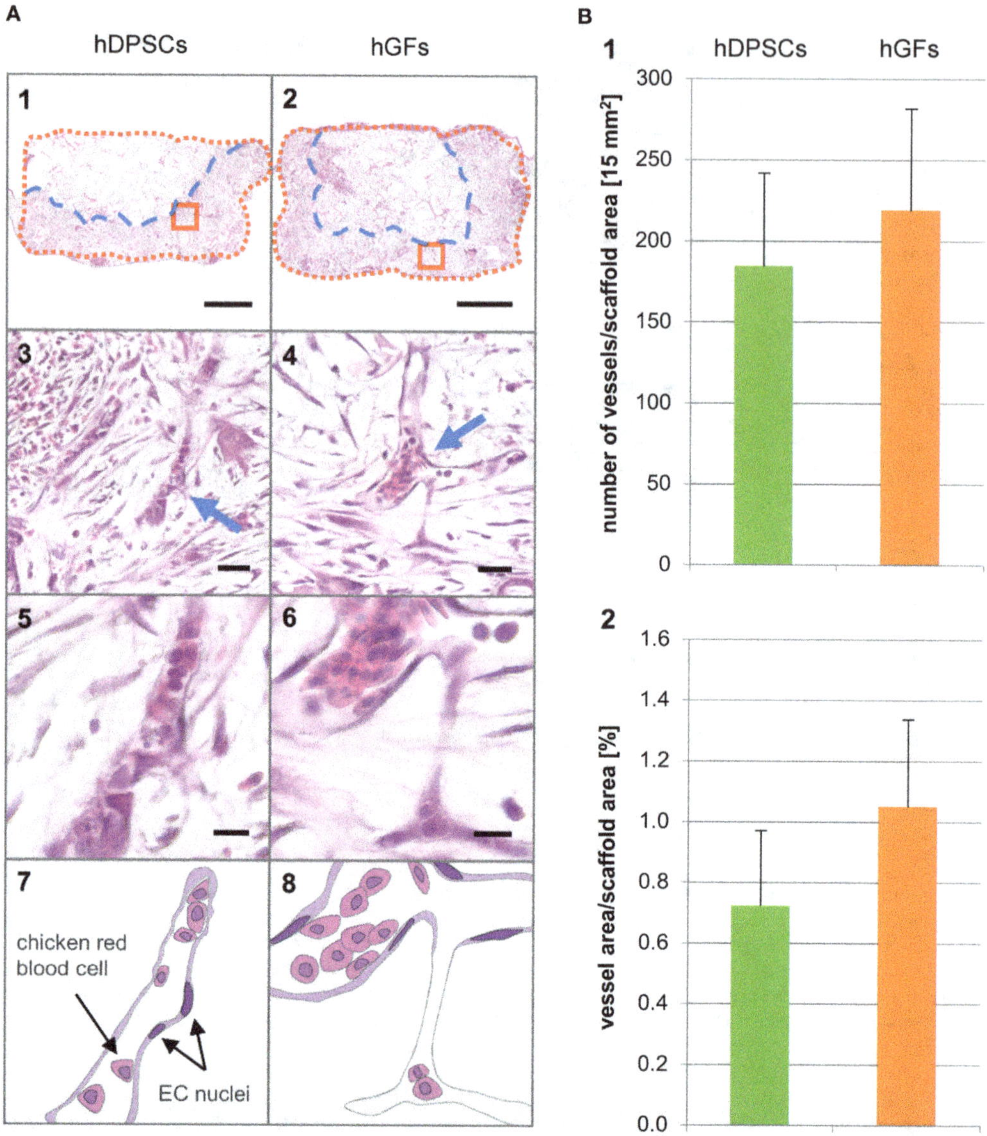


**FIGURE 2 | Hematoxylin and Eosin stainings of longitudinal sections and histomorphometric analysis. ($A_{1,3,5,7}$)** hDPSCs-seeded scaffolds. **($A_{2,4,6,8}$)** hGFs-seeded scaffolds. **($A_{1,2}$)** Scaffold section overview. Blue dashed line indicates the front line of the growing tissue. Red dotted line indicates the outline of the scaffold. Scale bar = 1 mm. **($A_{3,4}$)** Magnifications showing vascularization in the area marked with a red box in the corresponding overview picture. Arrows indicate capillaries. Scale bar = 25 μm. **($A_{5,6}$)** Magnifications showing single capillaries. Scale bar = 10 μm. **($A_{7,8}$)** Schematic representation of the capillaries shown in 5 and 6. **($B_1$)** Number of vessels per scaffold area. **($B_2$)** Percent vessel area per scaffold area. Values are given as mean ± standard deviation. No statistically significant differences were found. EC, endothelial cells; hDPSCs, human dental pulp stem cells; hGFs, human gingival fibroblasts.

the percent area occupied by the vessels within the three defined scaffold areas (**Figure 2B**). The corresponding graphs showed proportional values for scaffolds seeded with hDPSCs and hGFs. Although the average size of the counted vessels in both scaffolds was the same, a higher number of vessels was counted in hGFs-seeded scaffolds. This is due to the larger area occupied by the tissue in hGFs-seeded scaffolds when compared to the occupied tissue area in hDPSC-seeded scaffolds. The distribution of the vasculature along the horizontal axis of the scaffold was nearly homogeneous, whereas the vessel density decreased along the vertical axis following an interface-middle-surface gradient.

## DISCUSSION

The use of biomaterials combined with stem cells aims at the successful healing and regeneration of injured or pathological tissues and organs (Stock and Vacanti, 2001; Griffith and Naughton, 2002). An essential prerequisite for effective tissue repair is the integration of the grafted material into the host tissue and its fast and effective vascularization, which ensures the constant supply of nutrients and oxygen, thus preventing necrosis of the newly formed tissue (Novosel et al., 2011). Therefore, it is essential and vital in stem cell-based regenerative treatments to immediately attract blood vessels into the implanted cell-seeded scaffolds. Enhanced vascularization of the silk fibroin scaffolds has been achieved by integrating a mixture of endothelial cells with osteoblasts (Unger et al., 2010), but also by adding only one of these two cell populations (Unger et al., 2010; Ghanaati et al., 2011). Here we analyzed the capacity of human dental pulp stem cells (hDPSCs) and gingival fibroblasts (hGFs) seeded into silk fibroin scaffolds to attract vessels from the chicken embryo chorioallantoic membrane (CAM). Vascularization of the scaffolds was assessed with magnetic resonance imaging (MRI) and histomorphometric analyses demonstrating that both hDPSCs and hGFs have an equal capacity in attracting vessels within silk fibroin scaffolds. Small discrepancies between MRI and histomorphometric analysis data can be explained by the sample size that was evaluated: histomorphometry assesses only a part of the scaffold, whereas MRI measures the entire scaffold. The high perfusion capacity and the homogenous vessel distribution within hDPSC- or hGF-seeded silk fibroin scaffolds suggest an improved and faster regenerative outcome. The present results also indicate that a relatively long pre-incubation period (i.e., 1 week) of these cells is necessary for obtaining the homogeneous and abundant vascularization of the entire scaffold that favors its integration into the host tissue. Indeed, our previous studies based exclusively on MRI measurements have shown that a shorter pre-incubation period (i.e., 1 day) of hDPSCs is not leading to such a uniform distribution of vessels within silk scaffolds (Kivrak Pfiffner et al., 2015). Comparison between hDPSCs and hGFs seeded scaffolds did not result in obvious differences concerning the attraction of vessels. Similarly to the hDPSCs, hGFs are derived from cranial neural crest cells that possess stem cell properties (Xu et al., 2013; Chiquet et al., 2015; Mitsiadis et al., 2015) and exhibit a higher regenerative potential when compared to fibroblasts of non-oral origin (Eslami et al., 2009) that may explain the similarities observed in vessel attraction into the scaffolds by hDPSCs and hGFs. Previous studies based on gene expression analysis have compared the angiogenic properties of hDPSCs and hGFs and suggested that hDPSCs possess a stronger angiogenic potential (Hilkens et al., 2014). However, studies realized on the CAM have shown that the number of vessels growing into hDPSC- and hGF-containing Matrigel™ droplets was not variable (Hilkens et al., 2014). Vascular ingrowths have been observed into cell-free silk scaffolds after subcutaneous transplantation in mice, but these structures were mainly localized on the scaffold surface (Unger et al., 2010; Ghanaati et al., 2011).

Taken together the present findings clearly demonstrate that hDPSCs and hGFs possess equal capabilities in attracting vessels within silk fibroin scaffolds. Furthermore, these results show that the prolonged pre-incubation period of these two cell populations before their implantation, favors the homogeneous distribution of vessels within silk fibroin scaffolds, a process that guarantees successful tissue regeneration.

## AUTHOR CONTRIBUTIONS

AW: experimental design, performance of experiments, writing of the manuscript, editing, discussing; JB: experimental design, MRI-measurements and analysis, writing of the manuscript, editing, discussing; CW: MRI-measurements and analysis, writing of the manuscript, editing, discussing; BS: experimental design, writing of the manuscript, editing, discussing; TM: experimental design, writing of the manuscript, editing, discussing.

## FUNDING

This work was supported by the Swiss National Foundation (SNSF) grant 31003A_135633 (TM, AW), by institutional funds from University of Zurich (TM) and by the Matching Funds from the University of Zurich (JB, CW).

## ACKNOWLEDGMENTS

The authors thank KD Dr. Michael Locher, Dr. Katharina Filo, and Dr. Philipp Sahrmann of the Clinic for Dental Medicine for providing teeth and gingival tissue, Dr. Yinghua Tian for the injection of the contrast agent. We are thankful to Prof. Ralph Müller, Prof. Sandra Hofmann, and Dr. Jolanda Baumgartner (Institute of Biomechanics, ETH Zurich) for manufacturing the silk scaffolds and Trudel Silk Inc. (Zurich, Switzerland) is highly acknowledged for providing silk fibroin. This work was supported by the Swiss National Foundation (SNSF) grant 31003A_135633 (TM, AW), by institutional funds from University of Zurich (TM), and by the Matching Funds from the University of Zurich (JB, CW). All authors contributed to the planning, writing, critical reading, and editing of the present manuscript. The authors confirm that there are no conflicts of interest associated with this work. Imaging was performed with equipment maintained by the Center for Microscopy and Image Analysis, University of Zurich.

## REFERENCES

Altman, G. H., Diaz, F., Jakuba, C., Calabro, T., Horan, R. L., Chen, J. S., et al. (2003). Silk-based biomaterials. *Biomaterials* 24, 401–416. doi: 10.1016/S0142-9612(02)00353-8

Bluteau, G., Luder, H. U., De Bari, C., and Mitsiadis, T. A. (2008). Stem cells for tooth engineering. *Eur. Cells Mater.* 16, 1–9. doi: 10.5167/uzh-6570

Chiquet, M., Katsaros, C., and Kletsas, D. (2015). Multiple functions of gingival and mucoperiosteal fibroblasts in oral wound healing and repair. *Periodontology 2000* 68, 21–40. doi: 10.1111/prd.12076

Eslami, A., Gallant-Behm, C. L., Hart, D. A., Wiebe, C., Honardoust, D., Gardner, H., et al. (2009). Expression of integrin avb6 and TGF-Beta in scarless vs scar-forming wound healing. *J. Histochem. Cytochem.* 57, 543–557. doi: 10.1369/jhc.2009.952572

Ghanaati, S., Unger, R. E., Webber, M. J., Barbeck, M., Orth, C., Kirkpatrick, J. A., et al. (2011). Scaffold vascularization *in vivo* driven by primary human osteoblasts in concert with host inflammatory cells. *Biomaterials* 32, 8150–8160. doi: 10.1016/j.biomaterials.2011.07.041

Giannicola, G., Ferrari, E., Citro, G., Sacchetti, B., Corsi, A., Riminucci, M., et al. (2010). Graft vascularization is a critical rate-limiting step in skeletal stem cell-mediated posterolateral spinal fusion. *J. Tissue Eng. Regen. Med.* 4, 273–283. doi: 10.1002/term.238

Giuliani, A., Manescu, A., Langer, M., Rustichelli, F., Desiderio, V., Paino, F., et al. (2013). Three graft vascularization is a critical rate-limiting step in skeletal stem cell-mediated posterolateral spinal fusion. *Stem Cells Transl. Med.* 2, 316–324. doi: 10.5966/sctm.2012-0136

Griffith, L. G., and Naughton, G. (2002). Tissue engineering-current challenges and expanding opportunities. *Science* 295, 1009–1014. doi: 10.1126/science.1069210

Gronthos, S., Mankani, M., Brahim, J., Robey, P. G., and Shi, S. (2000). Postnatal human dental pulp stem cells (DPSCs) *in vitro* and *in vivo*. *Proc. Natl. Acad. Sci. U.S.A.* 97, 13625–13630. doi: 10.1073/pnas.240309797

Hilkens, P., Fanton, Y., Martens, W., Gervois, P., Struys, T., Politis, I., et al. (2014). Pro-angiogenic impact of dental stem cells *in vitro* and *in vivo*. *Stem Cell Res.* 12, 778–790. doi: 10.1016/j.scr.2014.03.008

Hofmann, S., Hagenmüller, H., Koch, A. M., Müller, R., Vunjak-Novakovic, G., Kaplan, D. L., et al. (2007). Control of *in vitro* tissue-engineered bone-like structures using human mesenchymal stem cells and porous silk scaffolds. *Biomaterials* 28, 1152–1162. doi: 10.1016/j.biomaterials.2006.10.019

Huang, G. T., Gronthos, S., and Shi, S. (2009). Mesenchymal stem cells derived from dental tissues vs. those from other sources: their biology and role in regenerative medicine. *J. Dent. Res.* 88, 792–806. doi: 10.1177/0022034509340867

Kivrak Pfiffner, F., Waschkies, C., Tian, Y., Woloszyk, A., Calcagni, M., Giovanoli, P., et al. (2015). A new *in vivo* magnetic resonance imaging method to noninvasively monitor and quantify the perfusion capacity of three-dimensional biomaterials grown on the chorioallantoic membrane of chick embryos. *Tissue Eng. Part C Methods* 2, 339–346. doi: 10.1089/ten.TEC.2014.0212

Koob, S., Torio-Padron, N., Stark, G. B., Hannig, C., Stankovic, Z., and Finkenzeller, G. (2011). Bone formation and neovascularization mediated by mesenchymal stem cells and endothelial cells in critical-sized calvarial defects. *Tissue Eng. A* 17, 311–321. doi: 10.1089/ten.tea.2010.0338

Kundu, B., Rajkhowa, R., Kundu, S. C., and Wang, X. (2013). Silk fibroin biomaterials for tissue regenerations. *Adv. Drug Deliv. Rev.* 65, 457–470. doi: 10.1016/j.addr.2012.09.043.

Lee, I.-K., Lee, M.-J., and Jang, H. S. (2013). The interrelationship between human gingival fibroblast differentiation and cultivating time. *Tissue Eng. Regener. Med.* 10, 60–64. doi: 10.1007/s13770-013-0371-y

Lloyd-Griffith, C., McFadden, T. M., Duffy, G. P., Unger, R. E., Kirkpatrick, C. J., and O'Brien, F. J. (2015). The pre-vascularisation of a collagen-chondroitin sulphate scaffold using human amniotic fluid-derived stem cells to enhance and stabilise endothelial cell-mediated vessel formation. *Acta Biomater.* 26, 263–273. doi: 10.1016/j.actbio.2015.08.030.

Mitsiadis, T. A., Orsini, G., and Jimenez-Rojo, L. (2015). Stem cell-based approaches in dentistry. *Eur. Cells Mater.* 30, 248–257.

Nazarov, R., Jin, H. J., and Kaplan, D. L. (2004). Porous 3-D scaffolds from regenerated silk fibroin. *Biomacromolecules* 5, 718–726. doi: 10.1021/bm034327e

Novosel, E. C., Kleinhans, C., and Kluger, P. J. (2011). Vascularization is the key challenge in tissue engineering. *Adv. Drug Deliv. Rev.* 63, 300–311. doi: 10.1016/j.addr.2011.03.004

Plock, J. A., Schnider, J. T., Zhang, W., Schweizer, R., Tsuji, W., Kostereva, N., et al. (2015). Adipose- and bone marrow–derived mesenchymal stem cells prolong graft survival in vascularized composite allotransplantation. *Transplantation* 99, 1765–1773. doi: 10.1097/TP.0000000000000731

d'Aquino, R., De Rosa, A., Laino, G., Caruso, F., Guida, L., Rullo, R., et al. (2009). Human dental pulp stem cells: from biology to clinical applications. *J. Exp. Zool. B Mol. Dev. Evol.* 312, 408–415. doi: 10.1002/jez.b.21263.

d'Aquino, R., Graziano, A., Sampaolesi, M., Laino, G., Pirozzi, G., De Rosa, A., et al. (2007). Human postnatal dental pulp cells co-differentiate into osteoblasts and endotheliocytes: a pivotal synergy leading to adult bone tissue formation. *Cell Death Differ.* 14, 1162–1171. doi: 10.1038/sj.cdd.4402121

Shi, S., Robey, P. G., and Gronthos, S. (2001). Comparison of human dental pulp and bone marrow stromal stem cells by cDNA microarray analysis. *Bone* 29, 532–539. doi: 10.1016/S8756-3282(01)00612-3

Sofia, S., McCarthy, M. B., Gronowicz, G., and Kaplan, D. L. (2001). Functionalized silk-based biomaterials for bone formation. *J. Biomed. Mater. Res.* 54, 139–148.doi: 10.1002/1097-4636(200101)54:1<139::AID-JBM17>3.0.CO;2-7

Stock, U. A., and Vacanti, J. P. (2001). Tissue engineering: current state and prospects. *Annu. Rev. Med.* 52, 443–451. doi: 10.1146/annurev.med.52.1.443

Tirino, V., Paino, F., De Rosa, A., and Papaccio, G. (2012). Identification, isolation, characterization, and banking of human dental pulp stem cells. *Methods Mol. Biol.* 879, 443–463. doi: 10.1007/978-1-61779-815-3_26

Unger, R. E., Ghanaati, S., Orth, C., Sartoris, A., Barbeck, M., Halstenberg, S., et al. (2010). The rapid anastomosis between prevascularized networks on silk fibroin scaffolds generated *in vitro* with cocultures of human microvascular endothelial and osteoblast cells and the host vasculature. *Biomaterials* 31, 6959–6967. doi: 10.1016/j.biomaterials.2010.05.057

Woloszyk, A., Holsten Dircksen, S., Bostanci, N., Müller, R., Hofmann, S., and Mitsiadis, T. A. (2014). Influence of the mechanical environment on the engineering of mineralised tissues using human dental pulp stem cells and silk fibroin scaffolds. *PLoS ONE* 9:e111010. doi: 10.1371/journal.pone.0111010

Xu, X., Chen, C., Akiyama, K., Chai, Y., Le, A. D., Wang, Z., et al. (2013). Gingivae contain neural-crest- and mesoderm-derived mesenchymal stem cells. *J. Dent. Res.* 92, 825–832. doi: 10.1177/0022034513497961

Zhang, W., Walboomers, X. F., Shi, S., Fan, M., and Jansen, J. A. (2006). Multilineage differentiation potential of stem cells derived from human dental pulp after cryopreservation. *Tissue Eng.* 12, 2813–2823. doi: 10.1089/ten.2006.12.2813

# 6

# Three-Dimensional Imaging of the Developing Vasculature within Stem Cell-Seeded Scaffolds Cultured *in ovo*

**Edited by:**
Sachiko Iseki,
Tokyo Medical and Dental University,
Japan

***Correspondence:**
Thimios A. Mitsiadis
thimios.mitsiadis@zzm.uzh.ch

*Anna Woloszyk*[1], *Davide Liccardo*[2] *and Thimios A. Mitsiadis*[1*]

[1] *Orofacial Development and Regeneration, Centre for Dental Medicine, Institute of Oral Biology, University of Zurich, Zurich, Switzerland,* [2] *Section of Biotechnology and Medical Histology and Embryology, Department of Experimental Medicine, Second University of Naples, Naples, Italy*

Successful tissue engineering requires functional vascularization of the three-dimensional constructs with the aim to serve as implants for tissue replacement and regeneration. The survival of the implant is only possible if the supply of oxygen and nutrients by developing capillaries from the host is established. The chorioallantoic membrane (CAM) assay is a valuable tool to study the ingrowth and distribution of vessels into scaffolds composed by appropriate biomaterials and stem cell populations that are used in cell-based regenerative approaches. The developing vasculature of chicken embryos within cell-seeded scaffolds can be visualized with microcomputed tomography after intravenous injection of MicroFil®, which is a radiopaque contrast agent. Here, we provide a step-by-step protocol for the seeding of stem cells into silk fibroin scaffolds, the CAM culture conditions, the procedure of MicroFil® perfusion, and finally the microcomputed tomography scanning. Three-dimensional imaging of the vascularized tissue engineered constructs provides an important analytical tool for studying the potential of cell seeded scaffolds to attract vessels and form vascular networks, as well as for analyzing the number, density, length, branching, and diameter of vessels. This *in ovo* method can greatly help to screen implants that will be used for tissue regeneration purposes before their *in vivo* testing, thereby reducing the amount of animals needed for pre-clinical studies.

**Keywords: chorioallantoic membrane (CAM), vascularization, stem cells, biomaterials, 3D imaging, MicroFil®, microcomputed tomography, regenerative medicine**

## INTRODUCTION

The formation of new networks of blood vessels (i.e., angiogenesis) is essential in embryonic development, tissue homeostasis, pathology, and regeneration. Hematopoietic cells circulating within the vasculature supply the surrounding tissues with oxygen and nutrients, transport hormones, remove waste products, and $CO_2$, and protect the body from infections (Carmeliet and Jain, 2011). Successful engineering of tissue substitutes and transplantable organs depends on their rapid and adequate angiogenesis, since the appropriate supply of oxygen and nutrients is crucial for their long-term survival (Mitsiadis and Harada, 2015; Mitsiadis et al., 2015). A dense network of capillaries is formed in most tissues of the body that regulates the diffusion limit of oxygen (Carmeliet and Jain, 2000; Novosel et al., 2011). Spontaneous vascular ingrowth from the host tissue to the transplanted devices (e.g., empty biodegradable implants) is very slow and limited to several tenths of micrometers per day (Rouwkema et al., 2008). Therefore, the improvement and acceleration of implant vascularization remains a key challenge in regenerative medicine.

Classical *in vivo* angiogenesis assays rely on small (e.g., mice, rats) and large (e.g., sheep, goats) animal models, where engineered constructs are most commonly implanted subcutaneously at their dorsal part (Staton et al., 2009; Jungraithmayr et al., 2013; Wang et al., 2015). However, these surgical procedures are time-consuming and often associated with high costs and repetitive animal sacrifice. The chorioallantoic membrane (CAM) is highly vascularized and serves as a transient gas exchange surface during the incubation period, similar to the lung (Romanoff, 1960). Originally, the CAM assay was used in order to study the developmental potential of embryonic tissue grafts (Rücker et al., 2006). As chicken embryos become immunocompetent only by day 18 of their development (Janković et al., 1975), various biological processes where vascularization plays a role can be studied without inducing an immune response, including insufficient vascularization (e.g., ischemic disorders) or excessive vessel formation (e.g., cancer), with the goal to either enhance or decrease vessel growth, respectively (Ribatti, 2014).

To visualize the three-dimensional (3D) development of the vasculature within implants cultured on the CAM, perfusion of the chicken embryos was performed with the radiopaque contrast agent MicroFil® followed by microcomputed tomography (microCT) of the implants. We demonstrate that this technique, which is commonly used in *in vivo* experiments performed in rodents (Bolland et al., 2008; Schmidt et al., 2009; Stoppato et al., 2013), can also successfully be applied in the CAM assay.

## MATERIALS AND METHODS

### Seeding of Human Dental Pulp Stem Cells

a. Defrost cryopreserved human dental pulp stem cells and culture in Dulbecco's Modified Eagle Medium: Nutrient Mixture F-12 (DMEM/F12) + 10% fetal bovine serum + 1% penicillin/streptamycin + 0.5 μg/mL fungizone in a humidified incubator at 37°C and 5% $CO_2$. Change the medium every 3–4 days.
b. At 80–90% confluency, trypsinize the cells, use a 70 μm strainer to obtain a single-cell suspension, centrifuge (1500 rpm, 5 min, RT), and resuspend the cell pellet at a concentration of $1 \times 10^6$ cells/50 μL.
c. Place the sterile cylindrical scaffold (silk fibroin, 5 mm diameter, 3 mm height) on a sterile filter paper to absorb any residual liquid and move the scaffold into the well of a 96-well-plate.
d. Seed the scaffold by pipetting 50 μL of the cell suspension on top of the scaffold, turn the scaffold, take up the cell suspension from the bottom of the well, and release it again on top of the scaffold.
e. For cell attachment, place the cell-seeded scaffolds in a humidified incubator for 1 h at 37°C and 5% $CO_2$. Wash the scaffold before placing it in a clean well of a 24-well-plate and adding 1 mL of medium. Culture for desired period of time and change medium every 3–4 days.

The procedure for anonymized cell collection was approved by the Kantonale Ethikkommission of Zurich and performed with written patients' consent.

### Preparation of the Chicken Eggs for the CAM Assay and Placing of the Cell-Seeded Samples

a. Pre-incubate fertilized Lohman white LSL (Lohman Selected Leghorn) chicken eggs in an egg incubator for 3 days at 38°C at a rotation speed of 360°/4 h.
b. On embryonic day 3 (ED 3), stop the rotation in the morning and let the eggs rest in this position for 3 h to ensure that the embryo is on the top.
c. Mark the top of the egg with a pencil and carefully wipe the egg-shell with 70% ethanol without turning it.
d. Inside a clean bench, place the egg in a 60 mm Petri dish on top of a piece of tape to stabilize the egg.
e. Make a small hole in the shell with the tip of sterile pointy scissors and remove 4 mL of albumen using a syringe and a needle to lower the developing embryo.
f. Put Scotch™ tape on the area where you want to make the window.
g. Make another small hole, insert the scissors carefully and start cutting an oval hole while turning the egg with the other hand.
h. Remove the shell and cover the opening with a second 60 mm Petri dish, which needs to be fixed to the bottom lid with tape, and incubate in a humidified incubator at 37°C and 0% $CO_2$.
i. On ED 7, the cell-seeded scaffolds can be placed on the vascularized CAM. Remove the Petri dish lid, place a silicone ring (taken from sterile cryovials) on the CAM to ensure a flat surface, and position the sample in the middle of this ring.
j. Incubate for 7 days until ED 14 in a humidified incubator at 37°C and 0% $CO_2$.

### Microfil® Perfusion and Microct Imaging

a. On ED 14, the chicken embryos are perfused with a mix of the MicroFil® components. Dilute the silicone rubber injection compound (yellow) 10-fold in MV-Diluent and add 10% (by weight) MV-Curing Agent right before use. Working time is at least 20 min and starts with the addition of curing agent.
b. Fill the MicroFil® mix into a 5 mL syringe and attach a three-way valve (Discofix® C) with a 10 cm tube for more flexibility between the 30G ½" needle and the syringe.
c. Using a stereoscope, fix a branch of the vitelline vasculature matching the diameter of the needle with blunt end tweezers and carefully insert the needle into the vessel. Apply a small drop of superglue where the needle enters the vasculature (**Figure 1**).
d. Inject the MicroFil® mix carefully into the vasculature until the pressure increases.

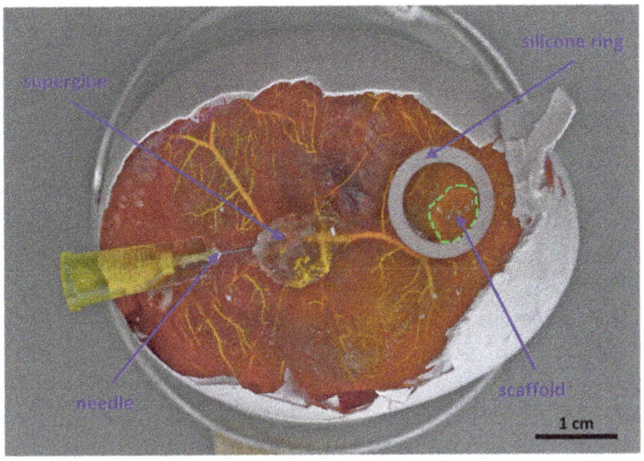


**FIGURE 1 | Setup for the perfusion of the chorioallantoic membrane vasculature.** The scaffold is placed in the middle of a silicone ring and cultured for 7 days *in ovo*. For proper perfusion a 30G ½" needle is fixed with a drop of superglue before MicroFil® (yellow) injection.

e. If filling of the vasculature is not sufficient, inject MicroFil® a second time into a non-perfused vessel. Remove the tube from the needle, which remains in the CAM, and attach a fresh needle to the tube. Repeat steps **c** and **d.**
f. Place the perfused chicken embryo overnight at 4°C for complete curing of the MicroFil®.
g. On the next day, remove the perfused scaffold samples from the CAM using scissors, wash in PBS, fix in 4% paraformaldehyde, wash in PBS, and place in 70% ethanol until microCT imaging.
h. Perform microCT scanning at an isotropic resolution of 20 μm, an energy level of 70 kVp, an intensity of 114 μA, and 300 ms integration time.

According to Swiss animal care guidelines experiments performed in chicken embryos until ED 14 do not need ethical approval (TSchV, Art. 112).

## RESULTS

We have used the CAM assay to study the vascularization of a 3D biomaterial when placed in a highly vascularized environment. The perfusion of the vascular system was performed without pre-perfusion with phosphate buffered saline, as the blood was forced out by the injected MicroFil®. The initial perfusion efficiency with MicroFil® diluted according to the manufacturer's recommendation was improved by using a higher dilution of the silicone rubber injection compound, which required an increased amount of the MV-Curing Agent of 10% instead of 5% (by weight). If the perfusion was not complete after one injection, a second injection site was chosen to fill non-perfused areas (**Figures 2A,B**). Immunohistological stainings can still be performed on sections of paraffin-embedded samples after perfusion and microCT analysis (**Figure 2C**).

The microCT scan showed the MicroFil® perfused 3D vascular structure growing into the scaffold (red area in

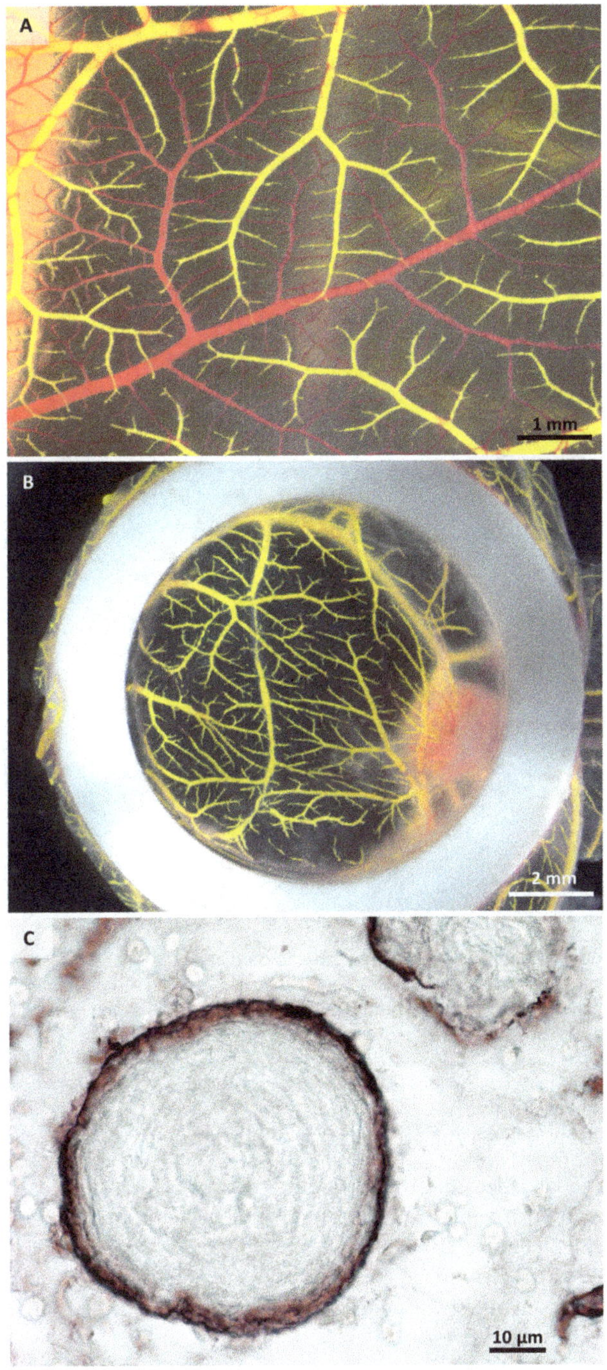


**FIGURE 2 | Macroscopical and microscopical view of perfused samples. (A)** Perfused (yellow) and non-perfused (red) vessels after one injection showing incomplete perfusion. **(B)** Exemplary sample after two injections of MicroFil®. **(C)** Histological section of a perfused sample showing vessels (brown) containing MicroFil®.

**Figure 2B**) from the bottom and from the sides within 7 days of *in ovo* culture. While the macroscopical image of the same sample *in ovo* (**Figure 3A**) provides only the information about the vascularization visible on the surface of the CAM, the microCT

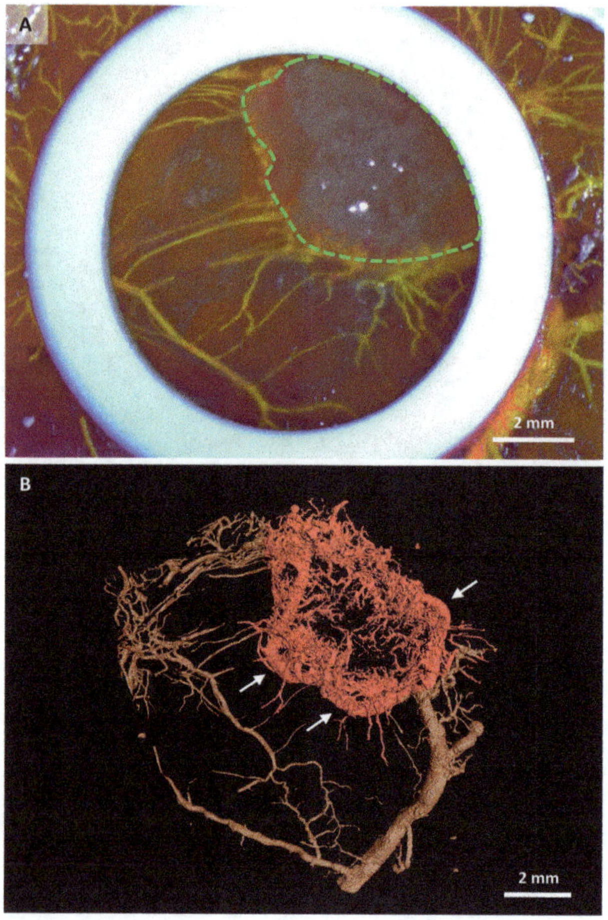


**FIGURE 3 | Stem cell-seeded scaffolds perfused with MicroFil® after their *in ovo* culture. (A)** Macroscopic view of a scaffold (green dashed line) immediately after perfusion with yellow MicroFil®. The silicone ring is seen in white, vasculature in yellow. **(B)** Microcomputed tomography image of the vascular cast within the scaffold (red color). Vasculature outside the scaffold area is marked in brown. New capillaries are sprouting from one large vessel that encircles the scaffold (white arrows).

image visualizes the whole vascular network. Interestingly, new capillaries are sprouting from one large vessel that encircles the scaffold, (**Figure 3B**, white arrows). The generated microCT data can be further used for complete morphometric characterization of the vascular network, including the number, length, branching, and diameter of vessels.

## DISCUSSION

The generation of vascularized tissues and organs remains one of the key challenges in regenerative medicine (Novosel et al., 2011; Mitsiadis et al., 2012; Dew et al., 2015). Visualization of angiogenesis within implanted engineered devices aiming at tissue replacement and/or regeneration is pivotal for predicting and understanding the outcome of new regenerative approaches before their application in clinics.

Several techniques have been extensively used to study the vascular architecture of the whole body, as well as the microvasculature of specific organs and tissues in both health and disease. The development of new visualization methods using microcomputed tomography (microCT) improved our knowledge on specific tissue anatomy, physiology, and pathology tremendously. Further, developments using perfusion of tissues and organs before microCT scanning allowed additional analyses at the histological level and generated a plethora of volumetric and quantitative data (Garcia-Sanz et al., 1998). Therefore, the combination of vascular perfusion with microCT imaging and analysis has been applied in many fields, including embryonic vascular development (Anderson-Berry et al., 2005), cancer research (Xuan et al., 2007), cardiac disease models (Sangaralingham et al., 2012), and tissue engineering (Bolland et al., 2008; Stoppato et al., 2013). For example, the combination of MicroFil® perfusion with microCT imaging has been used to study angiogenesis in tissue engineered constructs implanted subcutaneously into immunosuppressed mice. Both natural allografts and osteosynthetic [poly (D,L)-lactic acid; PDLLA] grafts seeded with human bone marrow stromal cells (BMSCs) have been used for this study. The presence of BMSCs was able to increase the number of vessels within the implants (Bolland et al., 2008). Similarly, MicroFil® perfusion and microCT scanning have been performed in VEGF-treated porous polyurethane scaffolds implanted subcutaneously into rats (Schmidt et al., 2009). A more recent study using MicroFil® perfusion and microCT scanning has demonstrated that silk fibroin fibers combined with a PDLLA salt-leached sponge promoted vascularization when implanted subcutaneously into rats (Stoppato et al., 2013).

However, all these previous studies are based on rodents and therefore necessitate extensive animal care-taking, ethical approvals, as well as surgical skills and equipment. Moreover, a minimum of 10 days incubation time is needed in order to analyze implant vasculature. In contrast, the CAM assay is a simple, cost-effective, and highly reproducible method, which does not require ethical approval when performing experiments in chicken embryos until embryonic day 14 (Swiss animal care guidelines, TSchV, Art. 112). Even though the incubation time on the CAM is limited to a period of 7 days, it constitutes an excellent screening method to study the early phase of angiogenesis within implanted scaffolds. Following the "3Rs" principles of replacement, refinement, and reduction of animal use in research, the CAM assay combined with MicroFil® perfusion and microCT analysis as described in this protocol provides a valuable intermediate platform for initial assessments prior to pre-clinical studies in mammals.

This technique could be applied for the direct comparison of scaffolds (ceramics, synthetic polymers, and natural polymers) seeded with stem cell populations of different origins [e.g., adipose-derived stem cells (ASCs), bone marrow stem cells (BMSCs), DPSCs, periodontal ligament stem cells]. For example, it has been shown that BMSCs possess angiogenic potential (Oswald et al., 2004), but little is known about their capability to attract vessels in engineered structures. In contrast, ASCs have been demonstrated to promote the neovascularization when seeded in different scaffolds (De Francesco et al., 2009; Chan et al., 2016; Guo et al., 2016). In conclusion, the present method can constitute a valuable tool for studying in detail cell-mediated vascularization efficiency.

## AUTHOR CONTRIBUTIONS

AW: experimental design, performance of experiments, writing of the manuscript, editing, discussing. DL: experimental design, writing of the manuscript, editing, discussing. TM: experimental design, writing of the manuscript, editing, discussing.

## FUNDING

This work was supported by the Swiss National Foundation (SNSF) grant 31003A_135633 (TM, AW), by institutional funds from University of Zurich (TM) and by funds from the Second University of Naples (SUN;DL).

## ACKNOWLEDGMENTS

The authors thank Dr. Bernd Stadlinger and Dr. Philipp Sahrmann of the Clinic for Dental Medicine for providing teeth for dental pulp stem cell extraction. Furthermore, Trudel Silk Inc. (Zurich, Switzerland) is highly acknowledged for providing silk fibroin and the Institute of Biomechanics, ETH for manufacturing the scaffolds. Further, we thank Dr. Johanna Buschmann for technical advice and valuable discussions.

## REFERENCES

Anderson-Berry, A., O'Brien, E. A., Bleyl, S. B., Lawson, A., Gundersen, N., Ryssman, D., et al. (2005). Vasculogenesis drives pulmonary vascular growth in the developing chick embryo. *Dev. Dyn.* 233, 145–153. doi: 10.1002/dvdy.20296

Bolland, B. J., Kanczler, J. M., Dunlop, D. G., and Oreffo, R. O. (2008). Development of *in vivo* μCT evaluation of neovascularisation in tissue engineered bone Constructs. *Biomaterials* 43, 195–202. doi: 10.1016/j.bone.2008.02.013

Carmeliet, P., and Jain, R. K. (2000). Angiogenesis in cancer and other diseases. *Nature* 407, 249–257. doi: 10.1038/35025220

Carmeliet, P., and Jain, R. K. (2011). Molecular mechanisms and clinical applications of angiogenesis. *Nature* 473, 298–307. doi: 10.1038/nature10144

Chan, E. C., Kuo, S. M., Kong, A. M., Morrison, W. A., Dusting, G. J., Mitchell, G. M., et al. (2016). Three dimensional collagen scaffold promotes intrinsic vascularisation for tissue engineering applications. *PLoS ONE* 11:e0149799. doi: 10.1371/journal.pone.0149799

De Francesco, F., Tirino, V., Desiderio, V., Ferraro, G., D'Andrea, F., Giuliano, M., et al. (2009). Human CD34+/CD90+ ASCs are capable of growing as sphere clusters, producing high levels of vegf and forming capillaries. *PLoS ONE* 4:e6537. doi: 10.1371/journal.pone.0006537

Dew, L., MacNeil, S., and Chong, C. K. (2015). Vascularization strategies for tissue engineers. *Regen. Med.* 10, 211–224. doi: 10.2217/rme.14.83

Garcia-Sanz, A., Rodriguez-Barbero, A., Bentley, M. D., Ritman, E. L., and Romero, J. C. (1998). Three-dimensional microcomputed tomography of renal vasculature in rats. *Hypertension* 31, 440–444. doi: 10.1161/01.HYP.31.1.440

Guo, L. Z., Kim, T. H., Han, S., and Kim, S. W. (2016). Angio-vasculogenic properties of endothelial-induced mesenchymal stem cells derived from human adipose tissue. *Circ. J.* 80, 998–1007. doi: 10.1253/circj.CJ-15-1169

Janković, B. D., Isaković, K., Lukić, M. L., Vujanović, N. L., Petrović, S., and Marković, B. M. (1975). Immunological capacity of the chicken embryo. I. Relationship between the maturation of lymphoid tissues and the occurrence of cell-mediated immunity in the developing chicken embryo. *Immunology* 29, 497–508.

Jungraithmayr, W., Laube, I., Hild, N., Stark, W. J., Mihic-Probst, D., Weder, W., et al. (2013). Bioactive nanocomposite for chest-wall replacement: cellular response in a murine model. *J. Biomater. Appl.* 29, 36–45. doi: 10.1177/0885328213513621

Mitsiadis, T. A., and Harada, H. (2015). Regenerated teeth: the future of tooth replacement. An update. *Regen. Med.* 10, 5–8. doi: 10.2217/rme.14.78

Mitsiadis, T. A., Orsini, G., and Jimenez-Rojo, L. (2015). Stem cell based approaches in dentistry. *Eur. Cell and Mat.* 30, 248–257.

Mitsiadis, T. A., Woloszyk, A., and Jiménez-Rojo, L. (2012). Nanodentistry: combining nanostructured materials and stem cells for dental tissue regeneration. *Nanomedicine (Lond).* 7, 1743–1753. doi: 10.2217/nnm.12.146

Novosel, E. C., Kleinhans, C., and Kluger, P. J. (2011). Vascularization is the key challenge in tissue engineering. *Adv. Drug Deliv. Rev.* 63, 300–311. doi: 10.1016/j.addr.2011.03.004

Oswald, J., Boxberger, S., Jørgensen, B., Feldmann, S., Ehninger, G., Bornhäuser, M., et al. (2004). Mesenchymal stem cells can be differentiated into endothelial cells *in vitro*. *Stem Cells* 22, 377–384. doi: 10.1634/stemcells.22-3-377

Ribatti, D. (2014). The chick embryo chorioallantoic membrane as a model for tumor biology. *Exp. Cell Res.* 328, 314–324. doi: 10.1016/j.yexcr.2014.06.010

Rouwkema, J., Rivron, N. C., and van Blitterswijk, C. A. (2008). Vascularization in tissue engineering. *Trends Biotechnol.* 26, 434–441. doi: 10.1016/j.tibtech.2008.04.009

Rücker, M., Laschke, M. W., Junker, D., Carvalho, C., Schramm, A., Mülhaupt, R., et al. (2006). Angiogenic and inflammatory response to biodegradable scaffolds in dorsal skinfold chambers of mice. *Biomaterials* 27, 5027–5038. doi: 10.1016/j.biomaterials.2006.05.033

Sangaralingham, S. J., Ritman, E. L., McKie, P. M., Ichiki, T., Lerman, A., Scott, C. G., et al. (2012). Cardiac micro-computed tomography imaging of the aging coronary vasculature. *Circ. Cardiovasc. Imaging* 5, 518–524. doi: 10.1523/JNEUROSCI.3593-07.2007.Omega-3

Schmidt, C., Bezuidenhout, D., Beck, M., Van der Merwe, E., Zilla, P., and Davies, N. (2009). Rapid three-dimensional quantification of VEGF-induced scaffold neovascularisation by microcomputed tomography. *Biomaterials* 30, 5959–5968. doi: 10.1016/j.biomaterials.2009.07.044

Staton, C. A., Reed, M. W., and Brown, N. J. (2009). A critical analysis of current *in vitro* and *in vivo* angiogenesis assays. *Int. J. Exp. Pathol.* 90, 195–221. doi: 10.1111/j.1365-2613.2008.00633.x

Stoppato, M., Stevens, H. Y., Carletti, E., Migliaresi, C., Motta, A., and Guldberg, R. E. (2013). Effects of Silk Fibroin Fiber Incorporation on Mechanical Properties, Endothelial Cell Colonization and Vascularization of PDLLA Scaffolds. *Biomaterials* 34, 4573–4581. doi: 10.1016/j.biomaterials.2013.02.009

Wang, K., Yu, L. Y., Jiang, L. Y., Wang, H. B., Wang, C. Y., and Luo, Y. (2015). The paracrine effects of adipose-derived stem cells on neovascularization and biocompatibility of a macroencapsulation device. *Acta Biomater.* 15, 65–76. doi: 10.1016/j.actbio.2014.12.025

Xuan, J. W., Bygrave, M., Jiang, H., Valiyeva, F., Dunmore-Buyze, J., and Holdsworth, D. W. (2007). Functional neoangiogenesis imaging of genetically engineered mouse prostate cancer using three-dimensional power doppler ultrasound. *Cancer Res.* 67, 2830–2839. doi: 10.1158/0008-5472.CAN-06-3944

7

# The Nervous System Orchestrates and Integrates Craniofacial Development

**Edited by:**
Thimios Mitsiadis,
University of Zurich, Switzerland

***Correspondence:**
Igor Adameyko
igor.adameyko@ki.se;
Kaj Fried
kaj.fried@ki.se

*Igor Adameyko [1,2]* and Kaj Fried [3]**

[1] Department of Physiology and Pharmacology, Karolinska Institutet, Stockholm, Sweden, [2] Department of Molecular Neurosciences, Center of Brain Research, Medical University of Vienna, Vienna, Austria, [3] Department of Neuroscience, Karolinska Institutet, Stockholm, Sweden

Development of a head is a dazzlingly complex process: a number of distinct cellular sources including cranial ecto- and endoderm, mesoderm and neural crest contribute to facial and other structures. In the head, an extremely fine-tuned developmental coordination of CNS, peripheral neural components, sensory organs and a musculo-skeletal apparatus occurs, which provides protection and functional integration. The face can to a large extent be considered as an assembly of sensory systems encased and functionally fused with appendages represented by jaws. Here we review how the developing brain, neurogenic placodes and peripheral nerves influence the morphogenesis of surrounding tissues as a part of various general integrative processes in the head. The mechanisms of this impact, as we understand it now, span from the targeted release of the morphogens necessary for shaping to providing a niche for cellular sources required in later development. In this review we also discuss the most recent findings and ideas related to how peripheral nerves and nerve-associated cells contribute to craniofacial development, including teeth, during the post- neural crest period and potentially in regeneration.

**Keywords: nervous system, craniofacial, development, glia, stem cell, tooth**

## INTEGRATION OF EARLY NEURAL DERIVATIVES WITH OTHER CELLULAR SOURCES DURING CRANIOFACIAL DEVELOPMENT

The involvement of neural structures in facial development begins as soon as Neural Crest cells (NCCs) emigrate from the dorsal neural tube (Simões-Costa and Bronner, 2015). The neural crest and its derivatives are keys to the understanding of the evolution and morphogenesis of the face (Green et al., 2015; see **Figure 1**). Thus, this transient cellular source contributes cartilage and bone, adipose tissue, tendons and fasciae, dermal fibroblasts and smooth muscles, pericytes, pigmentation, sensory neurons, peripheral glial cells and many more cell types to the developing head (Dupin et al., 2006). The vertebrate face is sculpted in a series of complex morphogenetic events. These involve neural crest coordination with other cellular sources such as mesoderm, endoderm and other ectodermal components (Couly et al., 2002; Rinon et al., 2007; Grenier et al., 2009; Marcucio et al., 2011; Van Ho et al., 2011).

More than 30 years ago, Gans and Northcutt proposed the hypothesis of "a new head." This suggested that the evolutionary success of vertebrates is attributed to the development of their facial compartment. The face has emerged with various separated sensory organs due to a coordinated

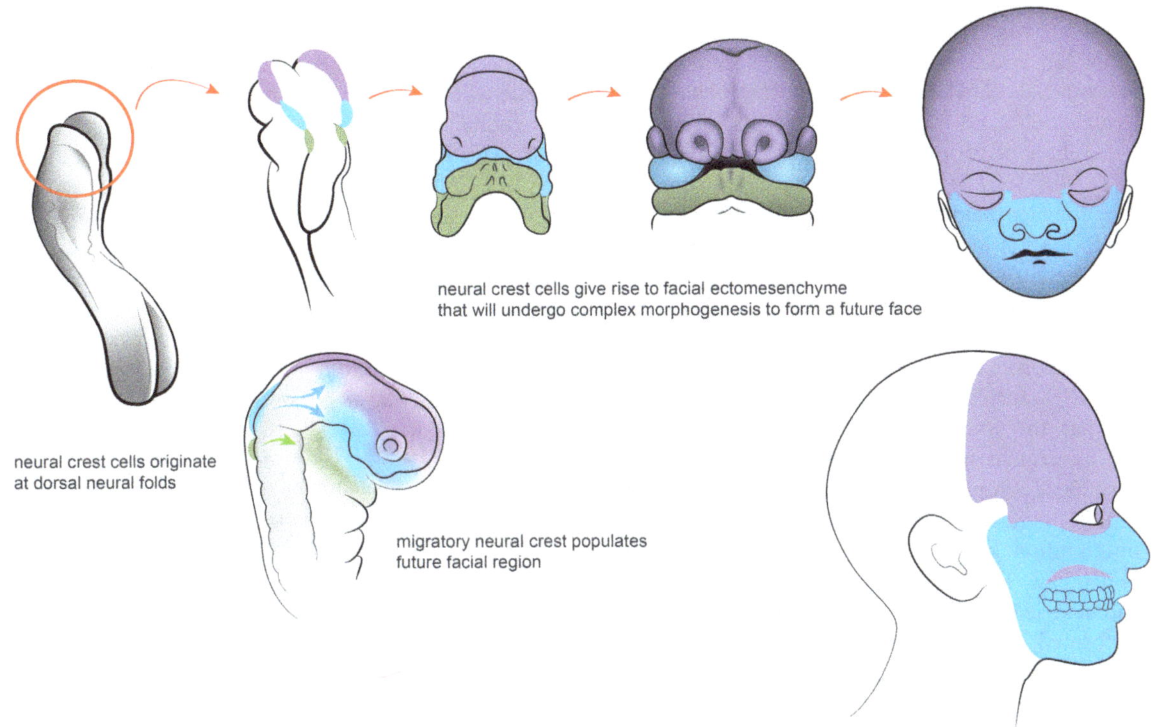


**FIGURE 1 | Neural crest cells migrate from dorsal neuroectoderm and organize the facial development in vertebrate embryos.** Colors highlights regions of the developing and adult face that correspond to different neural crest populations along the posterior axis.

activity of the neural crest, together with other neural and skeletal elements (Gans and Northcutt, 1983). Historically, views and theories have held that the vertebrate head has its evolutionary origins in a segmented structure. This inferred that the head has evolved from of a series of complete head segments (metameres), such as those seen in lower species. However, there is no obvious scientific support for this view (Noden and Trainor, 2005). Instead, segmentation in the vertebrate head has been interpreted as the division of one or more embryonic tissues, such as the paraxial mesoderm, neurectoderm or endoderm into a series of iterative structures in the anterior to posterior axis (Noden and Trainor, 2005; Northcutt, 2008). During early embryogenesis, NCCs arise at the margins between the ectoderm (the future skin) and the neural plate. The formation of the neural crest is governed by a regulatory gene network, that will endow the NCCs with their typical features. This includes multipotency and migratory capabilities (Sauka-Spengler et al., 2007). After neurulation, NCCs from the roof plate of the neural tube undergo an epithelial to mesenchymal transition. They delaminate from the neuroepithelium and migrate outwards to populate the pharyngeal arches and other locations corresponding to the future face. NCCs also invade a number of specific sites in other parts of developing body.

Eventually, NCCs differentiate into a wide range of structures and tissues along the anterior-posterior axis of the embryo (Trainor, 2005; Gitton et al., 2010; Minoux and Rijli, 2010). Those NCCs that enter the future frontonasal prominence as well as the first and second pharyngeal arches will initiate, organize and coordinate craniofacial development. Having arrived at their destinations, the NCCs that are responsible for craniofacial morphogenesis are regulated by complex actions of the genetic machinery that will determine tissue patterning and cell differentiation. This involves signaling by e.g., FGF, Shh, Wnt, BMP, PDGF, retinoic acid (RA), endothelin and other molecules (Kurihara et al., 1995; Clouthier et al., 2003; Macatee et al., 2003; Abzhanov and Tabin, 2004; Jiang et al., 2006; Abe et al., 2008). NCCs will mainly form the anterior compartment of the head, while the posterior part, including the cranial roof is created largely by mesoderm (see Noden and Trainor, 2005).The relative size and shape of the anterior neural tube probably plays an important role in facial shaping. Thus, these parameters, together with local physical forces, may influence the amount and spatial distribution of emigrating NCCs during early development. The logics of setting down the boundary between neural crest and mesoderm-derived parts may also be important for differences in bone geometry and facial modeling. Furthermore, it might be relevant for the evolutionary plasticity of a head in multiple vertebrate species (Gross and Hanken, 2008).

Coordination and integration are key features during both early and late head and neck development. For example, induction of tracheal cartilages as well as some skeletal components of upper face and jaws depends on the activity of the endoderm and Wnt signaling pathways (Couly et al., 2002; Snowball et al., 2015). Dental placodal epithelia influence the competence of underlying mesenchyme while producing teeth and vice versa (Thesleff, 2003).

One of the most striking concerted event during facial development is when the Frontonasal Ectodermal Zone (FEZ; Hu et al., 2003; Hu and Marcucio, 2009a), a specific region in the anterior facial ectoderm, regulates the behavior of ectomesenchymal cells and skeletogenesis. This occurs via regionalized secretion of various morphogens, including Shh, Fgf8, and BMPs. FEZ may be considered as a facial organizer, as evidenced by the fact that transplantation or rotation of FEZ causes ectopic formation of skeletal elements or altered dorso-ventral axis in the forming face, respectively; (see Marcucio et al., 2011) for in-depth discussion. On the other hand, the competence to create a particular, species-specific facial morphology in response to epithelial signals is attributed to the neural crest. Transplantation experiments have clearly demonstrated that the final facial shape in a host embryo is determined by cranial neural crest of the donor (Helms and Schneider, 2003; Schneider and Helms, 2003). In general, numerous studies converge on the possibility that NCCs, after their immigration from the anterior dorsal neural tube, coordinate with FEZ formation to produce the outline of the face (Marcucio et al., 2011). Not only skeletal elements become transformed according to the instructive cues and typical morphology of the donor neural crest. The facial muscles also change accordingly, although the skeletal muscles in the developing face are derived from the mesoderm of the host (Tokita and Schneider, 2009). Hence, NCCs pattern developing head muscles (Rinon et al., 2007).

The instructive competence of the neural crest is further illustrated by experiments where mouse neural crest was transplanted into chick embryos, which led to the formation of dental primordia in the developing jaws (Mitsiadis et al., 2003). This shows that mouse neural crest can unlock the potential of chick ectoderm to form teeth. Similarly, Eames and Schneider demonstrated that neural crest transplantations between duck and quail change the pattern of cranial feathers according to the donor's profile. This includes expression of key morphogens in developing feather placodes (Eames and Schneider, 2005). These experiments provide critical examples of the shared competence and intricate interplay between epithelium and underlying neural crest-derived mesenchyme in the complex morphogenetic events that occur in a forming head.

Being derived from neural ectoderm, NCCs signal back to the developing CNS and modulate Fgf8 expression in the Anterior Neural Ridge and the isthmus in the brain. Moreover, Foxg1 expression, which is vital for fore- and midbrain patterning, is regulated by Smad1 activity of NCCs (Creuzet et al., 2006; Le Douarin et al., 2007; Creuzet, 2009a,b; Aguiar et al., 2014). Hence, the neural crest acts as an important signaling center that controls brain development (Le Douarin et al., 2012).

Disturbances in the normal migration and subsequent actions of NCCs and other inductive cell sources may cause abnormal development, as seen in a number of human syndromes with craniofacial malformations (Noden and Trainor, 2005; Chai and Maxson, 2006; Walker and Trainor, 2006). Among those most commonly observed are congenital disorders of the lip and/or palate, but a range of other dysfunctions in the soft and mineralized tissues of the head and face are caused by genetic deviations. For obvious reasons, an understanding of the etiology of these aberrations is fundamental for basic and translational science. Thus, novel data of this kind may subsequently be applied in the clinic to treat or even prevent craniofacial congenital malformations.

Interestingly, recent studies have clearly demonstrated that the developing neural structures do not cease to influence the morphogenesis of other cranial tissues and organs after NCCs have finished their migration from the dorsal neural tube. A large body of evidence now points toward the fact that the brain, the neurogenic placodes as well as the peripheral nerves are important for correct facial shaping as well as for providing necessary cell types to multiple locations in the entire head, until late developmental stages or even in adulthood.

### Further Reading:

1. Molecular mechanisms of cranial NCCs migration and patterning in craniofacial development (Minoux and Rijli, 2010).
2. Neural crest and the origin of vertebrates: a new head (Gans and Northcutt, 1983).
3. Establishing neural crest identity: a gene regulatory recipe (Simões-Costa and Bronner, 2015).
4. Evolution of vertebrates as viewed from the crest (Green et al., 2015).

## BRAIN-DEPENDENT INTEGRATION IN THE CRANIAL COMPARTMENT

At post-neural crest developmental stages, the growing brain continues to play an important role in coordinating and assisting the development of other craniofacial parts and tissue types. In the past, numerous suggestions have been made regarding the developmental interaction between the brain and the facial compartment. Physical interactions with underlying mechanical forces should be of at least some significance in the coordination of brain and face morphogenesis and growth. Indeed, many cases of microcephaly or macrocephaly are associated with changes, often dramatic, in the function and shape of the facial compartment (Kivitie-Kallio and Norio, 2001; Chen et al., 2004; Vasudevan et al., 2005). Human trisomy may involve severe disturbances in the patterning of the skull base, accompanied by disruptions in cranial nerve development. This underpins the fact that knowledge of complex osteogenic–neural dynamics is integral for the understanding of the pathophysiology behind genetic craniofacial malformations (Demyer et al., 1964; Colleran et al., 2014; Reid et al., 2015). Pushing this line of reasoning further, one can speculate that the nervous system might and should be capable of influencing the size of its protective skeletal encasement with corresponding facial compartment. Such a developmental integration would have emerged over millennia of co-evolution, leading to a sophisticated brain-to-skeleton crosstalk. This, in turn, would allow for a coordinated volume increase over developmental or evolutionary time. This concept is not new and appears multiple times in the literature. Biegert and De Beer were among those that propagated the notion that increasing brain size would cause predictable changes in the cranium (De Beer, 1937; Biegert, 1963). Indeed, Hallgrimsson and co-authors demonstrated that experimentally induced changes in brain size co-vary with alterations in morphologies of the skull base. This is in agreement with predictions of Biegert's model (Hallgrímsson et al., 2007; Hallgrímsson and Lieberman, 2008; Lieberman et al., 2008). For a detailed discussion of the "spatial packing" hypothesis, the brain as the architectural foundation of the face and other relevant issues including synchronized changes in skull base, please see the review by Marcucio et al. (2011).

The mechanisms that mediate the coordination between the growing brain and its surrounding cartilage and bone may include so called "quasi-static strain" tension stress, and intracellular systems of tension sensing and response via proliferation and production of the extracellular matrix (Moss and Young, 1960; Henderson et al., 2005; Jaalouk and Lammerding, 2009; Temiyasathit and Jacobs, 2010). For an extensive discussion of cranial bone development matching brain growth (see Richtsmeier and Flaherty, 2013).

As mentioned above, physical interaction and integration in the developing head have been topics for research and discussion since long. However, more recently a signaling crosstalk between the developing brain and the face was identified. This crosstalk commences early, when NCCs influence the ongoing development of the anterior CNS in the embryo (Creuzet et al., 2006; Le Douarin et al., 2007; Creuzet, 2009a,b). It became obvious that Shh-based signaling coordinates the development of the brain and the face. It has been widely known that mutations in the Shh pathway cause a number of pathologies involving both facial and brain-related phenotypes (holoprosencephaly, Greig Cephalopolysyndactyly, Gorlin syndrome; Ming et al., 1998; Pan et al., 2013; Chaudhary et al., 2015). In line with this, it was recently shown that silencing of Shh signaling in the brain influences Shh expression in FEZ, and causes phenotypes similar to holoprosencephaly (Chong et al., 2012; see **Figure 2**). Further studies from the Hallgrimsson and the Marcucio laboratories established that a Shh-responsive signaling center in the anterior CNS controls facial development through actions on the FEZ organizer in the anterior facial ectoderm (Hu and Marcucio, 2009b). Experimental disruption of Shh in the brain distorted facial development, but it was possible to rescue facial shape to a large extent by early application of Shh to the embryos (Chong et al., 2012). Further studies also highlighted an important evodevo aspect: animals with different facial morphology demonstrate significant differences in the organization of Shh-releasing zones in the face and in the forebrain (Hu et al., 2015). For example, the spatial structure of FEZ is clearly different between mammals and birds. Moreover, it is possible to interfere and change that structure in chick embryos. This yields chick embryonic faces that bear resemblance to faces of mice embryos (Hu and Marcucio, 2009b). In addition, both FEZ and Shh-releasing regions in the forebrain appear to be different between avian species. Thus, when duck forebrain was transplanted into the chick embryo, the facial compartment started to develop according to the donor tissue (Hu et al., 2015; Smith et al., 2015). For a detailed discussion regarding the molecular dialogue between brain, FEZ and facial compartments (see Marcucio et al., 2011, 2015; Young et al., 2014).

The development of the pituitary gland, an endocrine gland with modular structure, provides another example of a complex

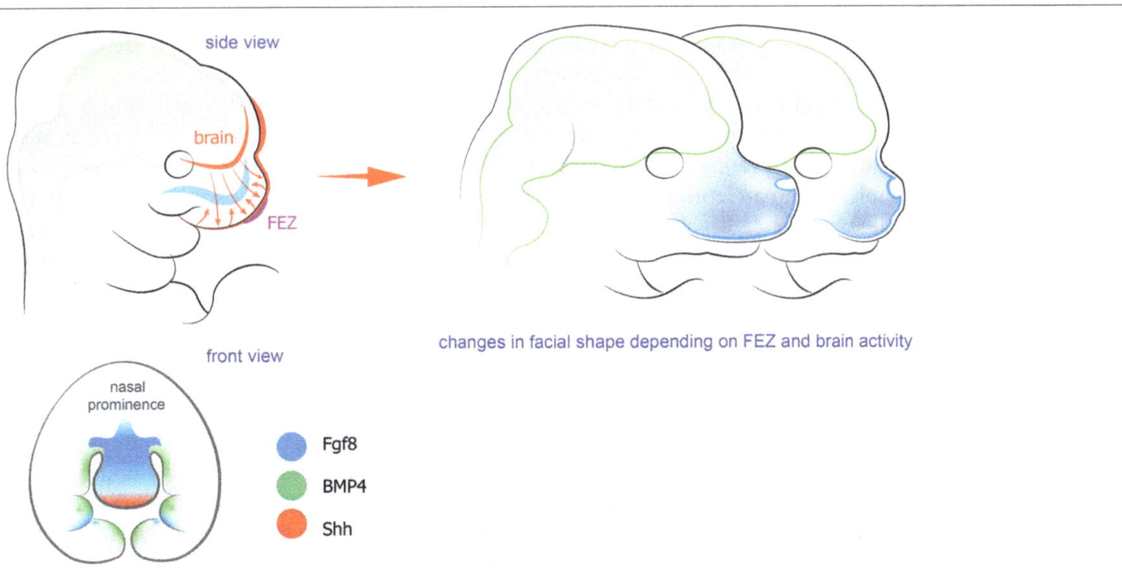


**FIGURE 2 | Forebrain and FEZ exchange signals to shape the facial compartment.** Factors produced by the epithelium in the frontal face (FEZ) control the formation of future skeletal elements together with signals coming from the developing forebrain. Manipulation of FEZ leads to changes in the shape of **Figure 5**. Peripheral nerves host and transport neural crest-derived associated glial cells that give rise to a number of cell types in developing body. Left: examples and position of nerve-derived cell types. A significant number of melanocytes (purple circles on a scheme) in a head-neck region is produced from recruited Schwann cell precursors. Additionally, some mesenchymal progenitors in developing teeth (shown as red ellipses) are also recruited from the peripheral nerves. At the same time all parasympathetic neurons in the head are derived from nerve-associated cells. Right: the spectrum of currently confirmed nerve-derived cell types in the developing face (right panel).

molecular dialogue between the brain and oral epithelium based on Shh, Fgf8, and BMP4 signaling. The pituitary gland originates in part from the most anterior neural ridge in the developing brain and in part from Rathke's pouch. Rathke's pouch formation begins as an invagination of oral ectoderm, which is initiated in response to BMP4 provided by the ventral diencephalon. Shh also plays a prominent role in this process (Zhu et al., 2007). The gland starts to develop prior to the formation of the surrounding *sella turcica*, a depression in the sphenoid bone. Some pathological cases related to hypo- or hyperthyroidism show that variations in size of the gland is reflected in the shape and volume of corresponding lacunae in *sella turcica* (Gopalakrishnan et al., 2015). This suggests the presence of at least a mechanical coordination in the development of the pituitary gland and the skeletal compartment that enclose it.

The eye is a prominent craniofacial organ derived from the developing brain. From an evolutionary standpoint, photosensory systems are products of neuroepithelium from different parts of embryonic or larval CNS. This explains the fact that the eyes or ocelli are located inside of the nervous system in a number of lower animals (Ivashkin and Adameyko, 2013). Ontogenetically and phylogenetically, the neural folds in what eventually will become the diencephalon form indentations, and these expand to create the optic vesicles and eventually the optic cups. The lens placode, the origin of the lens of the eye, arises from the extended anterior placodal area (Toro and Varga, 2007) and invaginates adjacent to the optic cup. Brain-derived optic vesicle interacts with future lens tissue to promote maturation and further transformations (signaling crosstalk in eye development is reviewed in Gunhaga (2011). Later on the lens cells will differentiate, elongate and become transparent. The outer and inner sheaths of the optic cup differentiate into the pigment and neural retinas, respectively. This process is, meanwhile, strictly coordinated with the formation and insertion of the extraocular muscles that surround the optic cup. This is indicated by observations of frequent anomalies of the extraocular muscles in patients with rather extreme craniofacial malformations. For example, in human fetuses with anencephaly or other grave skull deficits, absence or abnormalities of the extraocular muscles were found, including anomalous insertions. Similar feature may be present also in milder developmental disturbances of the craniofacial region (Plock et al., 2007).

Little is known about the integration of the eye and its muscles into the developing skeletal socket of the face, the orbit. The orbit is created through intramembranous ossification of different embryological structures that eventually will form seven bones. The concomitant incorporation of the visual organ into the orbit during this process must require an extremely complex synchronized mechanism. Eyes are sensory organs of utmost importance, and their position in a head, their direction and relative size are tightly selected by evolution in all animal species. This, in turn, depends on the evolutionary and ontogenetic interactions of the eyes with the forming cranium. Changes in orbit position and orientation, for example, enabled binocular vision—one of the factors that shaped human face (see **Figure 3**). This implicates that disturbances in craniofacial bone development might be accompanied by deficits in the eye or its appendages. It has been suggested that the developing eye, in addition to the forebrain and FEZ, is an important organizer of craniofacial development, including roles non-related to visual perception (Kish et al., 2011). Thus, the eye vesicle influences neural crest migration (Langenberg et al., 2008) as well as production of retinoic acid (Matt et al., 2005, 2008; White and Schilling, 2008) and Shh. Indeed, it is possible that eye-derived retinoic acid or Shh mediate a crosstalk with mesenchymal tissues of the future orbit, coordinate patterning of extraocular muscles and influence the geometry of periocular and other skeletal parts. There are no animals where eye development programs are completely aborted. All eyeless species of fish and salamander have early steps of eye development, which could well be necessary for proper integration of structures during craniofacial morphogenesis (personal communication William R. Jeffery, University of Maryland, as described in Kish et al., 2011).

The migrating orbits in developing flatfishes represent one of the best examples of coordination between orbit position, cranial bone structure and the eye (see **Figure 3**). In these fishes, one eye moves to the contralateral side as an adaptation to the lifestyle at the sea floor. The movement of an orbit is caused by proliferating periocular cell masses on the future ventral side of the head. The rotation of the cranial bones depends on the translocation of the eye. Inhibition of proliferation in the suborbital area causes an abrogated migration of the eye to the opposite side, and a changed structure of a skull (Bao et al., 2011). In line with this, the cave-dwelling fish *Astyanax mexicanus* demonstrates a variety of eye-dependent transformations of the cranium in different subspecies living in conditions with or without light. In addition, transplantations of embryonic lenses and removal of optic vesicles in *Astyanax* showed that six suborbital bones and cranial neuromasts partially depend on the presence of an eye (Yamamoto et al., 2003). The fact that it is possible to change the cranial bone size and geometry by manipulating eye development is indicative of a close combination and crosstalk between the developing eye and the skull during ontogeny. The nature of this crosstalk, though, is still not understood. Interestingly, in many groups of animals there are cartilages and bones that form what is called an ocular skeleton directly inside of the eyes. The ocular skeleton may include a ring of scleral ossicles, and a cartilage that supports the eyeball or join the ossicles together. The function of these skeletal elements that often attain a significant size is not clear (Franz-Odendaal, 2011).

Taken together, it seems that signaling crosstalk between the developing brain (including parts forming the pituitary gland and eyes) and surrounding tissues provides both for a coordinated general shaping of the facial compartment and for proper development of particular structures.

## Further Reading:

1. Mechanisms that underlie co-variation of the brain and face (Marcucio et al., 2011).
2. Embryonic bauplans and the developmental origins of facial diversity and constraint (Young et al., 2014).
3. The eye as an organizer of craniofacial development (Kish et al., 2011).

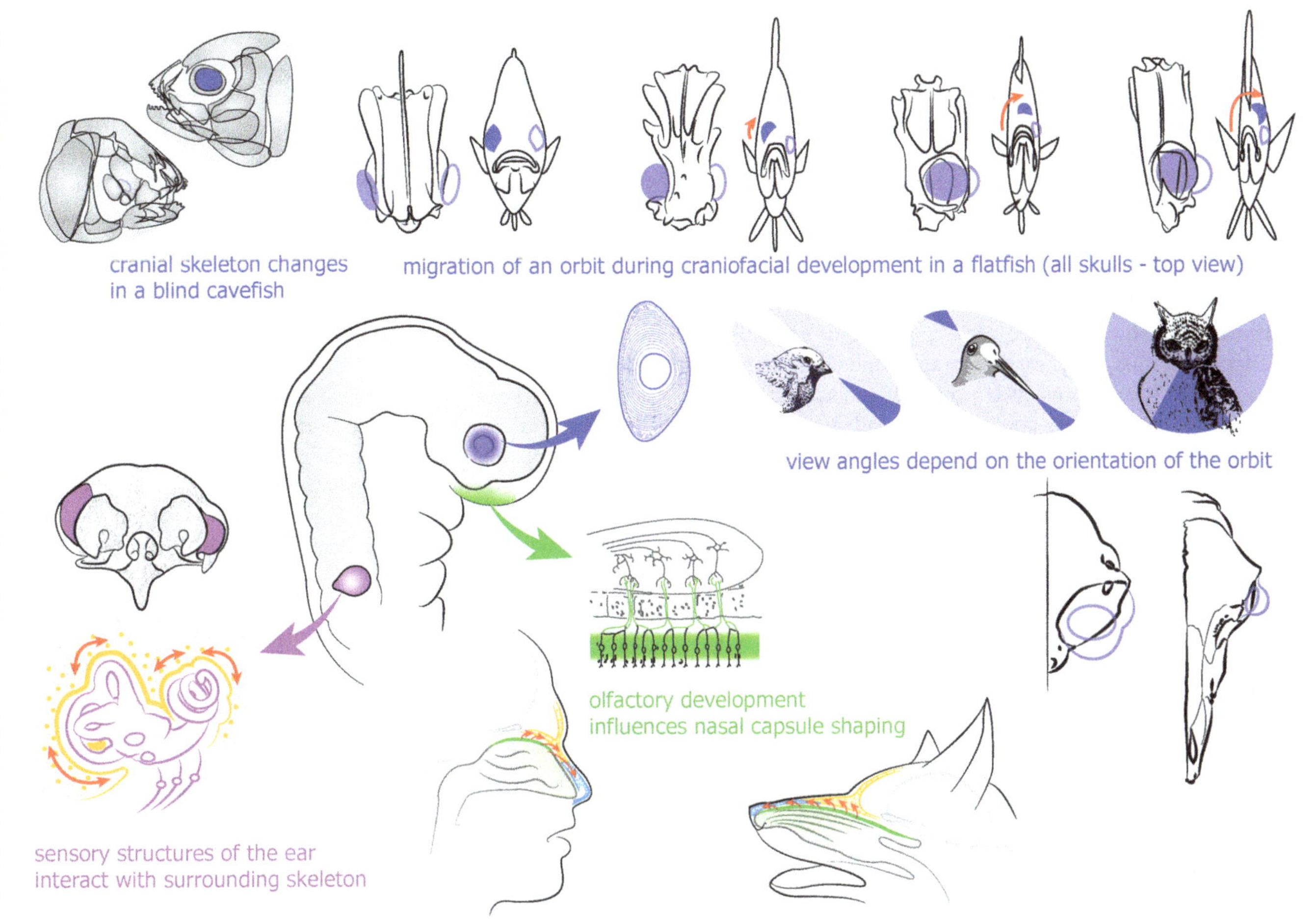


**FIGURE 3 | Developing eye and sensory placode-derived structures influence the development of surrounding skeletal and other tissues in the head.** Upper part (in blue): developing eye influences the formation of surrounding skeleton as evidenced in blind cavefish and observed in the development of a flatfish. Integration of an eye into orbit provides the specie-specific view angle and stands behind stereoscopic vision. Left (in purple): otic vesicle and sensory ear components induce and integrate surrounding cartilage and bone. Lower part (in green): olfactory epithelium development influences formation of surrounding skeletal parts.

## SENSORY NEUROGENIC PLACODES IN THE CRANIAL COMPARTMENT

Cranial neurogenic placodes originate as ectodermal thickenings from the anterior neural plate border area, the so-called pre-placodal region (Streit, 2007). Neural plate and mesoderm-derived FGFs act to induce the pre-placodal region concomitant with a local downregulation of BMPs and Wnts (Litsiou et al., 2005; Streit, 2007; Park and Saint-Jeannet, 2008; Grocott et al., 2012; Groves and LaBonne, 2014). Placodes contain clusters of progenitor cells that will give rise to an array of sensory and neurosecretory organs. With the exception of the nodose ganglia, the placode-derived structures occupy specifically designed skeletal lodges in the cranium. Some evidence point toward the fact that all neural placodes share a common evolutionary origin. This ancient origin was subsequently elaborated in different ways to produce a number of tools that are specified to gather information about the environment (Schlosser, 2015). From an evolutionary point of view, this would have enabled a profound change in lifestyle, from a passive feeding to an active search and hunt of prey (Lassiter et al., 2014; Schlosser, 2014). Such a dramatic change would inevitably cause modifications of the feeding system with further development of jaws, and also improve the protective encasements for CNS and sensory organs. However, the mechanisms behind the sophisticated interactive coordination during craniofacial sensory and skeletal co-evolution are not fully understood.

The otic placode is induced by extrinsic FGF signals from the pre-placodal region immediately bordering the anterior neural plate (Ohyama et al., 2007). It later develops into the inner ear, which eventually becomes enclosed in the densely mineralized petrous part of the temporal bone (Basch et al., 2016). The inner ear is connected to the other sections of the auditory system, the middle and the outer ear. These parts have different developmental origins. The middle ear is separated from the auditory canal by the tympanic membrane, which has an outer layer continuous with the ectoderm of the ear canal, and an inner layer that is assumed to be of endodermal origin.

The middle ear is a cavity in the temporal bone with a very complex anatomy. It is covered by endoderm- and neural crest-derived epithelium (Thompson and Tucker, 2013) and is bridged by the three middle ear ossicles, malleus, incus, and stapes, which are the result of endochondral ossification from neural crest of the first and second arches (reviewed by Anthwal and Thompson, 2016). The pinna, which gives rise to the auricle, is discerned as six small mounds, or hillocks, derived from the 1st and 2nd pharyngeal arches at E11.5 in the mouse, and 6 weeks gestation in humans. These hillocks grow and unite to form a cartilage-filled structure at the entrance of the auditory canal (reviewed by Anthwal and Thompson, 2016). The nature of organization between neural, glia or sensory cells and other different types of tissues during ear ontogeny is not well understood. It may be suggested that extrinsic co-regulation and active crosstalk between tissue types might not be necessary during development of an ear, since coordinated morphogenesis can be achieved due to autonomous behavior of every partaking tissue after millennia of a tight co-evolution. When considering the evolutionary history of the middle and outer ear in vertebrates, there will be some significant support for such logics, especially taking into account significant variations in middle ear structure without accompanying changes in the basic configuration of the inner ear (Maier and Ruf, 2015). However, despite possible autonomic control and congruence of different parts of a hearing system after a protracted co-evolution, there are clear examples that demonstrate a functional cross-talk between placode-derived and other structures that shape the hearing sensory organ. In the beginning of the twentieth century, Luther demonstrated that surgical removal of the otic capsule from frog embryos prevents formation of otic cartilage. However, this operation did not affect columella auris. Grafting of the otic vesicle into a head region could induce formation of surrounding cartilage, but this did not occur in cases of transplantations into the trunk (Luther, 1924). On the other hand, in mice with a conditional knockout of Dicer1, all major cranial sensory organs are severely impaired and a craniofacial phenotype occurs. These mice demonstrate a truncated development of the otic capsule and some changes in the craniofacial development associated with the loss of olfactory epithelium and forebrain (Kersigo et al., 2011). In agreement with this, Six1 knockout embryos with abnormally developed placode-derived sensory components show distorted cochlea morphologies (Laclef et al., 2003).

The olfactory and the vomeronasal epithelia are generated by the olfactory placode, and line bony skull parts of impressive sizes in many animal species with a highly developed sense of olfaction. It appears as if the geometry and the amount of necessary bone are proportional to the surface of olfactory epithelium in various animals. Moreover, the cribriform plate appears to have a size and structure that corresponds to the olfactory needs (Bird et al., 2014; Van Valkenburgh et al., 2014). In humans, with a poor sense of smell in comparison with for example dogs, the corresponding cranium parts are proportionally much smaller. The protracted co-evolution of skeletal and mesenchymal structures in the anterior head allowed a fusion of olfactory and respiratory passages (Jankowski, 2011). However, similar to what was discussed above, a perfect fit of various tissues in the nose can be achieved through evolutionary autonomic tuning of developmental dynamics. So far there is no clearly identified regulatory crosstalk between skeletal tissues and the olfactory epithelium that they host. However, more than 70 years ago, Schmalhausen demonstrated that the formation of the cartilaginous nasal capsule depends on olfactory epithelium development, using surgical methods in urodeles (Schmalhausen, 1939). Furthermore, Burr and Reiss showed the response of the facial skeleton after removal of the nasal placode (Burr, 1916; Reiss, 1998). In line with this, analyses of Six1 and conditional Dicer1 knockout animals indicated some degree of extrinsic signaling and synchronization, since the affected olfactory placodes in these animals yielded disturbances in facial shape (Laclef et al., 2003; Kersigo et al., 2011). It seems reasonable to assume that neural placode-derived structures destined to become e.g. olfactory or auditory or vestibular, interact with the cellular progenies that eventually will form their protective cartilage and bony cases, see **Figure 3**. Despite this, the detailed coordination of sensory organ and cartilage and bone formation in the head, in terms of molecular signaling, does not seem to have been the subject of much attention.

The ophthalmic and maxillary placode of the trigeminal nerve contributes sensory neurons to the trigeminal ganglion (see Schlosser, 2010). These cells, which coalesce with neural crest-derived neurons, convey sensory modalities such as e.g., touch, temperature and pain, from the exterior and interior of the head. The trigeminal ganglion, which harbors the trigeminal primary sensory neurons, is situated in a tightly sculpted bony furrow of the sphenoid bone in the middle cranial fossa. With regard to the sensory innervation of the facial mesenchymal derivatives and especially bone, not much is known to what extent it might convey secreted signals to affect developmental events there. However, the opposite is true: development of craniofacial non-neural structures influences the gene expression in trigeminal neurons. For instance, target-derived BMP4 helps to determine the phenotype of trigeminal ganglion nerve cells in mice (Hodge et al., 2007). In this way, neural crest- and placode-derived nervous system progenitors on the one hand, and ectomesenchymal ones on the other, adapt very different fates but then collaborate to control the ontogeny and evolution of the different systems they eventually will form.

## Further Reading:

1. Vertebrate cranial placodes as evolutionary innovations—the ancestor's tale (Schlosser, 2015).
2. Where hearing starts: the development of the mammalian cochlea (Basch et al., 2016).
3. The development of the mammalian outer and middle ear (Anthwal and Thompson, 2016).
4. Revisiting human nose anatomy: phylogenic and ontogenic perspectives (Jankowski, 2011).

## NERVE-ORGANOGENESIS INTERPLAY IN THE CRANIAL COMPARTMENT

Recently it became apparent that peripheral nerves play a number of non-canonical functions related to morphogenesis of innervated tissue, in addition to canonical action potential propagation (Kaucká and Adameyko, 2014). A striking example where peripheral innervation seems indispensable for proper tissue or organ generation/regeneration in vertebrates is provided by fish teeth (Tuisku and Hildebrand, 1994). Cichlids were used to perform unilateral denervation studies of the lower jaw, followed by extraction of mandibular teeth. Corresponding teeth were extracted from both sides of the jaw, and the unoperated side served as control for the denervated side. Cichlids have continuous tooth replacement under normal circumstances. Interestingly, after a one-year follow-up, it was found that the teeth on the side where the nerve was lesioned did not regenerate, in contrast to the control side with the intact nerve. This is a strong indication that there is a link between peripheral innervation and organ formation. Hypothetically, nerves may provide signals for tooth formation by presenting factors that influence the ectomesenchyme or dental epithelium. Organotypic *in vitro* and *ex vivo* cultures have shown that tooth development can proceed without nerve fibers (Lumsden and Buchanan, 1986). Tooth germs can develop in standard tissue culture conditions for 7–8 days, but eventually become flattened and disorganized. When using 3D culture systems, this period can be slightly extended (Sun et al., 2014). However, tooth explant cultures have been performed with tissues that may already be committed to a dental fate, and it cannot be altogether excluded that the actual initial tooth-determining signals to epithelium and mesenchyme are of neural or glial origin. Indeed, a recent study from Yang Chai's laboratory demonstrated that nerve-dependent cues are necessary for driving the activity in a mesenchymal stem cell niche associated with the neuro-vascular bundle in continuously growing mouse incisors. Thus, Shh released from trigeminal ganglion sensory endings proximal to Gli1$^{+}$ dental mesenchymal stem cells (MSCs) appears to be a key factor to ensure continuous tooth growth. Ablation of the sensory innervation of the incisor eventually led to the deterioration of the tooth (Zhao et al., 2014; see **Figure 4**).

The taste bud is another craniofacial sensory organ whose fate is intertwined with its innervation. Earlier transplantation studies in the axolotl have suggested that nerve fibers may not be necessary *per se* for the primary taste bud development, since very early donor embryo oropharyngeal tissue devoid innervation as well as taste buds develop taste buds when grafted to the trunk of a host embryo (Barlow et al., 1996). However, during subsequent development, it is since long well established that taste bud growth and maintenance is dependent on an intact innervation, originating from the VIIth and IXth cranial nerves (Oakley and Witt, 2004). The molecular regulation behind this phenomenon has been linked to the expression of Shh in taste bud basal cells. After chorda tympani denervation, taste buds appear reduced in size as compared to control side of the tongue (Li et al., 2015). Furthermore, long term application of the Shh inhibitor LDE225 results in a similar phenotype, with a severe size reduction of taste buds (Kumari et al., 2015). Shh expression is lost after denervation, which would explain why progenitor activity is hampered (Miura et al., 2006). Furthermore, artificially induced expression of Shh in lingual epithelium induces the formation of ectopic taste buds, which in contrast to normal taste buds

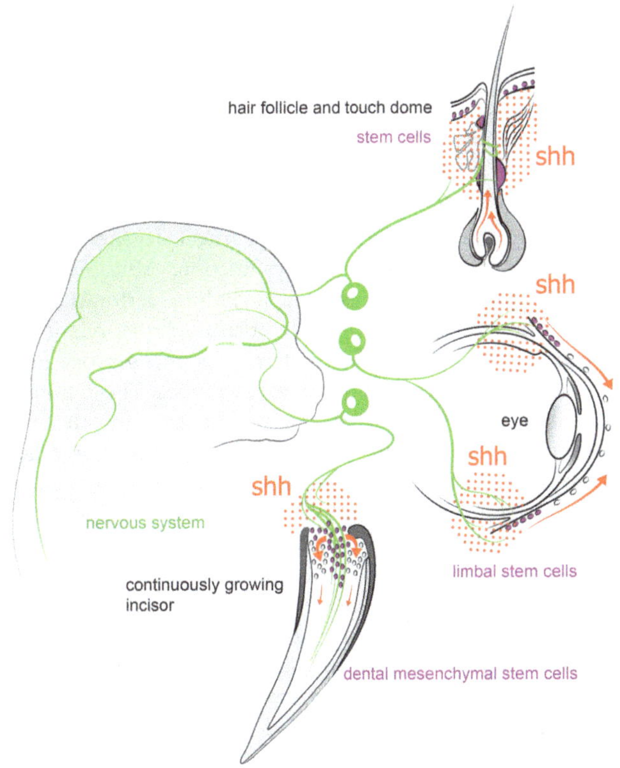


**FIGURE 4 | Peripheral sensory nerves inject Shh into variety of structures in the head and tune the activity of stem cell compartments.** For instance, nerve-derived Shh plays an important role in controlling stem cell niches in continuously growing incisor, hair follicle, touch dome, and limbal region of cornea in the eye.

seem to be independent of individual innervation (Castillo et al., 2014). Taken together, these data indicate that nerve-derived Shh maintains taste buds. Thus, neural Shh may control proliferation of adjacent progenitors, and is crucial for the regulation of taste bud density on the tongue. In addition to this coordinated development of neural and an epithelial sensory system, recent data indicate a common genetic ancestry between the gustatory system and teeth. In teleosts (cichlids), oral epithelium seems to possess an ancient inherent single regulatory gene system. This system, which may persist also in mammals, is suggested to be capable of co-patterning teeth and taste buds. Specifically, Wnt determines density (coordination) of teeth and taste buds, while BMP and Shh influence organ characteristics (Bloomquist et al., 2015). If, and if so to what extent this genetic pathway would be under the developmental influence of the ubiquitous innervation of the oral cavity has however not been addressed.

The touch dome (Merkel cell-neurite complex), a highly innervated epithelium-derived sensory structure in the skin, also depends on neural hedgehog signaling for self-renewal. Denervation experiments or ablations of Shh in sensory neurons showed that touch dome stem cells fully rely on the neural environment for their propagation and maintenance. Accordingly, an elevated production of Shh results in neoplastic proliferation of touch dome cells (Xiao et al., 2015). In line with this, Shh appears to be an important signal for some particular Gli1$^+$ hair follicle epithelial cells in the bulge region. Gli1$^+$ bulge cells are known to incorporate into healing skin lesions, and also to function as stem cells to restore hair follicles at each anagen phase (Brownell et al., 2011).

Another example of a nerve-dependent stem cell compartment in the face is represented by limbal stem cells in the cornea of the eye. Neurotrophic keratopathy (NK) is a disease manifested by a progressive corneal degeneration that is the result of corneal nerve dysfunction. Multiple defects eventually develop in the cornea, including perforations and corneal thinning. A recent study identified the relationship between corneolimbal epithelial stem cells and sensory nerves with the help of a mouse denervation model. The authors of this study electro-coagulated the ophthalmic branch of the trigeminal nerve, and after 7 days they observed a significant loss of corneolimbal stem cell markers as well as a reduction in the colony-forming efficiency of stem cells obtained from denervated corneas (Ueno et al., 2012).

The salivary gland has proved to be a good model system to address how local organogenesis can be directed by the peripheral nervous system. Sarah Knox and co-workers discovered that parasympathetic neurons that innervate salivary gland also control the organogenesis of the developing gland. Their studies demonstrated that during early salivary gland development, parasympathetic axons grow to surround the end buds of the ductal epithelium. Once there, vasoactive intestinal peptide (VIP) is being released from nerve endings and diffuses toward the epithelium. VIP then activates the cyclic AMP (cAMP)/protein kinase A (PKA) pathway, and helps to increase duct elongation and the subsequent formation of a single contiguous structure. Nerve depletion during this process causes a distorted tubulogenesis. When the lumen is established, VIP is also required for its enlargement through a cAMP/PKA/cystic fibrosis transmembrane conductance regulator (CFTR)-dependent pathway (Nedvetsky et al., 2014). This is *prima faciei* evidence for the necessity of an intact peripheral nervous system for correct craniofacial organ development, and underlines the need for more research into developmental interactions between nerves and other epithelial derivatives. For example, postganglionic sympathetic neurons that express a cholinergic/noradrenergic co-phenotype are present before the sweat glands that they will innervate are formed (Schütz et al., 2008). Thus, it is possible that these nerve fibers may influence target organ formation in an as yet unknown manner.

Diseases causing abnormal cranial nerve development often lead to aberrant growth of target organs and tissues. It is evident that the peripheral innervation in many cases is needed for proper development and function of orofacial structures (Pagella et al., 2014). The aetiologies behind congenital facial abnormalities vary. They can be caused by genetic or, most commonly, unknown factors. Deformations in facial growth can be environmentally influenced during embryogenesis and disruptions in the growth can also have metabolic, vascular and/or teratogenic causes. One example is Möbius syndrome that causes palsy and nerve weakness, which in turn gives facial asymmetry. This congenital disease is characterized by deficient innervation (abducens (VI) and facial (VII) nerves), and causes clinical symptoms such as deafness, tooth anomalies, and cleft palate (Rizos et al., 1998). Another example is hereditary sensory and autonomic neuropathy type IV (HSAN IV), a rare inherited disorder of the peripheral nervous system. It is the caused by mutations in the neurotrophic tyrosine kinase receptor 1 gene (*NTRK1*), which encodes the high-affinity nerve growth factor receptor TRKA. Affected patients of this multisystem syndrome have a severe peripheral nerve fiber loss and display a lack of reaction to pain stimuli, inability to sweat, and mental retardation. Interestingly, from a developmental point of view, oral and craniofacial manifestations include missing teeth, nasal malformation, cleft palate, dental caries and malocclusion (Gao et al., 2013). Furthermore, severe hemifacial atrophy is seen in Parry-Romberg syndrome. This disorder, which may be accompanied by a range of neurological pathologies, including trigeminal neuralgia, has an unclear etiology but has been linked to defects in innervation (Vix et al., 2015). Various problems in the cervical sympathetic trunk leading to dysfunctions in the sympathetic system seem to play important roles in the development of facial atrophy, and cause a number of additional symptoms including alopecia and scleroderma (Scope et al., 2004) Indeed, experimental animals with ablated superior cervical sympathetic ganglia develop manifestations similar to those seen in Parry-Romberg syndrome in humans (Resende et al., 1991).

A number of so called neuro-cutaneous diseases show manifestation in the face (Little et al., 2015). For example, pigmentation defects such as Nevus of Ota or vitiligo, which involve loss or overproduction of pigmentation in specific locations, are often associated with changes in facial neuroanatomy (Nelhaus, 1970). In the case of Nevus of Ota the affected locations correspond to areas supplied by branches of the trigeminal nerve (Jovovic-Dagovic et al., 2007; Trufant et al., 2009). Further, the development of vitiligo has been related to dysfunctions in the sympathetic nervous system (Wu et al., 2000; van Geel et al., 2012), since certain cases of segmental vitiligo were found to develop after sympathectomy in patients (Lerner et al., 1966). Parry-Romberg syndrome has also been associated with sympathetic nerves (Janowska et al., 2013), and in addition both Parry-Romberg syndrome and vitiligo are linked to immune system dysfunctions and local inflammatory processes (Creus et al., 1994; van Geel et al., 2012). Interestingly, several studies have already pointed out at a connection between sympathetic nerves and local inflammation. This might play a role in the autoimmune component of vitiligo, with a malfunction of the primary beta-adrenoceptor signaling system (Wu et al., 2000). Furthermore, adrenergic compounds that are released from sympathetic nerves may serve as initiating or facilitating factors for numerous Th1-sustained inflammatory skin diseases (Manni and Maestroni, 2008).

Yet another nerve-associated tissue defect is Neurofibromatosis, which manifests itself through benign tumors and pigmentation spots that originate from peripheral nerves (Abramowicz and Gos, 2014). This is somewhat similar to a malicious contagious facial Schwannoma cancer, which almost eradicated the population of Tasmanian devils (*Sarcophilus harrisii*; Murchison et al., 2010).

As seen from above, the spectrum and severity of craniofacial anomalies involving nerves differ widely, but all cause some degree of functional physiological impairment. If these embryonic defects are too extensive, they can drastically reduce fetus survival rate (Sperber et al., 2010). It may also be added that distortions due to congenital disease may not only gravely impair obvious physiological craniofacial activities such as e.g. feeding, breathing, hearing and vision, but also cause dysfunctions in complex social communications (Jack and Schyns, 2015), and in this way severely reduce the quality of life.

### Further Reading:

1. Non-canonical functions of the peripheral nerve (Kaucká and Adameyko, 2014).
2. Nerve dependence in tissue, organ, and appendage regeneration (Kumar and Brockes, 2012).
3. Roles of innervation in developing and regenerating orofacial tissues (Pagella et al., 2014).

## THE PERIPHERAL NERVE AS A PROVIDER OF NECESSARY CELL TYPES IN CRANIAL DEVELOPMENT

The timing of the activation of different cellular sources for coordinated cranial development is tightly controlled. It enables the impressive evolutionary flexibility of head development that underlies the heterochrony in multiple vertebrate species. Recently, a novel cellular source has emerged as a key factor in the formation of a complete and functional head: the nerve-associated neural crest-derived cells (Schwann cell precursors, SCPs). The latest discoveries in the field demonstrate that these nerve-dwelling glial cells can produce other cell types, and through this participate in developmental mechanisms that shape and integrate the cranial compartment. Peripheral nerves can be viewed as navigating routes and a stem cell niche from which various cell types, including myelinating and non-myelinating Schwann cells, endoneural fibroblasts, parasympathetic neurons, enteric neurons, bone marrow mesenchymal cells and melanocytes originate at different time points and in various locations (Joseph et al., 2004; Adameyko et al., 2009, 2012; Budi et al., 2011; Laranjeira et al., 2011; Nitzan et al., 2013; Dyachuk et al., 2014; Espinosa-Medina et al., 2014; Isern et al., 2014; Uesaka et al., 2015) (see **Figure 5**).

### Cranial Parasympathetic Neurons Originate from Nerve-Associated Embryonic Glial Progenitors

The nerve cells of the parasympathetic ganglia of the head send their axons to various adjacent structures that are of fundamental importance for normal homeostasis. These structures include salivary and lacrimal glands as well as ciliary muscles of the eye. It has long been assumed that the parasympathetic neurons of the head, similar to the sensory ganglia of the cranial nerves, are derived from migrating specified NCCs. This has remained somewhat of an enigma, since parasympathetic gangliogenesis does not occur in the developing embryo until time points when the short pulse of neural crest migration already has ceased. Remarkably, it was recently found that these neurons actually originate not from waves of migrating NCCs, but instead from cells that initially travel to their target areas on outgrowing nerve fibers. In most cases these precursors follow the preganglionic axon route to the target locations. At the sites of the different future ganglia, among them the ciliary, the submandibular, the sphenopalatine and the otic ganglia, SCPs detach and change fate into parasympathetic nerve cells (Dyachuk et al., 2014; Espinosa-Medina et al., 2014). This conversion from glial to neuronal phenotype seems to be triggered by a local induction of ASCL1, which in turn may be influenced by local secretion of BMPs and/or Wnts (Müller and Rohrer, 2002; Knosp et al., 2015). This both unanticipated and sophisticated process shows how the developing nervous system, using an intrinsic machinery, can both transport necessary nerve cells as precursors to the proper target site using matrices laid out by the preganglionic axons, and, when they subsequently have changed phenotype, connect these postganglionic neurons to the same preganglionic axons that they previously trekked on. Obviously, this raises a number of challenging questions related to the extremely detailed temporal coordination of gene expression that underlies this complex mechanism (Lleras-Forero and Streit, 2012). What signals induce the genes that specify parasympathetic neuronal fate in local SCPs in extremely restricted locations in the head? Are these signals coordinated with the genetic networks that induce the actual target organ formation? Do the peripheral neural components control the development of craniofacial elements?

To summarize, the development of parasympathetic ganglia requires a late progenitor cell source that can ensure a neural crest type of neurogenesis long after neural crest migration is over. This is solved by SCPs. The concept of using SCPs from presynaptic nerves facilitates navigation, and eventually establishes and warrants synaptic connectivity far away from the original neural crest source (Adameyko and Ernfors, 2014; Ivashkin et al., 2014).

### Cranial Pigment Cells, Melanocytes, are Derived in Part from Nerve-Associated Schwann Cell Precursors

Melanocytes, the pigment cells, are important not only for the color of the eyes or pigmentation of hairs and skin in the head, but they are also essential for hearing. Melanocytes residing in the inner ear are indeed an essential component of the integral inner ear environment that is necessary for survival of sensory hair cells. The melanocyte as a cell type is essential for proper cochlea development, since mutant mice without melanocytes develop impaired auditory structures (Hozumi et al., 2012; Ni et al., 2013). At the same time, melanin does not seem to be important for the sensory function of the ear (Tachibana, 1999). Additionally, melanocytes are abundant in brain meninges (Painter et al., 2000), but their function there is still unclear. All these extracutaneous cranial compartment melanocytes might be important points of origin for malignant melanomas (Hussein, 2008). Recently, a new origin of melanocytes has been revealed in a number of species, in particular in mouse, chick, and fish (Adameyko et al., 2009, 2012; Budi et al., 2011; Dooley et al.,

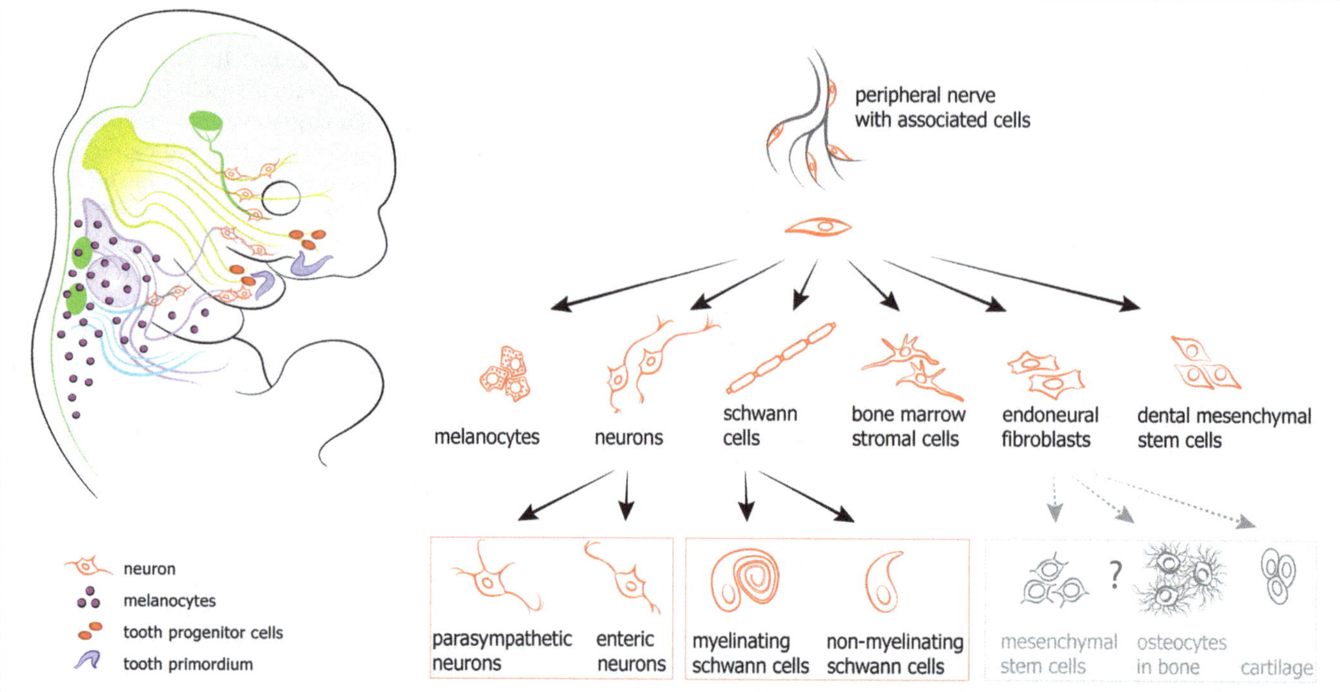


**FIGURE 5 | Peripheral nerves host and transport neural crest-derived associated glial cells that give rise to a number of cell types in developing body. Left:** examples and position of nerve-derived cell types. A significant number of melanocytes (purple circles on a scheme) in a head-neck region is produced from recruited Schwann cell precursors. Additionally, some mesenchymal progenitors in developing teeth (shown as red ellipses) are also recruited from the peripheral nerves. At the same time all parasympathetic neurons in the head are derived from nerve-associated cells. **Right:** the spectrum of currently confirmed nerve-derived cell types.

2013; Nitzan et al., 2013). In all of those cases melanocytes have been produced not only by NCCs directly, but also from nerve-associated glial cells: SCPs. In the mouse, the first melanoblasts appear inside of the IXth and Xth cranial nerves in the E9.5 embryo. These melanoblasts migrate outwards to subepithelial spaces 1 day later to extensively proliferate and populate all adjacent areas. Other facial nerves produce melanocytes as well. Edn3 and Kit ligand are essential signals for propagating these nerve-derived melanocytes in the head and neck (see Adameyko et al., 2012).

The close association of melanocyte progenitors with nerves may provide a logic for neural crest evolution (Ivashkin and Adameyko, 2013) and explain how melanocytes can find routes to the iris and interior of the cochlea, as well as to other locations deep inside of the head (Adameyko and Lallemend, 2010).

## Nerve-Derived Mesenchymal Stem Cells Participate in Tooth Development and Repair

Peripheral ganglia and nerves together with associated glia, to a large extent derived from migratory NCCs, develop and target all parts of the head, starting from relatively early embryonic stages. In mice the tooth pulp receives its nerve supply very late (P3-4) in comparison to the surrounding mesenchymal tissue, which is densely innervated already early (E12.5) when tooth placodes are formed (Fried et al., 2000). There has been substantial interest in the potential of SCPs to act as multipotent progenitor cells of the PNS. Considering the significant inherent plasticity of the niche containing SCPs, it could constitute a cellular reservoir during tooth organogenesis. Technically, it has been a daunting task to address this issue, since both ectomesenchymal cells and glial cells of the peripheral nerve are of neural crest origin. However, mouse strains that allow for selective genetic labeling of peripheral glial cells have provided a tool for this purpose (Adameyko et al., 2009, 2012). Results from studies on PLP-CreERT2 and Sox10-CreERT2 mice have demonstrated that SCP-derived cells in the surrounding area of developing teeth contribute with pulp cells as well as odontoblasts in a clonal pattern (Kaukua et al., 2014). This mechanism continues to operate also in the adult, as determined in the continuously growing mouse incisor. Furthermore, the generation of SCP-derived progeny of dental MSCs and odontoblasts is impaired after denervation (Kaukua et al., 2014).

It is interesting to consider the novel model of glial-assisted tooth development and growth (Kaukua et al., 2014) in light of earlier proposals that the tooth, from an evolutionary aspect, is a primary sensory organ. According to this view, dentin is a tissue that developed in order to protect and enhance the sensitivity of a pre-historical sensory organ (Gans and Northcutt, 1983). This fits well with the fact that matrix-producing odontoblasts are intimately associated with sensory nerve endings that transduce somatic signals (experienced as pain) in the mammalian tooth (Magloire et al., 2009, 2010). Odontoblasts could then be seen as adapted terminal glial cells, similar to the modified Schwann cells that enfold nerve fibers in sensory end-organs in the skin such as e.g. Meissner's and Pacinian corpuscles.

## Peripheral Glial Cells Might Mediate Important Signals during Development and Regeneration in the Head

The impact of the peripheral nervous system on wound healing and tissue regeneration in mammalian head has been under debate. Wounded pinna, the outer ear, serves as a model system to study regeneration in mammals. Mice from MRL/MpJ strain are capable of enhanced regeneration of the ear wounds as compared to the other strains, and such regenerative capacity is enhanced by the presence of the nerves densely surrounding regenerating tissue. Denervation of the ear leads to obliteration of regenerative capacity in this model system (Buckley et al., 2012).

In addition to this, genetic lineage tracing and clonal analysis of individual cells in denervated mouse limb tissues during regeneration demonstrated that cellular turnover, and differentiation from stem/progenitor cells remain functionally independent of nerve and nerve-derived factors. However, regenerated digit tips displayed patterning defects in bone and nail matrix. Interestingly, these nerve-depe ndent phenotypes mimic clinical observations of patients with nerve damage after spinal cord injury (Rinkevich et al., 2014). Recent discoveries from Jeremy Brockes' laboratory highlight the specific role of nerve-associated glial cells in regenerative blastema formation during regeneration of salamander tissues (Kumar et al., 2007; Kumar and Brockes, 2012). These studies demonstrated that the nerve-associated peripheral glial cells release nAG—anterograde signaling protein that initiates de-differentiation of multiple cell types in a wounded bodypart of salamander. Therefore, nerve-associated cells might be important integral components of the nerve that are responsible for the crosstalk between the nerve and innervated tissue during regeneration and healing. This is further supported by cellular and molecular mechanisms of neuro-vascular alignment, where embryonic peripheral glial cells release the signals that pattern and rebuild the vessels into arteries and arterioles during development of vertebrate embryos (Li et al., 2013).

The facts that nerves seem to be involved in the regeneration of injured mineralized mammalian limb tissue, and that nerve fiber glia is a reservoir of dental MSCs in the adult tooth, at least in the mouse incisor, could infer that nerve-borne cells might be mobilized after injury and contribute to regenerative and reparative events. Examinations in damaged mandibular incisors of adult PLP-CreERT2/R26YFP confirmed that SCP-derived cells were gathered at the site of damage, many of which had attained the characteristics of matrix-secreting odontoblasts. Pericytes, which have previously been shown to generate odontoblasts after injury (Feng et al., 2011), were excluded as an intermediate cell type in this case (Kaukua et al., 2014).

## Aligned Pericytes and Nerves: Strategies Converge

The vasculature of the dental pulp follows the same routes as the nerves, as in majority of locations in the head. A layer of loose connective tissue surrounds many arteries and nerves, forming a neurovascular bundle. This bundle constitutes a niche for MSCs that participate in both homeostasis and injury repair in teeth (Zhao et al., 2014). Previously, it has been shown that SCPs of peripheral nerves secrete CXCL12 that attracts the endothelial cells to align adjacent to the nerves during development (Li et al., 2013). This demonstrates the presence of a sophisticated system where nerves direct the development of an accompanying primary vessel network. A continued nerve-vessel crosstalk might also influence the neurovascular tissue homeostasis in the adult. This is indicated by studies of the development of the arterial innervation. Thus, in addition to vascular tone, sympathetic nerves also influence arterial maturation and growth through VEGF-dependent neurovascular synapses (Mukouyama et al., 2005).

Furthermore, the vasculature along peripheral nerves contains pericytes - contractile multifunctional cells that wrap around the endothelial cells of capillaries and venules within the vascular basement membrane (Sims, 1986). Cephalic pericytes in the forebrain seem to be neural crest-derived, as demonstrated in chick-quail chimeras (Etchevers et al., 2001; Korn et al., 2002) and in mice (Heglind et al., 2005). Pericytes in the other parts of the body are believed to be of mesodermal origin (Mills et al., 2013). It has been suggested that pericytes (also called adventitial or Rouget cells) may represent mesenchymal stem or progenitor cells (Crisan et al., 2008), since they can differentiate into a variety of MSC cell types, such as fibroblasts, chondroblasts, osteoblasts, odontoblasts, adipocytes, vascular smooth muscle cells, and myointimal cells (Díaz-Flores et al., 2006; Armulik et al., 2011; Feng et al., 2011). Some pericytes express markers characteristic for stem cells, such as Sca1 (Brachvogel et al., 2005) and STRO-1. STRO-1 is an early common marker for MSCs (Yoshiba et al., 2012). It has been demonstrated that upon tissue damage pericytes leave the perivascular space and generate myofibroblasts, thus playing a central role in organ fibrosis after injury. Ablating these cells ameliorates fibrosis and rescues organ function (Kramann et al., 2015). Moreover, a specific pericyte subtype gives rise to scar-forming stromal cells in CNS after the injury (Göritz et al., 2011). Ablation of these cells results in failure to seal the damaged CNS. In the continuously growing mouse incisor, pericytes play an important role in regeneration after the damage: they manage to leave the vessels and generate matrix-producing odontoblasts (Feng et al., 2011). Additionally, pericytes serve as a continuous cell source for matrix-laying cells at the very tip of the incisor. This region bears the maximum of the bite load, and wears out on a daily basis. In particular, pericytes generate streams of cells that obliterate the pulp cavity with hard matrix at the cutting surface of the tooth (Pang et al., 2015). Thus, pericytes play an important role in vascular development and homeostasis, are sources of fibrogenic cells in pathological situations, and may also serve as a reservoir of stem or progenitor cells for adult tissue repair in the cranial compartment.

The system of recruiting pericytes from vessels in development and regeneration strongly resembles the mechanism whereby peripheral glial cells are mobilized from nerves in the same processes. Here, we observe converging strategies that provide the developing or regenerating tissues with necessary progenitor cells. Thus, since craniofacial nerves and vessels usually are intimately associated, specific molecular signals may simultaneously engage both glial cells and pericytes for developmental and regenerative purposes in the head.

### Further Reading:

1. A paradigm shift in neurobiology: peripheral nerves deliver cellular material and control development (Ivashkin et al., 2014).
2. Nerves transport stem-like cells generating parasympathetic neurons (Adameyko and Ernfors, 2014).
3. Progenitors of the protochordate ocellus as an evolutionary origin of the neural crest (Ivashkin and Adameyko, 2013).
4. Glial versus melanocyte cell fate choice: Schwann cell precursors as a cellular origin of melanocytes (Adameyko and Lallemend, 2010).
5. A perivascular origin for mesenchymal stem cells in multiple human organs (Crisan et al., 2008).

## SUMMARY AND PERSPECTIVES

Recently, a growing amount of data has provided a deeper insight into how various cellular sources are coordinated and integrated during craniofacial development. The cranial nervous system, including the developing anterior neuroectoderm, brain, neurogenic placodes and peripheral nerves has appeared as an essential element in a number of regulatory interactions that result in a fully functional complex craniofacial organ.

Novel data on interactions between neurogenic placode-derived organs and their encasing cartilage or bone has improved the understanding of developmental coordination in a head. These processes are of utmost importance from an evolutionary perspective, since they will ensure the best functional outcome of cranial placode-derived sensory organs. A recently revealed brain-to-face interaction has highlighted a new degree of contribution of nervous system in the creation of the head. A plethora of functions of peripheral nerves in development was recently revealed. These nerves appear to serve as morphogenetic signal-releasing conduits as well as niches for multipotent glial cells that can be transformed into a spectrum of differentiated cell types in developing head. The importance of peripheral nerves in the cranial compartment is highlighted by a number of congenital or acquired pathologies associated with PNS development.

Taken together, it seems that neural components have co-evolved in tight coordination with other tissues and cell types in a head. Such a high degree of reciprocal influence should in principle increase developmental and evolutionary plasticity, and lead to optimal design and functional success. We anticipate that novel molecular interactions that aim to integrate various cell and tissue types soon will be discovered in craniofacial development. This will undoubtedly improve our fundamental understanding of coordinated growth strategies in this region of the body—an understanding that will benefit and empower the field of craniofacial regeneration.

## AUTHOR CONTRIBUTIONS

Both authors listed, have made substantial, direct and intellectual contribution to the work, and approved it for publication.

## ACKNOWLEDGMENTS

The authors received support from the Swedish Research Council and Karolinska Institutet (IA, KF), the Bertil Hållsten Research Foundation, the Åke Wiberg Foundation and ERC consolidator programme (IA). We thank Olga Kharchenko for illustrations.

## REFERENCES

Abe, M., Maeda, T., and Wakisaka, S. (2008). Retinoic acid affects craniofacial patterning by changing Fgf8 expression in the pharyngeal ectoderm. *Dev. Growth Differ.* 50, 717–729. doi: 10.1111/j.1440-169X.2008.01069.x

Abramowicz, A., and Gos, M. (2014). Neurofibromin in neurofibromatosis type 1—mutations in NF1gene as a cause of disease. *Dev. Period Med.* 18, 297–306.

Abzhanov, A., and Tabin, C. J. (2004). Shh and Fgf8 act synergistically to drive cartilage outgrowth during cranial development. *Dev. Biol.* 273, 134–148. doi: 10.1016/j.ydbio.2004.05.028

Adameyko, I., and Ernfors, P. (2014). Nerves transport stem-like cells generating parasympathetic neurons. *Cell Cycle* 13, 2805–2806. doi: 10.4161/15384101.2014.959854

Adameyko, I., and Lallemend, F. (2010). Glial versus melanocyte cell fate choice: Schwann cell precursors as a cellular origin of melanocytes. *Cell. Mol. Life Sci.* 67, 3037–3055. doi: 10.1007/s00018-010-0390-y

Adameyko, I., Lallemend, F., Aquino, J. B., Pereira, J. A., Topilko, P., Muller, T., et al. (2009). Schwann cell precursors from nerve innervation are a cellular origin of melanocytes in skin. *Cell* 139, 366–379. doi: 10.1016/j.cell.2009.07.049

Adameyko, I., Lallemend, F., Furlan, A., Zinin, N., Aranda, S., Kitambi, S. S., et al. (2012). Sox2 and Mitf cross-regulatory interactions consolidate progenitor and melanocyte lineages in the cranial neural crest. *Development* 139, 397–410. doi: 10.1242/dev.065581

Aguiar, D. P., Sghari, S., and Creuzet, S. (2014). The facial neural crest controls fore- and midbrain patterning by regulating Foxg1 expression through Smad1 activity. *Development* 141, 2494–2505. doi: 10.1242/dev.101790

Anthwal, N., and Thompson, H. (2016). The development of the mammalian outer and middle ear. *J. Anat.* 228, 217–232. doi: 10.1111/joa.12344

Armulik, A., Genové, G., and Betsholtz, C. (2011). Pericytes: developmental, physiological, and pathological perspectives, problems, and promises. *Dev. Cell* 21, 193–215. doi: 10.1016/j.devcel.2011.07.001

Bao, B., Ke, Z., Xing, J., Peatman, E., Liu, Z., Xie, C., et al. (2011). Proliferating cells in suborbital tissue drive eye migration in flatfish. *Dev. Biol.* 351, 200–207. doi: 10.1016/j.ydbio.2010.12.032

Barlow, L. A., Chien, C. B., and Northcutt, R. G. (1996). Embryonic taste buds develop in the absence of innervation. *Development* 122, 1103–1111.

Basch, M. L., Brown, R. M. II., Jen, H. I., and Groves, A. K. (2016). Where hearing starts: the development of the mammalian cochlea. *J. Anat.* 228, 233–254. doi: 10.1111/joa.12314

Biegert, J. (1963). "The evaluation of characteristics of the skull, hands, and feet, for primate taxonomy," in *Classification and Human Evolution,* ed S. Washburn (New Brunswick, NJ; London: Aldine transaction), 166–145.

Bird, D. J., Amirkhanian, A., Pang, B., and Van Valkenburgh, B. (2014). Quantifying the cribriform plate: influences of allometry, function, and phylogeny in Carnivora. *Anat. Rec.* 297, 2080–2092. doi: 10.1002/ar.23032

Bloomquist, R. F., Parnell, N. F., Phillips, K. A., Fowler, T. E., Yu, T. Y., Sharpe, P. T., et al. (2015). Coevolutionary patterning of teeth and taste buds. *Proc. Natl. Acad. Sci. U.S.A.* 112, E5954–E5962. doi: 10.1073/pnas.1514298112

Brachvogel, B., Moch, H., Pausch, F., Schlötzer-Schrehardt, U., Hofmann, C., Hallmann, R., et al. (2005). Perivascular cells expressing annexin A5 define a novel mesenchymal stem cell-like population with the capacity to differentiate into multiple mesenchymal lineages. *Development* 132, 2657–2668. doi: 10.1242/dev.01846

Brownell, I., Guevara, E., Bai, C. B., Loomis, C. A., and Joyner, A. L. (2011). Nerve-derived sonic hedgehog defines a niche for hair follicle stem cells capable of becoming epidermal stem cells. *Cell Stem Cell* 8, 552–565. doi: 10.1016/j.stem.2011.02.021

Buckley, G., Wong, J., Metcalfe, A. D., and Ferguson, M. W. (2012). Denervation affects regenerative responses in MRL/MpJ and repair in C57BL/6 ear wounds. *J. Anat.* 220, 3–12. doi: 10.1111/j.1469-7580.2011.01452.x

Budi, E. H., Patterson, L. B., and Parichy, D. M. (2011). Post-embryonic nerve-associated precursors to adult pigment cells: genetic requirements and dynamics of morphogenesis and differentiation. *PLoS Genet.* 7:e1002044. doi: 10.1371/journal.pgen.1002044

Burr, H. S. (1916). The effects of the removal of the nasal pits in Ambystoma embryos. *J. Exp. Zool.* 20, 27–57. doi: 10.1002/jez.1400200202

Castillo, D., Seidel, K., Salcedo, E., Ahn, C., de Sauvage, F. J., Klein, O. D., et al. (2014). Induction of ectopic taste buds by SHH reveals the competency and plasticity of adult lingual epithelium. *Development* 141, 2993–3002. doi: 10.1242/dev.107631

Chai, Y., and Maxson, R. E. Jr. (2006). Recent advances in craniofacial morphogenesis. *Dev. Dynamics* 235, 2353–2375. doi: 10.1002/dvdy.20833

Chaudhary, S. C., Tang, X., Arumugam, A., Li, C., Srivastava, R. K., Weng, Z., et al. (2015). Shh and p50/Bcl3 signaling crosstalk drives pathogenesis of BCCs in Gorlin syndrome. *Oncotarget* 6, 36789–36814. doi: 10.18632/oncotarget.5103

Chen, C. P., Lee, C. C., Chang, T. Y., Town, D. D., and Wang, W. (2004). Prenatal diagnosis of mosaic distal 5p deletion and review of the literature. *Prenat. Diagn.* 24, 50–57. doi: 10.1002/pd.794

Chong, H. J., Young, N. M., Hu, D., Jeong, J., McMahon, A. P., Hallgrimsson, B., et al. (2012). Signaling by SHH rescues facial defects following blockade in the brain. *Dev. Dynamics* 241, 247–256. doi: 10.1002/dvdy.23726

Clouthier, D. E., Williams, S. C., Hammer, R. E., Richardson, J. A., and Yanagisawa, M. (2003). Cell-autonomous and nonautonomous actions of endothelin-A receptor signaling in craniofacial and cardiovascular development. *Dev. Biol.* 261, 506–519. doi: 10.1016/S0012-1606(03)00128-3

Colleran, G. C., Hayes, R., Kearns, G., Kavanagh, P., Moylett, E., and Lynch, S. A. (2014). Craniofacial bony defect with developmental abnormality of facial bones, dental malalignment and ectopic neural tissue in the internal auditory meati—a new syndrome? *Eur. J. Med. Genet.* 57, 302–305. doi: 10.1016/j.ejmg.2014.03.013

Couly, G., Creuzet, S., Bennaceur, S., Vincent, C., and Le Douarin, N. M. (2002). Interactions between Hox-negative cephalic neural crest cells and the foregut endoderm in patterning the facial skeleton in the vertebrate head. *Development* 129, 1061–1073.

Creus, L., Sanchez-Regaña, M., Salleras, M., Chaussade, V., and Umbert, P. (1994). Parry-Romberg syndrome associated with homolateral segmental vitiligo. *Ann. Dermatol. Venereol.* 121, 710–711.

Creuzet, S. E. (2009a). Regulation of pre-otic brain development by the cephalic neural crest. *Proc. Natl. Acad. Sci. U.S.A.* 106, 15774–15779. doi: 10.1073/pnas.0906072106

Creuzet, S. E. (2009b). Neural crest contribution to forebrain development. *Semin. Cell Dev. Biol.* 20, 751–759. doi: 10.1016/j.semcdb.2009.05.009

Creuzet, S. E., Martinez, S., and Le Douarin, N. M. (2006). The cephalic neural crest exerts a critical effect on forebrain and midbrain development. *Proc. Natl. Acad. Sci. U.S.A.* 103, 14033–14038. doi: 10.1073/pnas.0605899103

Crisan, M., Yap, S., Casteilla, L., Chen, C. W., Corselli, M., Park, T. S., et al. (2008). A perivascular origin for mesenchymal stem cells in multiple human organs. *Cell Stem Cell* 3, 301–313. doi: 10.1016/j.stem.2008.07.003

De Beer, G. (1937). *The Development of the Vertebrate Skull.* Chicago, IL: University of Chicago Press.

Demyer, W., Zeman, W., and Palmer, C. G. (1964). The face predicts the brain: diagnostic significance of median facial anomalies for holoprosencephaly (Arhinencephaly). *Pediatrics* 34, 256–263.

Díaz-Flores, L. Jr., Madrid, J. F., Gutiérrez, R., Varela, H., Valladares, F., Alvarez-Argüelles, H., et al. (2006). Adult stem and transit-amplifying cell location. *Histol. Histopathol.* 21, 995–1027.

Dooley, C. M., Mongera, A., Walderich, B., and Nüsslein-Volhard, C. (2013). On the embryonic origin of adult melanophores: the role of ErbB and Kit signalling in establishing melanophore stem cells in zebrafish. *Development* 140, 1003–1013. doi: 10.1242/dev.087007

Dupin, E., Creuzet, S., and Le Douarin, N. M. (2006). The contribution of the neural crest to the vertebrate body. *Adv. Exp. Med. Biol.* 589, 96–119. doi: 10.1007/978-0-387-46954-6_6

Dyachuk, V., Furlan, A., Shahidi, M. K., Giovenco, M., Kaukua, N., Konstantinidou, C., et al. (2014). Neurodevelopment. Parasympathetic neurons originate from nerve-associated peripheral glial progenitors. *Science* 345, 82–87. doi: 10.1126/science.1253281

Eames, B. F., and Schneider, R. A. (2005). Quail-duck chimeras reveal spatiotemporal plasticity in molecular and histogenic programs of cranial feather development. *Development* 132, 1499–1509. doi: 10.1242/dev.01719

Espinosa-Medina, I., Outin, E., Picard, C. A., Chettouh, Z., Dymecki, S., Consalez, G. G., et al. (2014). Neurodevelopment. Parasympathetic ganglia derive from Schwann cell precursors. *Science* 345, 87–90. doi: 10.1126/science.12 53286

Etchevers, H. C., Vincent, C., Le Douarin, N. M., and Couly, G. F. (2001). The cephalic neural crest provides pericytes and smooth muscle cells to all blood vessels of the face and forebrain. *Development* 128, 1059–1068.

Feng, J., Mantesso, A., De Bari, C., Nishiyama, A., and Sharpe, P. T. (2011). Dual origin of mesenchymal stem cells contributing to organ growth and repair. *Proc. Natl. Acad. Sci. U.S.A.* 108, 6503–6508. doi: 10.1073/pnas.1015449108

Franz-Odendaal, T. A. (2011). The ocular skeleton through the eye of evo-devo. Journal of experimental zoology. *Part B Mol. Dev. Evol.* 316, 393–401. doi: 10.1002/jez.b.21415

Fried, K., Nosrat, C., Lillesaar, C., and Hildebrand, C. (2000). Molecular signaling and pulpal nerve development. *Crit. Rev. Oral Biol. Med.* 11, 318–332. doi: 10.1177/10454411000110030301

Gans, C., and Northcutt, R. G. (1983). Neural crest and the origin of vertebrates: a new head. *Science* 220, 268–273. doi: 10.1126/science.220.4594.268

Gao, L., Guo, H., Ye, N., Bai, Y., Liu, X., Yu, P., et al. (2013). Oral and craniofacial manifestations and two novel missense mutations of the NTRK1 gene identified in the patient with congenital insensitivity to pain with anhidrosis. *PLoS ONE* 8:e66863. doi: 10.1371/journal.pone.0066863

Gitton, Y., Heude, E., Vieux-Rochas, M., Benouaiche, L., Fontaine, A., Sato, T., et al. (2010). Evolving maps in craniofacial development. *Semin. Cell Dev. Biol.* 21, 301–308. doi: 10.1016/j.semcdb.2010.01.008

Gopalakrishnan, U., Mahendra, L., Rangarajan, S., Madasamy, R., and Ibrahim, M. (2015). The Enigma behind Pituitary and Sella Turcica. *Case Rep. Dent.* 2015:954347. doi: 10.1155/2015/954347

Göritz, C., Dias, D. O., Tomilin, N., Barbacid, M., Shupliakov, O., and Frisén, J. (2011). A pericyte origin of spinal cord scar tissue. *Science* 333, 238–242. doi: 10.1126/science.1203165

Green, S. A., Simoes-Costa, M., and Bronner, M. E. (2015). Evolution of vertebrates as viewed from the crest. *Nature* 520, 474–482. doi: 10.1038/nature14436

Grenier, J., Teillet, M. A., Grifone, R., Kelly, R. G., and Duprez, D. (2009). Relationship between neural crest cells and cranial mesoderm during head muscle development. *PLoS ONE* 4:e4381. doi: 10.1371/journal.pone.0004381

Grocott, T., Tambalo, M., and Streit, A. (2012). The peripheral sensory nervous system in the vertebrate head: a gene regulatory perspective. *Dev. Biol.* 370, 3–23. doi: 10.1016/j.ydbio.2012.06.028

Gross, J. B., and Hanken, J. (2008). Review of fate-mapping studies of osteogenic cranial neural crest in vertebrates. *Dev. Biol.* 317, 389–400. doi: 10.1016/j.ydbio.2008.02.046

Groves, A. K., and LaBonne, C. (2014). Setting appropriate boundaries: fate, patterning and competence at the neural plate border. *Dev. Biol.* 389, 2–12. doi: 10.1016/j.ydbio.2013.11.027

Gunhaga, L. (2011). The lens: a classical model of embryonic induction providing new insights into cell determination in early development. *Philos. Trans. R. Soc. Lond. B Biol. Sci.* 366, 1193–1203. doi: 10.1098/rstb.2010.0175

Hallgrímsson, B., and Lieberman, D. E. (2008). Mouse models and the evolutionary developmental biology of the skull. *Integr. Comp. Biol.* 48, 373–384. doi: 10.1093/icb/icn076

Hallgrímsson, B., Lieberman, D. E., Liu, W., Ford-Hutchinson, A. F., and Jirik, F. R. (2007). Epigenetic interactions and the structure of phenotypic variation in the cranium. *Evol. Dev.* 9, 76–91. doi: 10.1111/j.1525-142X.2006.00139.x

Heglind, M., Cederberg, A., Aquino, J., Lucas, G., Ernfors, P., and Enerbäck, S. (2005). Lack of the central nervous system- and neural crest-expressed forkhead gene Foxs1 affects motor function and body weight. *Mol. Cell. Biol.* 25, 5616–5625. doi: 10.1128/MCB.25.13.5616-5625.2005

Helms, J. A., and Schneider, R. A. (2003). Cranial skeletal biology. *Nature* 423, 326–331. doi: 10.1038/nature01656

Henderson, J. H., Chang, L. Y., Song, H. M., Longaker, M. T., and Carter, D. R. (2005). Age-dependent properties and quasi-static strain in the rat sagittal suture. *J. Biomech.* 38, 2294–2301. doi: 10.1016/j.jbiomech.2004.07.037

Hodge, L. K., Klassen, M. P., Han, B. X., Yiu, G., Hurrell, J., Howell, A., et al. (2007). Retrograde BMP signaling regulates trigeminal sensory neuron identities and the formation of precise face maps. *Neuron* 55, 572–586. doi: 10.1016/j.neuron.2007.07.010

Hozumi, H., Takeda, K., Yoshida-Amano, Y., Takemoto, Y., Kusumi, R., Fukuzaki-Dohi, U., et al. (2012). Impaired development of melanoblasts in the black-eyed white Mitf(mi-bw) mouse, a model for auditory-pigmentary disorders. *Genes Cells* 17, 494–508. doi: 10.1111/j.1365-2443.2012.01603.x

Hu, D., and Marcucio, R. S. (2009a). Unique organization of the frontonasal ectodermal zone in birds and mammals. *Dev. Biol.* 325, 200–210. doi: 10.1016/j.ydbio.2008.10.026

Hu, D., and Marcucio, R. S. (2009b). A SHH-responsive signaling center in the forebrain regulates craniofacial morphogenesis via the facial ectoderm. *Development* 136, 107–116. doi: 10.1242/dev.026583

Hu, D., Marcucio, R. S., and Helms, J. A. (2003). A zone of frontonasal ectoderm regulates patterning and growth in the face. *Development* 130, 1749–1758. doi: 10.1242/dev.00397

Hu, D., Young, N. M., Xu, Q., Jamniczky, H., Green, R. M., Mio, W., et al. (2015). Signals from the brain induce variation in avian facial shape. *Dev. Dynamics.* doi: 10.1002/dvdy.24284. [Epub ahead of print].

Hussein, M. R. (2008). Extracutaneous malignant melanomas. *Cancer Invest.* 26, 516–534. doi: 10.1080/07357900701781762

Isern, J., García-García, A., Martín, A. M., Arranz, L., Martín-Pérez, D., Torroja, C., et al. (2014). The neural crest is a source of mesenchymal stem cells with specialized hematopoietic stem cell niche function. *Elife* 3:e03696. doi: 10.7554/eLife.03696

Ivashkin, E., and Adameyko, I. (2013). Progenitors of the protochordate ocellus as an evolutionary origin of the neural crest. *Evodevo* 4:12. doi: 10.1186/2041-9139-4-12

Ivashkin, E., Voronezhskaya, E. E., and Adameyko, I. (2014). A paradigm shift in neurobiology: peripheral nerves deliver cellular material and control development. *Zoology* 117, 293–294. doi: 10.1016/j.zool.2014.08.001

Jaalouk, D. E., and Lammerding, J. (2009). Mechanotransduction gone awry. *Nat. Rev. Mol. Cell Biol.* 10, 63–73. doi: 10.1038/nrm2597

Jack, R. E., and Schyns, P. G. (2015). The Human Face as a Dynamic Tool for Social Communication. *Curr. Biol.* 25, R621–R634. doi: 10.1016/j.cub.2015.05.052

Jankowski, R. (2011). Revisiting human nose anatomy: phylogenic and ontogenic perspectives. *Laryngoscope* 121, 2461–2467. doi: 10.1002/lary.21368

Janowska, M., Podolec, K., Lipko-Godlewska, S., and Wojas-Pelc, A. (2013). Coexistence of Parry-Romberg syndrome with homolateral segmental vitiligo. *Postepy Dermatol. Alergol* 30, 409–411. doi: 10.5114/pdia.2013.39441

Jiang, R., Bush, J. O., and Lidral, A. C. (2006). Development of the upper lip: morphogenetic and molecular mechanisms. *Dev. Dynamics* 235, 1152–1166. doi: 10.1002/dvdy.20646

Joseph, N. M., Mukouyama, Y. S., Mosher, J. T., Jaegle, M., Crone, S. A., Dormand, E. L., et al. (2004). Neural crest stem cells undergo multilineage differentiation in developing peripheral nerves to generate endoneurial fibroblasts in addition to Schwann cells. *Development* 131, 5599–5612. doi: 10.1242/dev.01429

Jovovic-Dagovic, B., Ravic-Nikolic, A., Milicic, V., and Ristic, G. (2007). Bilateral nevus of Ota in a light-skinned woman. *Dermatol. Online J.* 13, 19.

Kaucká, M., and Adameyko, I. (2014). Non-canonical functions of the peripheral nerve. *Exp. Cell Res.* 321, 17–24. doi: 10.1016/j.yexcr.2013.10.004

Kaukua, N., Shahidi, M. K., Konstantinidou, C., Dyachuk, V., Kaucka, M., Furlan, A., et al. (2014). Glial origin of mesenchymal stem cells in a tooth model system. *Nature* 513, 551–554. doi: 10.1038/nature13536

Kersigo, J., D'Angelo, A., Gray, B. D., Soukup, G. A., and Fritzsch, B. (2011). The role of sensory organs and the forebrain for the development of the craniofacial shape as revealed by Foxg1-cre-mediated microRNA loss. *Genesis* 49, 326–341. doi: 10.1002/dvg.20714

Kish, P. E., Bohnsack, B. L., Gallina, D., Kasprick, D. S., and Kahana, A. (2011). The eye as an organizer of craniofacial development. *Genesis* 49, 222–230. doi: 10.1002/dvg.20716

Kivitie-Kallio, S., and Norio, R. (2001). Cohen syndrome: essential features, natural history, and heterogeneity. *Am. J. Med. Genet.* 102, 125–135. doi: 10.1002/1096-8628(20010801)102:2<125::AID-AJMG1439>3.0.CO;2-0

Knosp, W. M., Knox, S. M., Lombaert, I. M., Haddox, C. L., Patel, V. N., and Hoffman, M. P. (2015). Submandibular parasympathetic gangliogenesis requires sprouty-dependent Wnt signals from epithelial progenitors. *Dev. Cell* 32, 667–677. doi: 10.1016/j.devcel.2015.01.023

Korn, J., Christ, B., and Kurz, H. (2002). Neuroectodermal origin of brain pericytes and vascular smooth muscle cells. *J. Comp. Neurol.* 442, 78–88. doi: 10.1002/cne.1423

Kramann, R., Schneider, R. K., DiRocco, D. P., Machado, F., Fleig, S., Bondzie, P. A., et al. (2015). Perivascular gli1 progenitors are key contributors to injury-induced organ fibrosis. *Cell Stem Cell* 16, 51–66. doi: 10.1016/j.stem.2014.11.004

Kumar, A., and Brockes, J. P. (2012). Nerve dependence in tissue, organ, and appendage regeneration. *Trends Neurosci.* 35, 691–699. doi: 10.1016/j.tins.2012.08.003

Kumar, A., Godwin, J. W., Gates, P. B., Garza-Garcia, A. A., and Brockes, J. P. (2007). Molecular basis for the nerve dependence of limb regeneration in an adult vertebrate. *Science* 318, 772–777. doi: 10.1126/science.1147710

Kumari, A., Ermilov, A. N., Allen, B. L., Bradley, R. M., Dlugosz, A. A., and Mistretta, C. M. (2015). Hedgehog pathway blockade with the cancer drug LDE225 disrupts taste organs and taste sensation. *J. Neurophysiol.* 113, 1034–1040. doi: 10.1152/jn.00822.2014

Kurihara, Y., Kurihara, H., Maemura, K., Kuwaki, T., Kumada, M., and Yazaki, Y. (1995). Impaired development of the thyroid and thymus in endothelin-1 knockout mice. *J. Cardiovasc. Pharmacol.* 26(Suppl. 3), S13–S16. doi: 10.1097/00005344-199506263-00005

Laclef, C., Souil, E., Demignon, J., and Maire, P. (2003). Thymus, kidney and craniofacial abnormalities in Six 1 deficient mice. *Mech. Dev.* 120, 669–679. doi: 10.1016/S0925-4773(03)00065-0

Langenberg, T., Kahana, A., Wszalek, J. A., and Halloran, M. C. (2008). The eye organizes neural crest cell migration. *Dev. Dynam.* 237, 1645–1652. doi: 10.1002/dvdy.21577

Laranjeira, C., Sandgren, K., Kessaris, N., Richardson, W., Potocnik, A., Vanden Berghe, P., et al. (2011). Glial cells in the mouse enteric nervous system can undergo neurogenesis in response to injury. *J. Clin. Invest.* 121, 3412–3424. doi: 10.1172/JCI58200

Lassiter, R. N., Stark, M. R., Zhao, T., and Zhou, C. J. (2014). Signaling mechanisms controlling cranial placode neurogenesis and delamination. *Dev. Biol.* 389, 39–49. doi: 10.1016/j.ydbio.2013.11.025

Le Douarin, N. M., Brito, J. M., and Creuzet, S. (2007). Role of the neural crest in face and brain development. *Brain Res. Rev.* 55, 237–247. doi: 10.1016/j.brainresrev.2007.06.023

Le Douarin, N. M., Couly, G., and Creuzet, S. E. (2012). The neural crest is a powerful regulator of pre-otic brain development. *Dev. Biol.* 366, 74–82. doi: 10.1016/j.ydbio.2012.01.007

Lerner, A. B., Snell, R. S., Chanco-Turner, M. L., and McGuire, J. S. (1966). Vitiligo and sympathectomy. The effect of sympathectomy and alpha- melanocyte stimulating hormone. *Arch. Dermatol.* 94, 269–278. doi: 10.1001/archderm.1966.01600270019004

Li, W., Kohara, H., Uchida, Y., James, J. M., Soneji, K., Cronshaw, D. G., et al. (2013). Peripheral nerve-derived CXCL12 and VEGF-A regulate the patterning of arterial vessel branching in developing limb skin. *Dev. Cell* 24, 359–371. doi: 10.1016/j.devcel.2013.01.009

Li, Y. K., Yang, J. M., Huang, Y. B., Ren, D. D., and Chi, F. L. (2015). Shrinkage of ipsilateral taste buds and hyperplasia of contralateral taste buds following chorda tympani nerve transection. *Neural Regen Res.* 10, 989–995. doi: 10.4103/1673-5374.158366

Lieberman, D. E., Hallgrímsson, B., Liu, W., Parsons, T. E., and Jamniczky, H. A. (2008). Spatial packing, cranial base angulation, and craniofacial shape variation in the mammalian skull: testing a new model using mice. *J. Anat.* 212, 720–735. doi: 10.1111/j.1469-7580.2008.00900.x

Litsiou, A., Hanson, S., and Streit, A. (2005). A balance of FGF, BMP and WNT signalling positions the future placode territory in the head. *Development* 132, 4051–4062. doi: 10.1242/dev.01964

Little, H., Kamat, D., and Sivaswamy, L. (2015). Common neurocutaneous syndromes. *Pediatr. Ann.* 44, 496–504. doi: 10.3928/00904481-20151112-11

Lleras-Forero, L., and Streit, A. (2012). Development of the sensory nervous system in the vertebrate head: the importance of being on time. *Curr. Opin. Genet. Dev.* 22, 315–322. doi: 10.1016/j.gde.2012.05.003

Lumsden, A. G., and Buchanan, J. A. (1986). An experimental study of timing and topography of early tooth development in the mouse embryo with an analysis of the role of innervation. *Arch. Oral Biol.* 31, 301–311. doi: 10.1016/0003-9969(86)90044-0

Luther, A. (1924). Entwicklungsmekanische untersuchungen an labyrinth einiger Anuren. Comment. *Biol. Soc. Fenn.* 2, 1–24.

Macatee, T. L., Hammond, B. P., Arenkiel, B. R., Francis, L., Frank, D. U., and Moon, A. M. (2003). Ablation of specific expression domains reveals discrete functions of ectoderm- and endoderm-derived FGF8 during cardiovascular and pharyngeal development. *Development* 130, 6361–6374. doi: 10.1242/dev.00850

Magloire, H., Couble, M. L., Thivichon-Prince, B., Maurin, J. C., and Bleicher, F. (2009). Odontoblast: a mechano-sensory cell. *J. Exp. Zool.* 312b, 416–424. doi: 10.1002/jez.b.21264

Magloire, H., Maurin, J. C., Couble, M. L., Shibukawa, Y., Tsumura, M., Thivichon-Prince, B., et al. (2010). Topical review. Dental pain and odontoblasts: facts and hypotheses. *J. Orofac. Pain* 24, 335–349.

Maier, W., and Ruf, I. (2015). Evolution of the mammalian middle ear: a historical review. *J. Anat.* 228, 270–283. doi: 10.1111/joa.12379

Manni, M., and Maestroni, G. J. (2008). Sympathetic nervous modulation of the skin innate and adaptive immune response to peptidoglycan but not lipopolysaccharide: involvement of beta-adrenoceptors and relevance in inflammatory diseases. *Brain Behav. Immun.* 22, 80–88. doi: 10.1016/j.bbi.2007.06.016

Marcucio, R., Hallgrimsson, B., and Young, N. M. (2015). Facial morphogenesis: physical and molecular interactions between the brain and the face. *Curr. Top. Dev. Biol.* 115, 299–320. doi: 10.1016/bs.ctdb.2015.09.001

Marcucio, R. S., Young, N. M., Hu, D., and Hallgrimsson, B. (2011). Mechanisms that underlie co-variation of the brain and face. *Genesis* 49, 177–189. doi: 10.1002/dvg.20710

Matt, N., Dupé, V., Garnier, J. M., Dennefeld, C., Chambon, P., Mark, M., et al. (2005). Retinoic acid-dependent eye morphogenesis is orchestrated by neural crest cells. *Development* 132, 4789–4800. doi: 10.1242/dev.02031

Matt, N., Ghyselinck, N. B., Pellerin, I., and Dupé, V. (2008). Impairing retinoic acid signalling in the neural crest cells is sufficient to alter entire eye morphogenesis. *Dev. Biol.* 320, 140–148. doi: 10.1016/j.ydbio.2008.04.039

Mills, S. J., Cowin, A. J., and Kaur, P. (2013). Pericytes, mesenchymal stem cells and the wound healing process. *Cells* 2, 621–634. doi: 10.3390/cells2030621

Ming, J. E., Roessler, E., and Muenke, M. (1998). Human developmental disorders and the Sonic hedgehog pathway. *Mol. Med. Today* 4, 343–349. doi: 10.1016/S1357-4310(98)01299-4

Minoux, M., and Rijli, F. M. (2010). Molecular mechanisms of cranial neural crest cell migration and patterning in craniofacial development. *Development* 137, 2605–2621. doi: 10.1242/dev.040048

Mitsiadis, T. A., Cheraud, Y., Sharpe, P., and Fontaine-Pérus, J. (2003). Development of teeth in chick embryos after mouse neural crest transplantations. *Proc. Natl. Acad. Sci. U.S.A.* 100, 6541–6545. doi: 10.1073/pnas.1137104100

Miura, H., Kusakabe, Y., and Harada, S. (2006). Cell lineage and differentiation in taste buds. *Arch. Histol. Cytol.* 69, 209–225. doi: 10.1679/aohc.69.209

Moss, M. L., and Young, R. W. (1960). A functional approach to craniology. *Am. J. Phys. Anthropol.* 18, 281–292. doi: 10.1002/ajpa.1330180406

Mukouyama, Y. S., Gerber, H. P., Ferrara, N., Gu, C., and Anderson, D. J. (2005). Peripheral nerve-derived VEGF promotes arterial differentiation via neuropilin 1-mediated positive feedback. *Development* 132, 941–952. doi: 10.1242/dev.01675

Müller, F., and Rohrer, H. (2002). Molecular control of ciliary neuron development: BMPs and downstream transcriptional control in the parasympathetic lineage. *Development* 129, 5707–5717. doi: 10.1242/dev.00165

Murchison, E. P., Tovar, C., Hsu, A., Bender, H. S., Kheradpour, P., Rebbeck, C. A., et al. (2010). The Tasmanian devil transcriptome reveals Schwann cell origins of a clonally transmissible cancer. *Science* 327, 84–87. doi: 10.1126/science.1180616

Nedvetsky, P. I., Emmerson, E., Finley, J. K., Ettinger, A., Cruz-Pacheco, N., Prochazka, J., et al. (2014). Parasympathetic innervation regulates tubulogenesis in the developing salivary gland. *Dev. Cell* 30, 449–462. doi: 10.1016/j.devcel.2014.06.012

Nelhaus, G. (1970). Acquired unilateral vitiligo and poliosis of the head and subacute encephalitis with partial recovery. *Neurology* 20, 965–974. doi: 10.1212/WNL.20.10.965

Ni, C., Zhang, D., Beyer, L. A., Halsey, K. E., Fukui, H., Raphael, Y., et al. (2013). Hearing dysfunction in heterozygous Mitf(Mi-wh)/+ mice, a model for Waardenburg syndrome type 2 and Tietz syndrome. *Pigment Cell Melanoma Res.* 26, 78–87. doi: 10.1111/pcmr.12030

Nitzan, E., Pfaltzgraff, E. R., Labosky, P. A., and Kalcheim, C. (2013). Neural crest and Schwann cell progenitor-derived melanocytes are two spatially segregated populations similarly regulated by Foxd3. *Proc. Natl. Acad. Sci. U.S.A.* 110, 12709–12714. doi: 10.1073/pnas.1306287110

Noden, D. M., and Trainor, P. A. (2005). Relations and interactions between cranial mesoderm and neural crest populations. *J. Anat.* 207, 575–601. doi: 10.1111/j.1469-7580.2005.00473.x

Northcutt, R. G. (2008). Historical hypotheses regarding segmentation of the vertebrate head. *Integr. Comp. Biol.* 48, 611–619. doi: 10.1093/icb/icn065

Oakley, B., and Witt, M. (2004). Building sensory receptors on the tongue. *J. Neurocytol.* 33, 631–646. doi: 10.1007/s11068-005-3332-0

Ohyama, T., Groves, A. K., and Martin, K. (2007). The first steps towards hearing: mechanisms of otic placode induction. *Int. J. Dev. Biol.* 51, 463–472. doi: 10.1387/ijdb.072320to

Pagella, P., Jiménez-Rojo, L., and Mitsiadis, T. A. (2014). Roles of innervation in developing and regenerating orofacial tissues. *Cell. Mol. Life Sci.* 71, 2241–2251. doi: 10.1007/s00018-013-1549-0

Painter, T. J., Chaljub, G., Sethi, R., Singh, H., and Gelman, B. (2000). Intracranial and intraspinal meningeal melanocytosis. *Am. J. Neuroradiol.* 21, 1349–1353.

Pan, A., Chang, L., Nguyen, A., and James, A. W. (2013). A review of hedgehog signaling in cranial bone development. *Front. Physiol.* 4:61. doi: 10.3389/fphys.2013.00061

Pang, Y. W., Feng, J., Daltoe, F., Fatscher, R., Gentleman, E., Gentleman, M. M., et al. (2015). Perivascular stem cells at the tip of mouse incisors regulate tissue regeneration. *J. Bone Miner Res.* doi: 10.1002/jbmr.2717. [Epub ahead of print].

Park, B. Y., and Saint-Jeannet, J. P. (2008). Hindbrain-derived Wnt and Fgf signals cooperate to specify the otic placode in Xenopus. *Dev. Biol.* 324, 108–121. doi: 10.1016/j.ydbio.2008.09.009

Plock, J., Contaldo, C., and Von Lüdinghausen, M. (2007). Extraocular eye muscles in human fetuses with craniofacial malformations: anatomical findings and clinical relevance. *Clin. Anat.* 20, 239–245. doi: 10.1002/ca.20404

Reid, S. N., Ziermann, J. M., and Gondré-Lewis, M. C. (2015). Genetically induced abnormal cranial development in human trisomy 18 with holoprosencephaly: comparisons with the normal tempo of osteogenic-neural development. *J. Anat.* 227, 21–33. doi: 10.1111/joa.12326

Reiss, J. O. (1998). Anuran postnasal wall homology: an experimental extirpation study. *J. Morphol.* 238, 343–353.

Resende, L. A., Dal Pai, V., and Alves, A. (1991). Experimental study of progressive facial hemiatrophy: effects of cervical sympathectomy in animals. *Rev. Neurol. (Paris).* 147, 609–611.

Richtsmeier, J. T., and Flaherty, K. (2013). Hand in glove: brain and skull in development and dysmorphogenesis. *Acta Neuropathol.* 125, 469–489. doi: 10.1007/s00401-013-1104-y

Rinkevich, Y., Montoro, D. T., Muhonen, E., Walmsley, G. G., Lo, D., Hasegawa, M., et al. (2014). Clonal analysis reveals nerve-dependent and independent roles on mammalian hind limb tissue maintenance and regeneration. *Proc. Natl. Acad. Sci. U.S.A.* 111, 9846–9851. doi: 10.1073/pnas.14100 97111

Rinon, A., Lazar, S., Marshall, H., Büchmann-Møller, S., Neufeld, A., Elhanany-Tamir, H., et al. (2007). Cranial neural crest cells regulate head muscle patterning and differentiation during vertebrate embryogenesis. *Development* 134, 3065–3075. doi: 10.1242/dev.002501

Rizos, M., Negrón, R. J., and Serman, N. (1998). Mobius syndrome with dental involvement: a case report and literature review. *Cleft Palate Craniof. J.* 35, 262–268.

Sauka-Spengler, T., Meulemans, D., Jones, M., and Bronner-Fraser, M. (2007). Ancient evolutionary origin of the neural crest gene regulatory network. *Dev. Cell* 13, 405–420. doi: 10.1016/j.devcel.2007.08.005

Schlosser, G. (2010). Making senses development of vertebrate cranial placodes. *Int. Rev. Cell Mol. Biol.* 283, 129–234. doi: 10.1016/S1937-6448(10)83004-7

Schlosser, G. (2014). Development and evolution of vertebrate cranial placodes. *Dev. Biol.* 389, 1. doi: 10.1016/j.ydbio.2014.02.009

Schlosser, G. (2015). Vertebrate cranial placodes as evolutionary innovations—the ancestor's tale. *Curr. Top. Dev. Biol.* 111, 235–300. doi: 10.1016/bs.ctdb.2014.11.008

Schmalhausen, O. I. (1939). Role of the olfactory sac in the development of the cartilage of the olfactory organ in Urodela. *C.R. Acad. Sci. U.S.S.R.* 23, 395–398

Schneider, R. A., and Helms, J. A. (2003). The cellular and molecular origins of beak morphology. *Science* 299, 565–568. doi: 10.1126/science.1077827

Schütz, B., von Engelhardt, J., Gordes, M., Schafer, M. K., Eiden, L. E., Monyer, H., et al. (2008). Sweat gland innervation is pioneered by sympathetic neurons expressing a cholinergic/noradrenergic co-phenotype in the mouse. *Neuroscience* 156, 310–318. doi: 10.1016/j.neuroscience.2008.06.074

Scope, A., Barzilai, A., Trau, H., Orenstein, A., Winkler, E., and Haik, J. (2004). Parry-Romberg syndrome and sympathectomy—a coincidence? *Cutis* 73, 343–346.

Simões-Costa, M., and Bronner, M. E. (2015). Establishing neural crest identity: a gene regulatory recipe. *Development* 142, 242–257. doi: 10.1242/dev.105445

Sims, D. E. (1986). The pericyte—a review. *Tissue Cell* 18, 153–174. doi: 10.1016/0040-8166(86)90026-1

Smith, F. J., Percival, C. J., Young, N. M., Hu, D., Schneider, R. A., Marcucio, R. S., et al. (2015). Divergence of craniofacial developmental trajectories among avian embryos. *Dev. Dynamics* 244, 1158–1167. doi: 10.1002/dvdy.24262

Snowball, J., Ambalavanan, M., Whitsett, J., and Sinner, D. (2015). Endodermal Wnt signaling is required for tracheal cartilage formation. *Dev. Biol.* 405, 56–70. doi: 10.1016/j.ydbio.2015.06.009

Sperber, G., Sperber, S., and Guttmann, G. (2010). *Early Orofacial Development, Craniofacial Embryogenetics and Development.* Shelton, CT: People's Medical Publishing House.

Streit, A. (2007). The preplacodal region: an ectodermal domain with multipotential progenitors that contribute to sense organs and cranial sensory ganglia. *Int. J. Dev. Biol.* 51, 447–461. doi: 10.1387/ijdb.072327as

Sun, L., Yang, C., Ge, Y., Yu, M., Chen, G., Guo, W., et al. (2014). *In vitro* three-dimensional development of mouse molar tooth germs in a rotary cell culture system. *Inter. J. Paediatric Dentistry* 24, 175–183. doi: 10.1111/ipd.12057

Tachibana, M. (1999). Sound needs sound melanocytes to be heard. *Pigment Cell Res.* 12, 344–354. doi: 10.1111/j.1600-0749.1999.tb00518.x

Temiyasathit, S., and Jacobs, C. R. (2010). Osteocyte primary cilium and its role in bone mechanotransduction. *Ann. N. Y. Acad. Sci.* 1192, 422–428. doi: 10.1111/j.1749-6632.2009.05243.x

Thesleff, I. (2003). Epithelial-mesenchymal signalling regulating tooth morphogenesis. *J. Cell Sci.* 116, 1647–1648. doi: 10.1242/jcs.00410

Thompson, H., and Tucker, A. S. (2013). Dual origin of the epithelium of the mammalian middle ear. *Science* 339, 1453–1456. doi: 10.1126/science.1232862

Tokita, M., and Schneider, R. A. (2009). Developmental origins of species-specific muscle pattern. *Dev. Biol.* 331, 311–325. doi: 10.1016/j.ydbio.2009.05.548

Toro, S., and Varga, Z. M. (2007). Equivalent progenitor cells in the zebrafish anterior preplacodal field give rise to adenohypophysis, lens, and olfactory placodes. *Semin. Cell Dev. Biol.* 18, 534–542. doi: 10.1016/j.semcdb.2007.04.003

Ueno, H., Ferrari, G., Hattori, T., Saban, D. R., Katikireddy, K. R., Chauhan, S. K., et al. (2012). Dependence of corneal stem/progenitor cells on ocular surface innervation. *Invest. Ophthalmol. Vis. Sci.* 53, 867–872. doi: 10.1167/iovs.11-8438

Uesaka, T., Nagashimada, M., and Enomoto, H. (2015). Neuronal differentiation in schwann cell lineage underlies postnatal neurogenesis in the enteric nervous system. *J. Neurosci.* 35, 9879–9888. doi: 10.1523/JNEUROSCI.1239-15.2015

van Geel, N., Mollet, I., Brochez, L., Dutré, M., De Schepper, S., Verhaeghe, E., et al. (2012). New insights in segmental vitiligo: case report and review of theories. *Br. J. Dermatol.* 166, 240–246. doi: 10.1111/j.1365-2133.2011.10650.x

Van Ho, A. T., Hayashi, S., Bröhl, D., Auradé, F., Rattenbach, R., and Relaix, F. (2011). Neural crest cell lineage restricts skeletal muscle progenitor cell differentiation through Neuregulin1-ErbB3 signaling. *Dev. Cell* 21, 273–287. doi: 10.1016/j.devcel.2011.06.019

Van Valkenburgh, B., Smith, T. D., and Craven, B. A. (2014). Tour of a labyrinth: exploring the vertebrate nose. *Anat. Rec. (Hoboken).* 297, 1975–1984. doi: 10.1002/ar.23021

Vasudevan, P. C., Garcia-Minaur, S., Botella, M. P., Perez-Aytes, A., Shannon, N. L., and Quarrell, O. W. (2005). Microcephaly-lymphoedema-chorioretinal dysplasia: three cases to delineate the facial phenotype and review of the literature. *Clin. Dysmorphol.* 14, 109–116. doi: 10.1097/00019605-200507000-00001

Vix, J., Mathis, S., Lacoste, M., Guillevin, R., and Neau, J. P. (2015). Neurological manifestations in parry-romberg syndrome: 2 case reports. *Medicine* 94:e1147. doi: 10.1097/md.0000000000001147

Walker, M. B., and Trainor, P. A. (2006). Craniofacial malformations: intrinsic vs extrinsic neural crest cell defects in Treacher Collins and 22q11 deletion syndromes. *Clin. Genet.* 69, 471–479. doi: 10.1111/j.0009-9163.2006.00615.x

White, R. J., and Schilling, T. F. (2008). How degrading: Cyp26s in hindbrain development. *Dev. Dynamics* 237, 2775–2790. doi: 10.1002/dvdy.21695

Wu, C. S., Yu, H. S., Chang, H. R., Yu, C. L., Yu, C. L., and Wu, B. N. (2000). Cutaneous blood flow and adrenoceptor response increase in segmental-type vitiligo lesions. *J. Dermatol. Sci.* 23, 53–62. doi: 10.1016/S0923-1811(99)00090-0

Xiao, Y., Thoresen, D. T., Williams, J. S., Wang, C., Perna, J., Petrova, R., et al. (2015). Neural Hedgehog signaling maintains stem cell renewal in the sensory touch dome epithelium. *Proc. Natl. Acad. Sci. U.S.A.* 112, 7195–7200. doi: 10.1073/pnas.1504177112

Yamamoto, Y., Espinasa, L., Stock, D. W., and Jeffery, W. R. (2003). Development and evolution of craniofacial patterning is mediated by eye-dependent and -independent processes in the cavefish Astyanax. *Evol. Dev.* 5, 435–446. doi: 10.1046/j.1525-142X.2003.03050.x

Yoshiba, N., Yoshiba, K., Ohkura, N., Shigetani, Y., Takei, E., Hosoya, A., et al. (2012). Immunohistochemical analysis of two stem cell markers of alpha-smooth muscle actin and STRO-1 during wound healing of human dental pulp. *Histochem. Cell Biol.* 138, 583–592. doi: 10.1007/s00418-012-0978-4

Young, N. M., Hu, D., Lainoff, A. J., Smith, F. J., Diaz, R., Tucker, A. S., et al. (2014). Embryonic bauplans and the developmental origins of facial diversity and constraint. *Development* 141, 1059–1063. doi: 10.1242/dev.099994

Zhao, H., Feng, J., Seidel, K., Shi, S., Klein, O., Sharpe, P., et al. (2014). Secretion of shh by a neurovascular bundle niche supports mesenchymal stem cell homeostasis in the adult mouse incisor. *Cell Stem Cell* 14, 160–173. doi: 10.1016/j.stem.2013.12.013

Zhu, X., Gleiberman, A. S., and Rosenfeld, M. G. (2007). Molecular physiology of pituitary development: signaling and transcriptional networks. *Physiol. Rev.* 87, 933–963. doi: 10.1152/physrev.00006.2006

8

# The Perivascular Niche and Self-Renewal of Stem Cells

**Edited by:**
*Thimios Mitsiadis,*
*University of Zurich, Switzerland*

***Correspondence:**
*Jacques E. Nör*
*jenor@umich.edu*

*Min Oh* [1] *and Jacques E. Nör* [1,2,3]*

[1] *Department of Cariology, Restorative Sciences, Endodontics, University of Michigan School of Dentistry, Ann Arbor, MI, USA,* [2] *Department of Otolaryngology, University of Michigan School of Medicine, Ann Arbor, MI, USA,* [3] *Department of Biomedical Engineering, University of Michigan College of Engineering, Ann Arbor, MI, USA*

Postnatal stem cells are typically found in niches that provide signaling cues to maintain their self-renewal and multipotency. While stem cell populations may serve distinct purposes within their tissue of origin, understanding the conserved biology of stem cells and their respective niches provides insights to the behavior of these cells during homeostasis and tissue repair. Here, we discuss perivascular niches of two distinct stem cell populations (i.e., hematopoietic stem cells, mesenchymal stem cells) and explore mechanisms that sustain these stem cells postnatally. We highlight work that demonstrates the impact of cellular crosstalk to stem cell self-renewal and maintenance of functional perivascular niches. We also discuss the importance of the crosstalk within the perivascular niche to the biology of stem cells, and describe the regenerative potential of perivascular cells. We postulate that signaling events that establish and/or stabilize the perivascular niche, particularly through the modulation of self-renewing factors, are key to the long-term success of regenerated tissues.

**Keywords: regenerative endodontics, perivascular niche, inflammation, wound healing, tissue engineering**

## INTRODUCTION

Physiological stem cells enable tissue regeneration and repair. Vacanti and colleagues postulated that knowledge generated through research guided toward the regeneration of living tissues could lead to the cure of certain congenital and hereditary disorders, as well as to the development of strategies for tissue engineering that could address the shortage of donor tissues/organs (Vacanti and Langer, 1999). Successful regeneration of living tissues and/or organs that integrate functionally and properly within the host could also improve the quality of life of patients. Here, we highlight the role of postnatal stem cell populations in tissue repair and regeneration, with focus on their microenvironment (i.e., their niche). Stem cells are maintained in specialized niches, where they are relatively quiescent until external signals (e.g., wound) disrupt this equilibrium and drive their fate through downstream lineages that result in fully differentiated cells. Understanding the biology of these stem cell niches and mechanisms that drive stem cell fate can ultimately provide insights into potential signaling targets that can be exploited to regenerate functional tissues.

### Hematopoietic Stem Cells

Seminal work led to the identification of hematopoietic progenitor populations that are multipotent and self-renewing (Thomas et al., 1957; Till and McCulloch, 1961; Morrison et al., 1997). Thomas and colleagues introduced the concept of utilizing hematopoietic stem cells (HSC) for regenerative medicine when they infused intravenously suspensions of bone marrow-derived cells into patients that underwent radiation and chemotherapy

(Thomas et al., 1957, 1975a). These initial findings led to the development of therapies based on bone marrow transplantation that are now commonly utilized to repopulate lost hematopoietic stem cells (Thomas et al., 1957, 1975a,b). In association with the discovery of HSCs within the bone marrow, these findings contributed significantly to the use of multipotent and self-renewing cell populations for regenerative medicine (Till and McCulloch, 1961). The long-term survival rates of patients, and the existence of donor cells within the bone marrow of long-term survivors, provided compelling evidence that self-renewing cells reside within the bone marrow (Storb et al., 1969; Thomas et al., 1975b). Importantly, evidence of spleen colony-forming cells, derived from stem cell populations, suggested that stem cells reside in "niches" (Becker et al., 1963; Siminovitch et al., 1963; Schofield, 1978).

Several studies exhibited evidence of a perivascular niche for the maintenance of hematopoietic stem cells *in vitro* and *in vivo* (Cardier and Barberá-Guillem, 1997; Ohneda et al., 1998; Li et al., 2004; Kiel et al., 2005; Yao et al., 2005; Ding et al., 2012; Corselli et al., 2013). Kiel and colleagues concluded that hematopoietic stem cells within the spleen and bone marrow were associated with the sinusoidal endothelium, suggesting a perivascular niche (Kiel et al., 2005). Others demonstrated that hematopoietic stem cells localize to heterogeneous vascular niches in the bone marrow including arteries and arterioles, and suggested that these niches regulate their quiescence (Bourke et al., 2009; Kunisaki et al., 2013; Nombela-Arrieta et al., 2013). Indeed, the evidence illustrated that these perivascular niches are comprised of various cell types, each possessing a distinct function to contribute to the maintenance of hematopoietic stem cells. For instance, mesenchymal stromal cells secrete key factors including stem cell factor (SCF) and CXCL12 that contribute to the function of the perivascular niche, and the biology of hematopoietic stem cells (Sugiyama et al., 2006; Méndez-Ferrer et al., 2010; Greenbaum et al., 2013). Notably, emerging evidence suggests that endothelial cell-secreted factors play a critical role in the maintenance of hematopoietic stem cells.

Endothelial cell-secreted factors enabled hematopoietic stem cells to produce a significantly higher number of CFU-$S_8$ counts when compared to controls, suggesting that these factors enhance the proliferation and/or survival of the stem cell subpopulation (Li et al., 2004). Conditional knockout mice provided further support to the function of stem cell factor (SCF) to the survival of hematopoietic stem cells. When Ding and colleagues utilized a tamoxifen-inducible conditional knockout system for SCF (*Ubc-creER; Scf*$^{fl/fl}$), the hematopoietic stem cell population (CD150$^+$CD48$^-$Lin$^-$Sca1$^+$c-Kit$^+$) was depleted within the bone marrow and spleen postnatally (Ding et al., 2012). As SCF is a ligand for c-Kit, and inhibiting c-Kit resulted in the loss of hematopoietic progenitor cells, these results suggested that SCF is required for postnatal HSC maintenance (Zsebo et al., 1990; Ogawa et al., 1991; Ding et al., 2012). Furthermore, when they conditionally deleted *Scf* from endothelial cells (*Tie2-Cre; Scf*$^{fl/-}$), the fraction of hematopoietic stem cells decreased significantly (Ding et al., 2012). These observations were confirmed by selective deletion of gp130 expression in endothelial cells, utilizing Cre/*loxP*-mediated recombination (*Tie2-Cre;gp130*$^{flox/flox}$) (Yao et al., 2005). Collectively, several studies showed that endothelial cells are necessary for bone marrow homeostasis and regeneration, suggesting that signaling events mediated by endothelial cells play a major role in the maintenance of postnatal hematopoietic stem cells (Hooper et al., 2009; Butler et al., 2010; Kobayashi et al., 2010; Poulos et al., 2013).

## Mesenchymal Stem Cells

Friedenstein and colleagues discovered non-hematopoietic stem cells adherent to tissue culture conditions capable of forming fibroblastic colony forming units (CFU-F) (Friedenstein et al., 1970). Later coined as "mesenchymal stem cells" (MSC), these cell populations were self-renewing and were capable to give rise to multiple lineages (Caplan, 1991; Prockop, 1997; Pittenger et al., 1999; Bianco, 2007; Sacchetti et al., 2007). However, inconsistencies in defining mesenchymal stem cells presented various challenges to investigators within the field (Dominici et al., 2006). Emerging evidence showed that perivascular cells within the bone marrow exhibited characteristics of mesenchymal stem cells, forming a unique niche (Sacchetti et al., 2007; Méndez-Ferrer et al., 2010).

Perivascular cells were further investigated in various fetal and postnatal human tissues that identified these cell populations as mesenchymal stem cells (da Silva Meirelles et al., 2006; Crisan et al., 2008; Zannettino et al., 2008; Paul et al., 2012). Utilizing flow cell sorting, perivascular cells expressed mesenchymal stem cells markers (e.g., CD10, CD13, CD44, CD73, CD90, CD105) and did not express several markers for other cell types (e.g., CD56, CD106, CD133) (Crisan et al., 2008). Several studies proposed that pericytes exhibit the potential to commit to osteogenic, chondrogenic, and/or adipogenic lineages (Doherty et al., 1998; Farrington-Rock et al., 2004). Notably, long-term cultured perivascular cells possessed the ability to differentiate into mesenchymal stem cell lineages, including chondrocytes, multilocular adipocytes, and osteocytes (da Silva Meirelles et al., 2006; Crisan et al., 2008). Isolated pericytes formed mineralized nodules and structures resembling chondrocytes, and adipocytes both *in vitro* and *in vivo* (Doherty et al., 1998; Farrington-Rock et al., 2004). Furthermore, mRNA analysis of pericytes cultured in inductive conditions showed an upregulation of chondrogenic (i.e., Type II collagen, Sox9, aggrecan) and adipogenic (i.e., peroxisome proliferator-activated receptor gamma [PPAR-$\gamma$]) markers (Farrington-Rock et al., 2004). Further investigation into mesenchymal stem cell subpopulations in various tissues led to their identification and characterization within oral tissues, including teeth, periapical structures, and periodontal ligament.

Multipotent and self-renewing subpopulations of MSC-like cells was identified within the dental pulp of permanent (Gronthos et al., 2000) and primary teeth (Miura et al., 2003). Emerging evidence demonstrated that these dental stem cells are capable of differentiating into various other cell types, including osteoblasts (osteocytes), odontoblasts, and adipocytes (Gronthos et al., 2000; Miura et al., 2003). It has been also demonstrated that these cells can differentiate into neural cells (Nosrat et al., 2004; Sakai et al., 2012; De Berdt et al., 2015). Interestingly, these stem cells of dental origin have been implicated in partial recovery of movement when transplanted at spinal cord injury sites in laboratory animals (Sakai et al., 2012; De Berdt et al., 2015). And finally, work from our laboratory has demonstrated that dental pulp stem cells are capable of differentiating into vascular endothelial cells (Cordeiro et al., 2008; Sakai et al., 2010; Bento et al., 2013). Notably, these MSC-derived blood vessels are capable of forming anastomoses with the host vasculature to become functional, i.e., blood-carrying vessels (Cordeiro et al., 2008; Bento et al., 2013).

A perivascular niche was identified in postnatal mesenchymal stem cell populations within dental tissues, particularly the dental pulp (Shi and Gronthos, 2003; Machado et al., 2015). These cells residing near the dental pulp blood vessels exhibit hallmark features of stem cells, i.e., multipotency and self-renewal (**Figure 1**). Seminal work by Shi and colleagues utilized the putative marker STRO1 to identify mesenchymal stem cell subpopulations within the bone marrow and dental pulp, and to verify the potential existence of perivascular niches in these two tissues (Shi and Gronthos, 2003). When STRO1-positive bone marrow stem cells (BMSC) and DPSC were analyzed, they showed expression of pericyte markers ($\alpha$-smooth muscle actin, CD146) but not von Willebrand factor, a marker for platelets and endothelial cells (Shi and Gronthos, 2003). These findings suggested that these stem cell populations might reside in a perivascular niche and/or have the capacity to differentiate into other cell populations, such as pericytes.

As the origin and behavior of mesenchymal stem cell become better understood, more specific cellular markers can be identified and utilized to identify these cells for investigation or clinical application. Interestingly, recent studies explored potential markers that are more specific to mesenchymal stem cell populations. Lineage tracing studies on Gli1$^+$ cells within a murine incisor pulp suggested that Gli1 might be a possible marker for mesenchymal stem cells (Zhao et al., 2014). Utilizing an inducible tagging construct (*Gli1-CE;Zsgreen*) to follow Gli1$^+$ cells and their progenitors, ZsGreen$^+$ cells were expressed near the cervical loop of mouse incisors within 72 h. After 4-weeks, ZsGreen$^+$ cells populated the entire pulp mesenchyme up to the tip of the incisor suggesting that Gli1$^+$ cells were responsible for populating the dental pulp. Indeed, ZsGreen$^+$ cells were still detected when following Gli1$^+$ derivatives for up to 17.5 months, suggesting self-renewal of Gli1$^+$ mesenchymal cells (Zhao et al., 2014). Furthermore, Gli1$^+$ cells are found in networks around the vasculature, and Gli1$^+$PDGFR$\beta^+$ (platelet derived growth factor receptor-$\beta$) cells represent mesenchymal stem cell-like perivascular cells (Zhao et al., 2014; Kramann et al., 2015). The surface marker profile of these mesenchymal stem cell-like perivascular cells was maintained both in culture and *in vivo* (Kramann et al., 2015). Interestingly, as murine incisors develop continuously, dentinal development was severely stunted after vascular damage to the dental pulp, suggesting the functional relevance of the perivascular niche (Zhao et al., 2014). These findings further suggested that mesenchymal stem cell are located and maintained near the host vasculature.

Recent evidence further strengthened the hypothesis that DPSC reside in close proximity to blood vessels and nerves in the dental pulp tissue. These observations were derived from the identification of cells expressing the putative stem cell markers aldehyde dehydrogenase (ALDH)-1, CD90, and STRO1 in close proximity to pulp blood vessels (Machado

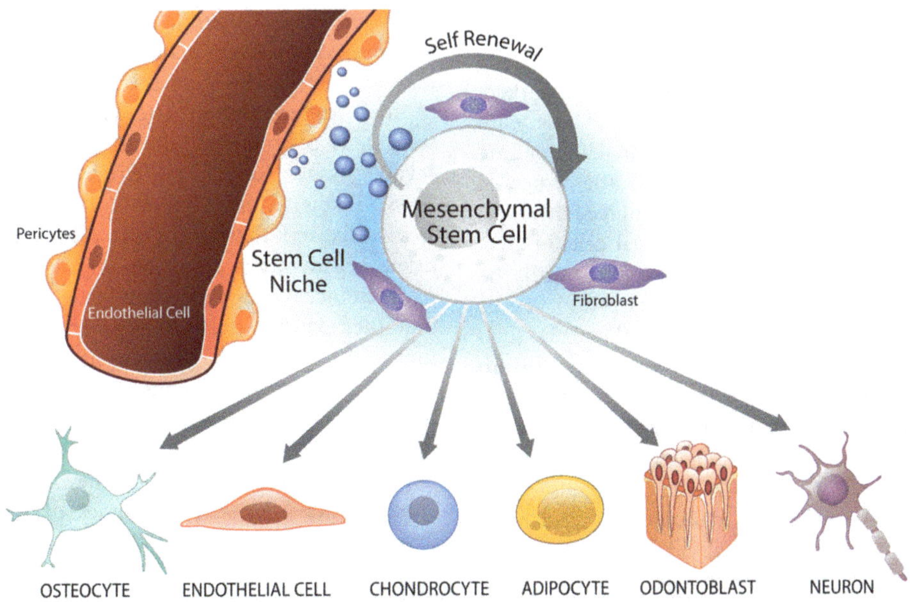


**FIGURE 1 | Perivascular niche and multipotency of mesenchymal stem cells (MSC).** Mesenchymal stem cells reside in perivascular niches where they undergo self-renewal and maintain the surrounding cells/tissue. Under specific signaling conditions, MSC can undergo differentiation into the osteoblastic (osteocytic), endothelial, chondrocytic, adipocytic, odontoblastic, and neural lineages.

et al., 2015). DPSC can generate spheroid bodies when cultured in ultra-low attachment conditions, suggesting the existence of a self-renewing subpopulation of cells within DPSC (Xiao et al., 2014). These self-renewing cells form and sustain growth of spheroid bodies in low attachment culture systems (Reynolds and Weiss, 1996; Weiss et al., 1996), particularly in presence of endothelial cell-derived factors. Collectively, these data demonstrated that endothelial cells serve as a source of factors that stimulate self-renewal of mesenchymal stem cells in the dental pulp, thus playing a critical role on the maintenance of the mesenchymal stem cell pool within perivascular niches.

## Stem Cell Niches and Dental Tissue Regeneration

While the presence of differentiated cells is critical for the function of tissues that have been regenerated, the ability to reconstitute the microenvironment that sustains stem cells is likely important for the successful long-term outcome of the tissue. In fact, it is possible that creation (or regeneration) of the stem cell niche might be sufficient for effective tissue regeneration. Targeting the perivascular niche via regeneration of the vasculature exhibited promising results in the context of dental pulp tissue engineering. A dentin/pulp-like complex was regenerated *in vivo* utilizing a tooth slice/scaffold model of dental pulp regeneration, where tooth slice/scaffolds from human third molars were seeded with SHED (stem cells from exfoliated deciduous teeth) cells and human dermal microvascular endothelial cells (HDMEC) and co-transplanted into the subcutaneous space of severe combined immunodeficient (SCID) mice (Cordeiro et al., 2008; Sakai et al., 2010; Bento et al., 2013). Interestingly, when SHED cells were treated with recombinant human vascular endothelial growth factor $(\text{rhVEGF})_{165}$ within tooth slice/scaffolds *in vitro*, they showed increased angiogenic potential and strong expression of endothelial cell markers (e.g., VEGFR2, PECAM1) (Sakai et al., 2010). These data suggested that these cells had the potential to differentiate into vascular endothelial cells in addition to the expected differentiation into odontoblasts. We observed that SHED cells have the potential to differentiate into endothelial cells *in vivo*, forming functional blood vessels that anastomized with the host vasculature becoming functional (blood-carrying) vessels (Cordeiro et al., 2008; Sakai et al., 2010; Bento et al., 2013). Such data suggested that a sub-population of the dental pulp stem cells could differentiate into tissue-specific odontoblasts while other sub-population may differentiate into vascular endothelial cells possibly recreating perivascular niches for stem cells in the regenerated tissue.

Recent evidence on the effects of endothelial cell-derived factors on head and neck squamous cell carcinoma (HNSCC) cells provided valuable insights on the cellular crosstalk within the perivascular niche. Endothelial cell-derived epidermal growth factor (EGF) promoted epithelial-mesenchymal transition (EMT) of HNSCC cells, endowing them with cancer stem cell characteristics (Zhang et al., 2014). As EMT has been linked to the acquisition of stem cell properties, it is without surprise that endothelial cell-derived EGF induced self-renewal via upregulation of Bmi-1 expression (Zhang et al., 2014). Interestingly, endothelial cells can also stimulate the self-renewal of neural stem cells (Shen et al., 2004). Neural stem cells co-cultured with endothelial cells exhibited delayed differentiation, shown by expression of neural progenitor markers (Nestin$^+$ and LeX$^+$) and an enhanced neural productive potential (Shen et al., 2004). These data further highlighted the significance of signaling within the perivascular niche for the biology of stem cells.

As stem cells are both, multipotent and self-renewing, a putative approach for tissue regeneration is based on the targeting of self-renewal factors to induce "stemness" of a sub-population of cells. Emulating the niche via controlled regulation of self-renewal pathways might allow stem cells to continue undergoing some level of asymmetric division, where one daughter cell would remain undifferentiated (i.e., self-renewal) while the other daughter cell would undergo differentiation (i.e., multipotency). Emerging evidence demonstrated the important role of self-renewal factors in dental tissue formation. For example, as Bmi-1 was shown to be a key regulator of neural stem cell self-renewal (Molofsky et al., 2003, 2005; Park et al., 2003) Bmi-1$^{-/-}$ mice incisors exhibited thinner dentinal and enamel layers (Biehs et al., 2013). These data illustrated that self-renewal is essential for odontogenesis, and suggested that this process is likely very important within the context of dental tissue engineering. We are currently designing experiments that will test this hypothesis.

## CONCLUSIONS

In summary, the interaction of stem cells with other cellular components of their niche is critical for self-renewal and the maintenance of the stem cell pool, and for the determination of their differentiation fate via multipotency. Mesenchymal stem cells play a vital role in the long-term maintenance of several tissues (da Silva Meirelles et al., 2006; Crisan et al., 2008). Likewise, emerging evidence suggest that mesenchymal stem cells and their niche are critically important for dental tissue regeneration by providing key molecular cues for the maintenance of diverse stem cells populations. We propose that therapeutic efforts to regenerate the stem cell niche are important for tissue engineering. Thus, studies focused on the understanding of conserved mechanisms regulating the biology of stem cell niches will provide valuable insights on the function and maintenance of stem cells, and may have a positive impact on the development of strategies that enhance the long-term outcomes of regenerated tissues and organs.

## ACKNOWLEDGMENTS

Funded by grant # T32-DE007057 (MO) and by R01-DE21410 from the NIH/NIDCR (JN).

## REFERENCES


Becker, A. J., McCulloch, E. A., and Till, J. E. (1963). Cytological demonstration of the clonal nature of spleen colonies derived from transplanted mouse marrow cells. *Nature* 197, 452–454. doi: 10.1038/197452a0

Bento, L. W., Zhang, Z., Imai, A., Nör, F., Dong, Z., Shi, S., et al. (2013). Endothelial differentiation of SHED requires MEK1/ERK signaling. *J. Dent. Res.* 1, 51–57. doi: 10.1177/0022034512466263

Bianco, P. (2007). Self-renewing mesenchymal progenitors in the bone marrow and in other mesodermal tissues. *J. Stem Cells Regen. Med.* 1, 44.

Biehs, B., Hu, J. K., Strauli, N. B., Sangiorgi, E., Jung, H., Heber, R. P., et al. (2013). BMI1 represses Ink4a/Arf and Hox genes to regulate stem cells in the rodent incisor. *Nat. Cell Biol.* 7, 846–852. doi: 10.1038/ncb2766

Bourke, V. A., Watchman, C. J., Reith, J. D., Jorgensen, M. L., Dieudonnè, A., and Bolch, W. E. (2009). Spatial gradients of blood vessels and hematopoietic stem and progenitor cells within the marrow cavities of the human skeleton. *Blood* 114, 4077–4080. doi: 10.1182/blood-2008-12-192922

Butler, J. M., Nolan, D. J., Vertes, E. L., Varnum-Finney, B., Kobayashi, H., Hooper, A. T., et al. (2010). Endothelial cells are essential for the self-renewal and repopulation of Notch-dependent hematopoietic stem cells. *Cell Stem Cell* 3, 251–264. doi: 10.1016/j.stem.2010.02.001

Caplan, A. I. (1991). Mesenchymal stem cells. *J. Orthop. Res.* 5, 641–650. doi: 10.1002/jor.1100090504

Cardier, J. E., and Barberá-Guillem, E. (1997). Extramedullary hematopoiesis in the adult mouse liver is associated with specific hepatic sinusoidal endothelial cells. *Hepatology* 1, 165–175. doi: 10.1002/hep.510260122

Cordeiro, M. M., Dong, Z., Kaneko, T., Zhang, Z., Miyazawa, M., Shi, S., et al. (2008). Dental pulp tissue engineering with stem cells from exfoliated deciduous teeth. *J. Endod.* 8, 962–969. doi: 10.1016/j.joen.2008.04.009

Corselli, M., Chin, C. J., Parekh, C., Sahaghian, A., Wang, W., Ge, S., et al. (2013). Perivascular support of human hematopoietic stem/progenitor cells. *Blood* 15, 2891–2901. doi: 10.1182/blood-2012-08-451864

Crisan, M., Yap, S., Casteilla, L., Chen, C. W., Corselli, M., Park, T. S., et al. (2008). A perivascular origin for mesenchymal stem cells in multiple human organs. *Cell Stem Cell* 3, 301–313. doi: 10.1016/j.stem.2008.07.003

da Silva Meirelles, L., Chagastelles, P. C., and Nardi, N. B. (2006). Mesenchymal stem cells reside in virtually all post-natal organs and tissues. *J. Cell Sci.* 11, 2204–2213. doi: 10.1242/jcs.02932

De Berdt, P., Vanacker, J., Ucakar, B., Elens, L., Diogenes, A., Leprince, J. G., et al. (2015). Dental apical papilla as therapy for spinal cord injury. *J. Dent. Res.* 11, 1575–1581. doi: 10.1177/0022034515604612

Ding, L., Saunders, T. L., Enikolopov, G., and Morrison, S. J. (2012). Endothelial and perivascular cells maintain haematopoietic stem cells. *Nature* 7382, 457–462. doi: 10.1038/nature10783

Doherty, M. J., Ashton, B. A., Walsh, S., Beresford, J. N., Grant, M. E., and Canfield, A. E. (1998). Vascular pericytes express osteogenic potential *in vitro* and *in vivo*. *J. Bone Miner. Res.* 5, 828–838. doi: 10.1359/jbmr.1998.13.5.828

Dominici, M., Le Blanc, K., Mueller, I., Slaper-Cortenbach, I., Marini, F., Krause, D., et al. (2006). Minimal criteria for defining multipotent mesenchymal stromal cells. The International society for cellular therapy position statement. *Cytotherapy* 4, 315–317. doi: 10.1080/14653240600855905

Farrington-Rock, C., Crofts, N. J., Doherty, M. J., Ashton, B. A., Griffin-Jones, C., and Canfield, A. E. (2004). Chondrogenic and adipogenic potential of microvascular pericytes. *Circulation* 15, 2226–2232. doi: 10.1161/01.CIR.0000144457.55518.E5

Friedenstein, A. J., Chailakhjan, R. K., and Lalykina, K. S. (1970). The development of fibroblast colonies in monolayer cultures of guinea-pig bone marrow and spleen cells. *Cell Tissue Kinet.* 4, 393–403. doi: 10.1111/j.1365-2184.1970.tb00347.x

Greenbaum, A., Hsu, Y. M., Day, R. B., Schuettpelz, L. G., Christopher, M. J., Borgerding, J. N., et al. (2013). CXCL12 in early mesenchymal progenitors is required for haematopoietic stem-cell maintenance. *Nature* 7440, 227–230. doi: 10.1038/nature11926

Gronthos, S., Mankani, M., Brahim, J., Robey, P. G., and Shi, S. (2000). Postnatal human dental pulp stem cells (DPSCs) *in vitro* and *in vivo*. *Proc. Natl. Acad. Sci. U.S.A.* 25, 13625–13630. doi: 10.1073/pnas.240309797

Hooper, A. T., Butler, J. M., Nolan, D. J., Kranz, A., Iida, K., Kobayashi, M., et al. (2009). Engraftment and reconstitution of hematopoiesis is dependent on VEGFR2-mediated regeneration of sinusoidal endothelial cells. *Cell Stem Cell* 3, 263–274. doi: 10.1016/j.stem.2009.01.006

Kiel, M. J., Yilmaz, O. H., Iwashita, T., Yilmaz, O. H., Terhorst, C., and Morrison, S. J. (2005). SLAM family receptors distinguish hematopoietic stem and progenitor cells and reveal endothelial niches for stem cells. *Cell* 7, 1109–1121. doi: 10.1016/j.cell.2005.05.026

Kobayashi, H., Butler, J. M., O'Donnell, R., Kobayashi, M., Ding, B. S., Bonner, B., et al. (2010). Angiocrine factors from Akt-activated endothelial cells balance self-renewal and differentiation of haematopoietic stem cells. *Nat. Cell Biol.* 11, 1046–1056. doi: 10.1038/ncb2108

Kramann, R., Schneider, R. K., DiRocco, D. P., Machado, F., Fleig, S., Bondzie, P. A., et al. (2015). Perivascular Gli1+ progenitors are key contributors to injury-induced organ fibrosis. *Cell Stem Cell* 1, 51–66. doi: 10.1016/j.stem.2014.11.004

Kunisaki, Y., Bruns, I., Scheiermann, C., Ahmed, J., Pinho, S., Zhang, D., et al. (2013). Arteriolar niches maintain haematopoietic stem cell quiescence. *Nature* 502, 637–643. doi: 10.1038/nature12612

Li, W., Johnson, S. A., Shelley, W. C., and Yoder, M. C. (2004). Hematopoietic stem cell repopulating ability can be maintained *in vitro* by some primary endothelial cells. *Exp. Hematol.* 12, 1226–1237. doi: 10.1016/j.exphem.2004.09.001

Machado, C. V., Passos, S. T., Campos, T. M., Bernardi, L., Vilas-Bôas, D. S., Nör, J. E., et al. (2015). The dental pulp stem cell niche based on aldehyde dehydrogenase 1 expression. *Int. Endod. J.* doi: 10.1111/iej.12511. [Epub ahead of print].

Méndez-Ferrer, S., Michurina, T. V., Ferraro, F., Mazloom, A. R., Macarthur, B. D., Lira, S. A., et al. (2010). Mesenchymal and haematopoietic stem cells form a unique bone marrow niche. *Nature* 466, 829–834. doi: 10.1038/nature09262

Miura, M., Gronthos, S., Zhao, M., Lu, B., Fisher, L. W., Robey, P. G., et al. (2003). SHED: stem cells from human exfoliated deciduous teeth. *Proc. Natl. Acad. Sci. U.S.A.* 100, 5807–5812. doi: 10.1073/pnas.0937635100

Molofsky, A. V., He, S., Bydon, M., Morrison, S. J., and Pardal, R. (2005). Bmi-1 promotes neural stem cell self-renewal and neural development but not mouse growth and survival by repressing the p16Ink4a and p19Arf senescence pathways. *Genes Dev.* 12, 1432–1437. doi: 10.1101/gad.1299505

Molofsky, A. V., Pardal, R., Iwashita, T., Park, I. K., Clarke, M. F., and Morrison, S. J. (2003). Bmi-1 dependence distinguishes neural stem cell self-renewal from progenitor proliferation. *Nature* 6961, 962–967. doi: 10.1038/nature02060

Morrison, S. J., Wandycz, A. M., Hemmati, H. D., Wright, D. E., and Weissman, I. L. (1997). Identification of a lineage of multipotent hematopoietic progenitors. *Development* 10, 1929–1939.

Nombela-Arrieta, C., Pivarnik, G., Winkel, B., Canty, K. J., Harley, B., Mahoney, J. E., et al. (2013). Quantitative imaging of haematopoietic stem and progenitor cell localization and hypoxic status in the bone marrow microenvironment. *Nat. Cell Biol.* 15, 533–543. doi: 10.1038/ncb2730

Nosrat, I. V., Smith, C. A., Mullally, P., Olson, L., and Nosrat, C. A. (2004). Dental pulp cells provide neurotrophic support for dopaminergic neurons and differentiate into neurons *in vitro*; implications for tissue engineering and repair in the nervous system. *Eur. J. Neurosci.* 9, 2388–2398. doi: 10.1111/j.0953-816X.2004.03314.x

Ogawa, M., Matsuzaki, Y., Nishikawa, S., Hayashi, S., Kunisada, T., Sudo, T., et al. (1991). Expression and function of c-kit in hemopoietic progenitor cells. *J. Exp. Med.* 1, 63–71. doi: 10.1084/jem.174.1.63

Ohneda, O., Fennie, C., Zheng, Z., Donahue, C., La, H., Villacorta, R., et al. (1998). Hematopoietic stem cell maintenance and differentiation are supported by embryonic aorta-gonad-mesonephros region-derived endothelium. *Blood* 3, 908–919.

Park, I. K., Qian, D., Kiel, M., Becker, M. W., Pihalja, M., Weissman, I. L., et al. (2003). Bmi-1 is required for maintenance of adult self-renewing haematopoietic stem cells. *Nature* 6937, 302–305. doi: 10.1038/nature01587

Paul, G., Özen, I., Christophersen, N. S., Reinbothe, T., Bengzon, J., and Visse, E. (2012). The adult human brain harbors multipotent perivascular mesenchymal stem cells. *PLoS ONE* 4:e35577. doi: 10.1371/journal.pone.0035577

Pittenger, M. F., Mackay, A. M., Beck, S. C., Jaiswal, R. K., Douglas, R., Mosca, J. D., et al. (1999). Multilineage potential of adult human mesenchymal stem cells. *Science* 5411, 143–147. doi: 10.1126/science.284.5411.143

Poulos, M. G., Guo, P., Kofler, N. M., Pinho, S., Gutkin, M. C., Tikhonova, A., et al. (2013). Endothelial Jagged-1 is necessary for homeostatic and regenerative hematopoiesis. *Cell Rep.* 5, 1022–1034. doi: 10.1016/j.celrep.2013.07.048

Prockop, D. J. (1997). Marrow stromal cells as stem cells for nonhematopoietic tissues. *Science* 5309, 71–74. doi: 10.1126/science.276.5309.71

Reynolds, B. A., and Weiss, S. (1996). Clonal and population analyses demonstrate that an EGF-responsive mammalian embryonic CNS precursor is a stem cell. *Dev. Biol.* 175, 1–13. doi: 10.1006/dbio.1996.0090

Sacchetti, B., Funari, A., Michienzi, S., Di Cesare, S., Piersanti, S., Saggio, I., et al. (2007). Self-renewing osteoprogenitors in bone marrow sinusoids can organize a hematopoietic microenvironment. *Cell* 2, 324–336. doi: 10.1016/j.cell.2007.08.025

Sakai, K., Yamamoto, A., Matsubara, K., Nakamura, S., Naruse, M., Yamagata, M., et al. (2012). Human dental pulp-derived stem cells promote locomotor recovery after complete transection of the rat spinal cord by multiple neuro-regenerative mechanisms. *J. Clin. Invest.* 1, 80–90. doi: 10.1172/JCI59251

Sakai, V. T., Zhang, Z., Dong, Z., Neiva, K. G., Machado, M. A., Shi, S., et al. (2010). SHED differentiate into functional odontoblasts and endothelium. *J. Dent. Res.* 8, 791–796. doi: 10.1177/0022034510368647

Schofield, R. (1978). The relationship between the spleen colony-forming cell and the haemopoietic stem cell. *Blood Cells* 4, 7–25.

Shen, Q., Goderie, S. K., Jin, L., Karanth, N., Sun, Y., Abramova, N., et al. (2004). Endothelial cells stimulate self-renewal and expand neurogenesis of neural stem cells. *Science* 5675, 1338–1340. doi: 10.1126/science.1095505

Shi, S., and Gronthos, S. (2003). Perivascular niche of postnatal mesenchymal stem cells in human bone marrow and dental pulp. *J. Bone Miner. Res.* 4, 696–704. doi: 10.1359/jbmr.2003.18.4.696

Siminovitch, L., McCulloch, E. A., and Till, J. E. (1963). The distribution of colony-forming cells among spleen colonies. *J. Cell. Physiol.* 62, 327–336. doi: 10.1002/jcp.1030620313

Storb, R., Epstein, R. B., Rudolph, R. H., and Thomas, E. D. (1969). Allogeneic canine bone marrow transplantation following cyclophosphamide. *Transplantation* 5, 378–386. doi: 10.1097/00007890-196905000-00007

Sugiyama, T., Kohara, H., Noda, M., and Nagasawa, T. (2006). Maintenance of the hematopoietic stem cell pool by CXCL12-CXCR4 chemokine signaling in bone marrow stromal cell niches. *Immunity* 6, 977–988. doi: 10.1016/j.immuni.2006.10.016

Thomas, E. D., Lochte, H. L. Jr., Lu, W. C., and Ferrebee, J. W. (1957). Intravenous infusion of bone marrow in patients receiving radiation and chemotherapy. *N. Engl. J. Med.* 11, 491–496. doi: 10.1056/NEJM195709122571102

Thomas, E. D., Storb, R., Clift, R. A., Fefer, A., Johnson, L., Neiman, P. E., et al. (1975b). Bone-marrow transplantation (second of two parts). *N. Engl. J. Med.* 17, 895–902.

Thomas, E., Storb, R., Clift, R. A., Fefer, A., Johnson, F. L., Neiman, P. E., et al. (1975a). Bone-marrow transplantation (first of two parts). *N. Engl. J. Med.* 16, 832–843.

Till, J. E., and McCulloch, E. A. (1961). A direct measurement of the radiation sensitivity of normal mouse bone marrow cells. *Radiat. Res.* 14, 213–222. doi: 10.2307/3570892

Vacanti, J. P., and Langer, R. (1999). Tissue engineering: the design and fabrication of living replacement devices for surgical reconstruction and transplantation. *Lancet* 1, S132–S134. doi: 10.1016/s0140-6736(99)90247-7

Weiss, S., Reynolds, B. A., Vescovi, A. L., Morshead, C., Craig, C. G., and van der Kooy, D. (1996). Is there a neural stem cell in the mammalian forebrain? *Trends Neurosci.* 19, 387–393.

Xiao, L., Kumazawa, Y., and Okamura, H. (2014). Cell death, cavitation and spontaneous multi-differentiation of dental pulp stem cells-derived spheroids *in vitro*: a journey to survival and organogenesis. *Biol. Cell* 12, 405–419. doi: 10.1111/boc.201400024

Yao, L., Yokota, T., Xia, L., Kincade, P. W., and McEver, R. P. (2005). Bone marrow dysfunction in mice lacking the cytokine receptor gp130 in endothelial cells. *Blood* 13, 4093–4101. doi: 10.1182/blood-2005-02-0671

Zannettino, A. C., Paton, S., Arthur, A., Khor, F., Itescu, S., Gimble, J. M., et al. (2008). Multipotential human adipose-derived stromal stem cells exhibit a perivascular phenotype *in vitro* and *in vivo*. *J. Cell. Physiol.* 2, 413–421. doi: 10.1002/jcp.21210

Zhang, Z., Dong, Z., Lauxen, I. S., Filho, M. S., and Nör, J. E. (2014). Endothelial cell-secreted EGF induces epithelial to mesenchymal transition and endows head and neck cancer cells with stem-like phenotype. *Cancer Res.* 10, 2869–2881. doi: 10.1158/0008-5472.CAN-13-2032

Zhao, H., Feng, J., Seidel, K., Shi, S., Klein, O., Sharpe, P., et al. (2014). Secretion of shh by a neurovascular bundle niche supports mesenchymal stem cell homeostasis in the adult mouse incisor. *Cell Stem Cell* 2, 160–173. doi: 10.1016/j.stem.2013.12.013

Zsebo, K. M., Williams, D. A., Geissler, E. N., Broudy, V. C., Martin, F. H., Atkins, H. L., et al. (1990). Stem cell factor is encoded at the Sl locus of the mouse and is the ligand for the c-kit tyrosine kinase receptor. *Cell* 1, 213–224. doi: 10.1016/0092-8674(90)90302-U

# 9

# Pulp Regeneration: Current Approaches and Future Challenges

**Edited by:**
Giovanna Orsini,
Università Politecnica delle Marche,
Italy

***Correspondence:**
Zhi Chen
zhichen@whu.edu.cn

*Jingwen Yang [1,2], Guohua Yuan [1,2] and Zhi Chen [1*]*

[1] *The State Key Laboratory Breeding Base of Basic Science of Stomatology (Hubei-MOST) and Key Laboratory of Oral Biomedicine Ministry of Education, School and Hospital of Stomatology, Wuhan University, Wuhan, China,* [2] *Department of Pediatric Dentistry, School and Hospital of Stomatology, Wuhan University, Wuhan, China*

Regenerative endodontics aims to replace inflamed/necrotic pulp tissues with regenerated pulp-like tissues to revitalize teeth and improve life quality. Pulp revascularization case reports, which showed successful clinical and radiographic outcomes, indicated the possible clinical application of pulp regeneration via cell homing strategy. From a clinical point of view, functional pulp-like tissues should be regenerated with the characterization of vascularization, re-innervation, and dentin deposition with a regulated rate similar to that of normal pulp. Efficient root canal disinfection and proper size of the apical foramen are the two requisite preconditions for pulp regeneration. Progress has been made on pulp regeneration via cell homing strategies. This review focused on the requisite preconditions and cell homing strategies for pulp regeneration. In addition to the traditionally used mechanical preparation and irrigation, antibiotics, irrigation assisted with EndoVac apical negative-pressure system, and ultrasonic and laser irradiation are now being used in root canal disinfection. In addition, pulp-like tissues could be formed with the apical foramen less than 1 mm, although more studies are needed to determine the appropriate size. Moreover, signaling molecules including stromal cell derived factor (SDF-1$\alpha$), basic Fibroblast Growth Factor (bFGF), Platelet Derived Growth Factor (PDGF), stem cell factor (SCF), and Granulocyte Colony-Stimulating Factor (G-CSF) were used to achieve pulp-like tissue formation via a cell homing strategy. Studies on the cell sources of pulp regeneration might give some indications on the signaling molecular selection. The active recruitment of endogenous cells into root canals to regenerate pulp-like tissues is a novel concept that may offer an unprecedented opportunity for the near-term clinical translation of current biology-based therapies for dental pulp regeneration.

**Keywords: regenerative endodontics, root canal disinfection, cell homing, stem cells, signaling molecules**

## INTRODUCTION

Infected dental pulp is traditionally removed and replaced with inorganic materials (paste and gutta percha) via root canal therapy (RCT). Dental pulp primarily provides nutrition and detects potential pathogens, and the loss of its vitality will increase fragility of the tooth. Therefore, RCT-treated teeth are destined to be devitalized, brittle, and susceptible to postoperative fracture. Thus, an effective treatment strategy is needed to regain vital dental pulp to treat dental pulp diseases. The emergence of modern tissue engineering and regenerative medicine has opened possibilities for regenerative endodontics (Nakashima and Iohara, 2011).

*In vitro* and *in vivo* animal studies have demonstrated great potential for pulp regeneration. Traditionally, three elements, namely (i) stem cells, (ii) scaffolds, and (iii) signaling molecules (e.g., growth factors), were used to achieve pulp regeneration. In the process of pulp regeneration, stem cells were first isolated and manipulated *in vitro*. Then, the cells were loaded onto scaffolds incorporated with signaling molecules and transplanted into the root canal of *ex vivo* tooth slides or *in situ* canine tooth. The formation of pulp-like tissues (connective tissues with blood vessel formation and dentin-like tissue deposition) was observed in many experimental studies (Nakashima and Iohara, 2011; Sun et al., 2014; Yang et al., 2015a,b).

Until now, both stem cell transplantation and cell homing strategies have been applied in pulp regeneration. In the strategy of cell transplantation, stem cells should first be isolated, expanded, seeded into the scaffold, and finally transplanted. Cell homing is aimed to achieve tissue repair/regeneration through recruiting of endogenous cells to injured tissue via signaling molecules. Compared with stem cell transplantation, cell homing strategies do not need to isolate and manipulate stem cells *in vitro*.

Pulp revascularization of immature teeth is a type of cell homing strategy for pulp regeneration in clinical application. It is a two-visit therapeutic approach, which has been proposed in clinical practice over the past decade (Thibodeau and Trope, 2007; Wigler et al., 2013). In this approach, the root canal system is filled with endodontic instrument-induced blood clot after disinfection with a combination of antibiotics. Some case reports have shown the blood flow and sensitiveness to cold or electric stimuli of the tissue are formed in the canal system. This supported the possible application of pulp regeneration strategy without stem cell transplantation for mature teeth in the clinic. However, histological studies have shown that most of the tissues formed in pulp revascularization cases were non-pulp-like tissues comprising cementum, periodontal, and bone-like tissues (Becerra et al., 2014). Moreover, the successful rate of pulp revascularization is low, mainly because of the difficulty in efficient disinfection or induction of blood clot in the canal. Therefore, further studies are needed to facilitate the formation of pulp-like tissues, to increase the success rate of pulp revascularization in immature teeth, and probably to apply this procedure or cell homing strategy in mature teeth.

Possible applications of pulp regeneration strategies continue to evolve, with significant prospects related to the regeneration of functional pulp tissues. The purpose of this review is to provide a detailed overview of present regenerative endodontic approaches aiming to revitalize teeth. From a clinical point of view, we focused on requisite preconditions (including root canal disinfection and enlargement of apical foramen) and cell homing strategies for pulp regeneration.

## REQUISITE PRECONDITIONS FOR PULP REGENERATION

Two preconditions are requisite to achieve pulp regeneration (**Figure 1**): (i) efficient root canal disinfection and (ii) proper size of the apical foramen.

During pulp inflammation, diverse oral and food-borne microorganisms invade the pulp space, form biofilm on canal walls, and infiltrate the dentinal tubules (Duggan et al., 2009). To promote regeneration, the pulp space and dentinal walls must be sufficiently disinfected before performing pulp regeneration procedures, and the required degree is possibly higher than that in traditional endodontic therapy (Fouad, 2011). Therefore, efficient root canal disinfection is required for pulp regeneration.

Mechanical preparation, sodium hypochlorite, and calcium hydroxide were the traditionally advocated substances to combat root canal infection in endodontics. However, these methods have been shown to be ineffective, mainly in cases of biofilm-related persistent infections. It was reported that 90% of the bacteria remain positive following irrigation with 10 ml 1.25%

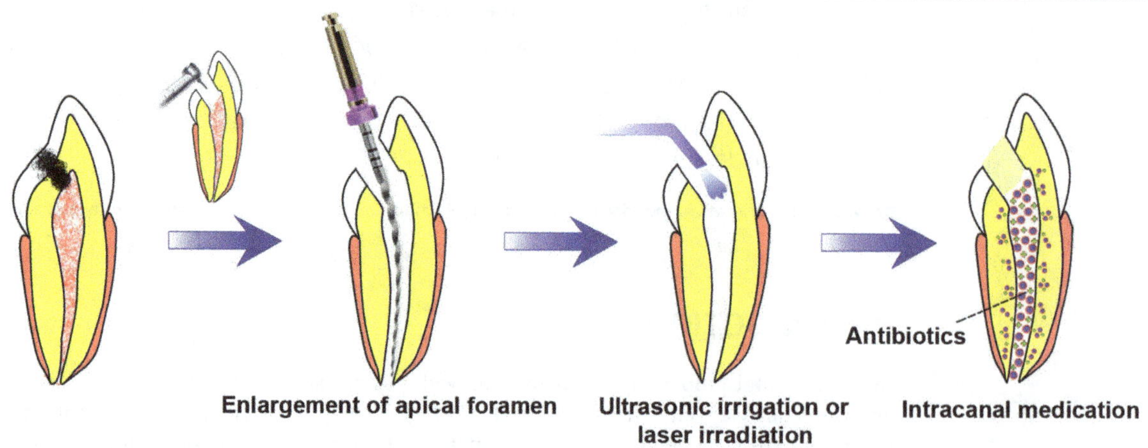


**FIGURE 1 | Requisite preconditions for pulp regeneration (root canal disinfection and enlargement of the apical foramen).** After mechanical preparation of the root canal combined with irrigation, the apical foramen should be enlarged to a proper size. Root canal disinfection could be achieved through intracanal medication combined with irrigation assisted with EndoVac apical negative-pressure system or ultrasonic and/or laser irradiation.

sodium hypochlorite (William et al., 2005). Recently, intracanal medication of antibiotics, EndoVac apical negative-pressure system of irrigation, ultrasonic-assisted irrigation, and laser irradiation have been introduced to disinfect root canals.

Clinical studies have proven the potency of triple antibiotic paste (TAP, a combination of metronidazole, ciprofloxacin, and minocycline) as the disinfectant during revascularization (Shivashankar et al., 2012; Vijayaraghavan et al., 2012). It was shown that only 30% of the bacteria remained positive after the application of the TAP for 2 weeks (William et al., 2005). However, there are close relationships between tooth discoloration and minocycline (Lenherr et al., 2012). Therefore, Yassen et al. (2014) suggested the use of double antibiotic paste (DAP, without minocycline) or substitution of minocycline with another antibiotic (clindamyxin, cefaclor, or amoxicillin) for pulp regeneration.

Appropriate use of antibiotics during endodontic regeneration should not only disinfect the root canal but also decrease the adverse effects of antibiotics on transplanted/recruited stem cells. Further, 0.125 mg/ml DAP or TAP has been indicated to exhibit significant antibacterial effects without cytotoxic effects on stem cells (Sabrah et al., 2015). Antibiotic-loaded nanofibrous scaffolds is another method to minimize the adverse effects of highly concentrated antibiotic pastes (Chen, 2010; Bottino et al., 2013; Albuquerque et al., 2015; Kamocki et al., 2015). As the scaffold degrades, antibiotics are released over time. However, the locally sustained release of antibiotics could develop resistant bacterial strains and induce allergic reactions (Lenherr et al., 2012). The application of EndoVac apical negative-pressure system of irrigation, ultrasonic-assisted irrigation, and laser irradiation in root canal disinfection are new methods of root canal disinfection (da Silva et al., 2010; Castelo-Baz et al., 2012; Sahar-Helft et al., 2013; Ghinzelli et al., 2014; Johns et al., 2014; Layton et al., 2015; Neelakantan et al., 2015).

The EndoVac apical negative-pressure system of irrigation, passive ultrasonic irrigation, and laser irradiation have been reported to render similar antibacterial effects to antibiotics (da Silva et al., 2010; Johns et al., 2014; Layton et al., 2015; Neelakantan et al., 2015). *In vitro* studies have shown that continuous ultrasonic-assisted irrigation and NaOCl and EDTA or $Ca(OCl)_2$ solutions could aid in chemomechanical preparation and significantly reduce microbial content during root canal treatment (Castelo-Baz et al., 2012). *In vitro* irrigation solutions combined with Er:YAG-laser irradiation are effective in removing Enterococcus faecalis biofilm from root canal walls (Sahar-Helft et al., 2013). In addition, ultrasonic activation could strengthen the elimination of E. faecalis from the root canal (Ghinzelli et al., 2014), although diode and Er:YAG-laser activation have been reported as superior to ultrasonic activation in dentinal tubule disinfection (Neelakantan et al., 2015). Therefore, ultrasonic irrigation and laser irradiation could be used as a substitute of or in combination with antibiotics for tooth disinfection.

Another indispensable precondition for pulp regeneration is the proper size of the apical foramen, especially in mature teeth with closed apex in adults. During tooth root development, the root apex reduces, finally closes, and forms a narrow foramen. This foramen is the only access through which the blood vessels, nerves, and cells inside the dental pulp communicate with surrounding tissues. If the apical foramen is too small in size, it will impact not only the migration of endogenous cells but also the neovascularization and re-innervation during regeneration. Kling et al. (1986) have shown that a minimum of 1.1 mm is necessary to obtain proper revascularization. They found that an apex smaller than 1.0 mm did not allow pulp revascularization in re-implanted permanent incisors. Another study on replantation of avulsed teeth also showed that apices smaller than 1.5 mm have the lowest rate of pulp healing (Andreasen et al., 1995). Size more than 1 mm would remove the majority of the dentin in the apex, which might be too large for teeth and lead to apical trauma or even fracture. Therefore, the apex should be as small as possible, without affecting cell migration, neo-vascularization, and re-innervation. Further, Laureys et al. (2013) reported that 0.32 mm apical foramen did not prevent the ingrowth of new tissue in two-thirds of the pulp chamber 90 days after tooth transplantation. Our previous research has shown that apices approximately 0.8 mm allowed the migration of endogenous cells and blood vessel formation in the root canal of mature dog teeth *in situ* (Yang et al., 2015a). Therefore, it is possible to achieve pulp regeneration through cell homing with the apical foramen less than 1 mm. However, further studies are needed to determine an appropriate size of apical foramen, especially for human teeth. Moreover, the instruments used to enlarge apical foramen should be modified, and a more proper method should be developed to enlarge the apex efficiently and reduce root-fracture risks.

## ESSENTIAL FEATURES OF THE REGENERATED PULP TISSUE

As known, dental pulp is a loosely connective tissue enclosed within rigid dentine walls. There are blood vessels, nerves, and odontoblasts lining the predentine in the dental pulp, which could help supply nutrients, react to infection, and form reactionary dentin, thus maintaining pulp homeostasis (Ricucci et al., 2014). Therefore, the regenerated tissues should be connective tissues that (i) produce new dentin with a controlled rate similar to the normal pulp, (ii) exhibit similar cell density and architecture to the natural pulp, (iii) are vascularized, and (iv) are innervated (Fawzy El-Sayed et al., 2015). Those functional characters of regenerated tissues are more important than the morphological characters are.

Dentinogenesis is an important character of the pulp. However, after being fully developed, the odontoblasts give rise to the secondary dentin at a regulated and low deposition rate (Magloire et al., 2001). Therefore, the regenerated dentin should be formed along the residual dentinal wall with a very low deposition rate similar to that of the normal pulp. No mineralized tissue should be formed in the center of the regenerated tissue. Extensive mineralization in the regenerated pulp will lead to pulp calcification, which will finally result in loss of pulp viability and block the root canal system. This situation will also cause difficulty in re-treatment. Therefore, too much and extensive mineralization should be prohibited.

Vascularization and innervation are the other two characteristics of the pulp. The regenerated blood vessels should have a connection with periapical or bone marrow tissues around the teeth, which could receive a regular blood flow from circulation and supply nutrient to the regenerated tissue and dentin. More importantly, the regenerated tissue should be innervated, so that the teeth are be able to sense hot/cold stimulation and pain during infection (Kökten et al., 2014). Until now, many published studies have examined the dentin deposition and vascularization of the regenerated tissue. However, few studies have been focused on the re-innervation of the tissue. This might be attributed to the limitation of the methods employed for the examination of innervation. Pagella et al. (2014) used the microfluidics co-culture systems to study tooth innervation. They found that microfluidics co-culture systems provided a valuable tool for investigating the innervation in developing or regenerating teeth. Such systems might also be used to analyze the innervation of regenerated dental pulp.

## CELL HOMING FOR PULP REGENERATION

Compared with cell transplantation strategy, the cell homing strategy might be easier to perform in clinic, as there is no need to isolate or manipulate stem cells *in vitro* (Kim et al., 2013; Huang and Garcia-Godoy, 2014; Xiao and Nasu, 2014). In addition to the pulp revascularization in immature teeth, cell homing strategy was introduced and applied in pulp regeneration in a series of studies (Kim K. et al., 2010; Suzuki et al., 2011; Yang et al., 2015a).

Mao's group showed the formation of vascularized connective tissues in the canal with collagen scaffold and a series of molecules (VEGF, PDGF, or bFGF with a basal set of NGF and BMP7). In Mao's study, extracted human canines and incisors were used and treated endodontically without root canal filling materials. After injection of the scaffold combined with molecules into the canal, the teeth were transplanted subcutaneously into mice. Three weeks later, cellularized and vascularized tissues with new dentin formation over the native dentin were observed in some teeth. This is the first study using an ectopic model to demonstrate the formation of pulp-like tissue through the migration, proliferation, and differentiation of host endogenous cells (Kim J. Y. et al., 2010). Pulp-like tissue formation was also found in another study of this group. In Kim's study, anatomically shaped tooth scaffolds mimicking human molar or rat incisor with an embedded mixture of SDF1, BMP7, and neutralized type-1 collagen solution were used to generate tooth-like structures (including pulp) *in vivo* (Kim K. et al., 2010). The scaffold was fabricated by three-dimensional (3D) bioprinting with 200 μm diameter interconnecting microchannels with polycaprolactone (PCL) and HA. This diameter allows for cell migration and proliferation. More importantly, besides formation of periodontal ligament-like tissues and new alveolar bone, vascularized connective tissues were observed in the canal-like space in the model (Kim K. et al., 2010).

Our published data have shown the formation of pulp-like tissues in an *in situ* model using canine mature teeth. In that study, only chemotaxis factor SDF-1α loaded silk fibroin scaffold (pore size 200 μm in diameter) was used. Canine premolars were selected and periapical lesions were first induced. After root canal disinfection, SDF-1α-loaded scaffolds were inserted into the canal following the induction of blood clot. Three months after surgery, formation of pulp-like tissues with neovascularization and dentin formation along the native dentinal wall were observed. The formation of pulp-like tissues in our study might be attributed to the role of SDF-1α in neovascularization and mineralization, as well as its chemotaxis function. Moreover, compared with the blood clot group, no mineralization was observed in the center of the tissues formed in the SDF-1α-loaded scaffold group. However, the innervation of the formed tissue must be further clarified (Yang et al., 2015a).

To initiate the healing potentials of endogenous cells, scaffolds incorporated with different types of signaling molecules should be added. Signal molecules associated with the formation of vessels, nerves, and dentin are used for pulp regeneration. For example, SDF-1α, bFGF and PDGF are molecules for chemotaxis; PDGF and VEGF for vasculogenesis/angiogenesis; NGF for neuronal growth and survival; and BMP-7 for odontoblast differentiation and mineralization (Yang et al., 2015a; Kim J. Y. et al., 2010). Besides those listed, some other signal molecules are indicated to act as a homing factor for pulp regeneration. Stem cell factor (SCF), a powerful chemokine capable of recruiting progenitor cells, has been shown to increase dental pulp cells proliferation and migration. When subcutaneously implanted with collagen sponges, SCF facilitates cell homing, angiogenesis, and tissue remodeling, which indicated suitability of SCF as a potent aid in the regeneration of dental pulp (Pan et al., 2013). G-CSF and bFGF were also employed for pulp regeneration through cell homing (Takeuchi et al., 2015). Both molecules showed similar effect in high migration, proliferation, anti-apoptotic, angiogenic, and neurite outgrowth stimulatory activities *in vitro*. Using an ectopic transplantation model, G-CSF and bFGF led to the regeneration of pulp-like tissues with dentin formation along the dentinal wall.

A major concern in pulp regeneration through cell homing strategy is stem cell sources. Until now, few studies have reported on this issue. The possible cell sources for pulp regeneration through cell homing include dental pulp stem cells (DPSCs), stem cells from apical papilla (SCAP), and bone marrow stem cells (BMSCs), and others.

DPSCs were traditionally used for pulp regeneration through a cell transplantation strategy, and could also be a cell source via cell homing. In infected immature teeth, efficient root canal disinfection could be achieved without mechanical preparation. In this case, some DPSCs with vitality could reside in the root canal system. Studies of Mitsiadis's group have shown that in seriously injured or carious teeth, stem cells residing in the dental pulp are responsible for the repair and regeneration of the damaged dental tissues (Mitsiadis et al., 2011; Mitsiadis and Woloszyk, 2015). In addition, DPSCs from inflamed dental pulp (DPSCs-IPs) have been identified and shown to exhibit similar mesenchymal stem cell properties to those from normal pulp (DPSCs-NPs) (Alongi et al., 2010). DPSCs-IPs could form pulp/dentin complexes when transplanted in immune-compromised mice. Moreover, they exhibit considerably lower osteo/dentinogenic potential than DPSCs-NPs do on the basis of mineral deposition in cultures. However, it is very difficult to get DPSCs-IPs in mature teeth after mechanical preparation and root canal disinfection. Therefore, DPSCs residual in the canal might contribute to pulp regeneration in immature teeth.

SCAP might be another possible cell source for pulp regeneration. Apical papilla is apical to the epithelial diaphragm of the immature teeth, and it has the collateral circulation. Moreover, there is an apical cell-rich zone lying between the apical papilla and the pulp (Saito et al., 2015). Therefore, the apical papilla is able to survive during the process of pulp necrosis. SCAPs were first identified by Sonoyama et al. Although, shown to have somewhat different characteristics compared with DPSCs, SCAPs have been highly proliferative in cultures and have a strong odontogenic differentiation capacity (Sonoyama et al., 2008). The *in vivo* implantation of SCAP with a scaffold allowed the formation of pulp-like tissues in the root canal (Huang et al., 2010). Na et al. (2013) have also reported the formation of heterotopic dental pulp/dentine complex in empty root canals using SCAP-cell sheet-derived pellet without a scaffold. In addition, SCAPs were shown to be chemoattracted via the SDF-1a/CXCR4 axis and were used as an exogenous cell source to regenerate pulp- and dentin-like tissues in root canal spaces in animal models (Liu et al., 2015). Therefore, SCAPs might be a cell source for pulp regeneration in immature teeth.

Cells homed from bone marrow could be another source for pulp regeneration. Bone marrow–derived progenitor cells have been reported to communicate with dental pulp in mature teeth and become tissue-specific mesenchymal progenitor cells to maintain pulp homeostasis (Zhou et al., 2011). This result indicated that bone marrow-derived cells were capable of migrating into the root canal and participating in pulp formation.

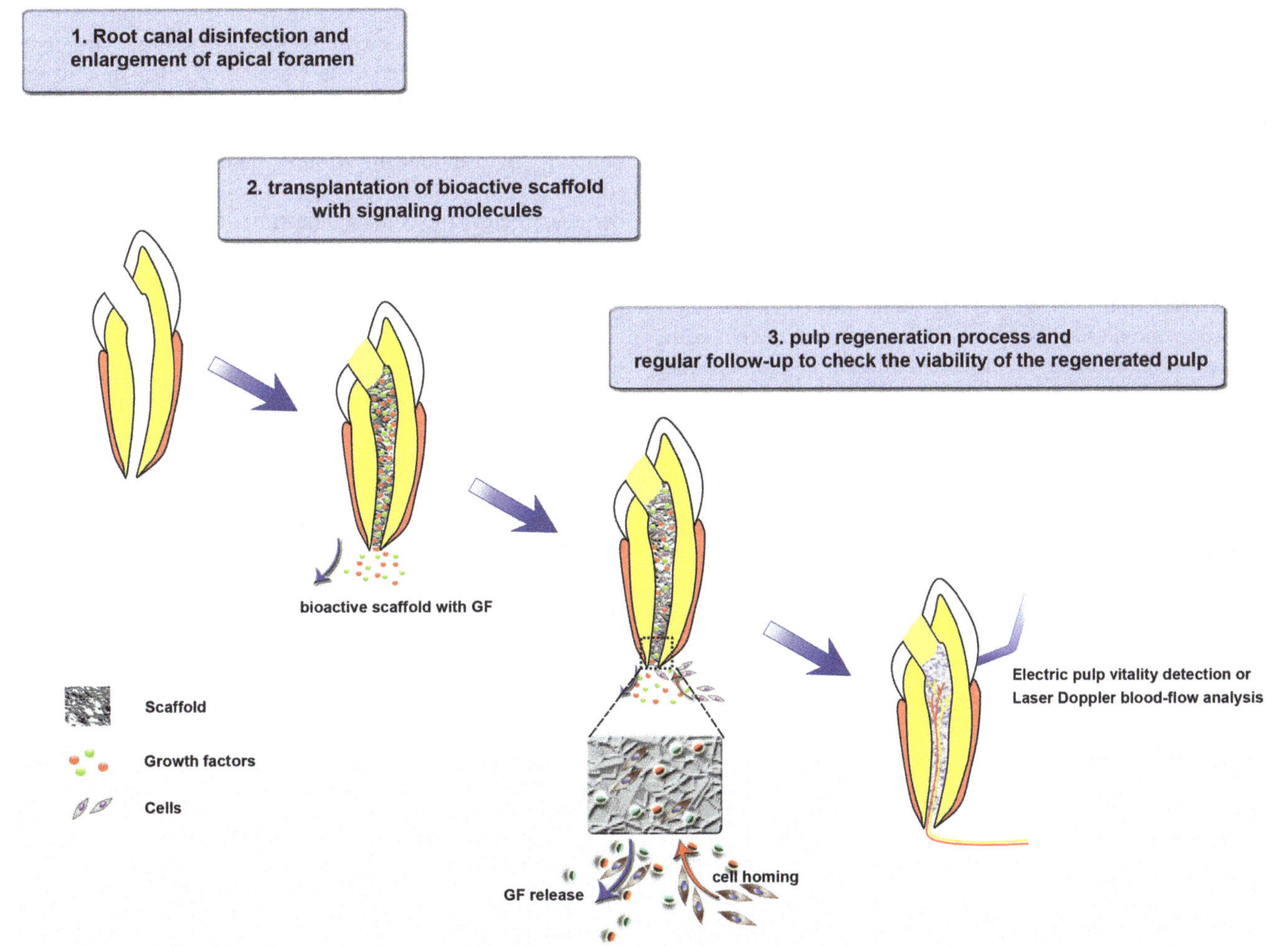


**FIGURE 2 | Tissue-engineering strategies for regenerative endodontics through a cell homing strategy.** Step 1. Root canal disinfection and enlargement of apical foramen. Step 2. Bioactive scaffold transplantation and tooth restoration. Load bioactive scaffold in the canal after cleaning the antibiotics effectively. The growth factors, which are released from the scaffold to the surrounding tissues, will recruit cells into the scaffold. Step 3. Pulp-formation process. Recruited cells migrate, proliferate, differentiate in the scaffold, and participate in the formation of blood vessels, nerves, and regulated dentin deposition. During this step, regular follow-up to check the viability of the regenerated pulp are needed.

Moreover, transplantations of CD31$^{-}$ SP BMSCs or G-CSF-mobilized BMSCs could induce pulp-like tissue formation in the pulpectomized root canal of dogs. In their studies, pulp-like connective tissues with vascularization, innervation, and collagenous matrix containing dentin sialophosphoprotein positive cells were formed (Ishizaka et al., 2013; Murakami et al., 2015).

In addition to the aforementioned possible cell sources, cells of periodontal ligament might be recruited to the root canal system by the chemokines. The periodontal ligament is a fibrous connective tissue structure that joins the cementum covering the root to the alveolar bone. Undifferentiated cells in the periodontal ligament could differentiate into the specialized cells that form bone (osteoblasts) and cementum (cementoblasts). When periodontal ligament stem cells are transplanted with HA/TCP into immune-compromised mice, cementum-like structures associated with periodontal ligament-like connective tissue are generated (Shi et al., 2005). Therefore, the presence of cementum and bone-like tissues in the root canals of some pulp revascularization cases might be attributed to the recruitment of periodontal ligament cells (Wang et al., 2010; Becerra et al., 2014). Thus, the recruitment of periodontal ligament cells should be prohibited to achieve the formation of pulp-like tissues.

In summary, although vascularized pulp-like tissues have been formed in some experimental and clinical studies, little has been known on the function of the regenerated tissue. Further, studies are needed to achieve functional pulp regeneration. Studies on the cell sources of pulp regeneration via cell homing strategy might reveal more information on the signaling molecular selection. The proper signaling molecules for pulp regeneration should facilitate the recruitment of stem cells with the vasculogenic and neurogenic differentiation potential, while inhibiting cells with osteogenic or cementogenic potential (e.g., periodontal ligament cells).

## FUTURE PROSPECT AND CHALLENGES IN PULP REGENERATION THROUGH CELL HOMING

Cell transplantation and cell homing are both scientifically meritorious approaches. However, the active recruitment of endogenous stem/progenitor cells into root canals to regenerate pulp tissues is a novel concept that may offer an unprecedented opportunity for the near-term clinical translation of current biology-based therapies for dental pulp regeneration. Three clinical procedures should be performed if cell homing is applied in endodontic treatment (**Figure 2**): (i) root canal disinfection and apical foramen enlargement; (ii) transplantation of bioactive scaffold with signaling molecules, and tooth restoration; (iii) regular follow-up to check the viability (neovascularization and re-innervation) of the regenerated pulp. Further, studies are needed to achieve clinical translation of pulp regeneration via cell homing strategy. First, for root canal disinfection, intracanal medication, irrigation assisted with EndoVac apical negative-pressure system, or ultrasonic and laser irradiation can be used, but the antibacterial efficiency, effects on cell viability, and dentin mechanical strength of each method or a combination of two or more of them must be further clarified. Meanwhile, the appropriate size of apical foramen should be determined. The size should be as small as possible without affecting cell migration and formation of blood vessels and nerves during pulp regeneration. Second, an appropriate combination of scaffold and growth factors must be selected. The signal molecules should recruit stem cells with the vasculogenic and neurogenic differentiation potential, but inhibit cells with osteogenic or cementogenic potential. In addition, the scaffold should be easily handled in clinical practice. Finally, long-term follow-up experiments will be necessary before the clinic application of cell homing strategy in humans.

## FUNDING

This work was supported by grants from the National Natural Science Foundation of China (81420108011, 31500788); the Fundamental Research Fund for the Central Universities (410500114).

## ACKNOWLEDGMENTS

We would like to thank Dr. Yangxi Chen (from School and Hospital of Stomatology, Wuhan University) for the drawing of the cartoons.

## REFERENCES

Albuquerque, M. T., Valera, M. C., Moreira, C. S., Bresciani, E., de Melo, R. M., and Bottino, M. C. (2015). Effects of ciprofloxacin-containing scaffolds on enterococcus faecalis biofilms. *J. Endod.* 41, 710–714. doi: 10.1016/j.joen.2014.12.025

Alongi, D. J., Yamaza, T., Song, Y., Fouad, A. F., Romberg, E. E., Shi, S., et al. (2010). Stem/progenitor cells from inflamed human dental pulp retain tissue regeneration potential. *Regen. Med.* 5, 617–631. doi: 10.2217/rme.10.30

Andreasen, J. O., Borum, M. K., Jacobsen, H. L., and Andreasen, F. M. (1995). Replantation of 400 avulsed permanent incisors. 4. Factors related to periodontal ligament healing. *Endod. Dent. Traumatol.* 11, 76–89. doi: 10.1111/j.1600-9657.1995.tb00464.x

Becerra, P., Ricucci, D., Loghin, S., Gibbs, J. L., and Lin, L. M. (2014). Histologic study of a human immature permanent premolar with chronic apical abscess after revascularization/revitalization. *J. Endod.* 40, 133–139. doi: 10.1016/j.joen.2013.07.017

Bottino, M. C., Kamocki, K., Yassen, G. H., Platt, J. A., Vail, M. M., Ehrlich, Y., et al. (2013). Bioactive nanofibrous scaffolds for regenerative endodontics. *J. Dent. Res.* 92, 963–969. doi: 10.1177/0022034513505770

Castelo-Baz, P., Martín-Biedma, B., Cantatore, G., Ruíz-Piñón, M., Bahillo, J., Rivas-Mundiña, B., et al. (2012). *In vitro* comparison of passive and continuous ultrasonic irrigation in simulated lateral canals of extracted teeth. *J. Endod.* 38, 688–691. doi: 10.1016/j.joen.2011.12.032

Chen, M. H. (2010). Update on dental nanocomposites. *J. Dent. Res.* 89, 549–560. doi: 10.1177/0022034510363765

da Silva, L., Nelson-Filho, P., da Silva, R. A., Flores, D. S., Heilborn, C., Johnson, J. D., et al. (2010). Revascularization and periapical repair after endodontic treatment using apical negative pressure irrigation versus conventional irrigation plus triantibiotic intracanal dressing in dogs' teeth with apical periodontitis. *Oral Surg. Oral Med. Oral Pathol. Oral Radiol. Endod.* 109, 779–787. doi: 10.1016/j.tripleo.2009.12.046

Duggan, D., Arnold, R. R., Teixeira, F. B., Caplan, D. J., and Tawil, P. (2009). Periapical inflammation and bacterial penetration after coronal inoculation of dog roots filled with RealSeal 1 or Thermafil. *J. Endod.* 35, 852–857. doi: 10.1016/j.joen.2009.03.050

Fawzy El-Sayed, K. M., Jakusz, K., Jochens, A., Dörfer, C., and Schwendicke, F. (2015). Stem Cell transplantaion for pulpal regeneration: a systematic review. *Tissue Eng. Part B Rev.* 21, 451–460. doi: 10.1089/ten.teb.2014.0675

Fouad, A. F. (2011). The microbial challenge to pulp regeneration. *Adv. Dent. Res.* 23, 285–289. doi: 10.1177/0022034511405388

Ghinzelli, G. C., Souza, M. A., Cecchin, D., Farina, A. P., and de Figueiredo, J. A. (2014). Influence of ultrasonic activation on photodynamic therapy over root canal system infected with Enterococcus faecalis–an *in vitro* study. *Photodiagnosis Photodyn. Ther.* 11, 472–478. doi: 10.1016/j.pdpdt.2014.07.004

Huang, G. T., and Garcia-Godoy, F. (2014). Missing Concepts in De Novo Pulp Regeneration. *J. Dent. Res.* 93, 717–724. doi: 10.1177/0022034514537829

Huang, G. T., Yamaza, T., Shea, L. D., Djouad, F., Kuhn, N. Z., Tuan, R. S., et al. (2010). Stem/progenitor cell-mediated de novo regeneration of dental pulp with newly deposited continuous layer of dentin in an *in vivo* model. *Tissue Eng. Part A* 16, 605–615. doi: 10.1089/ten.tea.2009.0518

Ishizaka, R., Hayashi, Y., Iohara, K., Sugiyama, M., Murakami, M., Yamamoto, T., et al. (2013). Stimulation of angiogenesis, neurogenesis and regeneration by side population cells from dental pulp. *Biomaterials* 34, 1888–1897. doi: 10.1016/j.biomaterials.2012.10.045

Johns, D. A., Shivashankar, V. Y., Krishnamma, S., and Johns, M. (2014). Use of photoactivated disinfection and platelet-rich fibrin in regenerative Endodontics. *J. Conserv. Dent.* 17, 487–490. doi: 10.4103/0972-0707.139850

Kamocki, K., Nör, J. E., and Bottino, M. C. (2015). Dental pulp stem cell responses to novel antibiotic-containing scaffolds for regenerative endodontics. *Int. Endod. J.* 48, 1147–1156. doi: 10.1111/iej.12414

Kim, J. Y., Xin, X., Moioli, E. K., Chung, J., Lee, C. H., Chen, M., et al. (2010). Regeneration of dental-pulp-like tissue by chemotaxis-induced cell homing. *Tissue Eng. Part A* 16, 3023–3031. doi: 10.1089/ten.tea.2010.0181

Kim, K., Lee, C. H., Kim, B. K., and Mao, J. J. (2010). Anatomically shaped tooth and periodontal regeneration by cell homing. *J. Dent. Res.* 89, 842–847. doi: 10.1177/0022034510370803

Kim, S. G., Zheng, Y., Zhou, J., Chen, M., Embree, M. C., Song, K., et al. (2013). Dentin and dental pulp regeneration by the patient's endogenous cells. *Endod. Topics* 28, 106–117. doi: 10.1111/etp.12037

Kling, M., Cvek, M., and Mejare, I. (1986). Rate and predictability of pulp revascularization in therapeutically reimplanted permanent incisors. *Endod. Dent. Traumatol.* 2, 83–89. doi: 10.1111/j.1600-9657.1986.tb00132.x

Kökten, T., Bécavin, T., Keller, L., Weickert, J. L., Kuchler-Bopp, S., and Lesot, H. (2014). Immunomodulation stimulates the innervation of engineered tooth organ. *PLoS ONE* 9:e86011. doi: 10.1371/journal.pone.0086011

Laureys, W. G., Cuvelier, C. A., Dermaut, L. R., and De Pauw, G. A. (2013). The critical apical diameter to obtain regeneration of the pulp tissue after tooth transplantation, replantation, or regenerative endodontic treatment. *J. Endod.* 39, 759–763. doi: 10.1016/j.joen.2013.02.004

Layton, G., Wu, W. I., Selvaganapathy, P. R., Friedman, S., and Kishen, A. (2015). Fluid dynamics and biofilm removal generated by syringe-delivered and 2 ultrasonic-assisted irrigation methods: a novel experimental approach. *J. Endod.* 41, 884–889. doi: 10.1016/j.joen.2015.01.027

Lenherr, P., Allgayer, N., Weiger, R., Filippi, A., Attin, T., and Krastl, G. (2012). Tooth discoloration induced by endodontic materials: a laboratory study. *Int. Endod. J.* 45, 942–949. doi: 10.1111/j.1365-2591.2012.02053.x

Liu, J. Y., Chen, X., Yue, L., Huang, G. T., and Zou, X. Y. (2015). CXC chemokine receptor 4 is expressed paravascularly in apical papilla and coordinates with stromal cell-derived factor-1α during transmigration of stem cells from apical papilla. *J. Endod.* 41, 1430–1436. doi: 10.1016/j.joen.2015.04.006

Magloire, H., Romeas, A., Melin, M., Couble, M. L., Bleicher, F., and Farges, J. C. (2001). Molecular regulation of odontoblast activity under dentin injury. *Adv. Dent. Res.* 15, 46–50. doi: 10.1177/08959374010150011201

Mitsiadis, T. A., Feki, A., Papaccio, G., and Catón, J. (2011). Dental pulp stem cells, niches, and notch signaling in tooth injury. *Adv. Dent. Res.* 23, 275–279. doi: 10.1177/0022034511405386

Mitsiadis, T. A., and Woloszyk, A. (2015). Odyssey of human dental pulp stem cells and their remarkable ability tosurvive in extremely adverse conditions. *Front. Physiol.* 6:99. doi: 10.3389/fphys.2015.00099

Murakami, M., Hayashi, Y., Iohara, K., Osako, Y., Hirose, Y., and Nakashima, M. (2015). Trophic effects and regenerative potential of mobilized mesenchymal stem cells from bone marrow and adipose tissue as alternative cell sources for pulp/dentin regeneration. *Cell Transplant.* 24, 1753–1765. doi: 10.3727/096368914X683502

Na, S., Zhang, H., Huang, F., Wang, W., Ding, Y., Li, D., et al. (2013). Regeneration of dental pulp/dentine complex with a three-dimensional and scaffold-free stem-cell sheet-derived pellet. *J. Tissue Eng. Regen. Med.* doi: 10.1002/term.1686. [Epub ahead of print].

Nakashima, M., and Iohara, K. (2011). Regeneration of dental pulp by stem cells. *Adv. Dent. Res.* 23, 313–319. doi: 10.1177/0022034511405323

Neelakantan, P., Cheng, C. Q., Mohanraj, R., Sriraman, P., Subbarao, C., and Sharma, S. (2015). Antibiofilm activity of three irrigation protocols activated by ultrasonic, diode laser or Er:YAG laser *in vitro*. *Int. Endod. J.* 48, 602–610. doi: 10.1111/iej.12354

Pagella, P., Neto, E., Jiménez-Rojo, L., Lamghari, M., and Mitsiadis, T. A. (2014). Microfluidics co-culture systems for studying tooth innervations. *Front. Physiol.* 5:326. doi: 10.3389/fphys.2014.00326

Pan, S., Dangaria, S., Gopinathan, G., Yan, X., Lu, X., Kolokythas, A., et al. (2013). SCF promotes dental pulp progenitor migration, neovascularization, and collagen remodeling-potential applications as a homing factor in dental pulp regeneration. *Stem Cell Rev.* 29, 655–667. doi: 10.1007/s12015-013-9442-7

Ricucci, D., Loghin, S., Lin, L. M., Spångberg, L. S., and Tay, F. R. (2014). Is hard tissue formation in the dental pulp after the death of the primary odontoblasts a regenerative or a reparative process? *J. Dent.* 42, 1156–1170. doi: 10.1016/j.jdent.2014.06.012

Sabrah, A. H., Yassen, G. H., Liu, W. C., Goebel, W. S., Gregory, R. L., and Platt, J. A. (2015). The effect of diluted triple and double antibiotic pastes on dental pulp stem cells and established Enterococcus faecalis biofilm. *Clin. Oral Investig.* 19, 2059–2066. doi: 10.1007/s00784-015-1423-6

Sahar-Helft, S., Stabholtz, A., Moshonov, J., Gutkin, V., Redenski, I., and Steinberg, D. (2013). Effect of Er:YAG laser-activated irrigation solution on Enterococcus Faecalis biofilm in an *ex-vivo* root canal model. *Photomed. Laser Surg.* 31, 334–341. doi: 10.1089/pho.2012.3445

Saito, M. T., Silvério, K. G., Casati, M. Z., Sallum, E. A., Nociti, F. H. Jr. (2015). Tooth-derived stem cells: update and perspectives. *World J. Stem Cells* 7, 399–407. doi: 10.4252/wjsc.v7.i2.399

Shi, S., Bartold, P. M., Miura, M., Seo, B. M., Robey, P. G., and Gronthos, S. (2005). The efficacy of mesenchymal stem cells to regenerate and repair dental structures. *Orthod. Craniofac. Res.* 8, 191–199. doi: 10.1111/j.1601-6343.2005.00331.x

Shivashankar, V. Y., Johns, D. A., Vidyanath, S., and Kumar, M. R. (2012). Platelet Rich Fibrin in the revitalization of tooth with necrotic pulp and open apex. *J. Conserv. Dent.* 15, 395–398. doi: 10.4103/0972-0707.101926

Sonoyama, W., Liu, Y., Yamaza, T., Tuan, R. S., Wang, S., Shi, S., et al. (2008). Characterization of the apical papilla and its residing stem cells from human immature permanent teeth: a pilot study. *J Endod.* 34, 166–1671. doi: 10.1016/j.joen.2007.11.021

Sun, H. H., Chen, B., Zhu, Q. L., Kong, H., Li, Q. H., Gao, L. N., et al. (2014). Investigation of dental pulp stem cells isolated from discarded human teeth extracted due to aggressive periodontitis. *Biomaterials* 35, 9459–9472. doi: 10.1016/j.biomaterials.2014.08.003

Suzuki, T., Lee, C. H., Chen, M., Zhao, W., Fu, S. Y., Qi, J. J., et al. (2011). Induced migration of dental pulp stem cells for *in vivo* pulp regeneration. *J. Dent. Res.* 90, 1013–1018. doi: 10.1177/0022034511408426

Takeuchi, N., Hayashi, Y., Murakami, M., Alvarez, F. J., Horibe, H., Iohara, K., et al. (2015). Similar *in vitro* effects and pulp regeneration in ectopic tooth transplantation by basic fibroblast growth factor and granulocyte-colony stimulating factor. *Oral Dis.* 21, 113–122. doi: 10.1111/odi.12227

Thibodeau, B., and Trope, M. (2007). Pulp revascularization of a necrotic infected immature permanent tooth: case report and review of the literature. *Pediatr. Dent.* 29, 47–50.

Vijayaraghavan, R., Mathian, V. M., Sundaram, A. M., Karunakaran, R., and Vinodh, S. (2012). Triple antibiotic paste in root canal therapy. *J. Pharm. Bioallied Sci.* 4, S230–S233. doi: 10.4103/0975-7406.100214

Wang, X., Thibodeau, B., Trope, M., Lin, L. M., and Huang, G. T. (2010). Histologic characterization of regenerated tissues in canal space after the revitalization/revascularization procedure of immature dog teeth with apical periodontitis. *J. Endod.* 36, 56–63. doi: 10.1016/j.joen.2009.09.039

Wigler, R., Kaufman, A. Y., Lin, S., Steinbock, N., Hazan-Molina, H., and Torneck, C. D. (2013). Revascularization: a treatment for permanent teeth with necrotic pulp and incomplete root development. *J. Endod.* 39, 319–326. doi: 10.1016/j.joen.2012.11.014

William, W. III., Teixeira, F., Levin, L., Sigurdsson, A., and Trope, M. (2005). Disinfection of immature teeth with a triple antibiotic paste. *J. Endod.* 31, 439–443. doi: 10.1097/01.don.0000148143.80283.ea

Xiao, L., and Nasu, M. (2014). From regenerative dentistry to regenerative medicine: progress, challenges, and potential applications of oral stem cells. *Stem Cells Cloning* 4, 89–99. doi: 10.2147/sccaa.s51009

Yang, J. W., Zhang, Y. F., Sun, Z. Y., Song, G. T., and Chen, Z. (2015b). Dental pulp tissue engineering with bFGF-incorporated silk fibroin scaffolds. *J. Biomater. Appl.* 30, 221–229. doi: 10.1177/0885328215577296

Yang, J. W., Zhang, Y. F., Wan, C. Y., Sun, Z. Y., Nie, S., Jian, S. J., et al. (2015a). Autophagy in SDF-1α-mediated DPSC migration and pulp regeneration. *Biomaterials* 44, 11–23. doi: 10.1016/j.biomaterials.2014.12.006

Yassen, G. H., Al-Angari, S. S., and Platt, J. A. (2014). The use of traditional and novel techniques to determine the hardness and indentation properties of immature radicular dentin treated with antibiotic medicaments followed by ethylenediaminetetraacetic acid. *Eur. J. Dent.* 8, 521–527. doi: 10.4103/1305-7456.143636

Zhou, J., Shi, S., Shi, Y., Xie, H., Chen, L., He, Y., et al. (2011). Role of bone marrow-derived progenitor cells in the maintenance and regeneration of dental mesenchymal tissues. *J. Cell. Physiol.* 226, 2081–2090. doi: 10.1002/jcp.22538

# 10

# Designing and testing regenerative pulp treatment strategies: modeling the trans-dentinal transport mechanisms

**Edited by:**
*Thimios Mitsiadis,*
*University of Zurich, Switzerland*

***Correspondence:**
*Spiros V. Paras,*
*Department of Chemical Engineering,*
*Aristotle University of Thessaloniki,*
*University Box 455, GR 54124*
*Thessaloniki, Greece*
*paras@auth.gr*

***Agathoklis D. Passos*** [1], ***Aikaterini A. Mouza*** [1], ***Spiros V. Paras*** [1*], ***Christos Gogos*** [2] ***and Dimitrios Tziafas*** [2]

[1] *Department of Chemical Engineering, Aristotle University of Thessaloniki, Thessaloniki, Greece,* [2] *Department of Endodontology, School of Dentistry, Aristotle University of Thessaloniki, Thessaloniki, Greece*

The need for simulation models to thoroughly test the inflammatory effects of dental materials and dentinogenic effects of specific signaling molecules has been well recognized in current dental research. The development of a model that simulates the transdentinal flow and the mass transfer mechanisms is of prime importance in terms of achieving the objectives of developing more effective treatment modalities in restorative dentistry. The present protocol study is part of an ongoing investigation on the development of a methodology that can calculate the transport rate of selected molecules inside a typical dentinal tubule. The transport rate of biological molecules has been investigated using a validated *CFD* code. In that framework we propose a simple algorithm that, given the type of molecules of the therapeutic agent and the maximum acceptable time for the drug concentration to attain a required value at the pulpal side of the tubules, can estimate the initial concentration to be imposed.

**Keywords: dentinal tubule, dentin regeneration, transdentinal diffusion, bioactive molecules, CFD, μ-LIF**

## Introduction

During the last decades the clinical practice has been oriented toward the design and development of modern dental treatment techniques that would ensure the long-term maintenance of vitality and function of the dentine–pulp complex (de Peralta and Nör, 2014). The traditional treatment strategies in vital pulp therapy have been mainly focused on protection of dental pulp from possible irritation presented by components released from dental materials and induction of replacement of diseased dentin by a dentin-like material (Tziafas et al., 2000). Furthermore, the fact that the pulp-dentin complex can be repaired and regenerated by forming tertiary dentin, has recently led the scientific community toward the development of novel optimal procedures and production of potential therapeutic agents for use in regenerative pulp therapies. There is a growing weight of evidence that bioactive molecules diffused through the dentinal tubules can regulate the biosynthetic activity of pulpal cells (Rutherford et al., 1995; Smith et al., 2001). In a previous experimental approach we reported that *TGF-b1* and, to a lesser extent, *BMP-7* provided evidence that stimulate tertiary dentin, while intratubular mineralization may occur when these growth factors are placed on deep dentine cavities (Kalyva et al., 2010).

Pre-clinical testing of dental materials to evaluate biologically their application includes studies in animals and humans. Human studies are most appropriate when investigating dentine-pulp reactions to various newly introduced substances and commercially available formulas. However, protection of patients from possible hazards presented by dental materials and the biological effects that they might have is needed (Murray et al., 2007). On the other hand, animals' studies have raised concerns of their capability to predict human dental pulp reactions because of the fact that there are possible species variations. Thus the numbers of both clinical and animal screening tests must be minimized to make this form of testing legally and ethically acceptable. Development of several *in vitro* approaches simulating clinical conditions that are helpful to control parameters concerning experimental conditions is in progress during the last two decades.

Parameters that have been implicated with pulpal injury, and therefore affect the pulp responses to materials placed in a dentinal cavity environment, have attracted attention. The numbers of odontoblasts surviving the injury caused by the cavity cutting and restoring procedures have been strongly correlated with cavity preparation technique and dimensions, the nature of tested materials including the diffusion rate of their components, and method of application (Smith et al., 2001). Previous data have showed that diffusion rate of dental material components exerting possible toxicity to the pulpal cells depends on the remaining dentin thickness. Murray et al. (2001); Murray et al. (2003) further reported that there is an inverse relation between the remaining dentin thickness and odontoblast survival. They concluded that an *RDT* greater or equal to 0.5 mm is necessary to protect the underlying odontoblasts form the operative trauma.

Since it is evident that a remaining dentin zone is necessary to protect the dental pulp survival and function, much has still to be learnt on the effect of potent toxic components or bioactive agents that are released from traditional and regenerative therapeutic approaches. Since it is reasonable to suggest that any toxic interruption or therapeutic up-regulation of the biosynthetic activity of odontoblasts (Smith, 2003) will probably reflect the molecular concentration of these constituents at the dentin-pulp interface area, a number of delivery considerations might be firstly addressed. Among other issues, the simulation of clinical conditions requires the development of an experimental methodology that can calculate the transport rate of selected molecules by employing advanced non-intrusive techniques. The experimental study of the diffusion rate of therapeutic molecules inside the dentin tubules is almost impossible using the established experimental techniques due to the minute dimensions of the dentinal tubules. On the other hand, the analytical solution of the governing mass and momentum transfer equations is practically infeasible due to the non-uniformity of the tubules cross section. Therefore, Computational Fluid Dynamics (*CFD*) seems to be the only feasible method for studying the problem under consideration. Recent studies confirmed that *CFD* is a powerful analytical tool in dental pulp research (Boutsioukis et al., 2009; Gao et al., 2009; Su et al., 2014). However, an up to date literature review has revealed that there is no significant progress interpretation of flow phenomena inside the dentinal tubules. It is, therefore, desirable to be able to suggest a new integrated computational approach that could adequately simulate both the fluid flow and diffusion characteristics inside the tubules.

The idea of using the dentinal tubules for drug transfusion in pulp was originally proposed by Pashley (1990), but there is limited information on the balance between the rate of internal diffusion of exogenous factors (e.g., drugs, molecules, bacterial byproducts) and the resistance of outward fluid flow inside a dentinal tubule. Later Pashley (1992a,b) suggested that the therapeutic agents must consist of small molecules or ions that exhibit relatively high diffusion coefficients, while high concentrations must be avoided due to the risk of increasing the rate of movement of dentinal fluid outwardly and thus prohibiting the internal diffusion of the drug. According to the dental clinical practice the resistance to the internal diffusion due to the fluid outflow could be considered to be minimal, if the application of the capping agent is followed by immediate covering the exposed dentinal surface with an adhesive dental material. It has been previously documented that large molecules such as endotoxins (1–30 kDa) or exotoxins (20–70 kDa) can dissolve in the dentinal fluid and diffuse to the pulp (Pashley and Matthews, 1993).

The present work is part of an ongoing investigation on phenomena related to the dental therapeutic practice and is expected to provide insights on the key issues of transdentinal regulation of the dentin-pulp complex functions. This article comprises the study of the diffusion of substances similar to dental materials components and bioactive agents used in today clinical practice and promising regenerative approaches respectively. Therefore, we describe the basic principles for the development of a model that would simulate the flow and mass transfer in the dentinal tubules and propose a numerical methodology for investigating the mass transfer characteristics in a microtube ($\mu$-tube) that closely resembles a typical dentinal tubule geometry. The *CFD* code is validated using the outcome of an analytical solution as well as with experimental data acquired using the non-intrusive experimental technique $\mu$-*LIF*.

The *CFD* simulations concerning mass transfer of chemical compounds confirm that:

- the diffusion is a very slow process, a fact verified by clinical observations,
- large molecules penetrate at a lower rate inside the dentinal tubules compared to smaller ones,
- the mass flux inside a tubule increases by increasing the initial concentration of the substance and
- the time required for the concentration of the signaling molecules to attain a *predefined* value at the pulp can be controlled by their *initial* concentration.

Thus, in the framework of developing more effective treatment modalities in restorative dentistry we are able to provide an algorithm that, given:

- the type, i.e., the size of the molecules of the therapeutic agent,
- the required drug concentration at the pulpal side of the tubules and
- the maximum *acceptable time* to attain the aforementioned concentration,

can estimate the *initial concentration* that must be imposed.

## Materials and Methods

The commercial *CFD* code *ANSYS CFX® 15.0* is employed for the simulations, i.e., for solving the incompressible *Navier-Stokes* and mass transfer equations (McCabe et al., 2005).This paper tackles the problem of the diffusion of substances through a conical μ-tube that simulates a typical dentinal tubule.

However, before proceeding to the computational simulations, is common practice the *CFD* code to be validated. As already mentioned, the theoretical and experimental study of the diffusion process inside the dentinal tubules is practically impossible. Therefore, at an initial stage the flow through a *cylindrical* μ-channel studied using the *CFD* code and the numerical results are compared with the analytical solution of *Fick's Second Law*. Experiments concerning the diffusion of a fluorescent dye in water are also performed in a glass capillary. The local dye concentration is measured by the non-intrusive *μ-LIF* measuring technique and the acquired experimental data are compared with the *CFD* results. It is therefore quite reasonable to assume that the validated computational code can be applied for studying the diffusion of substances similar to potential therapeutic agents through a typical dentinal tubule. In this stage and in accordance with the dental clinic practice, *no fluid outflow* from the μ-tube is assumed.

As already mentioned, for the experimental study of the diffusion in μ-channels and for validating the *CFD* code, the non-intrusive micro Laser Induced Fluorescence (*μ-LIF*) technique was employed. Laser-Induced Fluorescence (*LIF*) is an optical measuring technique used to measure instant whole-field concentration maps in liquid and gaseous flows. This can be done indirectly by measuring the light emitted (i.e., fluorescence) by the tracer compounds that are used to mark the fluids. The *LIF* experimental setup, available in our Lab, is shown in **Figure 1**. The experiments were performed in a glass capillary (*ID* = 580 μm, *L* = 3 cm). The measuring section was illuminated by a double cavity *Nd:YAG* Laser emitting at 532 nm. The fluid flux was measured by a high sensitivity *CCD* camera (*Hisense MkII*), connected to a Nikon (*Eclipse LV150*) microscope, which moves along the vertical axis with an accuracy of one micron. A *10X* air immersion objective with *NA* = 0.20 was used. For each measurement at least 20 images were acquired at a sampling rate of 5 Hz.

The experiments were performed using two liquids, namely distilled water as reference and distilled water marked with the fluorescent dye *Rhodamine B*, completely dissolved in water, whose diffusion coefficient in water is $4.5 \cdot 10^{-10}$ m$^2$/s (Gendron et al., 2008). *Rhodamine B* is a fluorescent dye with a quantum yield of up to $\varphi = 0.97$ at low concentrations. As reported by Bindhu and Harilal (2001) its quantum yield depends on the solvent and on the type of excitation (continuous, pulsed) and decreases weakly with increasing concentration. *Rhodamine B*, dissolved in water, is most effectively excited by green light and emits red light with the maximum intensity in the range 575–585 nm (Sakakibara and Adrian, 1999; Bindhu and Harilal, 2001). Image processing and concentration calculations were performed using appropriate software (*Flow Manager* by *Dantec Dynamics*).

A typical procedure for μ-LIF measurements consists of the following steps:

- Determination of the *relationship* between the measured fluorescence intensity field $I_{(x,t)}$ and the concentration field $C_{(x,y)}$.
- Calibration experiments prior to the actual measurements using a series of aqueous *Rhodamine B* solutions with known concentrations, namely $C$ = 0.05, 0.025, and 0.00 mg/L. For each concentration $C_i$ an image $C_{(x,y)}$ is taken.
- Image masking of the acquired images is also necessary in order to reduce noise and then an appropriate *Region of Interest* (*ROI*) is defined, at which the fluorescence intensity is measured.

For our experiments the optical system was set to have a *ROI* of 300*x*580 μm, while the lens was focused on the middle plane of the capillary. Care was taken to ensure that the experiments are conducted at identical conditions with the calibration procedure, so as to minimize the uncertainty of the experimental procedure.

After the calibration of the measuring system, the two liquids, namely water and the colored aqueous solution at $C$ = 0.05 mg/L, were successively inserted into the capillary. A syringe pump (*ALLADIN 2000*) was employed for the suction of the two liquids inside the capillary (**Figure 2**).

It is very important that the fluids enter the capillary at a very low velocity so as to avoid mixing due to convection, although a small initial concentration distribution of *Rhodamine B* inside the capillary is unavoidable. After the two liquids have entered the μ-channel, the syringe pump is turned off and the capillary is placed carefully under the microscope at a horizontal position for conducting the *LIF* measurements. The test-section remains connected to the syringe pump during the measurements to ensure constant pressure condition inside the μ-channel.

Finally, concentration measurements were performed at 10–15 locations on the middle plane, at 1 mm from each other along the axis of symmetry of the μ-tube. As there is no lateral diffusion, i.e., the process is *1D*, we can assume that the concentration is constant along the diameter of the μ-tube. Thus the *LIF* measurement corresponds to the concentration at a cross-section of the conduit. The axial length $x$ is normalized with respect to the tube length, $L$; thus $x/L = 0$ denotes the entrance of the capillary.

The image processing of the *LIF* images comprises the definition of the mean image out of the set of 20 images acquired and their processing according to the *LIF* calibration record that has been created. After the experimental measurements, appropriate numerical simulations that fully represent the initial experimental conditions are performed.

In **Figure 3A** a typical comparison of *CFD* data with the corresponding results from the *μ-LIF* technique is presented concerning the concentration inside the channel after $t$ = 4 h. The dashed line represents the calculated final concentration value $C_t$ inside the capillary for $t$ = 8. In **Figure 3B** the two methods are compared with respect to the temporal concentration variation at two locations inside the capillary ($x/L = 0.067$ and 0.330).

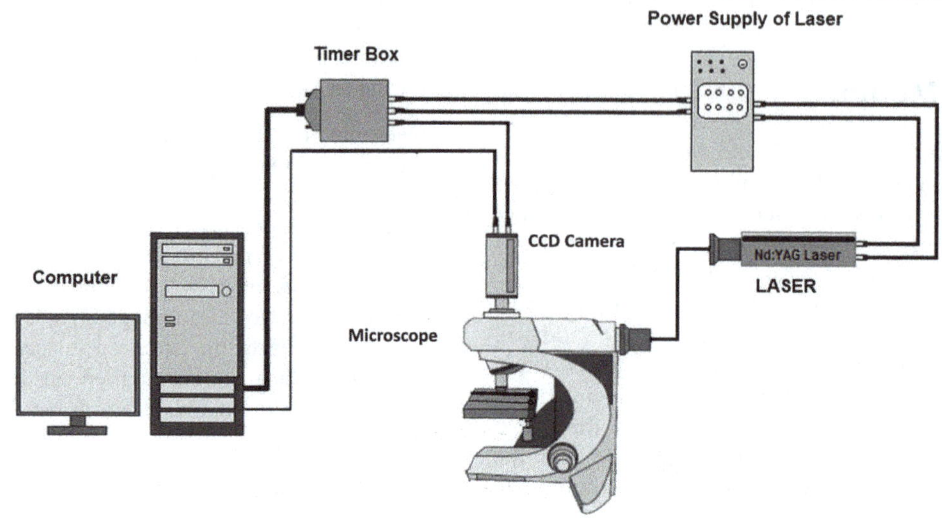


FIGURE 1 | μ-LIF experimental setup.

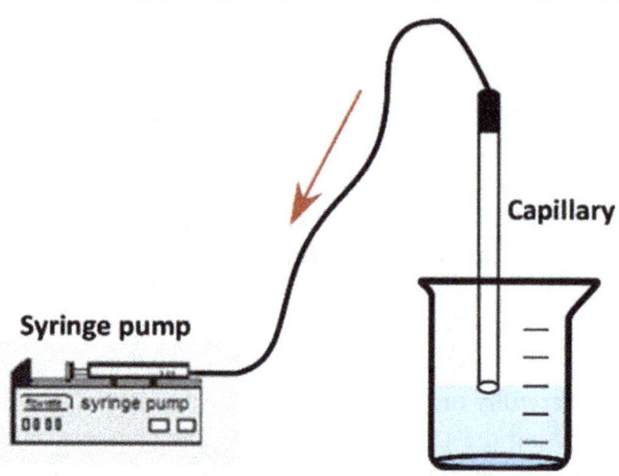


FIGURE 2 | Test-section connected with a syringe pump.

The experimental results are in fairly good agreement (<10%) with the *CFD* data. The discrepancy between the two methods may be attributed to the fact that the experimental data concern the mean concentration values that were measured at the applied *ROI*, while the corresponding values from the *CFD* results give the concentration at the center of a grid cell with an axial dimension of 5 μm. After comparing the data of the numerical simulations with the available experimental results from the *μ-LIF* technique we can come to the conclusion that the *CFD* code is able to predict diffusion of substances through liquids in such small diameter conduits.

## Theoretical Approach

The ability of the computational code to effectively simulate diffusional mass transfer in μ-conduits is confirmed by comparing the *CFD* results with analytical solutions of the governing equations for molecular mass transport. Diffusion is the net movement of a substance from a region of high concentration to a region of low concentration, i.e., it is the movement of a substance down a concentration gradient. In steady state conditions the diffusive flux $j$ of a substance driven by the concentration gradient in one dimension is given by the Fick's First Law (Equation 1):

$$j = -D\frac{\partial C}{\partial x} \tag{1}$$

where $j$ is the flux, $D$ is a diffusion coefficient, $\partial C/\partial x$ is the concentration gradient and $x$ is the distance in the direction of transfer. This equation follows the general rule that matter diffuses from a region of higher concentration to a region of lower concentration, hence the minus sign. The diffusion coefficient $D$ is a function of temperature, and its units are in length squared per unit time, provided that $j$, $C$ and $x$ are in consistent units.

Fick's Second law is used to predict how diffusion causes the concentration to change with time, i.e., unsteady conditions, and in one dimension is given by Equation (2):

$$\frac{\partial C}{\partial t} = D\frac{\partial^2 C}{\partial x^2} \tag{2}$$

where $t$ is the time, $C$ the concentration which is a function of both location $x$ and time $t$.

To comply with the actual case of transdentinal diffusion of substances, there is need to apply a rigorous analytical equation, originated from the Fick's Second Law, that incorporates a zero flux boundary condition at $x/L = 1$, i.e., the pulpal area. The new formulated analytical solution which is a sum of a cosine series is given by Equation (3):

$$C_{(x,t)} = \frac{2M}{L}\sum_{n=1}^{\infty} e^{-(n\pi/L)^2 tD}\cos(n\pi x/L) + M_t \tag{3}$$

where, $M$ is the total amount per area of the diffusing species, $x$ the distance from the source, $L$ the channel length and $M_t$ the final estimated concentration value inside the μ-channel.

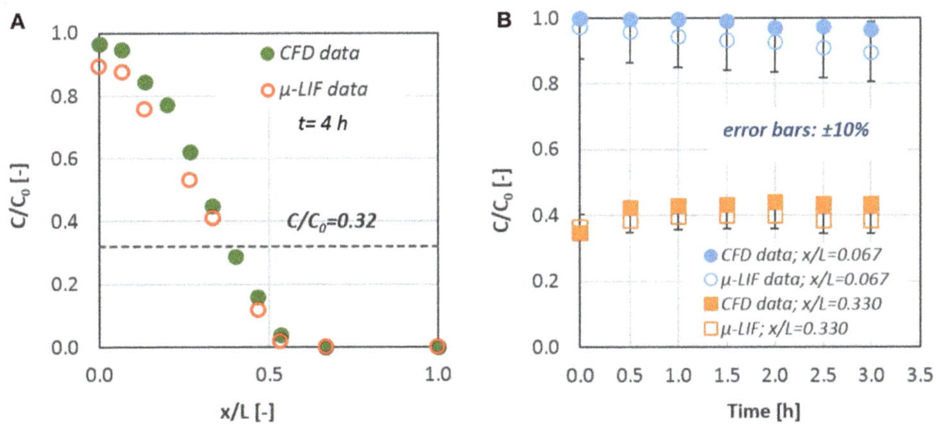


**FIGURE 3 | Comparison of CFD data with the corresponding results from the LIF technique: (A) mass concentration distribution inside the capillary after $t = 4$ h and (B) mass concentration values for x/L = 0.067 and 0.330; error bars: ±10%.**

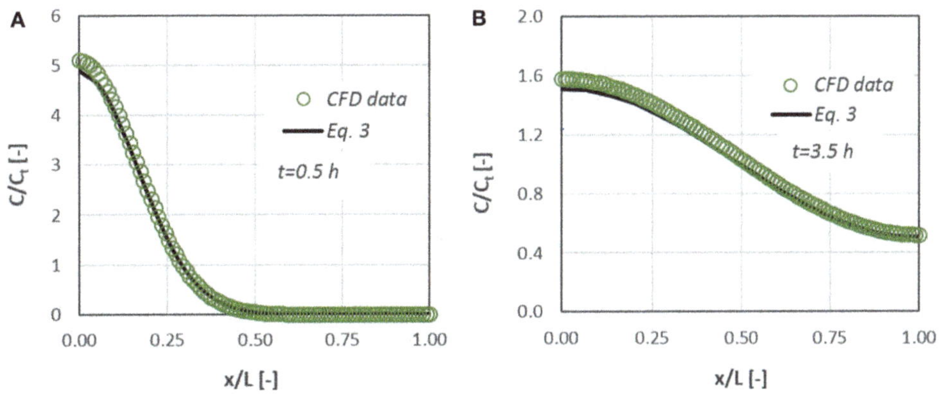


**FIGURE 4 | Concentration distribution of a diffusate in a cylindrical μ-tube.** Comparison between CFD data and the corresponding results from Equation (3) for: **(A)** $t = 0.5$ h and **(B)** $t = 3.5$ h after the diffusate release.

**Figure 4** presents the comparison between the results of Equation (3) and the data obtained from the *CFD* simulations for two time periods (i.e., 0.5 and 3.5 h). The initial mass of the diffusate is located at $x/L = 0$. A very good agreement (±10%) exists between the experiments and the analytical solution with the corresponding numerical ones. Consequently, we can conclude that the *CFD* code is capable of handling diffusion and mass transport phenomena in the microscale.

## Numerical Procedure

For studying the transdentinal diffusion, we use substances whose molecular sizes are the same as those of potential therapeutic agents that are used in dental clinic practice. The radius $R_{min}$ and the diffusion coefficient $D$ of a protein can be determined by Equations (4, 5) (Erickson, 2009).

$$R_{\min} = 0.066 M_w^{1/3} \tag{4}$$

where $R_{min}$ is given in nanometers and the molecular weight $M_w$ in Daltons (*Da*) and

$$D = \frac{kT}{6\pi \mu R_s} \tag{5}$$

where $k = 1.38 \times 10^{-16}$ g cm$^2$ s$^{-2}$ K$^{-1}$ is the *Boltzman's* constant and $T$ the absolute temperature. $k$ is given here in centimeter–gram–second units because $D$ is expressed in centimeter–gram–second, while $\mu$ that stands for the solute viscosity is in g/(cm·s). $R_s$, called *Stokes* radius, represents the radius of a smooth sphere that would have the same frictional coefficient $f$ with a protein and is expressed in centimeters in this equation. Assuming that $f$ equals $f_{min}$, i.e., the minimal frictional coefficient that a protein of a given mass would obtain if the protein was a smooth sphere of radius $R_{min}$, then $R_{min}$ could replace $R_s$ in Equation (5).

In **Table 1** some representative examples of substances or ions released from dental materials in use or experimentally designed bioactive agents are presented. Released monomers from resins (*TEGDMA*) or dental adhesives (*HEMA*) disturb cell functions including responses of the immune system, mineralization, and differentiation of dental pulp cells, or induce cell death via apoptosis (Schweikl et al., 2014). The role of bases and liners (zinc oxide-eugenol or calcium hydroxide or calcium silicate-based materials) indicated for pulp protection is still controversial in terms of molecules or ions diffusion through the exposed dentinal tubules. Furthermore biologically active molecules

**TABLE 1 | Representative traditional or experimental applications in the situation of exposed dentinal surfaces with the characteristics of released molecules or ions.**

| Material group for dental use | Released molecules/Ions | Molecular formula/Characteristics | Molecular/ Atomic weight (Da) | Diffusion coefficient ($m^2/s$) |
|---|---|---|---|---|
| Composite resins-tooth restoration | TEGDMA Triethylene glycol dimethacrylate | $CH_2{=}C(CH_3)COO(CH_2CH_2O)_3COC(CH_3){=}CH_2$ | 286 | $7.5{\cdot}10^{-10}$ |
| Bonding agents-tooth restoration | HEMA 2-Hydroxyethyl methacrylate | $CH_2{=}C(CH_3)COOCH_2CH_2OH$ Polymer absorbing up to 600% water. Basically it is hydrophobic but contains hydrophilic group. | 130 | $9.7{\cdot}10^{-10}$ |
| Glass ionomer cements- pulp protection | Fluoride ions | $F^-$ | 9 | $2.4{\cdot}10^{-09}$ |
| Zinc oxide-eugenol bases-pulp protection | Eugenol 4-Allyl-2-methoxyphenol | $C_{10}H_{12}O_2$hydrophobic | 164 | $8.9{\cdot}10^{-10}$ |
| Calcium hydroxide-based liners-pulp protection | Calcium ions | $Ca^{++}$ | 20 | $1.8{\cdot}10^{-09}$ |
| Calcium silicate-based bases -pulp protection | Silicon | $Si^{4-}$ | 14 | $2.1{\cdot}10^{-09}$ |
| EDTA-soluble dentinal constituents (experimental applications) Pulp protection | Transforming growth factor -beta | Polypeptide | 44,300 | $1.4{\cdot}10^{-10}$ |
| BMP7-containing capping agents (experimental applications) pulp protection | Bone morphogenetic protein 7 | Polypeptide | 50,000 | $1.3{\cdot}10^{-10}$ |

applied as possible therapeutic drugs with an appropriate delivery system (*BMP-7*) or endogenous growth factors released after dentin treatment with *EDTA* (*TGFbeta*) have shown important tissue specific activity for dentin-pulp complex regeneration.

In this computational study *three different substances* were used. The radius $R_s$ of their molecules is in the range of 2.2–22.0 nm and consequently the corresponding diffusion coefficient, *D*, in water at 37 C is in the range of $1.36–0.14{\cdot}10^{-10}$ $m^2/s$. The range of molecular sizes employed in this study corresponds to the size of actual bioactive molecules. For example, *BMP-7* is such a bioactive protein used in the dental clinic practice with approximately 50 kDa molecular weight and $R_s$ of 2.2 nm. To conduct a parametric study, three initial concentration values for each diffusing substance are also employed, namely 0.10, 0.05, and 0.01 mg/mL.

We studied the effect of:

- the initial diffusate concentration and
- the molecular size

on the transdentinal diffusion characteristics.

A grid dependence study has been also performed for the case involving the diffusate with the highest diffusion coefficient value. As the study comprises the time-dependent solution of diffusion, all simulations were run in *transient mode*. A time-step dependence study was also performed, to ensure that a suitable time step is selected for each simulation, i.e., the minimum number of calculation steps performed without jeopardizing the accuracy of the solution. The total simulation time for each run was set at 10 h as the diffusion process is expected to be extremely slow.

## Anticipated Results

The diffusion of a substance similar to the therapeutic agent *BMP-7*, through a dentinal tubule under different values of initial concentration has been studied. **Figure 5A**, which presents the therapeutic agent concentration at the bottom of the dentinal tubule, i.e., at the dentin-pulp junction, as a function of time, demonstrates the effect of initial substance concentration on the concentration change. **Figure 5B** shows the effect of the type of substance, i.e., its molecular size, on the concentration change at the pulpal area.

It is obvious that the diffusion rate is particularly low, since it takes more than 10 h for the concentration at the pulpal side to reach its final value, although after approximately 2 h, the first molecules of the substances do reach the bottom end. In addition, as the diffusion coefficient is a function of the size of the molecules, substances/proteins with larger molecules penetrate at a lower rate inside the dentinal tubules.

It is worth noting that the time required for the concentration of signaling molecules to attain a specific value at the pulp can be controlled by their initial concentration. By increasing the initial concentration of a potential therapeutic agent, the mass flux inside the dentinal tubule increases and as a result the signaling time of the molecules may also decrease. This is an important finding, especially for the dental community, since it gives the possibility to predict the behavior of each therapeutic agent prior to its application on the dental clinic practice.

Obviously it is important to be able to predict the final concentration of an applied therapeutic agent. In this case one must run the relevant *CFD* simulation to produce an appropriate curve like the one presented in **Figure 5**. However, this is not a trivial procedure to be used in every day practice. Thus, an effort was made to propose a simple correlation that could predict with reasonable accuracy the temporal concentration value at the pulp through the dentinal tubules, as a function of the diffusion coefficient of the substance, i.e., its molecular size. The proposed correlation can be then used to estimate the maximum required time for the diffusion process to reach steady state condition, i.e., when the concentration of the substance has the same value along the tubule, after calculating the term $L^2/D$. The

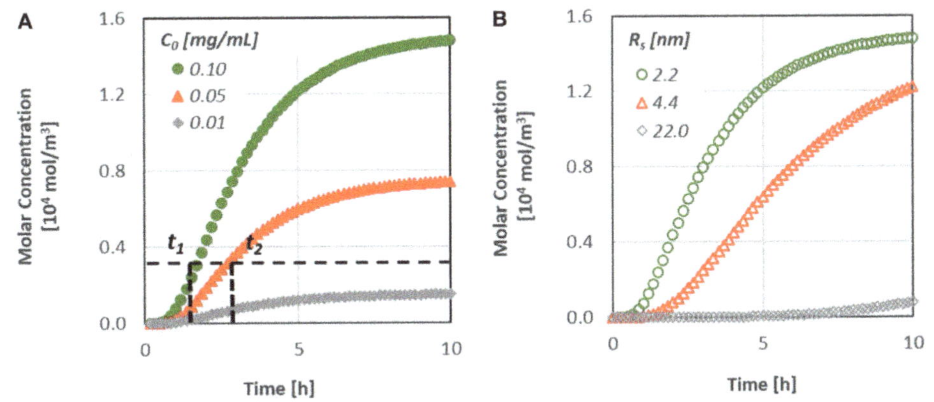


**FIGURE 5 | (A)** Effect of the initial substance concentration on the diffusion characteristics [$t_{(1,2)}$ time needed to reach a specified concentration value at the pulp] and **(B)** Effect of the molecular size on the diffusion characteristics.

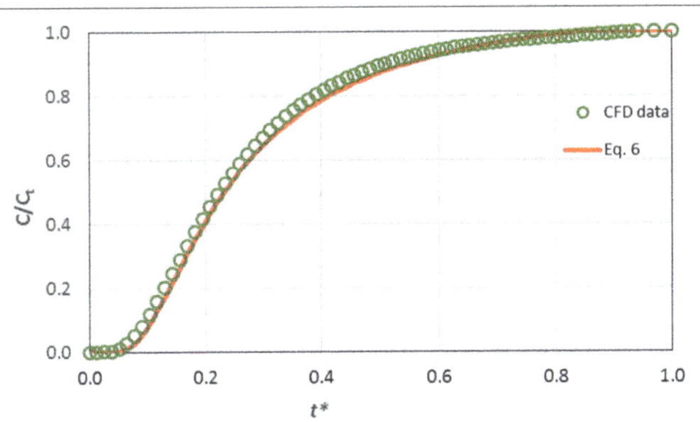


**FIGURE 6 | Comparison of CFD results on the transdentinal diffusion of a protein ($R_S$ = 2.2 nm, $C_0$ = 0.10 mg/mL) with the prediction of Equation (6).**

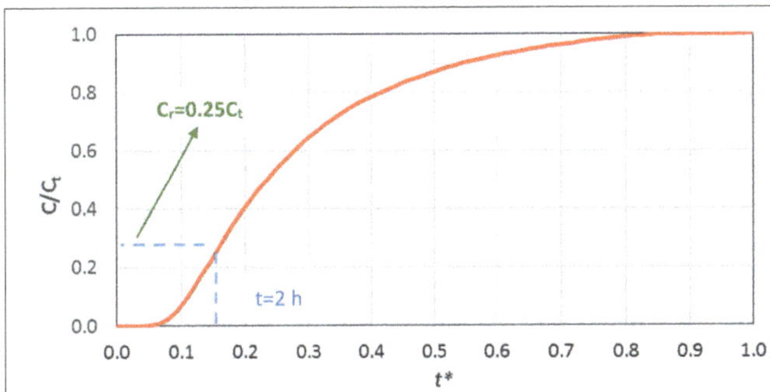


**FIGURE 7 | Graphical solution of Equation (6).**

proposed correlation, given in Equation (6), has been formulated by data fitting on the computational results and incorporates the dimensionless time $t^*$:

$$C/C_t = \exp\left(0.21 + \frac{0.115}{t^*} \cdot \ln\left(t^*\right)\right) \quad (6)$$

where $$t^* = Dt/L^2. \quad (7)$$

In **Figure 6** the computational results concerning the dimensionless concentration at the pulpal area vs. the dimensionless time $t^*$ are compared with the values predicted by Equation (6).

The data are in excellent agreement with the prediction of the proposed correlation and consequently one can draw the conclusion that Equation (6) is suitable for estimating the concentration at the pulp during the diffusion process. Obviously, the proposed correlation can be applied for substances with various molecular sizes $R_s$ and hence different diffusion coefficients, since diffusion in dentinal tubules can be safely considered one-dimensional.

## Stepwise Procedure

In the present protocol study a stepwise procedure for estimating the diffusate concentration to be imposed at the dentin-enamel junction so as the drug concentration to attain a *required value* at the pulpal side of the tubules is proposed given the geometrical characteristics of the dentinal tubules:

- Estimate the diffusion coefficient of the agent through Equations (4, 5), given its size or molecular weight.
- Choose the required value of the drug concentration, $C_r$, at the pulpal side of the tubules.
- Choose the maximum acceptable time, $t$, for the drug concentration to attain the required value $C_r$.
- Calculate the initial concentration $C_0$ of the substance by solving Equation (6) either numerically or graphically (**Figure 7**).

A detailed example concerning the application of this stepwise procedure, based on **Figure 7**, for the estimation of the initial concentration of the therapeutic agent ($C_o$), in order to achieve the required final concentration ($C_r$) after an acceptable time ($t$) is given hereafter.

- A typical protein with diameter $R_s$ = 2.2 nm is considered.

**TABLE 2 | Critical time for $C_t = C_r/0.25$ for various therapeutic agents.**

| Released molecules/Ions | Critical time $t_r$ (min) |
|---|---|
| TEGDMA Triethylene glycol dimethacrylate | 21 |
| HEMA 2-Hydroxyethyl methacrylate | 16 |
| Fluoride ions | 7 |
| Eugenol 4-Allyl-2-methoxyphenol | 17 |
| Calcium ions | 9 |
| Silicon | 8 |
| Transforming growth factor -beta | 113 |
| Bone morphogenetic protein 7 | 118 |

- The diffusion coefficient $D$ of the protein calculated by Equation (5) is $1.36 \cdot 10^{-10}$ m$^2$/s.
- A typical length ($L$) of a dentinal tubule can be considered to be 2.5 mm.
- Using the aforementioned values and Equation (6) one can plot the corresponding curve (**Figure 7**).
- If it is desirable for the required drug concentration value to reach the pulp within 2 h, the variable $t^* = 0.15$.
- From **Figure 7** the ratio $C_r/C_t = 0.25$ is determined.
- As the required effective drug concentration ($C_r$) is dictated by the dental clinic practice, the final concentration ($C_t$) can be calculated as $C_t = C_r/0.25$.
- Finally, for a given $C_t$ and the corresponding mass balance (drug quantity and tubule's dimensions one can easily estimate, from a mass balance (i.e., $C_0V_0 = C_tV_t$, where $V_t$ is the total volume of the tubulus and the drug), the initial concentration of the drug $C_0$ to be imposed at the *DEJ*.

Following the stepwise procedure and assuming that $C_t = C_r/0.25$ for the required effective concentration at the pulp for all the therapeutic substances of **Table 1**, the corresponding critical time are calculated through Equations (6, 7) and are presented in **Table 2**.

## Discussion on the Proposed Methodology

In the present study we propose a simple algorithm which, given the type of molecules of the therapeutic agent and the maximum acceptable time for the drug concentration to attain a required value at the pulpal side of the tubules, can estimate the initial concentration to be imposed. An example on the application of the proposed methodology is given in the stepwise procedure.

We must point out here that our study deals with a sole microtube that represents a typical dentin tubule that bears no obstructions of any type. The main assumptions made are:

- The geometry comprises a typical dentinal tubule 2.5 mm long and 1 and 3 μm in diameter at the dentin-enamel and the dentin-pulp junction respectively.
- The diffusion can be safely presumed one-dimensional.
- Molecules/ions that enter a dentinal tubule do not react with each other.
- The presence of large plasma proteins underlying the pulp, such as fibrinogen (Mw >300 kDa) or immunoglobulins (150 kDa) are not expected to impede the diffusion of therapeutic agents from the *DE* junction to the pulp.

However, the overall dentin permeability may be reduced due to occlusions of one or more dentin tubules and for this reason one must be able to apply a typical value (i.e., coefficient) of potential permeability, but this is beyond the scope of the present study. In the literature several factors that may lower the dentin permeability are introduced. Pashley and Tay (2012) mention that tubules in the dentin of mature teeth can be totally occluded, partially occluded and patent due to the presence of organic fibers and inorganic crystals or that smear layer and smear plugs that are produced during operative dental treatment may cover the exposed dentinal surface and seal the dentinal tubules.

Understanding the central role that fluid dynamics plays in the maintenance of vitality and function of the dentin-pulp complex, scientists can address the problems of delivery and control of potent toxic effects of molecules released from dental materials and of biologically active molecules used in tissue engineering approaches. Both advantages offer opportunities for development of new therapies in dental clinical practice.

## Acknowledgments

The authors would like to thank the Lab technician Mr. A. Lekkas for the construction and installation of the experimental setup. Prof. S. Yiantsios and Dr. I. A. Stogiannis are also kindly acknowledged for their valuable comments and suggestions. This research has been co-financed by the EU (ESF) and Hellenic National Funds Program "*Education and Lifelong Learning*" (NSRF)-Research Funding Program: "*ARISTEIA*"/"*EXCELLENCE*" (grant no 1904).

## References

Bindhu, C. V., and Harilal, S. S. (2001). Effect of the excitation source on the quantum-yield measurements of rhodamine B laser dye studied using thermal-lens technique. *Anal. Sci.* 17, 141–144. doi: 10.2116/analsci.17.141

Boutsioukis, C., Lambrianidis, T., and Kastrinakis, E. (2009). Irrigant flow within a prepared root canal using various flow rates: a Computational Fluid Dynamics study. *Int. Endod. J.* 42, 144–155. doi: 10.1111/j.1365-2591.2008.01503.x

de Peralta, T., and Nör, J. (2014). "Regeneration of the living pulp," in *The Dental Pulp*, ed M. Goldberg (Berlin; Heidelberg: Springer), 237–250.

Erickson, H. P. (2009). Size and shape of protein molecules at the nanometer level determined by sedimentation, gel filtration, and electron microscopy. *Biol. Proced. Online* 11, 32–51. doi: 10.1007/s12575-009-9008-x

Gao, Y., Haapasalo, M., Shen, Y., Wu, H., Li, B., Ruse, N. D., et al. (2009). Development and validation of a three-dimensional computational fluid dynamics model of root canal irrigation. *J. Endod.* 35, 1282–1287. doi: 10.1016/j.joen.2009.06.018

Gendron, P. O., Avaltroni, F., and Wilkinson, K. J. (2008). Diffusion coefficients of several rhodamine derivatives as determined by pulsed field gradient-nuclear magnetic resonance and fluorescence correlation spectroscopy. *J. Fluoresc.* 18, 1093–1101. doi: 10.1007/s10895-008-0357-7

Kalyva, M., Papadimitriou, S., and Tziafas, D. (2010). Transdentinal stimulation of tertiary dentine formation and intratubular mineralization by growth factors. *Int. Endod. J.* 43, 382–392. doi: 10.1111/j.1365-2591.2010.01690.x

McCabe, W. L., Smith, J. C., and Harriott, P. (2005). *Unit Operations of Chemical Engineering, 7th Edn.* Boston, MA: McGraw-Hill.

Murray, P. E., About, I., Franquin, J. C., Remusat, M., and Smith, A. J. (2001). Restorative pulpal and repair responses. *J. Am. Den. Ass.* 132, 482–491. doi: 10.14219/jada.archive.2001.0211

Murray, P. E., Garcia-Godoy, C., and Garcia-Godoy, F. (2007). How is the biocompatibility of dental biomaterials evaluated? *Med. Oral Patol. Oral Cir. Bucal* 12, E258–E266.

Murray, P. E., Smith, A. J., Windsor, L. J., and Mjör, I. A. (2003). Remaining dentine thickness and human pulp responses. *Int. Endod. J.* 36, 33–43. doi: 10.1046/j.0143-2885.2003.00609.x

Pashley, D. H. (1990). Dentin permeability: theory and practice. *Exp. Endodont.* 1, 19–49.

Pashley, D. H. (1992a). Dentin permeability and dentin sensitivity. *Proc. Finnish Den. Soc.* 88 (Suppl. 1), 31–37.

Pashley, D. H. (1992b). Smear layer: overview of structure and function. *Proc. Finnish Den. Soc.* 88 (Suppl. 1), 215–224.

Pashley, D. H., and Matthews, W. G. (1993). The effects of outward forced convective flow on inward diffusion in human dentin *in vitro*. *Arch. Oral Biol.* 38, 577–582. doi: 10.1016/0003-9969(93)90122-3

Pashley, D. H., and Tay, F. R. (2012). "Pulpodentin complex," in *Seltzer and Bender's Dental Pulp, 2nd Edn.*, eds K. M. Hargreaves, H. E. Goodis, and F. R. Tay (Chicago, IA: Quintessence Publishing Co), 47–66.

Rutherford, R. B., Spanberg, L., Tucker, M., and Charette, M. (1995). Transdentinal stimulation of reparative dentine formation by OP-1 in monkeys. *Arch. Oral Biol.* 40, 681–683. doi: 10.1016/0003-9969(95)00020-P

Sakakibara, J., and Adrian, R. J. (1999). Whole field measurement of temperature in water using two-color laser induced fluorescence. *Exp. Fluids* 26, 7–15. doi: 10.1007/s003480050260

Schweikl, H., Petzel, C., Bolay, C., Hiller, K. A., Buchalla, W., and Krifka, S. (2014). 2-Hydroxyethyl methacrylate-induced apoptosis through the ATM- and p53-dependent intrinsic mitochondrial pathway. *Biomaterials* 35, 2890–2904. doi: 10.1016/j.biomaterials.2013.12.044

Smith, A. J. (2003). Vitality of the dentin-pulp complex in health and disease: growth factors as key mediators. *J. Dent. Educ.* 67, 678–689.

Smith, A. J., Tobias, R. S., and Murray, P. E. (2001). Transdentinal stimulation of reactionary dentinogenesis in ferrets by dentine matrix components. *J. Dent.* 29, 341–346. doi: 10.1016/S0300-5712(01)00020-3

Su, K. C., Chuang, S. F., Ng, E. Y., and Chang, C. H. (2014). An investigation of dentinal fluid flow in dental pulp during food mastication: simulation of fluid-structure interaction. *Biomech. Model. Mechanobiol.* 13, 527–535. doi: 10.1007/s10237-013-0514-z

Tziafas, D., Smith, A. J., and Lesot, H. (2000). Designing new treatment strategies in vital pulp therapy. *J. Dent.* 28, 77–92. doi: 10.1016/S0300-5712(99)00047-0

# Human odontoblast-like cells produce nitric oxide with antibacterial activity upon TLR2 activation

**Edited by:**
*Giovanna Orsini, Polytechnic University of Marche, Italy*

***Correspondence:**
*Jean-Christophe Farges, Laboratoire de Biologie Tissulaire et Ingénierie Thérapeutique, Institut de Biologie et Chimie des Protéines, 7 Passage du Vercors, 69367 Lyon, France*
*jean-christophe.farges@univ-lyon1.fr*

***Jean-Christophe Farges[1,2,3,4]*, Aurélie Bellanger[1], Maxime Ducret[2,3,4], Elisabeth Aubert-Foucher[4], Béatrice Richard[1,2,3], Brigitte Alliot-Licht[5], Françoise Bleicher[1] and Florence Carrouel[1,2]***

*[1] Institut de Génomique Fonctionnelle de Lyon, UMR5242 Centre National de la Recherche Scientifique/ENS/Université Lyon 1, Equipe Physiopathologie des Odontoblastes, Lyon, France, [2] Faculté d'Odontologie, Université Lyon 1, Université de Lyon, Lyon, France, [3] Hospices Civils de Lyon, Service de Consultations et Traitements Dentaires, Lyon, France, [4] Laboratoire de Biologie Tissulaire et Ingénierie Thérapeutique, Institut de Biologie et Chimie des Protéines, UMR5305 Centre National de la Recherche Scientifique/Université Lyon 1, Lyon, France, [5] Faculté d'Odontologie, Centre de Recherche en Transplantation et Immunologie, INSERM UMR1064, Université de Nantes, Nantes, France*

The penetration of cariogenic oral bacteria into enamel and dentin during the caries process triggers an immune/inflammatory response in the underlying pulp tissue, the reduction of which is considered a prerequisite to dentinogenesis-based pulp regeneration. If the role of odontoblasts in dentin formation is well known, their involvement in the antibacterial response of the dental pulp to cariogenic microorganisms has yet to be elucidated. Our aim here was to determine if odontoblasts produce nitric oxide (NO) with antibacterial activity upon activation of Toll-like receptor-2 (TLR2), a cell membrane receptor involved in the recognition of cariogenic Gram-positive bacteria. Human odontoblast-like cells differentiated from dental pulp explants were stimulated with the TLR2 synthetic agonist Pam2CSK4. We found that *NOS1*, *NOS2,* and *NOS3* gene expression was increased in Pam2CSK4-stimulated odontoblast-like cells compared to unstimulated ones. *NOS2* was the most up-regulated gene. NOS1 and NOS3 proteins were not detected in Pam2CSK4-stimulated or control cultures. NOS2 protein synthesis, NOS activity and NO extracellular release were all augmented in stimulated samples. Pam2CSK4-stimulated cell supernatants reduced *Streptococcus mutans* growth, an effect counteracted by the NOS inhibitor L-NAME. *In vivo*, the *NOS2* gene was up-regulated in the inflamed pulp of carious teeth compared with healthy ones. NOS2 protein was immunolocalized in odontoblasts situated beneath the caries lesion but not in pulp cells from healthy teeth. These results suggest that odontoblasts may participate to the antimicrobial pulp response to dentin-invading Gram-positive bacteria through NOS2-mediated NO production. They might in this manner pave the way for accurate dental pulp healing and regeneration.

**Keywords: tooth, odontoblast, caries lesion, dental pulp regeneration, nitric oxide, toll-like receptor 2, *Streptococcus mutans***

## Introduction

Odontoblasts are neural crest-derived, highly specialized mesenchymal cells organized as a densely packed layer at the periphery of the loose connective tissue situated in the center of the tooth, the dental pulp. Their main functions are the synthesis, extracellular deposition and mineralization of a collagen-rich matrix to form the dentin tissue that surrounds the dental pulp and underlies the surface enamel. Recent data have indicated that odontoblasts may also have functions not related to dentinogenesis (Bleicher et al., 2015). Indeed, because of their specific location at the pulp-dentin interface and the entrapment of their long cell process in dentin, they become exposed to dentin-invading oral bacteria during the carious process (Love and Jenkinson, 2002). Odontoblasts are the first cells encountered by tooth-invading pathogens and they have been suggested to initiate pulp immune and inflammatory responses to these pathogens (Durand et al., 2006; Veerayutthwilai et al., 2007). These responses may eliminate the insult and block the route of infection. Unchecked, bacterial invasion results in irreversible pulp inflammation then necrosis, and dissemination of potentially lethal microorganisms may occur throughout the body (Farges et al., 2009). In parallel, dentin formation appears greatly disturbed (Bjorndal and Mjör, 2001; Durand et al., 2006). Several lines of evidence now support the notion that it is only when pulp infection and inflammation are under control that dentinogenesis-based pulp regeneration will occur. In this context, further studies are needed to elucidate the odontoblast response to cariogenic bacteria in order to design new antibacterial therapeutics that will reduce dental pulp inflammation while promoting tissue healing and regeneration (Farges et al., 2013; Cooper et al., 2014).

Studies that aimed at elucidating the triggering of dental pulp immunity by odontoblasts have mostly focused on gram-positive bacteria, because these largely dominate the microflora in initial and moderate dentin caries lesions (Love and Jenkinson, 2002; Hahn and Liewehr, 2007). In particular, odontoblast-like cells were found to be responsive to lipoteichoic acid (LTA), a Gram-positive bacteria component recognized at cell surface through the pattern recognition receptor (PRR) Toll-like receptor-2 (TLR2). Engagement of odontoblast TLR2 by LTA up-regulates TLR2 itself and nucleotide-binding oligomerization domain 2, a cytosolic PRR. It also stimulates the production of the proinflammatory chemokines and cytokines CCL2, CXCL1, CXCL2, CXCL8, CXCL10, and interleukin (IL)-6, and the recruitment of immature dendritic cells (Durand et al., 2006; Staquet et al., 2008, 2011; Farges et al., 2009, 2011; Keller et al., 2010, 2011). IL-10, a cytokine that plays a central role in limiting host immune responses to pathogens, was also up-regulated. Similar, effects were observed when using Pam2CSK4, a synthetic diacylated lipopeptide analog that specifically binds TLR2. Of note, the response obtained with Pam2CSK4 was always higher than with LTA. However, no additional cytokine was induced by Pam2CSK4 compared to LTA, suggesting that odontoblasts secrete a limited set of proinflammatory factors when challenged with Gram-positive bacteria. We also observed that the lipopolysaccharide (LPS)-binding protein (LBP) was up-regulated by Pam2CSK4 (our unpublished results) and that it decreased TLR2 activation and proinflammatory cytokine production in odontoblast-like cells (Carrouel et al., 2013).

If the role of odontoblasts in the triggering and control of dental pulp immunity begins to be elucidated, their involvement in the direct fight against dentin-invading bacteria is far less known. Among antibacterial agents putatively produced by odontoblasts, nitric oxide (NO) has recently received particular attention. NO is a highly diffusible, gaseous free radical generated by nitric oxide synthases (NOS) through the conversion of L-arginine to L-citrulline. Three NOS isoforms have been identified so far: two are constitutively expressed at low levels, NOS1 (neuronal NOS) and NOS3 (endothelial NOS), whereas one is produced upon cell stimulation by microorganisms or proinflammatory cytokines, NOS2 (inducible NOS). NOS1 and NOS3 participate to normal tissue functions by constitutively synthesizing very small amounts (picomolar to nanomolar levels) of short acting NO (seconds to minutes). NOS2 is the enzyme responsible for high NO production in infection settings (Arthur and Ley, 2013). It is predominantly regulated at the transcriptional level and is involved in antibacterial defense by producing large amounts of NO, up to micromolar levels, for sustained periods of time (hours to days) (Nathan, 1992; Nussler and Billiar, 1993; MacMicking et al., 1997; Bogdan, 2001; Coleman, 2001; Guzik et al., 2003). Previous studies indicated that the *NOS2* gene was not or weakly expressed in healthy dental pulps, but was sharply up-regulated in inflamed ones (Law et al., 1999; Di Nardo Di Maio et al., 2004; Kawashima et al., 2005; Korkmaz et al., 2011). Human odontoblasts showed a marked immunoreactivity for 3-nitrotyrosine (a biomarker for NO-derived peroxinitrite) in inflamed pulp, suggesting that these cells release NO upon NOS2 activation. NO production by odontoblasts might be an important defense mechanism against dentin-invading oral microorganisms because it inhibits *Streptococcus mutans* growth (Silva-Mendez et al., 1999). Despite these important findings, no direct evidence was brought so far that odontoblasts produce NO amounts bactericidal for caries-related, gram-positive microorganisms. Therefore, the aim of our study was to investigate, in a culture model of human odontoblasts differentiated *in vitro*, if these cells are able to produce NO with antibacterial activity upon TLR2 engagement. We first studied the effects of Pam2CSK4 stimulation on odontoblast *NOS1*, *NOS2*, and *NOS3* gene expression. We also examined NOS1, NOS2, and NOS3 protein synthesis, NOS intracellular activity and NO secretion upon Pam2CSK4 stimulation. We then assessed the antibacterial effect of odontoblast-derived NO by analyzing the growth of *Streptococcus mutans* bacteria in the presence of TLR2-activated or control odontoblast-like cell culture supernatants. Finally, expression of NOS2 transcript and protein was investigated *in vivo* in healthy and bacteria-challenged inflamed dental pulps.

## Materials and Methods

### Reagents

The synthetic diacylated lipopeptide analog Pam2CSK4 was from InvivoGen (San Diego, CA, USA). The mouse anti-NOS2 monoclonal antibody (clone 2D2-B2) was from R&D Systems Europe (Lille, France). Rabbit anti-NOS1 monoclonal (EP1855Y) and anti-NOS3 polyclonal antibodies were from Abcam (Cambridge, UK). The mouse anti-GAPDH monoclonal antibody (clone 8C2) was from Santa Cruz Biotechnology (Santa Cruz, CA USA). The mouse immunoglobulin G1 isotype control antibody (clone MOPC-21) and the arginine analog NOS inhibitor NG-nitro-L-arginine methyl ester (L-NAME) were from Sigma-Aldrich (St Louis, MO, USA).

## Dental Pulp Samples

Healthy and decayed human teeth were collected with informed consent of the patients or their parents, in accordance with the World Medical Association's Declaration of Helsinki and following a protocol approved by the local ethics committee. Healthy pulps were taken from impacted third molars. Inflamed pulps were taken from decayed erupted molars with clinical features of acute pulpitis (deep dentin caries lesions, severe spontaneous dental pain for 12–24 h, no sensitivity to vertical or horizontal percussion, lack of periapical lesions) and in the absence of anti-inflammatory treatment.

## Cell Culture and Treatments

Odontoblast-like cells were differentiated from dental pulp explants obtained from clinically healthy, impacted human third molars as previously described (Couble et al., 2000), then used for stimulation experiments. For detection of *NOS* gene expression, NOS protein production, NOS activity and NO extracellular levels, cells were cultured for the indicated times in the absence (controls) or in the presence of 10 μg/mL Pam2CSK4. To determine the antibacterial effect of odontoblast-like cell-derived NO on *Streptococcus mutans* bacteria, cells were treated with 10 μg/mL Pam2CSK4 for 24 h, and then culture media were collected and frozen until further use (see below). Some cultures were pretreated for 1 h with 0.5 or 1 mmol/L L-NAME prior to addition of Pam2CSK4 to confirm NO involvement in the effect observed.

## Reverse Transcription-Polymerase Chain Reaction

RNA extraction and reverse transcription were performed from Pam2CSK4-stimulated and control odontoblast-like cells and from healthy and inflamed dental pulp samples as described (Keller et al., 2010; Farges et al., 2011). Real-time polymerase chain reaction (PCR) was performed in a CFX96 Real-Time PCR Detection System with the Fast Start Master SYBR Green I kit (Bio-Rad Laboratories, Hercules, CA, USA) according to the manufacturer's specifications. The cyclophilin A housekeeping gene (*PPIA*) was used for sample normalization. Gene-specific primer sequences for *NOS1*, *NOS2*, *NOS3*, and *PPIA* are listed in **Table 1**. Annealing temperature was 65°C for all primer pairs. All runs were performed in duplicate. For each target gene, relative expression was determined after normalization using the Bio-Rad CFX Manager software. Results were expressed as fold change values relative to control odontoblast-like cell cultures for *in vitro* analyses and to healthy pulp samples for *in vivo* analyses.

## Protein Extraction and Western Blotting

Cells were washed twice with PBS and overlaid with ice-cold RIPA buffer (Sigma-Aldrich) supplemented with a protease inhibitor cocktail (P8340, dilution 1:100; Sigma-Aldrich). After 5 min on ice, cells were scraped and insoluble material was removed by centrifugation at 12,000 g for 10 min at 4°C. Total proteins were quantified by a Bradford assay (Coomassie Protein Assay Reagent; Pierce, Thermo Fischer Scientific Inc., Rockford, IL, USA). Proteins were concentrated by precipitation for NOS isoform detection. After addition of 4 volumes of cold acetone and incubation for at least 1 h at −20°C, pellets were collected by centrifugation at 12,000 g for 10 min at 4°C, air-dried and dissolved in reducing Laemmli sample buffer. Identical amounts of proteins were loaded for Pam2CSK4-stimulated and control samples. Positive controls for NOS1 (neuronal NOS) and NOS3 (endothelial NOS) were extracts from mouse whole brain and human umbilical vein endothelial cells (HUVEC), respectively. HUVEC were kindly provided by Dr Laurent Müller (CIRB CNRS UMR7241 - INSERM U1050, Collège de France, Paris). Proteins were resolved by 8.5% sodium dodecyl sulfate polyacrylamide gel electrophoresis and transferred to PVDF membranes (Millipore, Molsheim, France). Membranes were probed with anti-NOS1 (diluted 1:1000), anti-NOS2 (1:400), anti-NOS3 (1:1000) or anti-GAPDH (1:2000) and incubated with HRP- or alkaline phosphatase-conjugated anti-rabbit or anti-mouse IgGs (1:1000; Cell Signaling). Bound antibodies were detected on x-ray films by using Immunstar PA, Immunstar HRP or WesternC chemiluminescent substrates (Bio-Rad Laboratories).

## Detection of NOS Activity and Extracellular NO Production

NOS activity and NO production by Pam2CSK4-stimulated and control odontoblast-like cells were quantified in cell lysates and culture media by using an Ultrasensitive Colorimetric NOS Assay kit and a Nitric Oxide Colorimetric Assay kit (Oxford Biomedical

**TABLE 1 | Primers used for PCR analysis.**

| Gene | Forward primer | Reverse primer | Amplicon size (bp) |
|---|---|---|---|
| *NOS1* | CTGATACCAAAAGCCTCTCT | ATCTGAGCCTAACAATCTGG | 76 |
| *NOS2* | ACAGGCTCGTGCAGGACTCA | CACGGCTGGATGTCGGACTT | 126 |
| *NOS3* | CATGAGCACTGAGATCGGCA | CCAGGATGTTGTAGCGGTGA | 59 |
| *PPIA* | GGATTGCTTGAGCCTAGAGTGA | CCTCTGCCTACCTTTGAGACAC | 87 |

Research, Oxford, MI, USA), respectively, according to the manufacturer's specifications. Cells were lysed in Beadlyte® Cell Signaling Universal Lysis Buffer (Millipore). NO is highly labile, with a half-life in the order of seconds, and these kits are based on the colorimetric quantitation of nitrite ($NO_2^-$), the stable end product of NO oxidation, using Griess reagent. They include the conversion of nitrate to nitrite by NADH-dependent enzyme nitrate reductase before nitrite measurement, in order to provide for accurate determination of total NO production. Absorbance values were read at 540 nm using a microplate reader. NO/nitrite sample concentrations were determined from a sodium nitrite standard curve. Intracellular NO/nitrite concentration was expressed as μmoles/μg of proteins (determined using a Bradford protein assay).

### *Streptococcus mutans* Growth Assessment

The *Streptococcus mutans* strain (CIP 103220) was purchased from Institut Pasteur (Paris, France). Bacteria were cultured in Brain Heart Infusion broth (Biomérieux, Marcy-L'Etoile, France) at 37°C for 24 h. After centrifugation at 2500 rpm for 5 min, the supernatant was discarded and the bacterial pellet resuspended in water for determination of the bacteria number with McFarland Standard (Biomérieux). Samples containing $10^8$ bacteria were then taken and centrifuged at 15,000 rpm for 5 min. Bacterial pellets were resuspended in 100 μL odontoblast-like cell culture supernatants, then maintained at 37°C for 15, 30, 60, or 90 min, the later time being just before the end of the bacteria growth phase as determined by our preliminary experiments (not shown). Bacteria-containing samples were then plated onto Columbia agar supplemented with 5% defibrinated horse blood. Bacterial cultures were performed in anaerobic conditions (GENbox anaer, Biomérieux) for 5 days at 37°C, then *S. mutans* colonies were counted.

### Immunohistochemistry

Healthy teeth and carious ones with inflamed pulps were fixed in 4% paraformaldehyde-phosphate-buffered saline solution for 7 days, demineralized in 10% acetic acid for 4 months, and routinely treated for paraffin embedding. Eight-micrometer serial sections were then cut, deparaffinized, and rehydrated. Endogenous peroxidase was blocked by incubation in 0.3% hydrogen peroxide for 15 min at room temperature. Sections were incubated for antigen retrieval in 10 mmol/L citrate buffer (pH 6.0, 98°C) for 10 min and then blocked with normal horse serum for 45 min at room temperature. Sections were then incubated with 12.5 μg/mL anti-NOS2 antibody overnight at 4°C. Staining controls were performed by using a mouse immunoglobulin G1 isotype. Antibody detection was performed by using a Vectastain Elite ABC kit (Vector Laboratories, Burlingame, CA, USA) according to the manufacturer's protocol, peroxidase being localized with diaminobenzidine.

### Statistical Analysis

Results were expressed as mean values ± standard deviation obtained from different odontoblast-like cell cultures or tooth pulps originating from human third molars obtained from different donors. Statistical analysis was performed with a paired *t*-test. A $p < 0.05$ was considered significant.

## Results

### Pam2CSK4 Increases *NOS1, NOS2,* and *NOS3* Gene Expression and NOS2 Protein Synthesis in Odontoblast-Like Cells

We previously found that the synthetic lipoprotein analog Pam2CSK4 at a 10 μg/mL concentration was particularly efficient to activate TLR2 in odontoblast-like cells and induced the production of proinflammatory cytokines and chemokines (Keller et al., 2010, 2011; Farges et al., 2011; Staquet et al., 2011). Therefore we used, in the present study, the same concentration to assess Pam2CSK4 effect on the expression of *NOS1*, *NOS2,* and *NOS3* genes by these cells. We observed that Pam2CSK4 significantly up-regulated the three genes tested (**Figure 1A**). The gene coding for the inducible NOS, *NOS2,* was the most up-regulated one, the increase being maximal after 8 h of cell stimulation. At the protein level, NOS2 was strongly increased after 8 h of Pam2CSK4 stimulation compared to control unstimulated cells (**Figure 1B**). NOS1 and NOS3 were not detected in control or Pam2CSK4-stimulated samples stimulated for 8 or 16 h (not shown).

### Pam2CSK4 Increases NO Production by Odontoblast-like cells

To determine whether NOS2 up-regulation upon Pam2CSK4 stimulation was accompanied by an increase in NOS activity and NO production, intracellular and extracellular NO concentrations were assessed by the measure of the NO degradation end-product nitrite. We observed a strong intracellular nitrite increase that was maximal after 8 h (**Figure 2A**). To assess NO diffusion to the extracellular compartment, we measured nitrite concentration in supernatants of Pam2CSK4-stimulated odontoblast-like cells. We found a progressive accumulation of nitrite in the culture medium reaching a concentration of approximately 40 μmol/L after 24 h, the longest stimulation time tested (**Figure 2B**). In unstimulated samples, the nitrite concentration remained low and constant with time, of approximately 10 μmol/L.

### Odontoblast-Like Cell-Derived NO Reduces *Streptococcus mutans* Growth

Next, to evaluate the NO effect on the growth of cariogenic microorganisms, odontoblast-like cells were stimulated or not with 10 μg/mL Pam2CSK4 for 24 h with or without pretreatment with the NOS inhibitor L-NAME. Culture supernatants were collected and placed into contact with *Streptococcus mutans* bacteria for 15, 30, 60, or 90 min. In unstimulated samples, pretreatment with L-NAME increased the number of *Streptococcus mutans* colony-forming units, suggesting that NO from unstimulated odontoblast-like cells limits *Streptococcus mutans* growth (**Figure 3**). We observed that the number of *Streptococcus mutans* colony-forming units was clearly reduced in odontoblast-like cells stimulated with Pam2CSK4 compared to unstimulated ones, indicating a stronger antibacterial effect of culture supernatants from TLR2-activated cells. The decrease in NO production owing to increasing concentrations of L-NAME in Pam2CSK4-stimulated samples led to an augmentation of

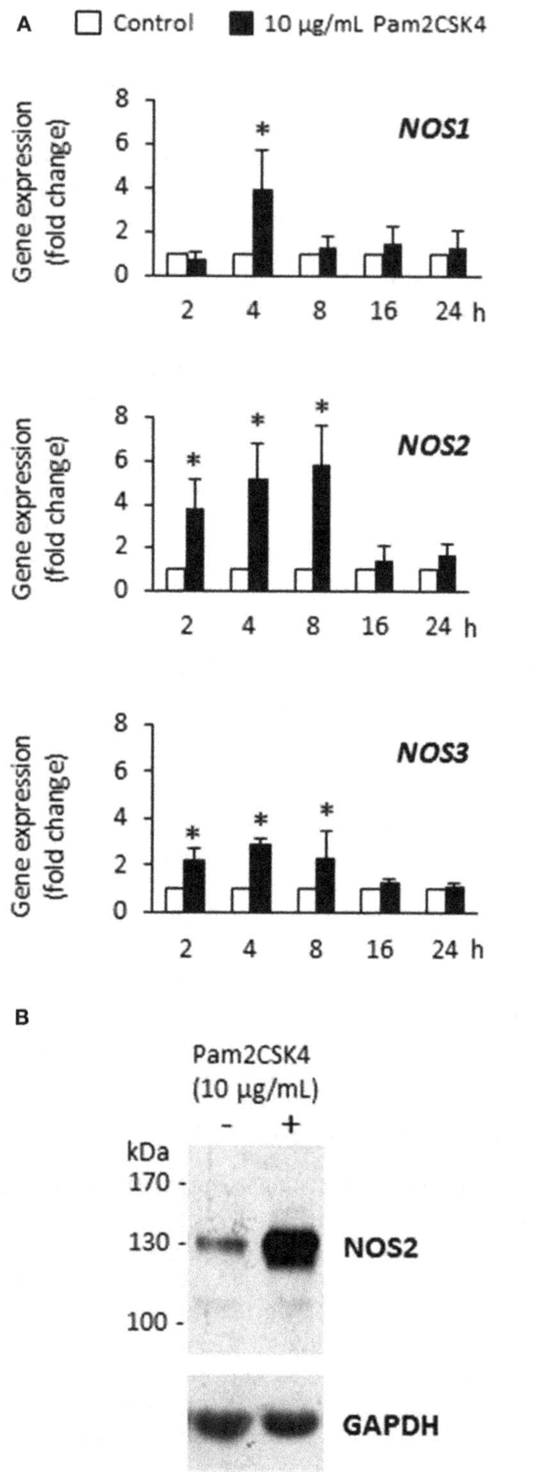


**FIGURE 1 | Pam2CSK4 increases *NOS1*, *NOS2*, and *NOS3* gene expression and NOS2 protein synthesis in odontoblast-like cells. (A)** Analysis of *NOS1*, *NOS2*, and *NOS3* gene expression after cell challenge with 10 µg/mL Pam2CSK4 for the indicated times. The three genes were significantly up-regulated upon Pam2CSK4 stimulation, *NOS2* being the most up-regulated one ($n = 4$). $^*p < 0.05$. **(B)** At the protein level, NOS2 synthesis was clearly increased after 8 h of odontoblast-like cell stimulation with 10 µg/mL Pam2CSK4. The gel shown is representative of three independent experiments.

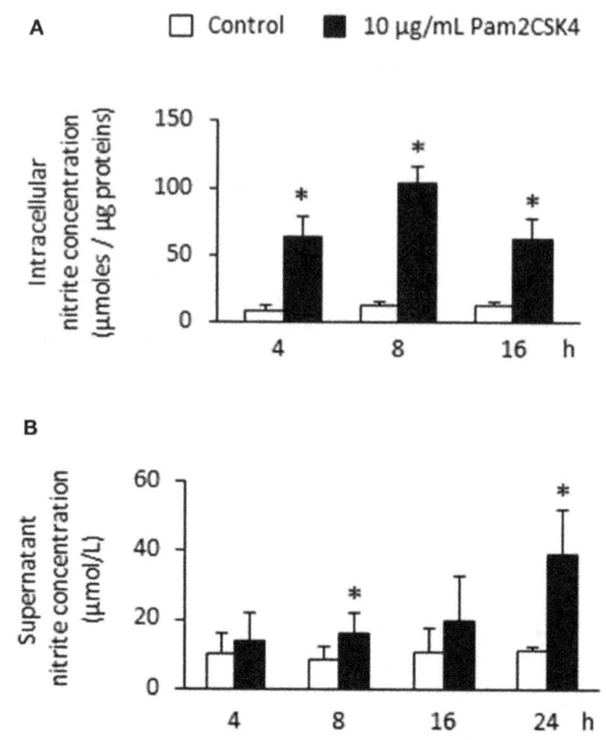


**FIGURE 2 | Pam2CSK4 increases NOS activity and extracellular NO production by odontoblast-like cells. (A)** Analysis of intracellular NO by the measurement of nitrite concentration in cells stimulated with 10 µg/mL Pam2CSK4 for the indicated times. Production of intracellular nitrite was strongly increased in PAM2CSK4-stimulated samples, being maximal after 8 h ($n = 5$). **(B)** Determination of NO concentration in culture supernatants of odontoblast-like cells stimulated with 10 µg/mL Pam2CSK4. Nitrite progressively accumulated in the culture medium, reaching a concentration of approximately 40 µmol/L after 24 h of stimulation ($n = 5$). $^*p < 0.05$.

the number of *Streptococcus mutans* colony-forming units, thus indicating that NO production by odontoblast-like cells was indeed responsible for the observed slowdown of bacterial growth.

## NOS2 Transcript and Protein are Up-Regulated in Inflamed Pulps from Decayed Teeth

To assess the *in vivo* relevance of these findings and determine whether NOS2 is expressed in odontoblasts, NOS2 transcript and protein were examined in healthy dental pulps and inflamed samples from carious teeth. We found that the *NOS2* gene was strongly up-regulated in inflamed pulps compared to healthy ones (**Figure 4A**). NOS2 protein was clearly detected by immunostaining in odontoblasts and subodontoblast cells in the inflamed area, but not in cells in the non-inflamed area far from the lesion (not shown) or in healthy pulps (**Figure 4B**). Staining controls performed by using the mouse immunoglobulin G1 isotype were negative.

## Discussion

Odontoblasts situated at the dental pulp periphery could play a role in the initiation of the tissue defense against

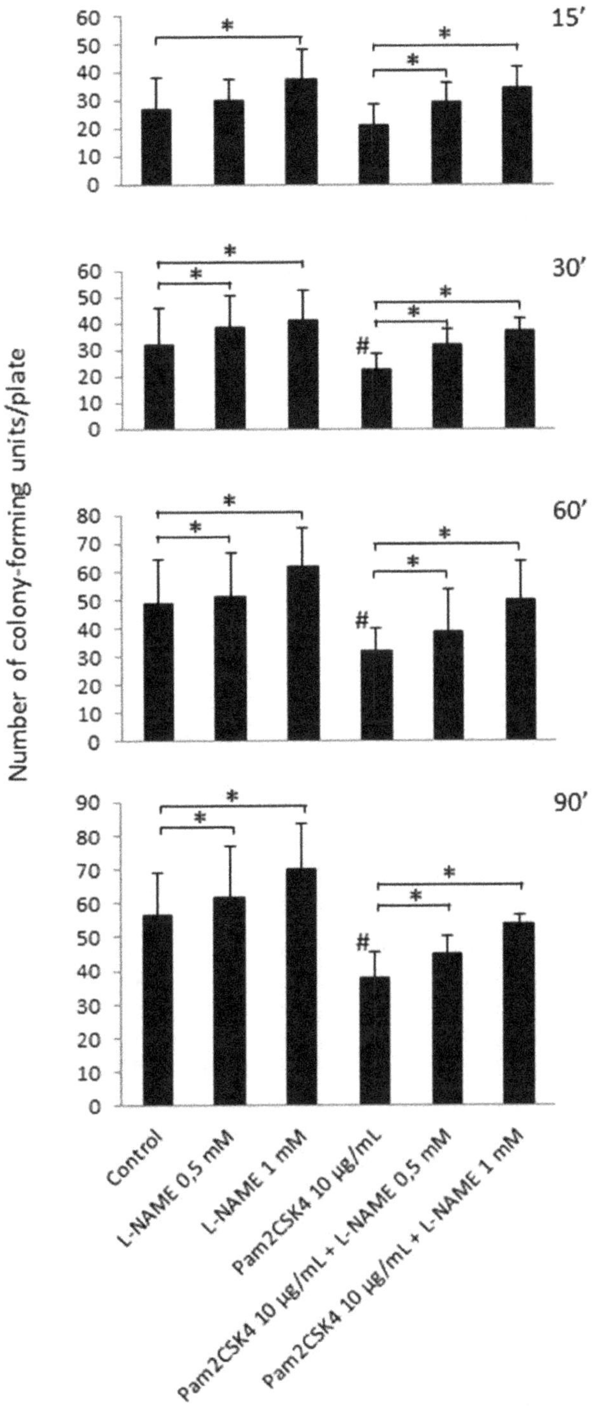


**FIGURE 3 | NO released from unstimulated or Pam2CSK4-stimulated odontoblast-like cells alters *Streptococcus mutans* viability.** Analysis of *Streptococcus mutans* growth after contact of bacteria for 15, 30, 60, or 90 min with culture supernatants of cells challenged with 10 µg/mL Pam2CSK4 for 24 h in the presence or in the absence of L-NAME. The number of *Streptococcus mutans* colony-forming units was reduced when odontoblast-like cells were stimulated with Pam2CSK4 compared to unstimulated ones. Pretreatment with the NOS inhibitor L-NAME increased the number of *Streptococcus mutans* colony-forming units in both unstimulated and Pam2CSK4-stimulated samples ($n = 6$). #$p < 0.05$ vs. control unstimulated cells. *$p < 0.05$ vs. cultures without L-NAME.

dentin-invading Gram-positive oral bacteria through their ability to recognize pathogens and to produce proinflammatory cytokines and chemokines (Farges et al., 2013). In this context, chemokine secretion from odontoblasts may induce accumulation of immune cells at the pulp-dentin interface, including antigen-presenting immature dendritic cells, to uptake bacterial by-products diffusing through dentin tubules and evolve pathogen-specific innate and adaptive responses (Durand et al., 2006). However, whether odontoblasts are able to directly destroy intradentinal or peripheral pulp-reaching microorganisms by producing antibacterial agents, without the intervention of immune cells, it is largely unknown. Nitric oxide is a highly diffusible, antimicrobial free radical generated and released by many cell types in inflammatory conditions to kill or inhibit the replication of a variety of microorganisms. NO antimicrobial activity is primarily due to NO reactivity with superoxide anion to form highly cytotoxic peroxynitrite, S-nitrosylation of thiol residues that changes protein conformation, inactivation of enzymes by disruption of iron centers, DNA damage, and membrane lipid peroxidation (Guzik et al., 2003). In this report we provide evidence that odontoblasts differentiated *in vitro* from human dental pulp explants are able to synthesize large amounts of NOS2 and produce NO with antibacterial activity upon TLR2 activation. We first observed that *NOS1*, *NOS2*, and *NOS3* gene expression was significantly increased in Pam2CSK4-stimulated cells compared to controls, *NOS2* being the most up-regulated gene. In agreement with this finding, NOS2 protein was clearly up-regulated in Pam2CSK4-stimulated cells, suggesting its involvement in NO production by these cells. Conversely, NOS1 and NOS3 isoforms, although clearly found in brain and endothelial cell extracts, respectively, were not detected in our Western blot analysis in stimulated or control samples. Accordingly, we speculate that most, if not all, of NO production by Pam2CSK4-stimulated odontoblast-like cells is due to the induction of NOS2, as shown in macrophages stimulated *in vitro* with lipopolysaccharide, another pattern recognition receptor ligand (Denlinger et al., 1996; MacMicking et al., 1997; Guzik et al., 2003).

We found that NO was produced to levels (several tenths of micromoles/liter) similar to those observed in macrophages *in vitro* stimulated with LPS or *Staphylococcus aureus* LTA, or with an association of *Streptococcus mutans* LTA and IFN-γ (Denlinger et al., 1996; Matsuno et al., 1998; Hong et al., 2014). This indicates that the responsivity of odontoblasts upon TLR2 activation, in terms of NO production, is comparable to that of specialized immune cells. To our knowledge, NO concentrations have not been reported in inflamed pulps. However, those we measured in Pam2CSK4-stimulated odontoblast-like cell supernatants were in the range of the concentrations found in periapical exudates from infected human root canals (Shimauchi et al., 2001). This indicated that NOS2-dependent NO amounts produced by TLR2-activated odontoblast-like cells is biologically relevant. We observed here that the number of *Streptococcus mutans* colony-forming units was significantly reduced by NO in stimulated odontoblast-like cells compared to control ones, suggesting the role of NO produced by odontoblasts in the fight against cariogenic bacteria.

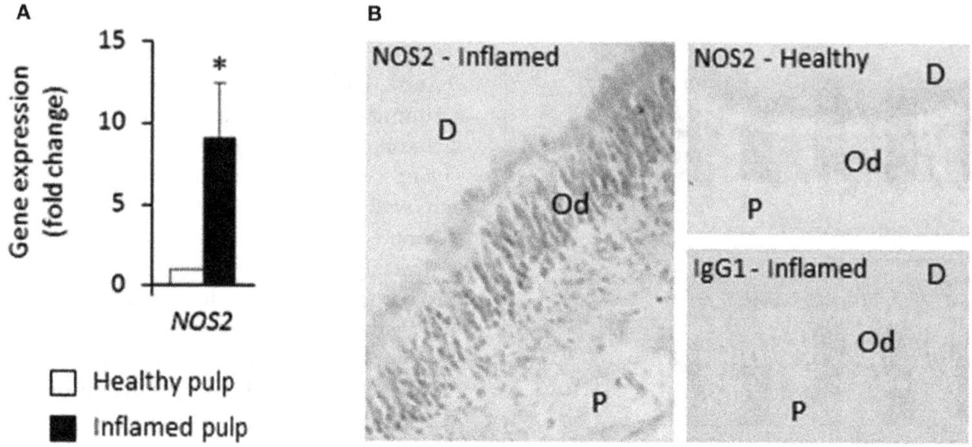


**FIGURE 4 | NOS2 transcript and protein are up-regulated in inflamed pulps from decayed teeth compared to healthy ones. (A)** Analysis of *NOS2* gene expression in healthy and inflamed pulps with real-time RT-PCR ($n = 3$). $^*p < 0.05$. **(B)** Immunohistochemical localization of NOS2 protein in healthy and bacteria-challenged inflamed pulps. No NOS2 staining was found in healthy sample, but odontoblasts and subodontoblast cells were stained in inflamed pulp beneath the caries lesion. D, dentin; Od, odontoblast layer; P, pulp. Data shown are representative of results obtained from independent experiments performed with two healthy and two carious teeth.

We then detected immunohistochemically the NOS2 protein in odontoblasts of inflamed pulps situated beneath dentin caries lesions, whereas it was not present in odontoblasts from healthy ones. This result is in accordance with the fact that NOS2 is not expressed in resting cells, but is only synthesized upon cell activation (Coleman, 2001). Odontoblasts from healthy teeth were also found to be negative for NOS2 (Kawanishi et al., 2004; Kawashima et al., 2005; Mei et al., 2007). NOS2 synthesis was increased in inflamed pulps beneath caries lesions or when inflammation was experimentally induced with bacterial by-products (Kawanishi et al., 2004; Kawashima et al., 2005; Mei et al., 2007; Korkmaz et al., 2011), underscoring the importance of this enzyme in NO production in pulp inflammatory conditions. We observed NOS2 immunoreactivity in odontoblast and subodontoblast cells of the peripheral inflamed pulp, as previously reported in human teeth (Korkmaz et al., 2011). This indicates that odontoblasts are not the only cells involved in the fight again dentin-invading microorganisms. Other cells might also include leukocytes, as previously shown (Guzik et al., 2003). We do not exclude that NOS1 and NOS3 could contribute to the high NO production in the odontoblast layer of bacteria-challenged inflamed pulps. However, several data suggests that such a contribution, if any, would be limited since NOS1 and NOS3 are only able to produce very low concentrations of NO (nanomolar range) compared to NOS2 (micromolar) (Coleman, 2001). The results presented here support the view that NOS2 is a key player in the production of physiologically relevant NO amounts by odontoblasts in bacteria-challenged inflamed pulps. NO could have deleterious effects on odontoblasts themselves. However, these effects might be limited since soluble guanylate cyclase, the receptor that mediates NO effects inside the cell, is decreased in odontoblasts in inflamed human pulps compared to healthy ones (Korkmaz et al., 2011). This indicates that the NO present in the odontoblast layer would rather act on neighboring cells and/or, as suggested by the present study, on dentin-invading bacteria. In this context, NO production by odontoblasts might modulate neurotransmission from deep dentin up to nerve endings present in the proximal dentin or the pulp periphery and/or might contribute to the regulation of the vascular tone of adjacent vessels. The large amount of NO synthesized by odontoblast NOS2 under pathological conditions might thus have an analgesic effect but might also dilate local blood vessels (McCormack and Davies, 1996; Di Nardo Di Maio et al., 2004).

NO has been recently proposed for a clinical use in the treatment of periodontal diseases, because of its drastic reduction of the viability of periodontopathogens (Backlund et al., 2014). Our results also demonstrated an antibacterial effect for NOS2-dependent production of NO by odontoblast-like cells. In the caries context, evidence of NO effects in animal models with cariogenic bacteria is warranted before envisaging the clinical use of NO to prevent dentin and pulp tissue colonization and subsequent irreversible pulpitis and necrosis.

Finally, studies have shown that NO can induce the differentiation of several cell types including osteoblastic, neuronal and endothelial cells (Beltran-Povea et al., 2015). It may also play a part in odontoblast differentiation and the subsequent formation of reparative dentin, notably by augmenting osteocalcin synthesis and alkaline phosphatase activity (Mei et al., 2007; Yasuhara et al., 2007). So NO donors could be use in regenerative dentistry as adjuvants to promote the mineralization events that lead to dentin or bone tissue formation. Additional studies using our culture model and others are required to test this hypothesis.

In summary, we report for the first time that NO with antibacterial activity is produced by TLR2-activated human odontoblast-like cells. Further studies are needed to determine the potential beneficial effect of this molecule on the reduction of human dental pulp inflammation and the promotion of tissue healing and regeneration.

## Acknowledgments

This work was supported by CNRS, University Lyon 1, the French Ministry of Higher Education and Research, and Expanscience Laboratories. Authors gratefully acknowledge Dr Laurent Müller (CIRB CNRS UMR7241 - INSERM U1050, Collège de France, Paris) for the generous gift of HUVEC.

## References

Arthur, J. S., and Ley, S. C. (2013). Mitogen-activated protein kinases in innate immunity. *Nat. Rev. Immunol.* 13, 679–692. doi: 10.1038/nri3495

Backlund, C. J., Sergesketter, A. R., Offenbacher, S., and Schoenfisch, M. H. (2014). Antibacterial efficacy of exogenous nitric oxide on periodontal pathogens. *J. Dent. Res.* 93, 1089–1094. doi: 10.1177/0022034514529974

Beltran-Povea, A., Caballano-Infantes, E., Salguero-Aranda, C., Martín, F., Soria, B., Bedoya, F. J., et al. (2015). Role of nitric oxide in the maintenance of pluripotency and regulation of the hypoxia response in stem cells. *World J. Stem Cells.* 7, 605–617. doi: 10.4252/wjsc.v7.i3.605

Bjorndal, L., and Mjör, I. A. (2001). Pulp-dentin biology in restorative dentistry. Part 4: dental caries—characteristics of lesions and pulpal reactions. *Quintessence Int.* 32, 717–736.

Bleicher, F., Richard, B., Thivichon-Prince, B., Farges, J.-C., and Carrouel, F. (2015). "Odontoblasts and dentin formation," in *Stem Cell Biology and Tissue Engineering in Dental Sciences*, eds A. Vishwakarma, P. Sharpe, S. Songtao, and M. Ramalingam (London: Elsevier), 379–395.

Bogdan, C. (2001). Nitric oxide and the immune response. *Nat. Immunol.* 2, 907–916. doi: 10.1038/ni1001-907

Carrouel, F., Staquet, M. J., Keller, J. F., Baudouin, C., Msika, P., Bleicher, F., et al. (2013). Lipopolysaccharide-binding protein inhibits Toll-like receptor 2 activation by lipoteichoic acid in human odontoblast-like cells. *J. Endod.* 39, 1008–1014. doi: 10.1016/j.joen.2013.04.020

Coleman, J. W. (2001). Nitric oxide in inmmunity and inflammation. *Int. Immunopharmacol.* 1, 1397–1406. doi: 10.1016/s1567-5769(01)00086-8

Cooper, P. R., Holder, M. J., and Smith, A. J. (2014). Inflammation and regeneration in the dentin-pulp complex: a double-edged sword. *J. Endod.* 40, S46–S51. doi: 10.1016/j.joen.2014.01.021

Couble, M. L., Farges, J. C., Bleicher, F., Perrat-Mabillon, B., Boudeulle, M., and Magloire, H. (2000). Odontoblast differentiation of human dental pulp cells in explant cultures. *Calcif. Tissue Int.* 66, 129–138. doi: 10.1007/pl000 05833

Denlinger, L. C., Fisette, P. L., Garis, K. A., Kwon, G., Vazquez-Torres, A., Simon, A. D., et al. (1996). Regulation of inducible nitric oxide synthase expression by macrophage purinoreceptors and calcium. *J. Biol. Chem.* 21, 337–442.

Di Nardo Di Maio, F., Lohinai, Z., D'Arcangelo, C., De Fazio, P. E., Speranza, L., De Lutiis, M. A., et al. (2004). Nitric oxide synthase in healthy and inflamed human dental pulp. *J. Dent. Res.* 83, 312–316. doi: 10.1177/1544059104083 00408

Durand, S. H., Flacher, V., Roméas, A., Carrouel, F., Colomb, E., Vincent, C., et al. (2006). Lipoteichoic acid increases TLR and functional chemokine expression while reducing dentin formation in in vitro differentiated human odontoblasts. *J. Immunol.* 176, 2880–2887. doi: 10.4049/jimmunol.176.5.2880

Farges, J. C., Alliot-Licht, B., Baudouin, C., Msika, P., Bleicher, F., and Carrouel, F. (2013). Odontoblast control of dental pulp inflammation triggered by cariogenic bacteria. *Front. Physiol.* 4:326. doi: 10.3389/fphys.2013. 00326

Farges, J. C., Carrouel, F., Keller, J. F., Baudouin, C., Msika, P., Bleicher, F., et al. (2011). Cytokine production by human odontoblast-like cells upon Toll-like receptor-2 engagement. *Immunobiology* 216, 513–517. doi: 10.1016/j.imbio.2010.08.006

Farges, J. C., Keller, J. F., Carrouel, F., Durand, S. H., Romeas, A., Bleicher, F., et al. (2009). Odontoblasts in the dental pulp immune response. *J. Exp. Zool. Mol. Dev. Evol.* 312B, 425–436. doi: 10.1002/jez.b.21259

Guzik, T. J., Korbut, R., and Adamek-Guzik, T. (2003). Nitric oxide and superoxide in inflammation and immune regulation. *J. Physiol. Pharmacol.* 54, 469–487. doi: 10.1177/154405910408300408

Hahn, C. L., and Liewehr, F. R. (2007). Innate immune responses of the dental pulp to caries. *J. Endod.* 33, 643–651. doi: 10.1016/j.joen.2007.01.001

Hong, S. W., Baik, J. E., Kang, S. S., Yun, C. H., Seo, D. G., and Han, S. H. (2014). Lipoteichoic acid of Streptococcus mutans interacts with Toll-like receptor 2 through the lipid moiety for induction of inflammatory mediators in murine macrophages. *Mol. Immunol.* 57, 284–291. doi: 10.1016/j.molimm.2013. 10.004

Kawanishi, H. N., Kawashima, N., Suzuki, N., Suda, H., and Takagi, M. (2004). Effects of an inducible nitric oxide synthase inhibitor on experimentally induced rat pulpitis. *Eur. J. Oral Sci.* 112, 332–337. doi: 10.1111/j.1600-0722.2004.00139.x

Kawashima, N., Nakano-Kawanishi, H., Suzuki, N., Takagi, M., and Suda, H. (2005). Effect of NOS inhibitor on cytokine and COX2 expression in rat pulpitis. *J. Dent. Res.* 84, 762–767. doi: 10.1177/00220345990780100301

Keller, J. F., Carrouel, F., Colomb, E., Durand, S. H., Baudouin, C., Msika, P., et al. (2010). Toll-like receptor 2 activation by lipoteichoic acid induces differential production of pro-inflammatory cytokines in human odontoblasts, dental pulp fibroblasts and immature dendritic cells. *Immunobiology* 215, 53–59. doi: 10.1016/j.imbio.2009.01.009

Keller, J. F., Carrouel, F., Staquet, M. J., Kufer, T. A., Baudouin, C., Msika, P., et al. (2011). Expression of NOD2 is increased in inflamed human dental pulps and lipoteichoic acid-stimulated odontoblast-like cells. *Innate Immun.* 17, 29–34. doi: 10.1177/1753425909348527

Korkmaz, Y., Lang, H., Beikler, T., Cho, B., Behrends, S., Bloch, W., et al. (2011). Irreversible inflammation is associated with decreased levels of the alpha1-, beta1-, and alpha2-subunits of sGC in human odontoblasts. *J. Dent. Res.* 90, 517–522. doi: 10.1177/0022034510390808

Law, A. S., Baumgardner, K. R., Meller, S. T., and Gebhart, G. F. (1999). Localization and changes in NADPH-diaphorase reactivity and nitric oxide synthase immunoreactivity in rat pulp following tooth preparation. *J. Dent. Res.* 78, 1585–1595. doi: 10.1177/00220345990780100301

Love, R. M., and Jenkinson, H. F. (2002). Invasion of dentinal tubules by oral bacteria. *Crit. Rev. Oral Biol. Med.* 13, 171–183. doi: 10.4049/jimmunol.176.5.2880

MacMicking, J., Xie, Q. W., and Nathan, C. (1997). Nitric oxide and macrophage function. *Annu. Rev. Immunol.* 15, 323–350. doi: 10.1146/annurev.immunol.15.1.323

Matsuno, R., Aramaki, Y., Arima, H., Adachi, Y., Ohno, N., Yadomae, T., et al. (1998). Contribution of CR3 to nitric oxide production from macrophages stimulated with high-dose of LPS. *Biochem. Biophys. Res. Commun.* 244, 115–119. doi: 10.1006/bbrc.1998.8231

McCormack, K., and Davies, R. (1996). The enigma of potassium ion in the management of dentine hypersensitivity: is nitric oxide the elusive second messenger? *Pain* 68, 5–11. doi: 10.1016/s0304-3959(96)03142-9

Mei, Y. F., Yamaza, T., Atsuta, I., Danjo, A., Yamashita, Y., Kido, M. A., et al. (2007). Sequential expression of endothelial nitric oxide synthase, inducible nitric oxide synthase, and nitrotyrosine in odontoblasts and pulp cells during dentin repair after tooth preparation in rat molars. *Cell Tissue Res.* 328, 117–127. doi: 10.1007/s00441-005-0003-5

Nathan, C. (1992). Nitric oxide as a secretory product of mammalian cells. *FASEB J.* 6, 3051–3064. doi: 10.1016/j.niox.2014.09.040

Nussler, A. K., and Billiar, T. R. (1993). Inflammation, immunoregulation, and inducible nitric oxide synthase. *J. Leukoc. Biol.* 54, 171–178.

Shimauchi, H., Takayama, S. I., Narikawa-Kiji, M., Shimabukuro, Y., and Okada, H. (2001). Production of interleukin-8 and nitric oxide in human periapical lesions. *J. Endod.* 27, 749–752. doi: 10.1097/00004770-200112000-00009

Silva-Mendez, L. S., Allaker, R. P., Hardie, J. M., and Benjamin, N. (1999). Antimicrobial effect of acidified nitrite on cariogenic bacteria. *Oral Microbiol. Immunol.* 14, 391–392.

Staquet, M. J., Carrouel, F., Keller, J. F., Baudouin, C., Msika, P., Bleicher, F., et al. (2011). Pattern-recognition receptors in pulp defense. *Adv. Dent. Res.* 23, 293–301. doi: 10.1177/0022034511405390

# 12

# Intercellular Odontoblast Communication via ATP Mediated by Pannexin-1 Channel and Phospholipase C-coupled Receptor Activation

**Edited by:**
*Thimios Mitsiadis,*
*University of Zurich, Switzerland*

***Correspondence:**
*Yoshiyuki Shibukawa*
*yshibuka@tdc.ac.jp*

***Masaki Sato*** [1], ***Tadashi Furuya*** [1,2], ***Maki Kimura*** [1], ***Yuki Kojima*** [1], ***Masakazu Tazaki*** [1], ***Toru Sato*** [2] ***and Yoshiyuki Shibukawa*** [1*]

[1] *Department of Physiology, Tokyo Dental College, Tokyo, Japan,* [2] *Department of Crown and Bridge Prosthodontics, Tokyo Dental College, Tokyo, Japan*

Extracellular ATP released via pannexin-1 channels, in response to the activation of mechanosensitive-TRP channels during odontoblast mechanical stimulation, mediates intercellular communication among odontoblasts in dental pulp slice preparation dissected from rat incisor. Recently, odontoblast cell lines, such as mouse odontoblast lineage cells, have been widely used to investigate physiological/pathological cellular functions. To clarify whether the odontoblast cell lines also communicate with each other by diffusible chemical substance(s), we investigated the chemical intercellular communication among cells from mouse odontoblast cell lines following mechanical stimulation. A single cell was stimulated using a glass pipette filled with standard extracellular solution. We measured intracellular free $Ca^{2+}$ concentration ($[Ca^{2+}]_i$) by fura-2 in stimulated cells, as well as in cells located nearby. Direct mechanical stimulation to a single odontoblast increased $[Ca^{2+}]_i$,which showed sensitivity to capsazepine. In addition, we observed increases in $[Ca^{2+}]_i$ not only in the mechanically stimulated odontoblast, but also in nearby odontoblasts. We could observe mechanical stimulation-induced increase in $[Ca^{2+}]_i$ in a stimulated human embryo kidney (HEK) 293 cell, but not in nearby HEK293 cells. The increase in $[Ca^{2+}]_i$ in nearby odontoblasts, but not in the stimulated odontoblast, was inhibited by adenosine triphosphate (ATP) release channel (pannexin-1) inhibitor in a concentration- and spatial-dependent manner. Moreover, in the presence of phospholipase C (PLC) inhibitor, the increase in $[Ca^{2+}]_i$ in nearby odontoblasts, following mechanical stimulation of a single odontoblast, was abolished. We could record some inward currents evoked from odontoblasts near the stimulated odontoblast, but the currents were observed in only 4.8% of the recorded odontoblasts. The results of this study showed that ATP is released via pannexin-1, from a mechanically stimulated odontoblast, which transmits a signal to nearby odontoblasts by predominant activation of PLC-coupled nucleotide receptors.

**Keywords: odontoblast, transient receptor potential channel, pannexin-1, adenosine triphosphate, P2Y, paracrine**

## INTRODUCTION

Odontoblasts are dentin-forming cells that secrete dentin matrix proteins during physiological and pathological tooth formation. In the pathological setting, such as an enamel lesion, reactionary dentin is formed by various external stimuli applied to the dentin surface. The thermal, chemical, mechanical, and osmotic stimuli applied to the exposed dentin surface increase the hydrodynamic force and the velocity of dentinal fluid movement inside dentinal tubules (Andrew and Matthews, 2000; Charoenlarp et al., 2007). This increase in fluid movement induces deformation of plasma membrane of the odontoblast processes within the dentinal tubules (Magloire et al., 2010; Lin et al., 2011). Recent studies have indicated that odontoblasts express mechanosensitive ionic channels such as transient receptor potential (TRP) channel-vanilloid subfamily member-1, -2, and -4 (TRPV1, TRPV2, TRPV4) and TRP-ankyrin subfamily member-1 (TRPA1) (Magloire et al., 2010; Sato et al., 2013; Tsumura et al., 2013). Odontoblast cell membrane deformation activates various mechanosensitive-TRP channels as mechanosensors (Son et al., 2009; Tsumura et al., 2012; Shibukawa et al., 2015).

We have previously reported functional expression of G-protein- and phospholipase C (PLC)-coupling nucleotide receptor in odontoblasts (Shibukawa and Suzuki, 2003). These receptors are responsible for receipt of extracellular ATP released not only by dental pulp tissue damage (Cook et al., 1997; Liu et al., 2015), but also from other cells in the dental pulp, so as to establish intercellular communication. Most recently, we have reported that extracellular ATP released via pannexin-1 channels, in response to the activation of mechanosensitive-TRP channels during odontoblast mechanical stimulation, mediates intercellular chemical communication between odontoblasts and trigeminal ganglion (TG) neurons, to drive the sensory transduction mechanism for dental pain. We refer to this mechanism as "odontoblast hydrodynamic receptor theory" (Shibukawa et al., 2015). In addition, odontoblasts also established intercellular communication with each other via ATP/ADP and their nucleotide receptors, $P2Y_1$ and $P2Y_{12}$, expressed on these cells. This previous research was conducted by using primary cultured TG neurons and odontoblasts. The odontoblasts were obtained from dental pulp slice preparation from rat tissues (Shibukawa et al., 2015). Although the dental pulp slice preparations have been well established (Okumura et al., 2005; Son et al., 2009; Magloire et al., 2010; Tsumura et al., 2010, 2012, 2013; Shibukawa et al., 2015), odontoblast cell lines, such as mouse odontoblast lineage cells (OLCs; Arany et al., 2006; Fujisawa et al., 2012) or human dental pulp cells with odontoblastic differentiation (HDPs; Kitagawa et al., 2007), have also been widely used to investigate physiological/pathological odontoblast cellular functions (Ichikawa et al., 2012; Sato et al., 2013). Cooperative cellular function via intercellular signal communication plays an important role in the formation of hard tissues, including teeth (Iwamoto et al., 2010). Therefore, to clarify whether the odontoblast cell lines communicate with each other by diffusible chemical substance(s), we investigated the intercellular odontoblast signal communication when direct and focal mechanical stimulation was applied to single living odontoblasts.

## MATERIALS AND METHODS

### Cell Culture

Mouse odontoblast lineage cells (OLC) (Arany et al., 2006; Fujisawa et al., 2012) were cultured in an alpha-minimum essential medium containing 10% fetal bovine serum, 1% penicillin-streptomycin, and 1% fungizone (Life technologies, Carlsbad, CA, USA) at 37°C with 5% $CO_2$. The cells were positive for various odontoblast representative transcripts of dentin sialophosphoprotein, dentin matrix protein-1, and nestin, generously provided by Dr. Masayuki Tokuda, Kagoshima University, Kagoshima, Japan. HEK293 cells were cultured in Dulbecco's modified Eagle's medium containing 10% fetal bovine serum, 1% penicillin-streptomycin, and 1% fungizone at 37°C with 5% $CO_2$.

### Solutions and Reagents

Standard extracellular solution (standard ECS) was composed of 135 mM NaCl, 5 mM KCl, 2.5 mM $CaCl_2$, 0.5 mM $MgCl_2$, 10 mM $NaHCO_3$, 10 mM 4-(2-hydroxyethyl)-1-piperazineethanesulfonic acid (HEPES), and 10 mM glucose and pH was adjusted to 7.4 by tris (hydroxymethyl) aminomethane (Tris) (328.5 mOsm/L). For $Ca^{2+}$-free ECS, we removed extracellular $Ca^{2+}$ (0 mM) from the standard ECS. Mefloquine and U73122 were obtained from TOCRIS Cookson (Bristol, UK). Capsazepine was obtained from Wako pure chemical (Osaka, Japan). All stock solutions were prepared in dimethyl sulfoxide. These stock solutions were diluted with standard ECS to the appropriate concentration before use. Except where indicated, all reagents were obtained from Sigma Chemical Co. (St. Louis, MO, USA).

### Direct Mechanical Stimulation of a Single Odontoblast

Direct mechanical stimulation was applied using a fire-polished glass micropipette with a tip diameter of 2–3 μm. The stimulation micropipettes were pulled from glass pipette tubes (Harvard apparatus, UK) by using a DMZ Universal Puller (Zeitz instruments, Martinsried, Germany) and the micropipettes were filled with standard ECS. The micropipette was operated using a micromanipulator (NHW-3, Narishige, Tokyo, Japan). The micropipette was placed at a site just above the cell attachment position and was gently moved by 4.3, 8.5, or 12.8 μm in the vertically downward direction at 2.2 μm/s velocity to depress the cell membrane, to generate a focused mechanical stimulation.

### Measurement of Peripheral Cell Length

Detached odontoblasts resuspended in standard ECS were placed into culture dishes at 37°C and 5% $CO_2$ for 1 h. Images of odontoblasts in standard ECS were acquired using an intensified charge-coupled device camera (Hamamatsu Photonics, Shizuoka, Japan) mounted on a microscope (Olympus, Tokyo, Japan). The odontoblast radius was determined from the images obtained

(AQUACOSMOS, HCImage, Hamamatsu Photonic, Shizuoka, Japan). Changes in peripheral cell length by mechanical stimulation were normalized to that found without any stimulation in the standard ECS.

### Measurement of $Ca^{2+}$-Sensitive Dye Fluorescence

Odontoblasts were incubated for 60 min (37°C) in standard ECS containing 10 μM fura-2 acetoxymethyl ester (Dojindo Laboratories, Kumamoto, Japan) and 0.1% (w/v) F-127 pluronic acid (Life technologies), followed by rinsing with fresh standard ECS. $[Ca^{2+}]_i$ was measured using an AQUACOSMOS and HCImage system with an excitation wavelength selector and an intensified charge-coupled device camera incorporated onto a microscope. Fura-2 fluorescence emission was measured at 510 nm in response to alternating excitation wavelengths of 340 nm (F340) and 380 nm (F380). $[Ca^{2+}]_i$ was measured as the fluorescence ratio ($R_{F340/F380}$) at two excitation wavelengths of 380 nm and 340 nm, and then expressed as $F/F_0$ units; the $R_{F340/F380}$ value ($F$) was normalized to the resting value ($F_0$).

### Whole-cell Patch-clamp Recording

Patch-clamp recordings of the whole-cell configuration were performed under voltage-clamp conditions. Patch pipettes (2–5 MΩ) were pulled from capillary tubes by using a DMZ Universal Puller (Zeitz Instruments, Martinsried, Germany), and the pipettes were filled with an intracellular solution. The intracellular solution contained 140 mM KCl, 10 mM NaCl, and 10 mM HEPES (pH adjusted to 7.2 by Tris). Whole-cell currents were measured using a patch-clamp amplifier (L/M-EPC-7+; Heka Elektronik, Lambrecht, Germany), and were monitored and stored using pCLAMP software (Molecular Devices, Sunnyvale, CA, USA), after digitizing the analog signals at 1 kHz (DigiData 1440A, Molecular Devices) and filtering the signals digitally at 100 Hz using pCLAMP. The data were analyzed offline by using pCLAMP and the technical graphics/analysis program ORIGIN (MicroCal Software, Northampton, MA, USA). All experiments were conducted at room temperature (30 ± 1.0°C).

### Statistical Analysis

Data are expressed as the mean ± standard deviation (SD) or standard error (SE) of the mean of $N$ observations, where $N$ represents the number of tested cells or separate experiments, respectively. Statistical differences were evaluated using analysis of variance (ANOVA) and the Steel-Dwass *post-hoc* test, and $P<0.05$ was considered to be significant.

## RESULTS

### Direct Mechanical Stimulation Induces $Ca^{2+}$ Influx in the Odontoblasts

Cell peripheral length was calculated to measure changes in cell size with or without exposure by penetration of a glass micropipette at three different depths (4.3, 8.5, and 12.8 μm). The normalized peripheral length of cells significantly increased as the glass pipette depth was measured from 0 to 8.5 μm (**Figure 1A**, $P<0.05$), indicating that direct mechanical stimulation using a glass pipette induced stretching of the odontoblast plasma membrane. The peripheral length of cells without mechanical stimulation was found to be 46.2 ± 1.4 μm ($N$=11).

A series of direct mechanical stimulations (4.3–12.8 μm) elicited transient increases in intracellular free $Ca^{2+}$ concentration ($[Ca^{2+}]_i$) (**Figure 1B**, black lines) in the presence of extracellular $Ca^{2+}$, while in the absence of extracellular $Ca^{2+}$ ($Ca^{2+}$-free extracellular solution; $Ca^{2+}$-free ECS), mechanical stimulation-induced $[Ca^{2+}]_i$ increases were completely abolished (**Figure 1B**, red line), indicating that mechanical stimulation of the odontoblasts elicited $Ca^{2+}$ influx. The linear plot in **Figure 1C** shows $F/F_0$ values as a function of applied direct mechanical stimulation. Dependence of $[Ca^{2+}]_i$ on mechanical stimulation by the pipette was confirmed by fitting the data to the following function:

$$A = (A_{min} - A_{max})/(1 + e^{(x-K/dx)}) + A_{max} \ldots \quad (1)$$

where $K$ is the half-maximal depth of a mechanical stimulation applied on the odontoblast (8.3 μm), $A_{max}$ is maximal and $A_{min}$ is minimal $F/F_0$ response. The x indicates applied depth of the glass pipette.

### Nonselective TRPV1 Channel Antagonist Inhibits Direct Mechanical Stimulation–induced $Ca^{2+}$ Influx in Odontoblast

To further investigate the $Ca^{2+}$ influx pathway activated by direct mechanical stimulation, the effects of nonselective TRPV1 and TRP Melastatin subfamily member 8 (TRPM8) channel antagonist, capsazepine (CZP), on direct mechanical stimulation-induced $Ca^{2+}$ influx were examined. In the presence of extracellular $Ca^{2+}$ (2.5 mM), $[Ca^{2+}]_i$ in odontoblasts showed a rapid and transient increase during direct mechanical stimulation (8.5 μm), which was significantly and reversibly inhibited by 1 μM CZP to 32.4 ± 12.1% ($N$=3) (**Figures 1D,E**).

### Direct Mechanical Stimulation Also Induces $[Ca^{2+}]_i$ Increase in Odontoblasts Around the Stimulated Odontoblast

We measured the increase in $[Ca^{2+}]_i$ by direct mechanical stimulation not only in the single odontoblast, but also in the neighboring odontoblasts. Direct mechanical stimulation of the single odontoblast increased $[Ca^{2+}]_i$ transiently. We also observed an increase in nearby odontoblasts (**Figure 2A**). The increase in $[Ca^{2+}]_i$ in nearby odontoblasts was reduced by increasing their distance from the stimulated odontoblast (**Figure 2A**). The plot in **Figure 2B** shows $F/F_0$ values as a function of distance from stimulated odontoblast to nearby odontoblasts. The spatial constant (τ), was obtained by fitting the data to the exponential decay function. The spatial constant was 30.1 μm. Direct mechanical stimulation of a human embryonic

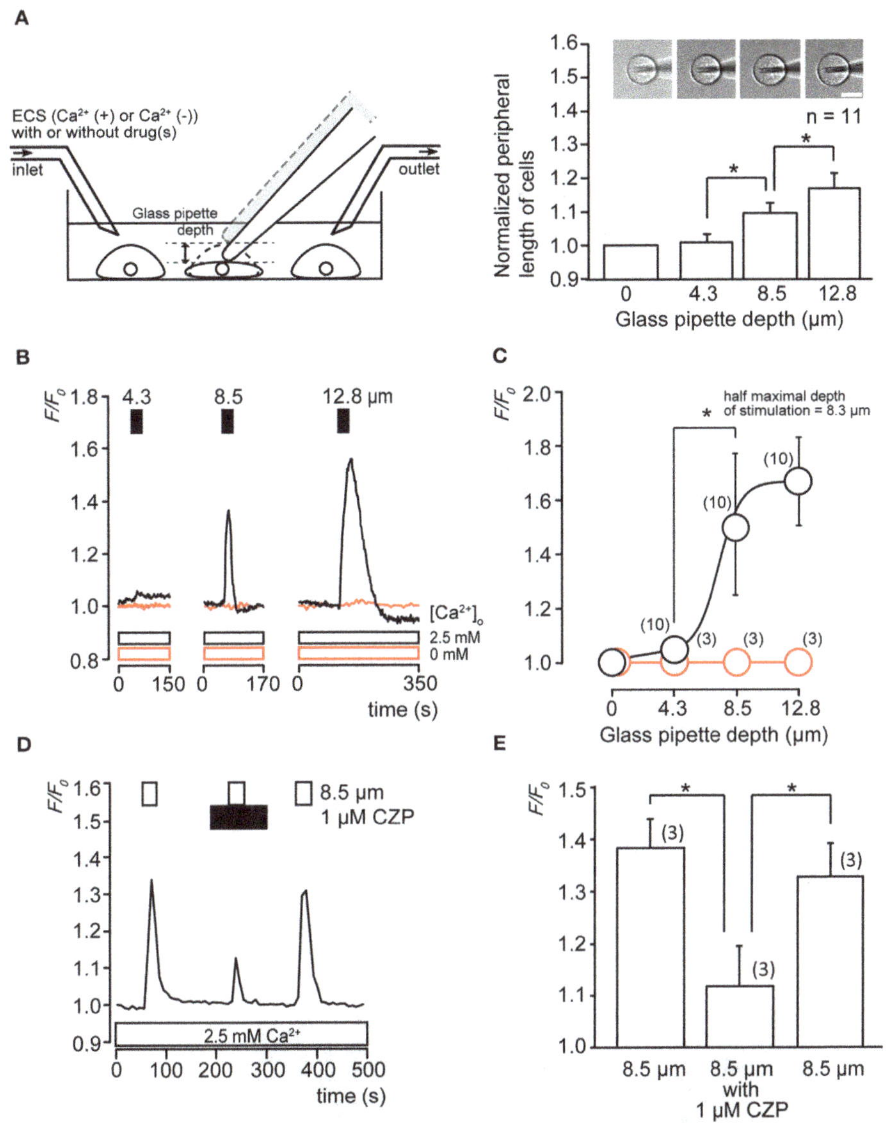


**FIGURE 1 | Cell deformation by direct stimulation induces increase in $[Ca^{2+}]_i$ (A)** Single-cell direct mechanical stimulation with glass micropipette in the recording bath. The relationship between changes in the peripheral length of cells and intensity of mechanical stimulation in terms of depth reached by the pipette. Normalized cell size increased with increasing mechanical stimulation, each normalized cell size was 1.02 ± 0.03-fold by 4.3 μm, 1.10 ± 0.03-fold by 8.5 μm, and 1.16 ± 0.05-fold by 12.8 μm of the vertical downward displacement of the pipette. Bars represent mean ± SD of 11 cells. Statistically significant differences between values are indicated by asterisks. *$P < 0.05$ (**A** right). Top panel shows images of cells during each stimulation. Bar indicates 10 μm. **(B)** Traces of transient increase in $[Ca^{2+}]_i$ during a series of mechanical stimulations induced by vertical micropipette displacements at depths of 4.3, 8.5, and 12.8 μm (upper filled boxes) in standard ECS with extracellular 2.5 mM $Ca^{2+}$ (black lines and black line boxes) or without extracellular $Ca^{2+}$ (0 mM) (red lines and red line boxes). **(C)** Linear plot of $F/F_0$ value against direct mechanical stimulation intensity with extracellular 2.5 mM $Ca^{2+}$ (black) or without extracellular $Ca^{2+}$ (red). The numbers in parentheses indicate the number of tested cells. **(D)** Mechanical stimulation-induced $Ca^{2+}$ influx was inhibited by TRPV1 antagonist (upper black box). $[Ca^{2+}]_i$ increase was elicited by 8.5 μm direct mechanical stimulation (upper white boxes). **(E)** Summary bar graphs of the increase in $[Ca^{2+}]_i$ induced by mechanical stimulation (to 8.5 μm) without (left column) or with (middle column) application of TRP channel antagonist. Recovery effect is shown in the right column. The resting value, $F/F_0 = 1.0$. Each bar indicates the mean ± SD for three cells. Statistically significant differences between columns (shown by solid lines) are indicated by asterisks. *$P<0.05$.

kidney (HEK) 293 cell increased $[Ca^{2+}]_i$ transiently, whereas $[Ca^{2+}]_i$ increase in HEK293 cells near the stimulated cell was not observed (**Figure 2C**). The plot in **Figure 2D** shows $F/F_0$ values as a function of distance from stimulated HEK293 cells to nearby HEK293 cells. The spatial constant could not be measured for HEK293 cells.

## Odontoblasts Release ATP into the Extracellular Space via Pannexin-1 Channel and Receive It via Phospholipase C-coupled Receptor

Using 10 μM mefloquine, which is an inhibitor of the pannexin-1 channel, mechanical-stimulation-induced $[Ca^{2+}]_i$

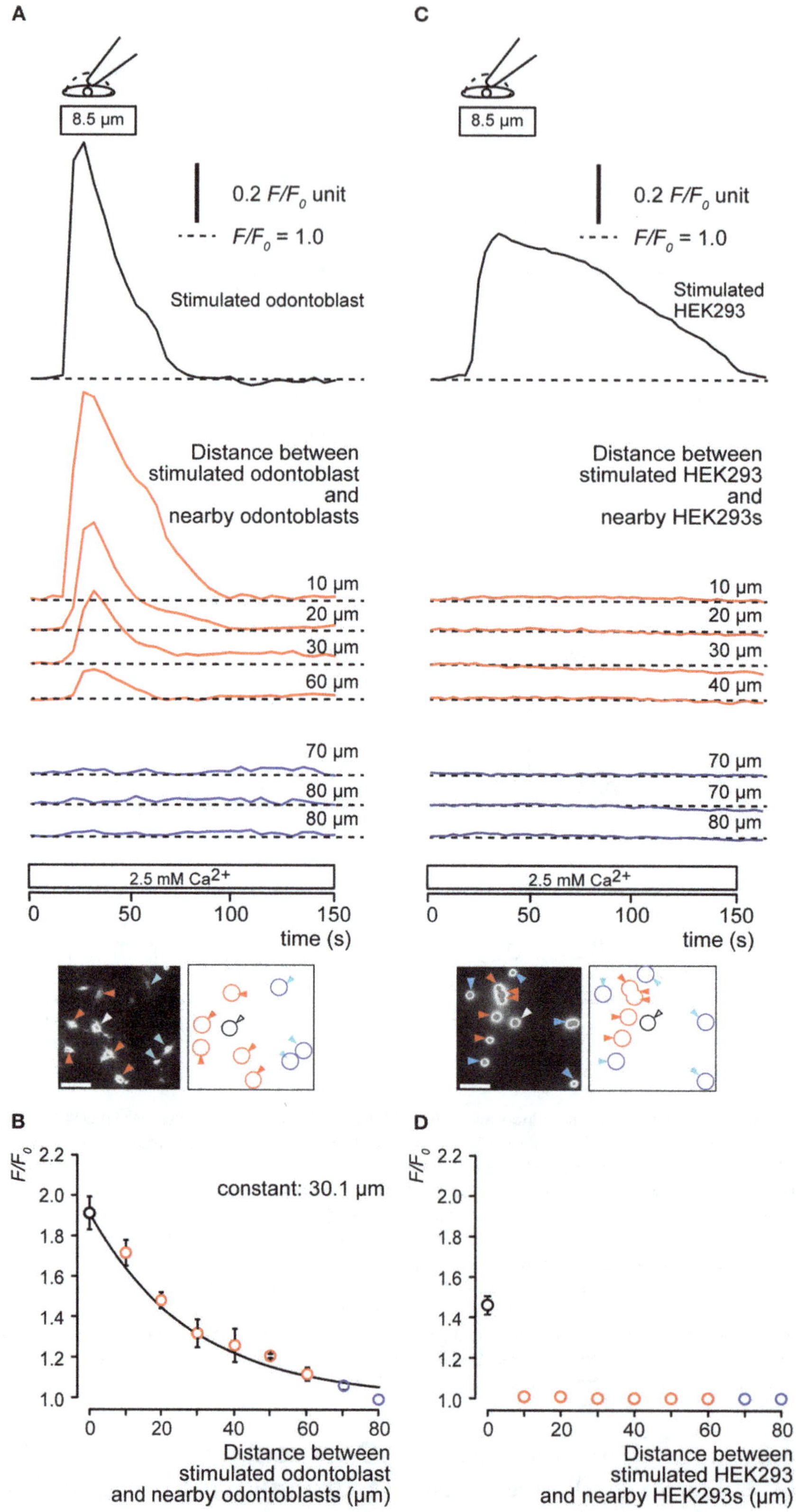


**FIGURE 2 | Communication between a mechanical stimulated odontoblast and nearby odontoblasts. (A,C)** Representative traces showing transient increase in $[Ca^{2+}]_i$ from a mechanically stimulated cell (upper black traces), nearby (middle red traces) and distant cells (lower blue cells) in odontoblast **(A)** and

*(Continued)*

**FIGURE 2 | Continued**
HEK293 cell **(C)** during focal, direct mechanical stimulation of a single cell. Cell deformation was induced by displacement of a micropipette to a depth of 8.5 μm (upper open boxes and drawings) in a single cell in standard ECS (2.5 mM $Ca^{2+}$). Bottom in **(A,C)** show images of relative fluorescence ratio ($F_0$) before recordings (white bars show 50 μm), and their schematic representations. Stimulated cells are shown by white arrowhead and black lines, nearby cells are indicated by red arrowheads and red lines, and distant cells are represented by blue arrowheads and blue lines. Each horizontal dotted line shows base line (as $F/F_0 = 1.0$) for each response. Responses from nearby (four red traces) or distant cells (three blue traces) were recorded 10–80 μm away from stimulated cells. **(B,D)** $F/F_0$ values (data points) as a function of the distance from the stimulated cell (0 μm) to nearby (red symbols) or distant cells (blue symbols) for odontoblasts **(A)** and HEK293 cells **(D)**. The superimposed lines denote the best fit of a single exponential function. This analysis yielded spatial constants (τ) for the distance-dependent decrease in $[Ca^{2+}]_i$. The increase of $[Ca^{2+}]_i$ was observed in neither nearby nor distant HEK293 cells. Data points represent the mean ± SE from 3 to 32 cells in 3 separate experiments in **(B)** and 3 to 25 cells in 3 separate experiments in **(D)**.

increase was observed in stimulated odontoblast, whereas in nearby odontoblasts no significant increase in $[Ca^{2+}]_i$ was observed (**Figure 3A**). In addition, mefloquine (0.1, 1.0, and 10 μM) inhibited $[Ca^{2+}]_i$ response in nearby odontoblasts in a concentration- and spatial-dependent manner (**Figures 3B,C**). The administration of 1.0 μM U73122, an inhibitor of phospholipase C, significantly suppressed mechanical stimulation-induced increase in $[Ca^{2+}]_i$ in nearby odontoblasts, but not the stimulated cell (**Figure 3D**). U73122 (0.01, 0.1, and 1.0 μM) inhibited $[Ca^{2+}]_i$ responses in nearby odontoblasts in a concentration- and spatial-dependent manner (**Figures 3E,F**). The decrease in $[Ca^{2+}]_i$ in nearby odontoblasts with increasing distance from stimulated odontoblasts occurred rapidly (**Figures 3B,E**) in a dose-dependent manner on mefloquine (**Figure 3C**) and U73122 treatment (**Figure 3F**), showing significant decrease in spatial constants.

## Evoked Inward Currents in Neighboring Odontoblasts Following Mechanical Stimulation of a Single Odontoblast

The whole-cell patch-clamp method was used to record membrane currents that are activated by intercellular transmitter released from mechanically stimulated odontoblasts (**Figure 4**). We recorded an evoked inward current in only 2 out of 42 tested odontoblasts located 5 μm from the mechanically stimulated cell (in 42 experiments). These currents had delay times of 7–10 s in their activation.

# DISCUSSION

In this study, we demonstrated that intercellular signal transduction between mechanically stimulated and neighboring odontoblasts occurs via activation of mechanosensitive TRP channels, release of ATP from the pannexin-1 channel, and activation of PLC-coupled receptors. Since we previously reported that TRPM8 channels are not expressed in mouse odontoblasts, CPZ-sensitive mechanical stimulation-induced $[Ca^{2+}]_i$ response in the present study is mediated by TRPV1 channels. Activation of TRPV1 channels, acting as sensor proteins (Magloire et al., 2010; Sato et al., 2013; Tsumura et al., 2013), induces the release of ATP via pannexin-1 channels from mechanically stimulated odontoblasts. ATP released from mechanically stimulated odontoblasts, as an intercellular transmitter in the extracellular medium, then activates PLC-coupled ATP/ADP receptors in neighboring odontoblasts. These results are in line with our previous results showing that mechanically stimulated odontoblasts release ATP via pannexin-1 channels to the neighboring odontoblasts, which activates the $P2Y_1$ and $P2Y_{12}$ receptors (Shibukawa et al., 2015).

The changes in the peripheral length and the increase in $[Ca^{2+}]_i$ depended on the intensity of the direct mechanical stimulation applied to odontoblasts. In the previous and present study, repeated mechanical stimulation to the odontoblasts induced increase in $[Ca^{2+}]_i$ repeatedly (Shibukawa et al., 2015). Although these results suggested that the stimuli did not induce any unfavorable effects to the cells, application of mechanical stimulation was limited to three times in the present study to avoid cell damage.

Treatment of the culture medium with an inhibitor of ATP-releasing pannexin-1 channels abolishes the increase in $[Ca^{2+}]_i$ in neighboring odontoblasts, but not in mechanically stimulated odontoblasts, indicating that ATP released via pannexin-1 acts as an intercellular transmitter for odontoblast–odontoblast chemical communication. In previous immunohistochemical studies, pannexin-1 was found to be localized throughout the cell body of odontoblasts (Shibukawa et al., 2015). In addition, TRPV4 and TRPA1 channel activation also elicits ATP release in odontoblasts (Egbuniwe et al., 2014). When direct mechanical stimulation was applied to HEK293 cells, internal $Ca^{2+}$ was increased in the mechanically stimulated cells, but not in the neighboring cells. This is consistent with previous results showing that pannexin-1 is not expressed in HEK293 cells (Langlois et al., 2014), and suggests that intercellular communication via diffusible substances (i.e., intercellular transmitters) is established specifically in inter-odontoblast cellular networks in the dental pulp.

Odontoblasts express connexin (Cx) hemi-channels, forming a gap junction and establishing cell–cell communication (Goldberg et al., 1981; Sasaki et al., 1982; Callé, 1985; Goldberg and Sasaki, 1985; About et al., 2001; Muramatsu et al., 2004; Ikeda and Suda, 2013). Connexin 43, a gap junction protein, is expressed in odontoblasts (Ikeda and Suda, 2013; Muramatsu et al., 2013), and seems to play a role in electrical communication between odontoblasts. It has been reported that connexin 43 also releases ATP extracellularly in the pathological setting, such as low (almost 0 mM) extracellular $Ca^{2+}$ circumstance or high (c.a. +60 mV) membrane potential. Since we did not expose the odontoblast to such extracellular conditions, contribution of connexin 43 to intercellular odontoblasts chemical communication is unlikely (Shibukawa et al., 2015).

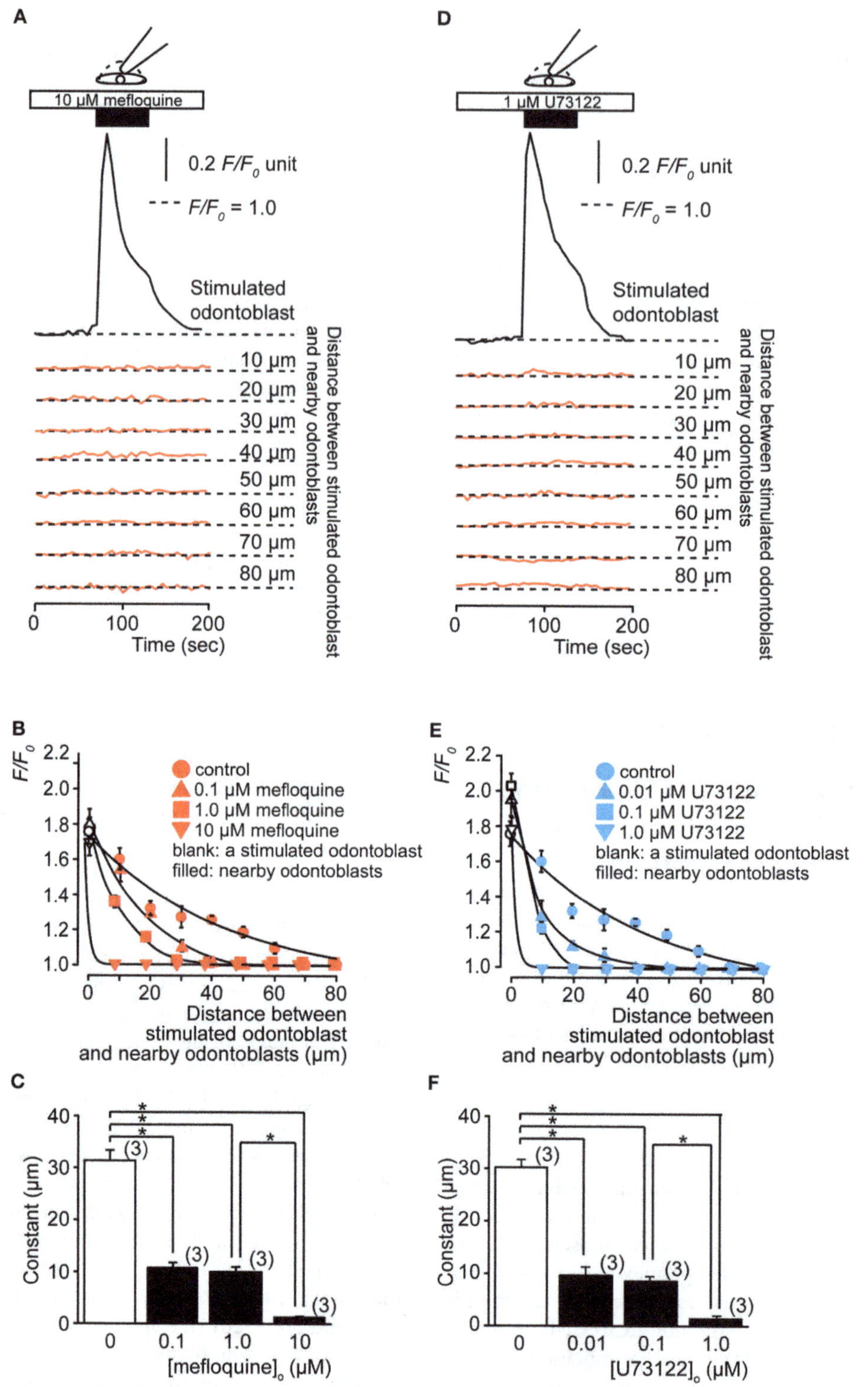


**FIGURE 3 | Intercellular odontoblast communication via ATP.** Effects of pannexin-1 inhibitor, mefloquine, and phospholipase C (PLC) inhibitor, U73122, on the increase in $[Ca^{2+}]_i$ following focal and direct mechanical stimulation of a single odontoblast. **(A,D)** Transient increase in $[Ca^{2+}]_i$ from a mechanically stimulated odontoblast (upper black traces), nearby and distant odontoblasts (lower red traces), during single odontoblast stimulation in the presence of mefloquine **(A)** or U73122 **(D)**. Mechanical stimulation was applied by displacement of a micropipette to a depth of 8.5 μm (upper filled boxes and drawings) in standard ECS (2.5 mM $Ca^{2+}$). Horizontal dotted lines show the baseline ($F/F_0 = 1.0$) for each response. Responses from nearby and distant odontoblast were recorded from cells located 10 to 80 μm away from the stimulated odontoblast. This distance is indicated on the right side of each trace. **(B,E)** $F/F_0$ values (data points) as a function of the distance

*(Continued)*

**FIGURE 3 | Continued**
from a stimulated odontoblast (0 μm) to nearby odontoblast, with or without pannexin-1 inhibitor (0.1–10 μM mefloquine; red symbols in **B**) and phospholipase C inhibitor (0.01–1 μM U73122; blue symbols in **E**). Each mechanical stimulation induced $[Ca^{2+}]_i$ increase in the stimulated odontoblast is shown by open symbols with each concentration of mefloquine or U73122. This response was not affected by treatment with mefloquine or U73122. The superimposed lines denote the best fit of a single exponential function. This analysis yielded spatial constants (τ) of the distance-dependent decreases in $[Ca^{2+}]_i$ (solid lines in **B,E**) with or without (filled circles) mefloquine **(B)** and U73122 **(E)**. Data points represent the mean ± SD from 3 to 41 cells in **(B,E)** from each three separate experiment. **(C,F)** Summary bar graphs of the mean τ values of the distance-dependent decrease in $[Ca^{2+}]_i$, measured from stimulated to nearby odontoblast, with pannexin-1 inhibitor **(C)** or phospholipase C inhibitor **(F)**. Each bar indicates mean ± SD. The numbers in parentheses in **(C,F)** indicate the number of tested cells. Statistically significant differences between spatial constant values are indicated by asterisks. *$P<0.05$.

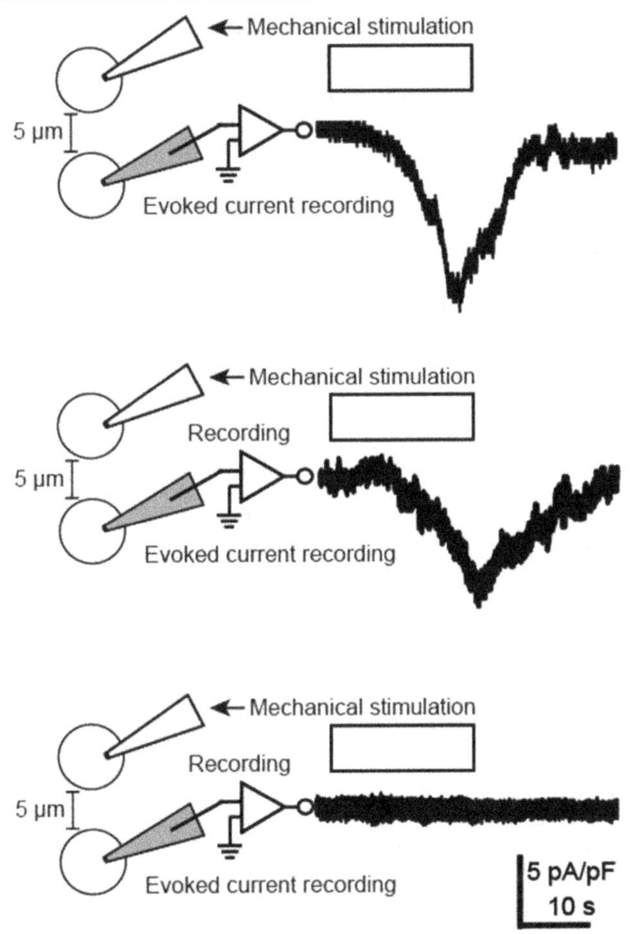


**FIGURE 4 | Evoked inward currents in neighboring odontoblasts following mechanical stimulation of a single odontoblast.** Traces of inward currents (upper two traces) were recorded by using whole-cell patch-clamp recordings of the cells located 5 μm away from a stimulated odontoblast, following mechanical stimulation (the white boxes and the drawings on the left). Pictures of the whole-cell patch-clamp recording are also shown. Note that we could record evoked inward currents in only 2 out of 42 tested odontoblasts. Lower trace shows current from cell which did not elicit inward current, following mechanical stimulation. The recording was obtained from three separated cells.

Use of U73122, an inhibitor of phospholipase C, did not affect calcium response in the mechanically stimulated odontoblast, but abolish it in the neighboring odontoblasts. P2Y receptors are coupled with PLC and activated principally by endogenous nucleotides, ATP, and ADP (Burnstock, 2007). A specific enzyme, nucleoside triphosphate diphosphohydrolase-2 (NTPDase2) (Liu et al., 2012), is expressed in the Schwann cells of the dental pulp and/or the odontoblast membrane, and has been reported to hydrolyze extracellular ATP to ADP. Thus, both, released ATP and ADP from degradation of the ATP by NTPDase2, activate P2Y receptors in nearby odontoblasts. In addition, an ATP derivative, 2-methylthio-ATP, mobilizes $[Ca^{2+}]_i$ in the odontoblasts (Shibukawa and Suzuki, 2003), showing expression of the $P2Y_1$ and $P2Y_{12}$ receptors. We previously reported that $P2Y_1$ and $P2Y_{12}$ receptor activation in odontoblasts established inter-odontoblast communication (Shibukawa et al., 2015).

On the other hand, as shown in **Figure 4**, we could successfully record evoked inward currents in the odontoblast located 5 μm away from the stimulated odontoblast. The evoked inward currents via intercellular transmitters were likely mediated by the activation of ionotropic receptors and/or ionic channels. Mechanical stimulation of the odontoblasts induces a release of intercellular transmitters, not only of ATP (as in the present study and in Shibukawa et al., 2015), but also of glutamate (our personal communication). However, the present results indicate that the ionotropic receptors (such as ionotropic ATP (P2Xs) and/or glutamate receptors) and ionic channel activation are hardly involved in the inter-odontoblast communication, since the evoked currents elicited by mechanical stimulation could be observed in only 4.8% of the odontoblasts recorded (2/42 cells) in the present study. We previously reported that the $P2X_3$ receptor is not expressed in odontoblasts, while the $P2X_3$ receptor in the TG neurons plays an important role in the sensory transduction sequence by receiving ATP from mechanically stimulated odontoblasts (Shibukawa et al., 2015). Although, we observed several P2X subtype expressions, except for the $P2X_3$ receptor, in odontoblasts (personal communication), these P2X receptor subtypes need a relative high concentration of extracellular ATP to be activated. Therefore, ATP released in response to TRPV1 channel activation during mechanical stimulation predominantly activates P2Y receptors on neighboring odontoblasts to mediate intercellular odontoblasts communication.

We previously showed that accumulated $[Ca^{2+}]_i$ following TRPV1 channel activation is extruded by $Na^+$-$Ca^{2+}$ exchangers (NCXs) in odontoblasts (Tsumura et al., 2012). Our results suggest that communication between odontoblasts mediated by ATP plays an important role in reactionary dentin formation following dentin stimulation by increased intracellular $Ca^{2+}$ signaling by TRPV-mediated $Ca^{2+}$ influx and P2Y receptor-mediated $Ca^{2+}$ mobilization as well as subsequent $Ca^{2+}$ extrusion by NCXs.

## CONCLUSION

The results from this study show that ATP is released from a mechanically stimulated odontoblast via pannexin-1 by TRP channel activation, and it transmits a signal to nearby odontoblasts by activating P2Y receptors. The results also strongly suggest that odontoblasts communicate with each other to drive their cellular functions such as enhancement of dentin formation. Our results also indicate that odontoblasts are sensory receptor cells (Shibukawa et al., 2015) that detect hydrodynamic force within dentinal tubules (Liu et al., 2015) via mechanosensitive TRP channels. Additionally, ATP released from odontoblasts via pannexin-1 pathway acts as the intercellular transmitter between odontoblasts by activating the P2Y receptors. Taken together with our previous results (Tsumura et al., 2010, 2012, 2013; Sato et al., 2013; Shibukawa et al., 2015), the present study also strongly suggests that the intercellular signaling via released ATP in response to activation of odontoblasts as mechano-sensitive sensory receptor cells are capable of activating two specific and separate pathways underlying odontoblast function: (1) the selective activation of P2Y receptors in odontoblasts establishes inter-odontoblast network that may drive dentin formation, and (2) specific activation of $P2X_3$ receptors in TG neurons mediates the sensory transduction sequence for dentin (Shibukawa et al., 2015). In addition, the results also prove that odontoblast cell lines are useful in studying the cellular functions that are mediated by intercellular signaling.

## AUTHOR CONTRIBUTIONS

MS, TF, MK, and YK carried out the measurement intracellular $Ca^{2+}$ signaling. YS, TS, and MT participated in the design of the study. MS and TF performed the statistical analysis. YS conceived of the study, and participated in its design and coordination and helped to draft the manuscript. All authors read and approved the final manuscript.

## FUNDING

This research was supported by a Grant-in-Aid (No. 26861559/15K11129/15K11056) for Scientific Research from the MEXT of Japan.

## REFERENCES

About, I., Proust, J. P., Raffo, S., Mitsiadis, T. A., and Franquin, J. C. (2001). *In vivo* and *in vitro* expression of connexin 43 in human teeth. *Connect. Tissue Res.* 43, 232–237. doi: 10.1080/03008200290000952

Andrew, D., and Matthews, B. (2000). Displacement of the contents of dentinal tubules and sensory transduction in intradental nerves of the cat. *J. Physiol.* 529(Pt 3), 791–802. doi: 10.1111/j.1469-7793.2000.00791.x

Arany, S., Nakata, A., Kameda, T., Koyota, S., Ueno, Y., and Sugiyama, T. (2006). Phenotype properties of a novel spontaneously immortalized odontoblast-lineage cell line. *Biochem. Biophys. Res. Commun.* 342, 718–724. doi: 10.1016/j.bbrc.2006.02.020

Burnstock, G. (2007). Physiology and pathophysiology of purinergic neurotransmission. *Physiol. Rev.* 87, 659–797. doi: 10.1152/physrev.00043.2006

Callé, A. (1985). Intercellular junctions between human odontoblasts. a freeze-fracture study after demineralization. *Acta Anat.* 122, 138–144. doi: 10.1159/000145995

Charoenlarp, P., Wanachantararak, S., Vongsavan, N., and Matthews, B. (2007). Pain and the rate of dentinal fluid flow produced by hydrostatic pressure stimulation of exposed dentine in man. *Arch. Oral Biol.* 52, 625–631. doi: 10.1016/j.archoralbio.2006.12.014

Cook, S. P., Vulchanova, L., Hargreaves, K. M., Elde, R., and McCleskey, E. W. (1997). Distinct ATP receptors on pain-sensing and stretch-sensing neurons. *Nature* 387, 505–508. doi: 10.1038/387505a0

Egbuniwe, O., Grover, S., Duggal, A. K., Mavroudis, A., Yazdi, M., Renton, T., et al. (2014). TRPA1 and TRPV4 activation in human odontoblasts stimulates ATP release. *J. Dent. Res.* 93, 911–917. doi: 10.1177/0022034514544507

Fujisawa, M., Tokuda, M., Morimoto-Yamashita, Y., Tatsuyama, S., Arany, S., Sugiyama, T., et al. (2012). Hyperosmotic stress induces cell death in an odontoblast-lineage cell line. *J. Endod.* 38, 931–935. doi: 10.1016/j.joen.2012.03.023

Goldberg, M., Escaig, F., and Septier, D. (1981). Freeze fracturing and thin-section study of intercellular junctions between odontoblasts and the rat incisor. changes induced by vinblastine. *J. Biol. Buccale* 9, 141–153.

Goldberg, M., and Sasaki, T. (1985). Intramembrane particle distribution on the plasma membrane of ruffle-ended and smooth ended maturation ameloblasts of the rat incisors. *J. Biol. Buccale* 13, 251–260.

Ichikawa, H., Kim, H.-J., Shuprisha, A., Shikano, T., Tsumura, M., Shibukawa, Y., et al. (2012). Voltage-dependent sodium channels and calcium-activated potassium channels in human odontoblasts *in vitro*. *J. Endod.* 38, 1355–1362. doi: 10.1016/j.joen.2012.06.015

Ikeda, H., and Suda, H. (2013). Odontoblastic syncytium through electrical coupling in the human dental pulp. *J. Dent. Res.* 92, 371–375. doi: 10.1177/0022034513478430

Iwamoto, T., Nakamura, T., Doyle, A., Ishikawa, M., de Vega, S., Fukumoto, S., et al. (2010). Pannexin 3 regulates intracellular ATP/cAMP levels and promotes chondrocyte differentiation. *J. Biol. Chem.* 285, 18948–18958. doi: 10.1074/jbc.M110.127027

Kitagawa, M., Ueda, H., Iizuka, S., Sakamoto, K., Oka, H., Kudo, Y., et al. (2007). Immortalization and characterization of human dental pulp cells with odontoblastic differentiation. *Arch. Oral Biol.* 52, 727–731. doi: 10.1016/j.archoralbio.2007.02.006

Langlois, S., Xiang, X., Young, K., Cowan, B. J., Penuela, S., and Cowan, K. N. (2014). Pannexin 1 and pannexin 3 channels regulate skeletal muscle myoblast proliferation and differentiation. *J. Biol. Chem.* 289, 30717–30731. doi: 10.1074/jbc.M114.572131

Lin, M., Luo, Z. Y., Bai, B. F., Xu, F., and Lu, T. J. (2011). Fluid mechanics in dentinal microtubules provides mechanistic insights into the difference between hot and cold dental pain. *PLoS ONE* 6:e18068. doi: 10.1371/journal.pone.0018068

Liu, X., Wang, C., Fujita, T., Malmstrom, H. S., Nedergaard, M., Ren, Y. F., et al. (2015). External dentin stimulation induces ATP release in human teeth. *J. Dent. Res.* 94, 1259–1266. doi: 10.1177/0022034515592858

Liu, X., Yu, L., Wang, Q., Pelletier, J., Fausther, M., Sévigny, J., et al. (2012). Expression of ecto-ATPase NTPDase2 in human dental pulp. *J. Dent. Res.* 91, 261–267. doi: 10.1177/0022034511431582

Magloire, H., Maurin, J. C., Couble, M. L., Shibukawa, Y., Tsumura, M., Thivichon-Prince, B., et al. (2010). Topical review. dental pain and odontoblasts: facts and hypotheses. *J. Orofac. Pain* 24, 335–349.

Muramatsu, T., Hamano, H., Ogami, K., Ohta, K., Inoue, T., and Shimono, M. (2004). Reduction of connexin 43 expression in aged human dental pulp. *Int. Endod. J.* 37, 814–818. doi: 10.1111/j.1365-2591.2004.00880.x

Muramatsu, T., Hashimoto, S., Shibukawa, Y., Yuasa, K., Furusawa, M., and Shimono, M. (2013). Immunoelectron microscopic observation of connexin43 in rat odontoblasts. *Microsc. Res. Tech.* 76, 988–991. doi: 10.1002/jemt.22271

Okumura, R., Shima, K., Muramatsu, T., Nakagawa, K.-I., Shimono, M., Suzuki, T., et al. (2005). The odontoblast as a sensory receptor cell? the expression of TRPV1 (VR-1) channels. *Arch. Histol. Cytol.* 68, 251–257. doi: 10.1679/aohc.68.251

Sasaki, T., Nakagawa, K., and Higashi, S. (1982). Ultrastructure of odontoblasts in kitten tooth germs as revealed by freeze-fracture. *Arch. Oral Biol.* 27, 897–904. doi: 10.1016/0003-9969(82)90048-6

Sato, M., Sobhan, U., Tsumura, M., Kuroda, H., Soya, M., Masamura, A., et al. (2013). Hypotonic-induced stretching of plasma membrane activates transient receptor potential vanilloid channels and sodium-calcium exchangers in mouse odontoblasts. *J. Endod.* 39, 779–787. doi: 10.1016/j.joen.2013.01.012

Shibukawa, Y., Sato, M., Kimura, M., Sobhan, U., Shimada, M., Nishiyama, A., et al. (2015). Odontoblasts as sensory receptors: transient receptor potential channels, pannexin-1, and ionotropic ATP receptors mediate intercellular odontoblast-neuron signal transduction. *Pflügers Arch.* 467, 843–863. doi: 10.1007/s00424-014-1551-x

Shibukawa, Y., and Suzuki, T. (2003). $Ca^{2+}$ signaling mediated by $IP_3$-dependent $Ca^{2+}$ releasing and store-operated $Ca^{2+}$ channels in rat odontoblasts. *J. Bone Miner. Res.* 18, 30–38. doi: 10.1359/jbmr.2003.18.1.30

Son, A. R., Yang, Y. M., Hong, J. H., Lee, S. I., Shibukawa, Y., and Shin, D. M. (2009). Odontoblast TRP channels and thermo/mechanical transmission. *J. Dent. Res.* 88, 1014–1019. doi: 10.1177/0022034509343413

Tsumura, M., Okumura, R., Tatsuyama, S., Ichikawa, H., Muramatsu, T., Matsuda, T., et al. (2010). $Ca^{2+}$ extrusion via $Na^{+}$-$Ca^{2+}$ exchangers in rat odontoblasts. *J. Endod.* 36, 668–674. doi: 10.1016/j.joen.2010.01.006

Tsumura, M., Sobhan, U., Muramatsu, T., Sato, M., Ichikawa, H., Sahara, Y., et al. (2012). TRPV1-mediated calcium signal couples with cannabinoid receptors and sodium-calcium exchangers in rat odontoblasts. *Cell Calcium* 52, 124–136. doi: 10.1016/j.ceca.2012.05.002

Tsumura, M., Sobhan, U., Sato, M., Shimada, M., Nishiyama, A., Kawaguchi, A., et al. (2013). Functional expression of TRPM8 and TRPA1 channels in rat odontoblasts. *PLoS ONE* 8:e82233. doi: 10.1371/journal.pone.0082233

13

# Dentin phosphophoryn in the matrix activates AKT and mTOR signaling pathway to promote preodontoblast survival and differentiation

**Edited by:**
*Victor E. Arana-Chavez, University of São Paulo, Brazil*

*Asha Eapen* [†] *and Anne George* [*]

*Brodie Tooth Development Genetics and Regenerative Medicine, Department of Oral Biology, University of Illinois at Chicago, Chicago, IL, USA*

***Correspondence:**
*Anne George, Department of Oral Biology, University of Illinois at Chicago, 801 S. Paulina, Chicago, IL 60612, USA*
*anneg@uic.edu*

[†] **Present Address:**
*Asha Eapen, Department of Growth, Development and Structure, School of Dental Medicine, Southern Illinois University-Edwardsville, Alton, IL, USA*

Dentin phosphophoryn (DPP) is an extracellular matrix protein synthesized by odontoblasts. It is highly acidic and the phosphorylated protein possesses a strong affinity for calcium ions. Therefore, DPP in the extracellular matrix can promote hydroxyapatite nucleation and can regulate the size of the growing crystal. Besides its calcium binding property, DPP can initiate signaling functions from the ECM (Extracellular matrix). The signals that promote the cytodifferentiation of preodontoblasts to fully functional odontoblasts are not known. In this study, we demonstrate that preodontoblasts on a DPP matrix, generates mechanical and biochemical signals. This is initiated by the ligation of the integrins with the RGD containing DPP. The downstream biochemical response observed is the activation of the AKT(protein kinase B) and mTOR (mammalian target of rapamycin) signaling pathways leading to the activation of the transcription factor NF- κB (Nuclear factor κB). Terminal differentiation of the preodontoblasts was assessed by identifying phosphate and calcium deposits in the matrix using von Kossa and Alizarin red staining respectively. Identifying the signaling pathways initiated by DPP in the dentin matrix would help in devising strategies for dentin tissue engineering.

**Keywords: dentin phosphophoryn, cell proliferation, pereodontoblasts, signaling, odontoblasts, differentiation**

## Introduction

Odontoblasts are post-mitotic neural crest-derived mesenchymal cells that are responsible for the production of dentin (Hao et al., 2004). The major acidic NCPs (non-collagenous proteins) are the dentin phosphophoryn (DPP) and the dentin sialoprotein (DSP). The parent protein DSPP has been reported to be a compound protein that encodes DSP at the amino end and DPP at the carboxyl end. Earlier work by Stetler-Stevenson and Veis (1983) and Butler (1998) has shown based on protein isolation and amino acid sequencing the inherent differences that exist between DPP and DSP (Butler, 1998; Butler et al., 2002). Recently, we provided evidence to demonstrate that DSPP (Dentin sialophosphoprotein) gene contains an internal ribosome entry site (IRES) that directs the synthesis of DPP (Zhang et al., 2013). This mechanism should account for unequal amounts of DPP and DSP.

Apart from its role in mineralization, DPP has also been shown to actively participate in cell signaling events leading to differentiation of precursor mesenchymal cells. DPP contains a conserved integrin-binding RGD domain. We and others have shown that binding of DPP to integrins on the cell surface could activate intracellular signals (Jadlowiec et al., 2004, 2006; Eapen et al., 2012a,b). These signals when translocated to the nucleus altered gene functions in undifferentiated mesenchymal cells.

DPP is predominantly present at the mineralization front of the developing dentin matrix (Hao et al., 2004, 2009; Suzuki et al., 2009). However, the signaling response of preodontoblasts to DPP in the ECM and the functional readout has not been investigated yet. The objective of this study was to investigate the signaling function of DPP in the matrix by which T4-4 (Hao et al., 2002) preodontoblast cells promote cell proliferation and cell survival.

## Materials and Methods

### Cell Culture

Rat immortalized pre-odontoblast cells (T4-4) (Hao et al., 2002) were cultured in DMEM/F-12 medium (growth media) supplemented with 10% FBS and 1% penicillin-streptomycin. Twelve to sixteen hours before the start of the experiment, the cells were cultured in growth medium supplemented with 1% FBS. Non-tissue culture grade six well plates were coated with recombinant DPP (750 ng/ml) in carbonate buffer. The cells were rinsed with PBS, trypsinized, and seeded at 80% confluency. T4-4 cells seeded on 6 well plates coated with carbonate buffer served as control (Eapen et al., 2012a).

### DPP Coating on Non Tissue Culture Plates

Non tissue culture plates coated with DPP were prepared by soaking the plate with 750 ng/ml of DPP as described earlier (Eapen et al., 2012a).

### Quantitative Real Time PCR

RNA was extracted according to the manufacturer's recommended protocol by using Trizol (Invitrogen). RT-qPCR was performed with DNase I (Promega) treated RNA. A total of 1 μg of total RNA was reverse transcribed for 90 min at 50°C with Superscript III (GIBCO) (Eapen et al., 2012a). After RNA extraction, quantitative real-time PCR (qPCR) analysis were carried out using ABI Step One Plus machine. Expression for Cyclin A1, Cyclin D1, Cyclin B1, CDK4, and GAPDH transcripts were analyzed by qPCR during its linear phase. The relative gene expression level was estimated by using the $2_T^{-\Delta\Delta C}$ method where $C_T$ value = log-linear plot of PCR signal versus the cycle number. $\Delta C_T = C_T$ value of target gene-$C_T$ value of GAPDH (Eapen et al., 2012a). Primers were obtained from Qiagen.

### Identification of Integrins

RNA was extracted from T4-4 cells seeded on DPP coated plates at 4 and 24 h time points. The samples were then subjected to genomic DNA contamination removal using elimination mixture (Qiagen), and first strand cDNA synthesis was carried out using the RT$^2$ Easy First Strand Kit (Qiagen) as described by the manufacturer's protocol. PCR array analysis was performed on the predesigned Focal Adhesion Profiler™ array of 96 genes (Super Array Bioscience Corporation). RT-qPCR was performed on ABI Step One Plus machine. For data analysis, the ΔΔCt method was used; for each gene fold-changes were calculated as difference in gene expression between untreated controls and treated cell cultures. The result from the array was interpreted using software provided by Qiagen.

### Identification of Cell Surface Receptor

Integrin receptors from T4-4 cells were isolated as published earlier (Eapen et al., 2012a). Briefly, the cell membrane proteins were extracted after treating T4-4 cells with GST-DPP. The membrane proteins were eluted with glutathione, lyophilized and western blotting performed with anti-α4 and anti-β1 antibody (1:500).

### Cell Cycle Analysis by Flow Cytometry

The effect of DPP on the different phases of the cell cycle in T4-4 cells was determined by flow cytometry. Cells were plated on DPP substrate for 24 h, harvested and fixed in ice cold 70% ethanol. The pellet was washed in ice-cold PBS followed by staining with propidium iodide (PI) at room temperature for 40 min. Cells were then rinsed with PBS and the cell cycle profiles were analyzed by flow cytometry using CellQuest software used for cell cycle analysis.

### Immunofluorescence

T4-4 cells were cultured on rDPP coated non-tissue culture grade glass cover slips for various time points. Cells were fixed in 4% paraformaldehyde, then permeabilized with 0.1% Triton X-100 in PBS for 5 min and rinsed twice with wash buffer (Eapen et al., 2012a). After blocking for 30 min, the cells were then incubated overnight in primary antibody namely, Integrin β1 (kind gift from S. Carbonetto, McGill University, Montreal, Quebec), anti-FAK and anti-Paxillin followed by incubation with a Cy3-conjugated secondary antibody for 1 h. The cells were washed three times with PBS and the cover glass was mounted using mounting media (Vector shield, CA) and imaged using confocal microscopy (Zeiss). The cytoskeleton of the cells were stained with actin (1:100) at different time points followed by DAPI staining for the nucleus and visualized with an Axio Observer D1 Fluorescence Microscope (Zeiss, NY) equipped with Axiovision imaging software (Zeiss, NY).

### Western Blot Analysis

Activation of the focal adhesion components, survival pathways (mTOR, AKT, and NF-κB), cyclins and odontoblast differentiation markers were determined by western blot analysis. Total proteins were extracted from T4-4 cells grown on DPP coated plates with or without mineralization media using M-per reagent (Pierce, IL) (Eapen et al., 2012a). A total of 35 μg of the protein was resolved on a 10% SDS-PAGE gel under reducing conditions. After electrophoresis, the proteins were electro-transferred onto nitrocellulose membrane (Bio-Rad Laboratories, CA), blocked with 3% BSA in 1X PBS, probed with either anti-FAK (1:500) (Santa cruz, CA), anti-paxillin, anti-phospho FAK (1:500) (Santa Cruz, CA), anti-phospho paxillin (1:500) (Cell signaling, MA), anti- phospho AKT(1:500) (Cell signaling, MA), anti-AKT (1:500) (Cell signaling, MA), anti-phospho mTOR (1:500) (Cell signaling, MA), anti-mTOR (1:500) (Cell signaling, MA), anti-phospho NFkB (1:500) (Cell signaling, MA), anti- NF-kB (1:5000) (Chemicon), anti-cyclin D1 (1:500) (Santa Cruz, CA), anti CDK4 (1:500) (Santa Cruz, CA), anti-DMP1 (1:500) anti-DPP (1:500) and anti-DSP (1:2000). HRP-conjugated goat anti-rabbit IgG were used for detection (Chemicon International, CA). Lightening chemiluminescence reagent (Perkin-Elmer Life Sciences, MA) was used as substrate for HRP. Each membrane was then carefully washed, treated for 5 min with a stripping buffer (Pierce, IL), washed with PBS and processed as above with anti- tubulin (1:10,000, Sigma, MO) antibody and HRP conjugated goat anti-mouse IgG (Eapen et al., 2012a).

### *In vitro* Assay to Determine Cell Differentiation

Mineralization microenvironment was induced by the addition of 10 mM β-glycerophosphate and 100 μg/ml ascorbic acid (CitySigma–Aldrich., MO) along with 10 nM dexamethasone (CitySigma–Aldrich., MO) in the growth media as published (Eapen et al., 2012a). Total proteins were extracted at 7, 14, and 21 days from T3 cells grown on DPP coated plates (Eapen et al., 2012a).

### von Kossa Staining for Phosphates in the Mineralized Nodule

von Kossa staining was performed as published (Eapen et al., 2012a) to determine the presence of phosphate in the mineralized nodules. T4-4 cells were grown to 60% confluency on DPP coated plates and the growth media was then replaced with mineralization media for 7, 14, and 21 days. The cells were fixed in formalin for 20 min, washed twice with distilled water and then stained with 1% silver nitrate solution (Sigma–Aldrich., MO) for 30 min and photographed. Cells grown on DPP coated plates without mineralization media and cells on tissue culture plate with mineralization media served as controls.

### Alizarin Red S Staining for Calcium in the Mineralized Nodule

T4-4 cells were grown to 60% confluency on DPP coated plates. The growth media was replaced with mineralization media for 7, 14, and 21 days. The cells were fixed in formalin for 20 min at room temperature and washed with distilled water. 2% Alizarin Red solution was added to fixed cells and incubated for 10–20 min (Eapen et al., 2012a). The cells were then rinsed with distilled water and were imaged.

### Statistical Analysis

PCR-array analysis was performed for both experimental groups ($n = 3$). Means and standard deviations (SE) were calculated, and the statistical significance of differences among each group was examined by student $t$-test between both groups ($p < 0.05$).

## Results

### DPP Mediates Cell Adhesion

T4-4 cells were seeded on DPP-coated non-tissue culture cover glass as published before (Eapen et al., 2012a) and cultured for 8 and 24 h. Actin staining was performed on the fixed cells.

A

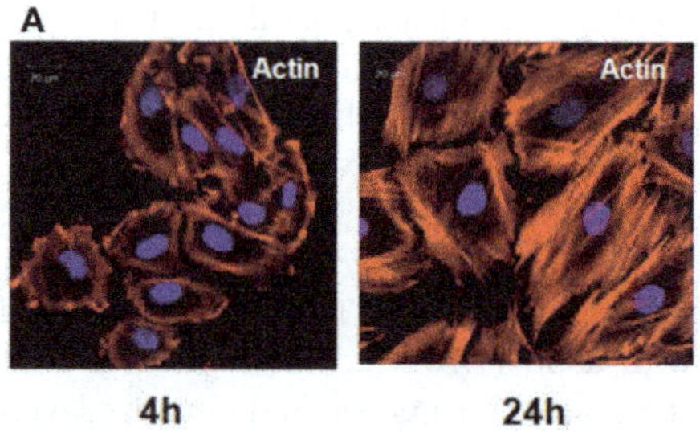


B

| Gene Symbol | Description | Fold Change 4h | p- value (t test) 4h | Fold Change 24h | p-value (t test) 24h |
|---|---|---|---|---|---|
| ITGA4 | Integrin, alpha 4 | 12.4 | 0.006115 | 21.01 | 0.02595 |
| ITGAL | Integrin, alpha L | 12.47 | 0.1486 | 0.67 | 0.8793 |
| ITGB1 | Integrin, beta 1 | 38.1 | 0.00697 | 41.42 | 0.00008 |
| ITGB6 | Integrin, beta 6 | 39.33 | 0.00002 | 33.4 | 0.00040 |

C D

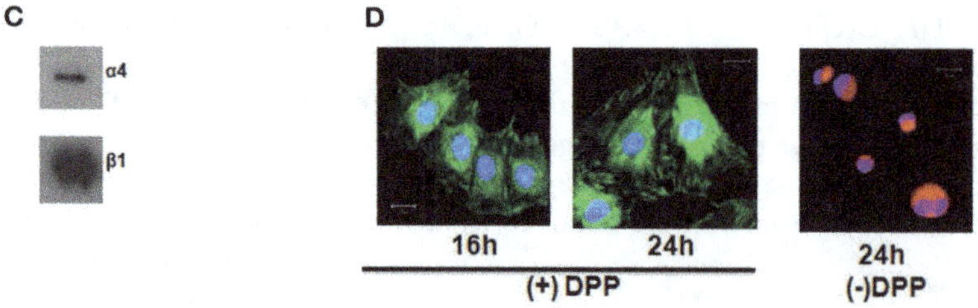


**FIGURE 1 | T4-4 preodontoblasts adheres to DPP substrate by α4β1intergrin and activates the cytoskeletal elements. (A)** T4-4 cells were seeded on DPP-coated non-tissue culture cover glass and cultured for 4 and 24 h time point. Immunofluorescences staining with Texas-red phalloidin show accumulation of actin filaments at the membrane surface at 4 h and polarized filaments at 24 h. No cell attachment was observed in the absence of DPP. **(B)** Identification of Integrin receptors. Expression of alpha and beta subunits of integrins present on T4-4 cells at 4 and 24 h when plated on DPP substrate. Total RNA was isolated and Focal Adhesion Profiler™ PCR array analysis was performed at 4 and 24 h on the DPP adherent T4-4 cells. Fold change increase of the integrin receptors is represented in **(B)**. **(C)** Total membrane proteins were isolated from T4-4 cells adhered to DPP substrate and Western Blot analysis was performed with anti-alpha 4 and anti-beta 1 integrin antibodies. **(D)** Confocal imaging show the localization of β1 integrin on the membrane of T4-4 cells adhered to DPP substrate. Cells seeded on plates coated with carbonate buffer (absence of DPP) served as the control.

Confocal microscopy image clearly showed the dynamic nature of the actin cytoskeleton in the cells attached on DPP substrate at 4 and 24 h (**Figure 1A**). Cells seeded on cover glass without DPP failed to adhere.

## Identification of Integrin Receptors

In order to identify the integrins specific for the binding of T4-4 cells on DPP coated plates we performed PCR-based integrin pathway-specific super array. RNA was isolated at 4 and 24 h from T4-4 cells that were seeded on the DPP coated substrate and real time super array was performed. Analysis revealed an increase in the expression of integrin αL, α4, β1, and β6 genes from the pathway-specific array containing several alpha and beta integrin receptors in the presence of DPP substrate (**Figure 1B**). T4-4 cells seeded on tissue culture plates served as controls. Specifically, the expression of integrin αL, α4, β1, and β6 genes were up regulated at 4 h time point respectively. Intracellular proteins responsible for transducing DPP mediated extracellular signals use integrins as a mediator molecule. These results suggest that the preodontoblasts utilize these integrins in DPP mediated cell adhesion and signaling. Interestingly, α4 and β1 was observed to be up-regulated at 4 and 24 h time points suggesting that α4β1 integrin might be involved during early stages of DPP mediated adhesion. Having identified the possible alpha and beta integrin receptors and in order to validate the array data we performed immunoblot analysis with membrane proteins isolated from adherent cells on DPP substrate. Results from the western blot clearly showed an up-regulation of α4 and β1 integrins in the presence of DPP (**Figure 1C**). **Figure 1D** shows the expression of β1 integrin at the focal adhesion points of T4-4 cells when plated on DPP substrate at 16 and 24 h. Cells seeded on plates coated with carbonate buffer served as control and failed to spread.

## DPP Facilitates Formation of Focal Adhesion Complex

Focal adhesion kinase (FAK) has been shown to regulate integrin mediated survival signaling. We therefore examined if DPP substrate would induce association of FAK and paxillin in preodontoblast cells. Confocal microscope images clearly indicated the co- localization of FAK and paxillin at the focal points on the cell membrane of adherent T4-4 cells at 24 h (**Figure 2A**). Cells plated on DMP1 and fibronectin substrates were used as positive controls. Interestingly, DPP mediated nuclear translocation of FAK was observed in adherent cells at 24 h time point. Control cells on carbonate buffer coated slides failed to express FAK and Paxillin and were rounded in morphology (**Figure 2A**). Therefore, we next determined whether protein expression for FAK and Paxillin were up regulated in T4-4 cells in the presence or absence of DPP. Immunoblot analysis confirmed that DPP adherent cells showed significant expression of FAK and Paxillin with increasing time (**Figure 2B**).

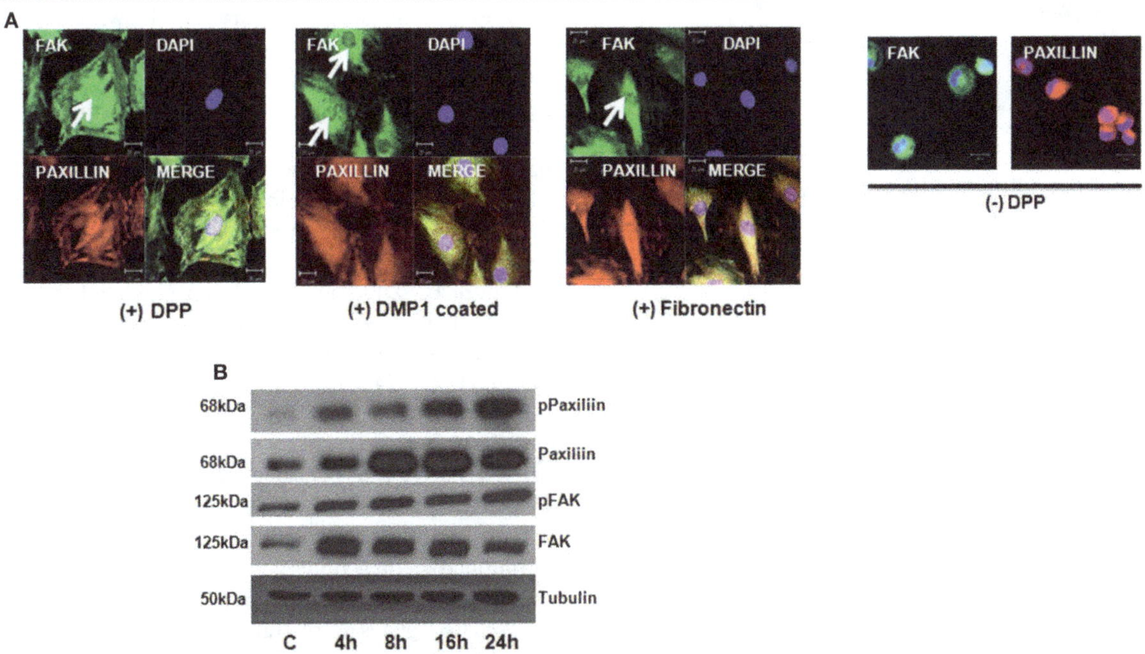


**FIGURE 2 | DPP matrix induces the activation of Focal adhesion complex in T4-4 adhered cells. (A)** Immunofluorescence staining of FAK and Paxillin in T4-4 cells cultured on DPP coated non-tissue culture slides for 24 h at 37°C. Nuclear localization of FAK (white arrow) and membrane localization of Paxillin was observed in the DPP mediated T4-4 adherent cells. Absence of nuclear localization of FAK was seen in cells seeded on DMP1 and Fibronectin coated substrates (white arrow) which were positive controls. Cells were rounded in the absence of DPP. Scale bar = 20 μm. **(B)** Western blot analysis of active FAK, total FAK, active Paxillin and total Paxillin showed DPP mediated activation of focal adhesion complexes in T4-4 cells at the specified time points. Experiments were repeated three times and similar results were obtained.

## DPP Mediates the Activation of AKT-mTOR-NF-kB Signaling Pathway

To assess the role of AKT in DPP mediated adhesion, we first determined if adherent T4-4 cells can induce AKT phosphorylation at serine residues (Ser473 and 308), Studies have shown that phosphorylation at Ser 473 is important for the activation of the enzymatic function of AKT kinases (Toker and Newton, 2000). Significant increase in AKT phosphorylation at Ser 473 was observed at 8 and 16 h when compared to control T4-4 cells cultured on tissue culture plates (**Figure 3A**). AKT phosphorylation at Ser 473 declined at 24 h time point suggesting the role of AKT during early events of cell adhesion and survival. To further corroborate the above results T4-4 cells were pre-treated with LY294002 and then seeded on DPP substrate. LY294002 is a well-known inhibitor of PI3K, which inhibits activation of AKT (Borgatti et al., 2000). As shown in **Figure 3B**, LY294002 treatment repressed AKT expression in preodontoblasts.

We next investigated if the activation of the AKT pathway by DPP could lead to cell survival by activation of mTOR (mammalian target of rapamycin) and NF-kB activation. mTOR is an important downstream target of AKT signaling pathway leading to its phosphorylation (Harris and Lawrence, 2003; Guertin and Sabatini, 2005; Rosner et al., 2008). To understand whether mTOR was activated by DPP, western blotting analysis was performed on cells plated on the DPP substrate. Results in **Figure 3C** show an upregulation of phosphorylated mTOR expression from 8 to 24 h time point.

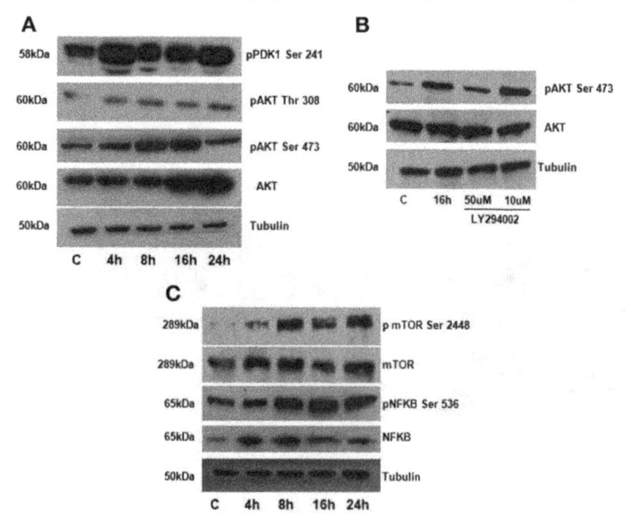


**FIGURE 3 | (A)** DPP activates AKT, mTOR and NFκB signaling pathways in T4-4 cells. T4-4 cells were cultured on DPP coated non tissue culture plates for 4,8,16, and 24 h. Cells were lysed and equal amounts of proteins were separated by SDS-PAGE, transferred to PVDF membrane, and immunoblotted with antibodies against AKT, p-AKT (Ser 473), p-AKT (Thr 308), p-PDK1 (ser 241), and Tubulin **(A)**. **(B)** Inhibitor LY294002 causes in-activation of AKT in DPP mediated adhered T4-4 cells. T4-4 cells were pre-treated with LY294002 10 and 50 μm for 30 min and then seeded on DPP substrate for 16 h. After 16 h, cells were lysed and equal amounts of proteins were separated by SDS-PAGE, transferred to PVDF membrane, and immunoblotted with antibodies against p-AKT, total AKT and tubulin. **(C)** DPP mediated activation of activation of NFκB and mTOR pathways. Total proteins were isolated from the T4-4 adhered cells, lysed and equal amounts of proteins were separated by SDS-PAGE, transferred to PVDF membrane, and immunoblotted with antibodies against p- NFκB, p-mTOR, total NFκB and total mTOR antibodies. Equal loading of the proteins were confirmed by stripping and reprobing the blot with tubulin antibody.

As NF-κB is a transcription factor considered to play a key role in both cell proliferation and apoptosis, therefore, we examined if NF-κB is activated downstream of signaling induced by DPP. In order to validate NF-kB activation, we isolated total proteins from cells seeded on DPP coated plates at 4, 8, 16, and 24 h respectively. A significant increase in the phosphorylated NF-kB (Ser 536) was observed from 8 to 24 h time points respectively (**Figure 3C**). Taken together, these results strengthened the finding that DPP stimulates the activation of cell adhesion mediated by AKT-mTOR-NF-kB signaling.

## DPP Regulates Cell Cycle Controlling Proteins

We next investigated the regulation of cell-cycle proteins by DPP. For this, T4-4 cells grown on DPP coated plates in the absence of serum for 24 h were harvested and flow cytometric analysis was performed. Cells grown on tissue culture plates were used as control. In contrast to G1 phase growth arrest in differentiated cells, proliferating T4-4 cells stimulated with DPP at 24 h showed a significant increase in the cell population in S phase (**Figure 4A**). As cell cycle regulation is controlled by a combination of cyclins, cdks, and cdk inhibitors, we therefore examined changes in gene expression for cyclins using Real-Time PCR. Cells seeded on DPP showed significant up regulation of cyclin A1 and D1 and a down regulation of cyclin B1 gene expression at 4 h (**Figure 4B**). However, Cyclin B1 was upregulated at 24 h. Interestingly, the gene expression level of Cdk4, which is the kinase regulatory partner of cyclin D1, was seen to be up regulated at 4 h when compared with control (**Figure 4B**). The complex, Cyclin D1 along with its catalytic partner Cdk4 may play a vital role in propelling the cell cycle through the G1/S checkpoint, a critical phase of cell proliferation. We then sought to determine the protein expression levels of cyclin D1 and CDK4 using western blot analysis. As revealed in **Figure 4C**, DPP significantly up regulated the expression of Cyclin D1 and CDK4 at 4 and 8 h. These results suggest that DPP promotes survival and proliferation of T4-4 cells by activating cyclin D1-CDK4 complex which in turn regulates the G1/S transition.

## DPP Promotes Terminal Differentiation of Preodontoblasts

As the preodontoblasts differentiate to polarized functional odontoblasts, they undergo a change in cellular morphology with the formation of mineralized matrix. Cells grown on DPP-coated plates were subjected to mineralization for 7, 14, and 21 days, and their morphology was assessed by light microscopy. Distinct morphological changes were observed when cells were cultured in the presence of mineralization medium for 21 days (**Figure 5A**). Differentiation was assessed by identifying odontoblastic differentiation markers. Data obtained from Western blots showed a significant increase in DSP, DMP1(dentin matrix protein 1) and DPP from day 7 to

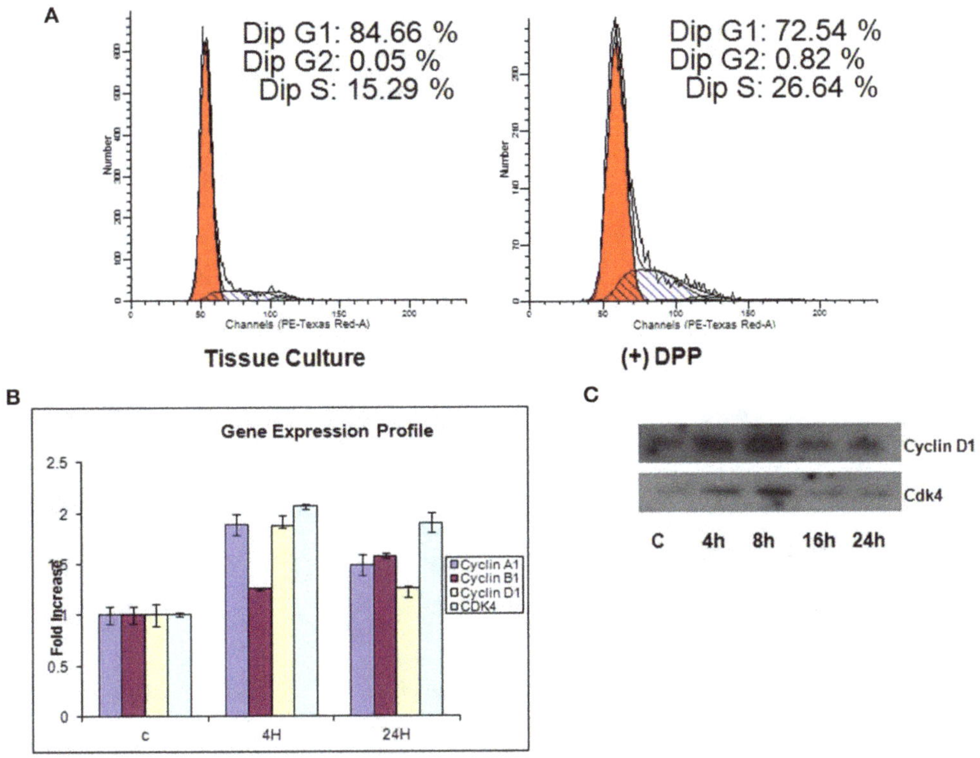


**FIGURE 4 | Illustration of DNA measurement by flow cytometry in cells cultured on tissue culture or DPP coated non-tissue culture plates.** **(A)** Cells were stained by PI solution, and the cell cycle distribution (G0/G1, S, and G2/M) was analyzed by flow cytometry. The distribution and percentage of cells in $G_1$, S, and $G_2$/M are indicated. T4-4 cells grown on tissue culture plates were used as controls. Flow cytometry analysis showed that 26.6% of cells cultured on DPP coated substrate were seen to be in the S-phase when compared to the cells that were cultured on tissue culture plates. **(B)** Total RNA was isolated from the T4-4 adhered cells at 4 and 24 h and real time PCR was performed for Cyclin A1, Cyclin D1, Cyclin B1, and CDK4. **(C)** Western blot analysis of Cyclin D1, and CDK4 proteins were perfomed with the total proteins isolated from the DPP substrate adhered T4-4 at the specified time points.

day 21 when compared with the control cells, which were obtained at 21 days in the absence of differentiation medium (**Figure 5B**). In order to determine whether DPP could influence the differentiation of preodontoblasts to fully differentiated cells *in vitro*, von-Kossa and Alizarin Red staining was performed at 7, 14, and 21 days time points under mineralization conditions on cells grown on DPP substrate. von Kossa staining showed dark nodules in the extracellular matrix, demonstrating the presence of phosphate in the calcified matrix. Odontogenic terminal differentiation of preodontoblsts was further confirmed by Alizarin Red staining. Results showed staining of the mineralized matrix at 7, 14, and 21 days demonstrating the presence of calcium deposits (**Figure 5C**).

## Discussion

Mechanisms involved in the terminal differentiation of preodontoblasts to functional odontoblasts are not well-defined. DPP is highly expressed by odontoblasts, however, early on in development expression has been observed in undifferentiated ameloblasts (Begue-Kirn et al., 1998; Bleicher et al., 1999; Paine et al., 2005). Earlier, studies have shown that the intact predentin was unable to promote physiological terminal differentiation of odontoblasts (Karcher-Djuricic et al., 1985). However, non-collagenous fractions from rabbit dentin facilitated the formation of polarized odontoblast-like cells. This suggests that the changing dentin extracellular matrix is not just an inert supporting material but a dynamic vector of information. Therefore, the dentin matrix plays an important role during terminal differentiation of odontoblasts. In this study, we demonstrate that DPP, a major component of the dentin ECM initiates a signaling program that is necessary for the terminal differentiation of preodontoblasts to functional odontoblasts.

We first showed that the preodontoblasts contain $\alpha4\beta1$ specific cell surface integrins that can interact with DPP in the matrix. In fact $\beta1$ interaction with DPP in the matrix was predominant. Absence of DPP resulted in cell death.

Terminal differentiation of odontoblasts requires structural integrity of the cytoskeleton. Studies have shown that the cytoskeleton of eukaryotic cells play an important role in cellular functions such as motility, mitosis, morphology and anchorage-adherent growth. At 4 h apical accumulation of actin was observed and alignment of actin was observed at 24 h inT4-4 cells on DPP substrate. Published studies have shown that colchisin, vinblastin as well as cytochalasin B were found to inhibit polarization of odontoblasts (Miake et al., 1982; Ruch et al.,

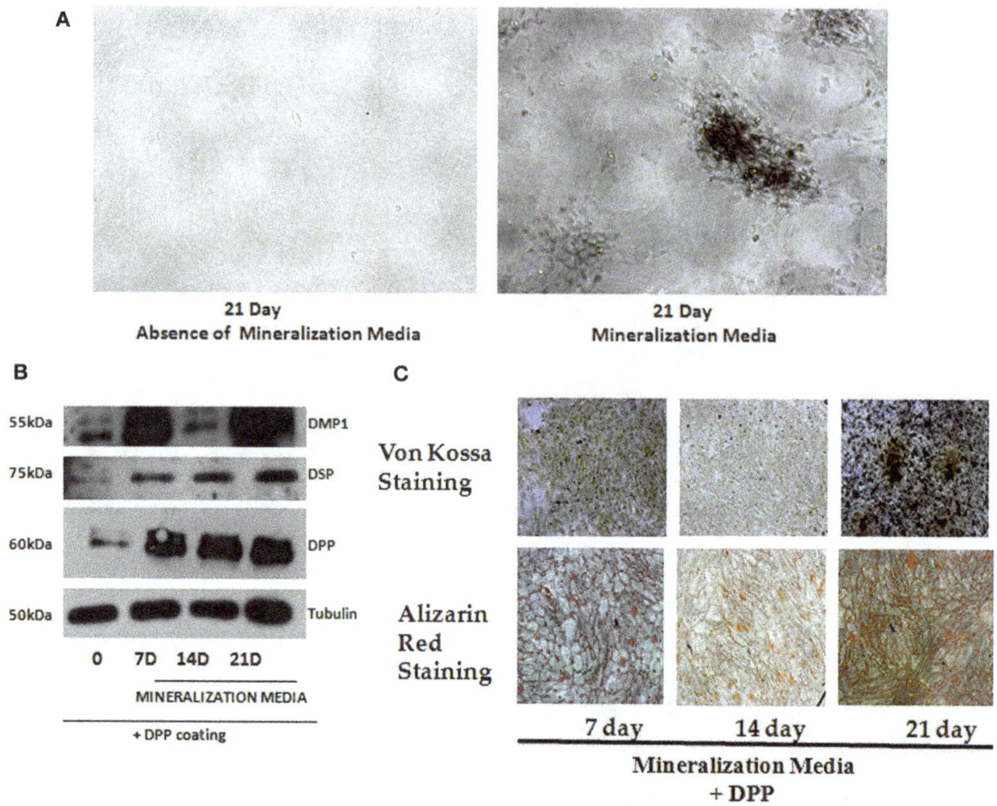


**FIGURE 5 | Role of DPP in terminal differentiation of T4-4 cells. (A)** T4-4 cells were cultured on DPP-coated plates in mineralization medium for 7, 14, and 21 days. Light microscopic images of the cells in the presence and absence of mineralization medium at 21 days were taken. Morphological changes in the cells were noticed in the presence of DPP and mineralization medium. **(B)** Total proteins were isolated from the DPP substrate adherent T4-4 cells and grown under mineralization conditions for 7, 14, and 21 days. Immunoblot analysis was performed for DPP, DSP and DMP1. **(C)** Alizarin Red and von Kossa staining were performed on T4-4 cells cultured on DPP substrate for 7, 14, and 21 days, respectively.

1995). Thus, cytoskeleton plays an important role in odontoblast polarization. Interestingly, within 24 h, phosphorylation of focal adhesion kinase (FAK) and paxillin were observed, suggesting the importance of the focal adhesion components activated by DPP. Focal adhesions are sites of cell attachment to the extracellular matrix where transmembrane integrins link the ECM to the cytoskeleton (Tureckova et al., 2009). Published reports suggest that FAK is activated through integrin receptors and gets recruited to integrins by paxillin, vinculin, and talin (Tureckova et al., 2009). This suggests that DPP in the matrix can influence the polarized alignment of actin, probably generating a mechanical force required for activation of paxillin and FAK. Published studies have shown that uniaxial mechanical stretch can stimulate the activation of ERK, p38MAPK and Akt pathways in dental pulp stem cells (Hata et al., 2013).

This led us to investigate the role of PDK1 a master kinase and Akt as a mediator of preodontoblast differentiation. Phosphorylation of PDK1 phosphorylation at Ser241 and Akt phosphorylation at Ser 473 were observed at early time points when T4-4 cells were cultured on DPP substrate. Interestingly, Akt phosphorylation levels declined at 24 h, suggesting that Akt activation is mainly required during early events of cell adhesion and survival. The inhibitor LY294002 which inhibits activation of AKT, downregulated DPP-induced AKT activation. These findings confirm the specificity of DPP in activating the AKT signaling pathway in preodontoblasts.

A key effector of AKT-induced signaling is the regulatory protein mTOR. mTOR regulates a number of functions stimulated by Akt activation such as cell cycle, proliferation, cytoskeletal organization and cell differentiation (Hayden et al., 2006; Skeen et al., 2006; Laplante and Sabatini, 2013). Previous studies have shown that mTOR plays an important role in odontoblast differentiation (Kim et al., 2011). Our data showed an increase in mTOR expression at the specified time points when plated on DPP substrate. mTOR exists in two different conformations in mammalian cells; mTOR complex-1 (mTORC1;mTOR-Raptor complex) and mTOR complex-2 (mTORC2; mTORC2; mTOR-Rictor complex) (Laplante and Sabatini, 2013). In this study mTOR is phosphorylated on Ser 2448 suggesting mTORC2 as the predominant form. Thus, DPP in the matrix can upregulate p-AKT and p-mTOR, predominantly mTORC2 which suggests that DPP mediated activation of AKT-mTOR signaling is required for preodontoblast differentiation.

In this study, we also demonstrate that the AKT-mTOR signaling pathway can also activate NF-κB (phosphorylation

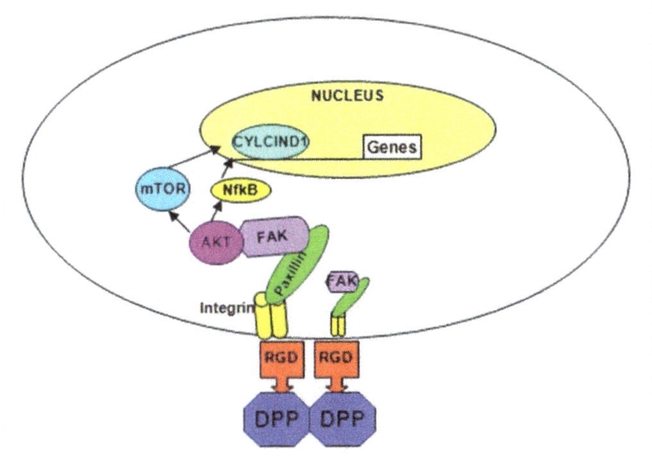


**FIGURE 6 | Hypothetical model.** The hypothetical model depicts the integrin-mediated anchorage of T4-4 cells on DPP substrate and the subsequent activation of focal adhesion complexes, survival and differentiation pathway in T4-4cells.

of Ser 538). The NF-κB family is comprised of five closely related members: p65/RelA, c-Rel, RelB, NF-κB1/p50, and NF-κB2/p52 (Hayden et al., 2006). This transcription factor, when inactive, resides in the cytoplasm as a heterotrimeric complex comprised of p50/p52, p65 and inhibitory kappa B (IκB). Upon phosphorylation of IκB through the activation of upstream kinases, this complex is disrupted. Dissociated p-IkB is ubiquitinated and degrades, whereas the remaining heterodimeric complexes comprised of p50/p65 and p52/p65 translocate to the nucleus to perform transcriptional functions. Results show that the serine 536 of NF- κBp65 can be activated by DPP during the differentiation process.

The cell cycle is controlled by cyclins, cyclin-dependent kinases (Cdks) and cyclin-dependent kinase inhibitors. Cyclins and cdks activate cell cycle factors essential for the start of the next cycle phase. Cells passing through the the G1 phase and following S phase entry requires the activities of the D-type cyclins and the cyclin D-dependent kinases. In this study, we observed increased expression levels of cyclin D1 and Cdk4 when cells were on DPP substrate at early time points. Lower expression levels of these cell cycle factors at 16 and 24 h suggest that after the proliferation phase DPP can promote cell differentiation.

Terminal differentiation of preodontoblasts was confirmed by the synthesis of major odontoblastic ECM proteins such as DMP1, DSP, and DPP. Formation of a mineralized matrix as assessed by von Kossa and Alizarin Red staining confirmed the functional nature of the odontoblast-like cells.

Overall, we have shown that DPP on the matrix can activate the cytoskeletal elements resulting in increased phosphorylation of AKT, mammalian target of rapamycin and the transcription factor NF-κB leading to cell survival and increased proliferation (**Figure 6**). In the presence of differentiation medium, the DPP substrate could promote terminal differentiation of preodontoblasts. These data strongly suggest that DPP could be a suitable target for therapeutic interventions for the proliferation and differentiation of preodontoblasts to fully functional odontoblasts. Dental pulp cells and preodontoblasts are responsive to the DPP signal from the matrix. Therefore, for regenerating or tissue engineering dentin, scaffolds could be immobilized with DPP for facilitating proliferation of stem cells or preodontoblasts based on the AKT-mTOR -cyclin D1 signaling pathway. DPP stimulus in the presence of a mineralization microenvironment can switch the proliferating cells into an odontoblast differentiation pathway. Such a strategy could be used for regenerating damaged dentin using preodontoblasts or stem cells.

## Author Contributions

AE Conceptualized, planned, performed all the experiments and wrote part of the manuscript. AG Was involved in conceptualization and planning with AE. Contributed toward writing, editing, and proofreading the manuscript along with AE.

## Funding

This project was funded by the NIH grant DE 19633 and the Brodie Endowment fund.

## References

Bègue-Kirn, C., Ruch, J. V., Ridall, A. L., and Butler, W. T. (1998). Comparative analysis of mouse DSP and DPP expression in odontoblasts, preameloblasts, and experimentally induced odontoblast-like cells. *Eur. J. Oral Sci.* 106(Suppl. 1), 1254–259. doi: 10.1111/j.1600-0722.1998.tb02184.x

Bleicher, F., Couble, M. L., Farges, J. C., Couble, P., and Magloire, H. (1999). Sequential expression of matrix protein genes in developing rat teeth. *Matrix Biol.* 18, 133–143. doi: 10.1016/S0945-053X(99)00007-4

Borgatti, P., Martelli, A. M., Bellacosa, A., Casto, R., Massari, L., Capitani, S., et al. (2000). Translocation of Akt/PKB to the nucleus of osteoblast-like MC3T3-E1 cells exposed to proliferative growth factors. *FEBS Lett.* 477, 27–32. doi: 10.1016/S0014-5793(00)01758-0

Butler, W. T. (1998). Dentin matrix proteins. *Eur. J. Oral Sci.* 106(Suppl. 1), 204–210. doi: 10.1111/j.1600-0722.1998.tb02177.x

Butler, W. T., Brunn, J. C., Qin, C., and McKee, M. D. (2002). Extracellular matrix proteins and the dynamics of dentin formation. *Connect. Tissue Res.* 43, 301–307. doi: 10.1080/713713518

Eapen, A., Ramachandran, A., and George, A. (2012a). Dentin phosphoprotein (DPP) activates integrin-mediated anchorage-dependent signals in undifferentiated mesenchymal cells. *J. Biol. Chem.* 287, 5211–5224. doi: 10.1074/jbc.M111.290080

Eapen, A., Ramachandran, A., and George, A. (2012b). DPP in the matrix mediates cell adhesion but is not restricted to stickiness: a tale of signaling. *Cell Adh. Migr.* 6, 307–311. doi: 10.4161/cam.20627

Guertin, D. A., and Sabatini, D. M. (2005). An expanding role for mTOR in cancer. *Trends Mol. Med.* 11, 353–361. doi: 10.1016/j.molmed.2005.06.007

Hao, J., Narayanan, K., Ramachandran, A., He, G., Almushayt, A., Evans, C., et al. (2002). Odontoblast cells immortalized by telomerase produce mineralized dentin-like tissue both *in vitro* and *in vivo*. *J. Biol. Chem.* 277, 19976–19981. doi: 10.1074/jbc.M112223200

Hao, J., Ramachandran, A., and George, A. (2009). Temporal and spatial localization of the dentin matrix proteins during dentin biomineralization. *J. Histochem. Cytochem.* 57, 227–237. doi: 10.1369/jhc.2008.952119

Hao, J., Zou, B., Narayanan, K., and George, A. (2004). Differential expression patterns of the dentin matrix proteins during mineralized tissue formation. *Bone* 34, 921–932. doi: 10.1016/j.bone.2004.01.020

Harris, T. E., and Lawrence, J. C. Jr. (2003). TOR signaling. *Sci. STKE* 2003:re15. doi: 10.1126/stke.2122003re15

Hata, M., Naruse, K., Ozawa, S., Kobayashi, Y., Nakamura, N., Kojima, N., et al. (2013). Mechanical stretch increases the proliferation while inhibiting the osteogenic differentiation in dental pulp stem cells. *Tissue Eng. A* 19, 625–633. doi: 10.1089/ten.tea.2012.0099

Hayden, M. S., West, A. P., and Ghosh, S. (2006). SnapShot: NF-kappaB signaling pathways. *Cell* 127, 1286–1287. doi: 10.1016/j.cell.2006.12.005

Jadlowiec, J., Koch, H., Zhang, X., Campbell, P. G., Seyedain, M., and Sfeir, C. (2004). Phosphophoryn regulates the gene expression and differentiation of NIH3T3, MC3T3-E1, and human mesenchymal stem cells via the integrin/MAPK signaling pathway. *J. Biol. Chem.* 279, 53323–53330. doi: 10.1074/jbc.M404934200

Jadlowiec, J. A., Zhang, X., Li, J., Campbell, P. G., and Sfeir, C. (2006). Extracellular matrix-mediated signaling by dentin phosphophoryn involves activation of the Smad pathway independent of bone morphogenetic protein. *J. Biol. Chem.* 281, 5341–5347. doi: 10.1074/jbc.M506158200

Karcher-Djuricic, V., Staubli, A., Meyer, J. M., and Ruch, J. V. (1985). Acellular dental matrices promote functional differentiation of ameloblasts. *Differentiation* 29, 169–175. doi: 10.1111/j.1432-0436.1985.tb00311.x

Kim, J. K., Baker, J., Nor, J. E., and Hill, E. E. (2011). mTor plays an important role in odontoblast differentiation. *J. Endod.* 37, 1081–1085. doi: 10.1016/j.joen.2011.03.034

Laplante, M., and Sabatini, D. M. (2013). Regulation of mTORC1 and its impact on gene expression at a glance. *J. Cell. Sci.* 126(Pt 8), 1713–1719. doi: 10.1242/jcs.125773

Paine, M. L., Luo, W., Wang, H. J., Bringas, P. Jr., Ngan, A. Y., Miklus, V. G., et al. (2005). Dentin sialoprotein and dentin phosphoprotein overexpression during amelogenesis. *J. Biol. Chem.* 280, 31991–31998. doi: 10.1074/jbc.M502991200

Rosner, M., Hanneder, M., Siegel, N., Valli, A., Fuchs, C., and Hengstschläger, M. (2008). The mTOR pathway and its role in human genetic diseases. *Mutat. Res.* 659, 284–292. doi: 10.1016/j.mrrev.2008.06.001

Ruch, J. V., Lesot, H., and Begue-Kirn, C. (1995). Odontoblast differentiation. *Int. J. Dev. Biol.* 39, 51–68.

Skeen, J. E., Bhaskar, P. T., Chen, C. C., Chen, W. S., Peng, X. D., Nogueira, V., et al. (2006). Akt deficiency impairs normal cell proliferation and suppresses oncogenesis in a p53-independent and mTORC1-dependent manner. *Cancer Cell* 10, 269–280. doi: 10.1016/j.ccr.2006.08.022

Stetler-Stevenson, W. G., and Veis, A. (1983). Bovine dentin phosphophoryn: composition and molecular weight. *Biochemistry* 22, 4326–4335. doi: 10.1021/bi00287a025

Suzuki, S., Sreenath, T., Haruyama, N., Honeycutt, C., Terse, A., Cho, A., et al. (2009). Dentin sialoprotein and dentin phosphoprotein have distinct roles in dentin mineralization. *Matrix Biol.* 28, 221–229. doi: 10.1016/j.matbio.2009.03.006

Toker, A., and Newton, A. C. (2000). Akt/protein kinase B is regulated by autophosphorylation at the hypothetical PDK-2 site. *J. Biol. Chem.* 275, 8271–8274. doi: 10.1074/jbc.275.12.8271

Turecková, J., Vojtechová, M., Krausová, M., Sloncová, E., and Korínek, V. (2009). Focal adhesion kinase functions as an akt downstream target in migration of colorectal cancer cells. *Transl. Oncol.* 2, 281–290. doi: 10.1593/tlo.09160

Zhang, Y., Song, Y., Ravindran, S., Gao, Q., Huang, C. C., Ramachandran, A., et al. (2013). DSPP contains an IRES element responsible for the translation of dentin phosphophoryn. *J. Dent. Res.* 93, 155–161. doi: 10.1177/0022034513516631

# 14

# Malformations of the tooth root in humans

**Edited by:**
*Victor E. Arana-Chavez,*
*University of São Paulo, Brazil*

***Correspondence:***
*Hans U. Luder*
*bhdk.luder@bluewin.ch*

***Hans U. Luder*** *

*Center of Dental Medicine, Institute of Oral Biology, University of Zurich, Zurich, Switzerland*

The most common root malformations in humans arise from either developmental disorders of the root alone or disorders of radicular development as part of a general tooth dysplasia. The aim of this review is to relate the characteristics of these root malformations to potentially disrupted processes involved in radicular morphogenesis. Radicular morphogenesis proceeds under the control of Hertwig's epithelial root sheath (HERS) which determines the number, length, and shape of the root, induces the formation of radicular dentin, and participates in the development of root cementum. Formation of HERS at the transition from crown to root development appears to be very insensitive to adverse effects, with the result that rootless teeth are extremely rare. In contrast, shortened roots as a consequence of impaired or prematurely halted apical growth of HERS constitute the most prevalent radicular dysplasia which occurs due to trauma and unknown reasons as well as in association with dentin disorders. While odontoblast differentiation inevitably stops when growth of HERS is arrested, it seems to be unaffected even in cases of severe dentin dysplasias such as regional odontodysplasia and dentin dysplasia type I. As a result radicular dentin formation is at least initiated and progresses for a limited time. The only condition affecting cementogenesis is hypophosphatasia which disrupts the formation of acellular cementum through an inhibition of mineralization. A process particularly susceptible to adverse effects appears to be the formation of the furcation in multirooted teeth. Impairment or disruption of this process entails taurodontism, single-rooted posterior teeth, and misshapen furcations. Thus, even though many characteristics of human root malformations can be related to disorders of specific processes involved in radicular morphogenesis, precise inferences as to the pathogenesis of these dysplasias are hampered by the still limited knowledge on root formation.

**Keywords: tooth root, abnormalities, humans, root dilaceration, taurodontism, odontodysplasia, dentin dysplasia type I, hypophosphatasia**

## INTRODUCTION

Owing to the belief that periodontal regeneration is a recapitulation of the processes involved in root formation, these processes have recently gained increased attention from researchers (Luan et al., 2006; Huang and Chai, 2012; Xiong et al., 2013; Bosshardt et al., 2015). There is complete agreement that radicular development is controlled by Hertwig's epithelial root sheath (HERS) which is derived from the cervical loop of the enamel organ and determines root number, shape, and length. The end of crown morphogenesis comprising the cessation of enamel formation and the development of HERS is associated with the disappearance of the expression of mesenchymal fibroblast growth factor 10 (Fgf10) and of epithelial growth factor (Egf) receptor (Tummers and Thesleff, 2003; Yokohama-Tamaki et al., 2006; Fujiwara et al., 2009). Subsequently, HERS proliferates in an apical direction and induces the differentiation of odontoblasts and dentinogenesis. Other than during crown development, radicular dentinogenesis critically depends on nuclear factor Ic (Nfic) and transforming growth factor β (Tgfβ) signaling mediated by Smad4 (Huang and Chai, 2012; Xiong et al., 2013). On the first layer of root dentin, HERS cells deposit enamel matrix proteins (Xiong et al., 2013; Bosshardt et al., 2015). As far as the ultimate fate of HERS and its contribution to cementogenesis are concerned, opinions differ. There is general consensus that HERS disintegrates, thus forming the epithelial cell rests of Malassez and allowing mesenchymal cells of the dental follicle to gain access to the surface of the outermost dentin layer, where they differentiate into cementoblasts and form radicular cementum (Diekwisch, 2001; Luan et al., 2006; Huang et al., 2009; Huang and Chai, 2012; Xiong et al., 2013; Bosshardt et al., 2015). In addition, several researchers attribute to HERS a more active role in cementogenesis. There is evidence to suggest that some HERS cells undergo epithelial mesenchymal transition and differentiate into cementoblasts (Huang and Chai, 2012; Xiong et al., 2013; Bosshardt et al., 2015). HERS cells may even participate directly in cementogenesis and be embedded in the matrix of cellular cementum (Huang et al., 2009; Huang and Chai, 2012; Xiong et al., 2013). In the cervical root areas, cementoblasts incorporate a dense fringe of collagen fibers into the outer dentin and thus deposit the first layer of acellular cementum (Xiong et al., 2013; Bosshardt et al., 2015). Fringe fibers are subsequently elongated and mineralized under the control of tissue-nonspecific alkaline phosphatase (TNALP), while cementoblasts retreat from the advancing mineralization front (Bosshardt et al., 2015). In more apical root areas, cellular cementum comprising a mixture of predominantly intrinsic and scattered extrinsic collagen fibers (Shapey's fibers) is laid down. Other than during acellular cementum formation, cementoblasts, similar to osteoblasts, occasionally are embedded in the collagenous matrix as cementocytes (Xiong et al., 2013). Thus, the basic processes of root formation appear to comprise (1) the development of HERS associated with the transition from crown to root development, (2) apical growth of HERS associated with root elongation, (3) the induction of odontoblast differentiation and radicular dentinogenesis, (4) the disintegration of HERS and the initiation of cementogenesis as well as (5) formation of acellular and cellular cementum.

A special process confined to the development of multirooted teeth is the formation of the bi- or trifurcation. The critical structures for furcation formation seem to be tongue-shaped epithelial projections from the cervical loop of the enamel organ, which are already present but remain inactive during crown formation. Only when the root trunk is about to divide, these tongues proliferate and unite to form a continuous bridge. Similar to HERS in the periphery of the root, the epithelium of the bridges induces the differentiation of odontoblasts which subsequently produce the dentin at the floor of the pulp cavity, while bridge cells proliferate and grow apically in concert with the peripheral HERS (Schroeder, 1991). Even though epithelial bridges in the furcation area thus seem to behave similarly to HERS, it is not known whether bridge formation proceeds under the control of HERS. In this context a recent study of Kim et al. (2015) is notable. It indicated that other than in the crown, the induction of root odontoblast differentiation and particularly the formation of dentin in and subjacent to the furcation critically depends on osterix. Hence the developmental processes involved in furcation formation could well be subject to specific regulatory mechanisms.

Short and/or misshapen roots are most often due to hard tissue resorption. Such secondary abnormalities which usually affect single teeth or small groups of teeth are a frequent consequence of dento-periodontal traumas, local periodontal inflammation, or orthodontic tooth movement using excessive forces (Andreasen, 1985; Tronstad, 1988). Irrespective of the cause, root resorption constitutes an inflammatory reaction. Therefore, its consequences can hardly be considered a malformation and will not be dealt with further in this review. The most common true human root malformations can be subdivided into (1) disorders of root development alone and (2) disorders of root development associated with a general tooth dysplasia. Disorders of root development alone comprise:

- Premature arrest of root formation due to an extrinsic adverse effect
- Root dilaceration
- Root malformation associated with a cervical mineralized diaphragm/molar incisor malformation
- Short root anomaly
- Taurodontism

Disorders of root development associated with a general tooth dysplasia include:

- Double teeth
- Regional odontodysplasia
- Hypophosphatasia
- Dentin dysplasia type I

The same extrinsic adverse effects that entail root resorption can also lead to true developmental disorders, if they affect teeth during root morphogenesis. Most of these disorders are due to a premature arrest of radicular development as a consequence of a direct mechanical dento-periodontal trauma (Andreasen and Flores, 2007), local infection, radiation, or chemotherapy during the period of root morphogenesis (Jaffe et al., 1984; Sonis et al., 1990; Zarina and Nik-Hussein, 2005; Barbería et al., 2008). A local trauma can also indirectly affect developing permanent teeth when the insult primarily impacts on the primary predecessor. The effects of such indirectly acting traumas usually comprise enamel and (hidden) dentin hypoplasias in

**Abbreviations:** DDI, dentin dysplasia type I; HERS, Hertwig's epithelial root sheath; HPP, hypophosphatasia; MIM, molar incisor malformation; RM-CMD, Root malformation associated with a cervical mineralized diaphragm; RO, regional odontodysplasia; SRA, short root anomaly; TNALP, tissue-nonspecific alkaline phosphatase.

the crown, but in severe cases so-called root dilaceration, i.e., a serious root malformation, can ensue (Jafarzadeh and Abbott, 2007; Topouzelis et al., 2010). Root malformation associated with a cervical mineralized diaphragm (Witt et al., 2014), also designated as molar-incisor malformation (Lee et al., 2014, 2015), constitutes a recently described condition which is probably due to an extrinsic although so far unknown cause and affects all permanent first molars. Two additional malformations confined to the roots in only part of the dentition are the so-called short root anomaly (Lind, 1972) and taurodontism (Haskova et al., 2009; Dineshshankar et al., 2014). Short root anomaly is mainly observed in permanent maxillary central incisors, while taurodontism, i.e., a disorder of furcation formation, affects only multirooted teeth. In both conditions at least a genetic component has been presumed, but taurodontism also occurs as a sequel of radiotherapy, i.e., an extrinsic cause (Barbería et al., 2008). In mice primary disruption of the processes of root formation affecting all teeth has been observed as a consequence of various genetic defects, for example in the *Nfic* (Steele-Perkins et al., 2003; Park et al., 2007), *Ptc* (patched; Nakatomi et al., 2006), *Dkk1* (dickkopf-related protein 1; Han et al., 2011), *Osx* (osterix; Kim et al., 2015), *Smad4* (Huang and Chai, 2012), and *Wls* (wntless; Bae et al., 2015) genes. In humans, however, only two forms of clearly hereditary malformations of the roots alone seem to exist. The first one is associated with osteopetrosis due to genetic defects of *CLCN7* (encoding a chloride channel component; Xue et al., 2012), the second one is related to a defective *PLG* gene (encoding plaminogen; Tananuvat et al., 2014). In the absence of confirming evidence, both conditions thus far constitute isolated cases.

Among the disorders of root development associated with a general tooth malformation, those observed in cases of double teeth, i.e., geminated and fused teeth (Schuurs and van Loveren, 2000), as well as in regional odontodysplasia (Crawford and Aldred, 1989; Hamdan et al., 2004; Tervonen et al., 2004; Al-Tuwirqi et al., 2014) are due to unknown causes. In agreement with the designation, double teeth involve only two teeth, whereas regional odontodysplasia affects at least a group of contiguous teeth in a quadrant of the dentition. Generalized dysplastic roots occur as a result of hypophosphatasia (McKee et al., 2013) and in dentin dysplasia type I (O Carroll et al., 1991; Ansari and Reid, 1997; Toomarian et al., 2010), both of which are hereditary. The aim of the present review is to analyze the characteristic features of these root malformations in an attempt to derive which basic processes of root morphogenesis potentially are disrupted.

## DISORDERS OF ROOT DEVELOPMENT ALONE

### Premature Arrest of Root Formation

Premature arrest of root formation most frequently results from a direct trauma to a developing tooth (Andreasen and Flores, 2007). If the traumatic insult irreversibly damages the apical periodontal ligament including HERS and the neurovascular supply, these tissues as well as the pulp become necrotic. This occurs particularly in cases of traumatic intrusion and less frequently due to lateral luxations and extrusions (Andreasen and Kahler, 2015). As a consequence root elongation and radicular dentinogenesis stop, leaving a shortened root with thin dentinal walls and a wide open apex. Such teeth are at increased risk of fractures and pose a challenge for the endodontic treatment. Therefore, efforts are made to close the apex using a so-called apexification (Shabahang, 2013) or even pulp revascularization (Wigler et al., 2013; Palit et al., 2014). In fact there is radiographic evidence indicating that root elongation and dentinogenesis can be resumed, forming a complete root with a closed apex (Kottoor and Velmurugan, 2013).

Treatment of childhood cancer using radio- or chemotherapy also entails developmental tooth alterations (Jaffe et al., 1984; Sonis et al., 1990; Minicucci et al., 2003; Zarina and Nik-Hussein, 2005; Barbería et al., 2008; Pedersen et al., 2012). Owing to their non-selective potential to destroy proliferating cells, the therapeutic agents affect developing teeth as well. Depending on the dosage of the therapy and the age of the patients, the resulting dental abnormalities range from agenesis of individual teeth over microdontia to shortened roots as a result of premature arrest of root formation. Interestingly, unlike short roots in cases of mechanical trauma, those due to early cancer therapy always exhibit closed apices. Thus, even if root elongation is halted prematurely, dentinogenesis seems to progress and to complete the root tip.

### Root Dilaceration

Dilaceration is most appropriately defined as a sharp bend of either the crown or root axis (Andreasen et al., 1971). This definition discriminates dilaceration from flexion which denotes a smooth physiologic or abnormal curvature of the root (Jafarzadeh and Abbott, 2007). Varying definitions of the condition might account for the wide range of percentages (0.42–98%) reported for the prevalence of dilaceration. Rather unexpectedly posterior teeth are more frequently affected than front teeth (Jafarzadeh and Abbott, 2007; Topouzelis et al., 2010). The cause of root dilaceration in molars and premolars is not entirely clear, although it is often seen in cases of eruption disorders when the forming roots of retained teeth encounter a cortical bone structure and subsequently are deflected (Marks and Cahill, 1984; Larson et al., 1994). In permanent front teeth dilaceration most often is a consequence of an indirect trauma to the primary predecessors (Jafarzadeh and Abbott, 2007; Topouzelis et al., 2010). The type of injury depends on the age of the patient. At early ages of 2–3 years the developing crown of the permanent tooth lies in a lingual position relative to the root of the primary predecessor. As a result, a luxation injury to the latter most likely hits the labial part of the permanent dental crown and causes enamel and (hidden) dentin hypoplasias. At the worst the formed part of the crown is dislocated to the lingual side, thus causing a crown dilaceration with a lingual angulation (Topouzelis et al., 2010). Root dilaceration occurs at later ages of 4–5 years, when the crown of the permanent successor is largely complete. At this stage of development, physiologic resorption of the primary tooth root has already started and the germ of the permanent tooth has moved to a position approximately in the axis of the predecessor. If the primary tooth at this stage is hit by an intrusive trauma, the crown as well as already formed radicular parts of the permanent tooth can be dislocated to the labial side (Topouzelis et al., 2010). As a consequence, a root dilaceration with a labial angulation ensues as is illustrated in **Figure 1**. In this example, the incisal edge of the affected central incisor pointed to the nasal floor (**Figure 1A**) and the formed root was hook-shaped (**Figure 1B**). As revealed by gaps in the enamel, the end of crown morphogenesis was temporarily disorganized, but coronal hard tissue formation apparently was resumed and completed (**Figures 1C,D**). Likewise the transition from crown to root development as well as the subsequent root elongation, dentinogenesis, and cementogenesis obviously progressed unaffected (**Figures 1C,D**). However, root morphogenesis appears to have followed the neuro-vascular supply which is derived from the infraorbital artery and nerve and runs down more or less vertically. As a consequence the flexed root developed (Topouzelis et al., 2010).

## Root Malformation Associated with a Cervical Mineralized Diaphragm/molar Incisor Malformation

At about the same time, an own study (Witt et al., 2014) and a report from South Korea (Lee et al., 2014) described a new type of root malformation which consistently affects the permanent first molars. Based on the observed distinguishing feature, we termed it root malformation associated with a cervical mineralized diaphragm (RM-CMD), while Lee et al. (2014) called it molar-incisor malformation (MIM), because these authors noted also involvement of primary second molars and permanent maxillary central incisors in some cases. Affected permanent molars exhibit inconspicuous crowns, short, tapered roots and slit-shaped pulp cavities of markedly reduced height (**Figures 2A,D**). The distinguishing microscopic feature is a roughly lens-shaped mineralized plate at the level of the cemento-enamel junction, which we called a cervical mineralized diaphragm (CMD; **Figures 2B,C,E**). It comprises densely calcified, sometimes coalesced globules embedded in a moderately mineralized collagenous matrix as well as a network of soft tissue canals containing large blood vessels and connective tissue resembling periodontal ligament (**Figures 2F,G**). On the basis of these microscopic features, we proposed that the CMD developed in response to an as yet unknown external insult and was derived from the dental follicle (Witt et al., 2014). In contrast, Lee et al. (2015) based on the immunohistochemical demonstration of dentin sialoprotein, collagen type XII, and osteocalcin concluded that the CMD originated mainly from the apical pulp, i.e., a derivative of the apical papilla, and partially from the dental follicle.

The course of the tubules in the cervical coronal dentin suggested that the CMD already existed when dentinogenesis approached the cemento-enamel junction. It seemed to constitute a mechanical obstacle interfering with the normal retraction of the odontoblasts (Witt et al., 2014). Similarly, it also affected the formation of the root canals which curved around the margins of the CMD and were markedly constricted (**Figures 2B,C**). Nevertheless, the outer parts of the root stumps were comprised of regular tubular dentin covered by a layer of acellular cementum (**Figure 2I**), whereas the roof of the furcation immediately subjacent to the CMD contained only cellular cementum and interspersed soft tissue canals (**Figure 2H**). Thus, the transition from crown to root development, the initial apical growth of HERS, and the induction of dentinogenesis and cementogenesis along the root periphery seem to have progressed more or less unaffected. However, in the furcation area dentinogenesis was completely disrupted and replaced by excessive formation of cellular cementum, although the epithelial tongues of HERS might have fused.

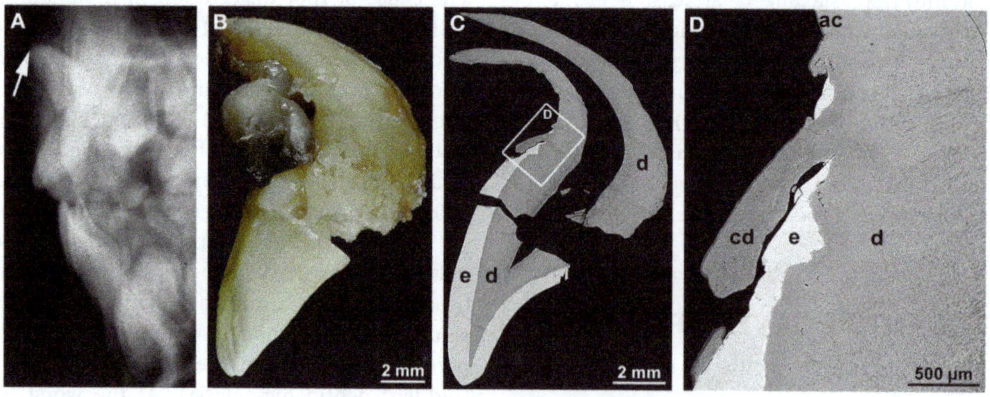


**FIGURE 1 | Radiographic, macroscopic, and microscopic appearance of root dilaceration. (A)** A lateral cephalogram shows the position of the incisal edge of a permanent maxillary central incisor (arrow) approximately 3 years after an intrusive trauma to the primary predecessor at the age of about 4.5 years. **(B)** A mesial macroscopic view of the reassembled permanent incisor reveals a sharp bend of the tooth axis in the cervical region and a curved hook-shaped root. **(C,D)** Corresponding overview **(C)** and detail **(D)** backscattered electron micrographs from a labio-lingual ground section depict normal enamel (e) and dentin (d), a tongue of cellular dentin (cd) which probably resulted from a local disorganization of the enamel organ, and normal acellular cementum (ac). Original magnifications **(B)** 4x, **(C)** 45x, **(D)** 350x.

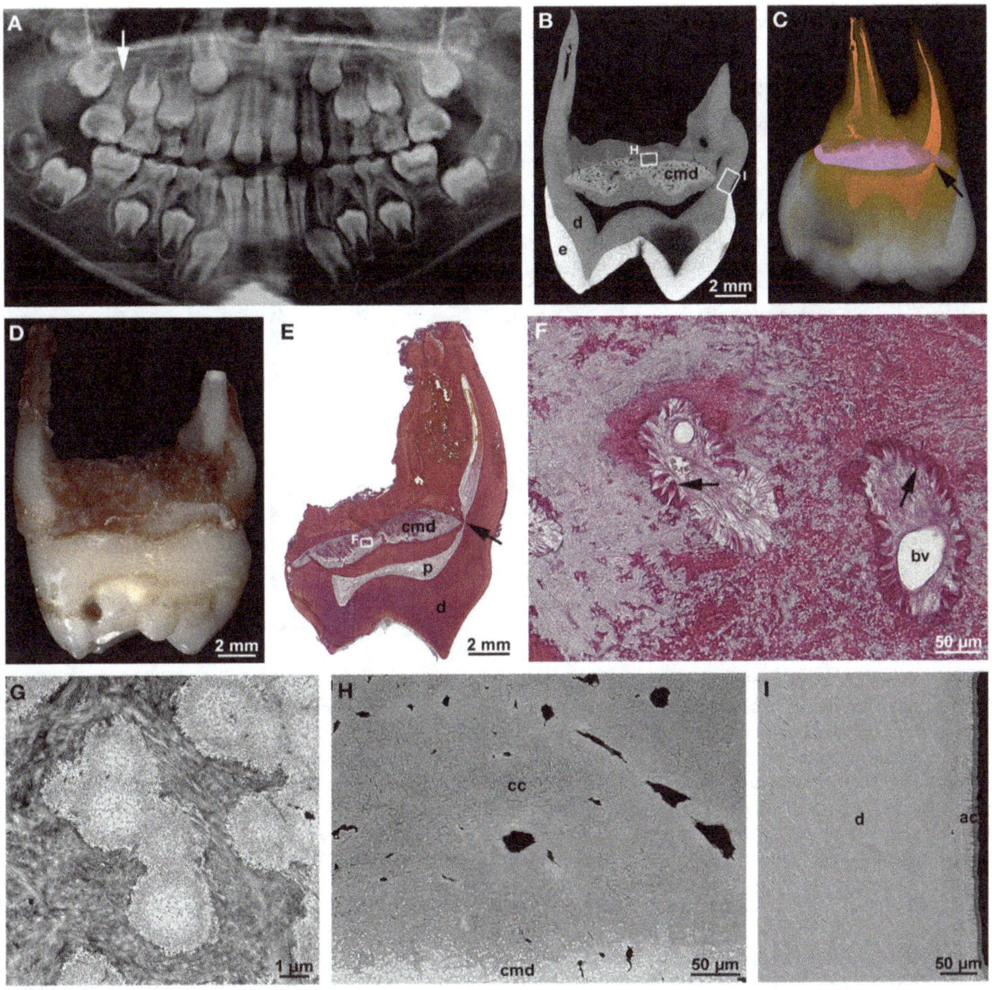


**FIGURE 2 | Radiographic and microscopic characteristics of root malformation associated with a cervical mineralized diaphragm/molar incisor malformation. (A)** A panoramic radiograph taken from a boy at the age of 8 years 1 month reveals rudimentary roots of all four permanent first molars, of which the maxillary right one (arrow) served for the microCT and microscopic evaluation. **(B)** Bucco-lingual microCT section depicting normal enamel (e) and dentin (d) as well as the cervical mineralized diaphragm (cmd). **(C)** A buccal view of a three-dimensional microCT reconstruction shows enamel (white), dentin (orange), the CMD (violet), and the pulp (red); note the constricted lingual root canal (arrow) curving around the margin of the CMD. **(D)** Mesial macroscopic view of the extracted permanent maxillary right first molar. **(E)** An overview micrograph from a bucco-lingual section stained with resorcin-fuchsin reveals dentin (d), the pulp (p), and the lingual root canal (arrow) curving around the margin of the CMD. **(F)** A detail of the CMD from the same section shows two soft tissue canals containing blood vessels (bv) and connective tissue resembling periodontal ligament (arrows). **(G)** A transmission electron micrograph of the CMD depicts fine-granular, partly coalesced globules embedded in a collagenous matrix. **(H,I)** Backscattered electron micrographs from the roof of the furcation **(H)** and the outer surface of the lingual root **(I)** display the margin of the CMD, dentin (d) as well as cellular (cc) and acellular (ac) cementum. Original magnifications **(D)** 3.2x, **(E)** 4x, **(F)** 200x, **(G)** 13000x, **(H,I)** 1500x. **(A)** is reprinted from Witt et al. (2014) with permission from Elsevier.

## Taurodontism

The term taurodontism denotes a feature of multirooted teeth characterized by apical displacement of the bi- or trifurcation (**Figures 3A–C**; Haskova et al., 2009; Dineshshankar et al., 2014). This is accompanied by a reduced or absent constriction at the cemento-enamel junction and an increased occluso-apical height of the pulp cavity (**Figure 3D**). Taurodontism is seen in both permanent and primary teeth, although less commonly in the latter (**Figure 3A**; Bafna et al., 2013). Its overall prevalence ranges from about 0.25 to 11.3% (Haskova et al., 2009). Depending on the severity it is classified as hypo- (mild), meso- (moderate), and hypertaurodontism (severe; Dineshshankar et al., 2014). Taurodontism arises when the formation of the epithelial bridges in the area of the future furcation is delayed (Haskova et al., 2009; Dineshshankar et al., 2014). The condition has been considered an atavistic trait, possibly because it was widespread in teeth of Neanderthals (Kupczik and Hublin, 2010). However, it also occurs as a consequence of childhood cancer treatment (Barbería et al., 2008). This is not particularly surprising when considering that both radiotherapy and chemotherapy are aimed at destroying proliferating tissues and, therefore, conceivably also impair growth of the epithelial

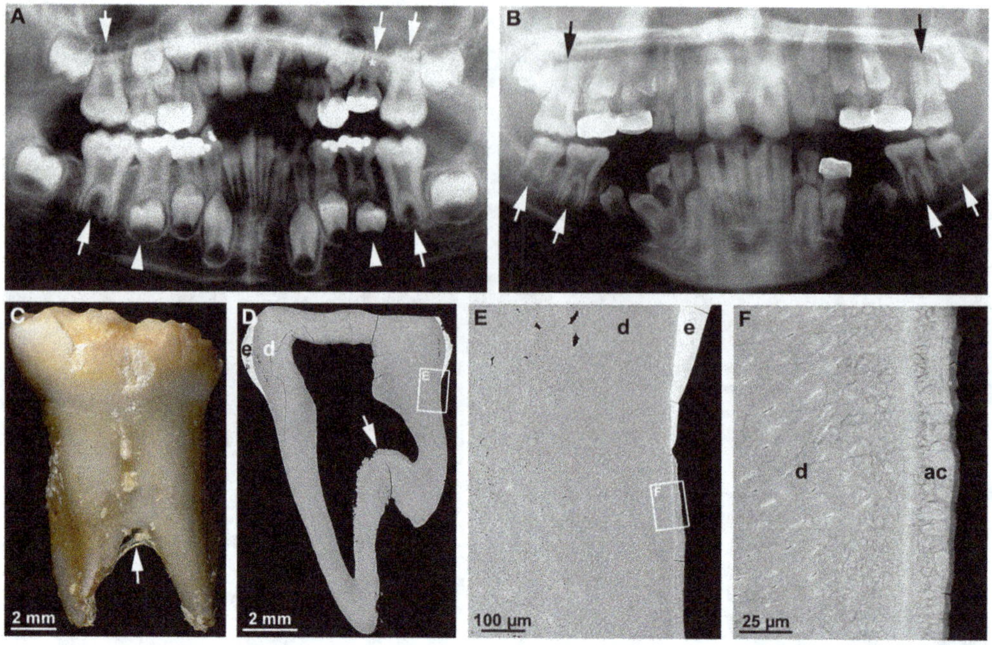


**FIGURE 3 | Radiographic, macroscopic, and microscopic features of taurodontism. (A)** A panoramic radiograph from a case of isolated taurodontism reveals mesotaurodontism of all permanent first molars and primary maxillary second molars (arrows), hypertaurodontism of the primary mandibular second molars (arrow-heads), and agenesis of the permanent maxillary left second premolar (asterisk). **(B)** The panoramic radiograph from an 11 year-old boy affected by tricho-dento-osseous syndrome due to a mutation in the *DLX3* gene reveals hypotaurodontism of all permanent first and mandibular second molars (arrows). Note the low contrast between enamel and dentin as a consequence of amelogenesis imperfecta. **(C)** A buccal macroscopic view of the primary mandibular left second molar extracted from the same boy several years earlier shows the markedly apical location of the bifurcation (arrow) and the brittle, partially chipped enamel. **(D–F)** Overview **(D)** and detail **(E,F)** backscattered electron micrographs from a mesio-distal ground section of the primary molar depict the apical position of the floor of the pulp cavity (arrow), hypoplastic-hypomaturated enamel (e), normal dentin (d), and normal acellular cementum (ac). Original magnifications **(C)** 6x, **(D)** 50x, **(E)** 800x, **(F)** 4000x.

tongues of HERS. Several associations between taurodontism and other dental and non-dental conditions reveal that a genetic component is involved in the etiology. Thus, taurodontism is a key feature of tricho-dento-osseous syndrome (TDO; [1]OMIM#190320) which besides is characterized by kinky, curly hair during childhood and adolescence, hypoplastic-hypomaturation type amelogenesis imperfecta, and increased bone density due to dominant mutations of the homeobox gene *DLX3* (**Figures 3B–F**; Wright et al., 1997, 2008; Price et al., 1998). A *DLX3* mutation has also been reported to account for amelogenesis imperfecta hypoplastic-hypomaturation with taurodontism (AIHHT; OMIM#104510; Dong et al., 2005), although it has been disputed whether the described condition really constituted AIHHT or rather TDO with only minor hair and bone involvement (Price et al., 1999).

A microscopic examination of a primary mandibular second molar from a case of TDO demonstrates that apart from the apical location of the floor of the pulp cavity (**Figure 3D**), all components of the root including dentin and cementum are normal (**Figures 3E,F**). Thus, in humans *DLX3* does not seem to be involved in any process of root development except the formation of the furcation. This contrasts with the phenotype entailed by a neural crest deletion of *Dlx3* in mice, which revealed short molar roots and enlarged pulp chambers with thin dentinal walls but no obvious taurodontism (Duverger et al., 2012). Since the features associated with the *Dlx3* deletion were shown to be due to down-regulation of dentin sialophosphoprotein (Dspp), they appear to rather phenocopy the so-called shell teeth observed in dentinogenesis imperfecta type III (OMIM#125500) which is caused by mutations in the *DSPP* gene (MacDougall et al., 2006; Kim and Simmer, 2007). Concordance of the phenotypes in knock-out mice and humans, at least with respect to taurodontism, was observed as a result of defects of the *WNT10A* gene (Yang et al., 2015). Yang et al. (2015) speculated that loss-of-function mutations of *WNT10A* in Neanderthals could account for the widespread occurrence of taurodontism in these ancestors. Apart from taurodontism, genetic defects of *WNT10A* in modern humans cause also tooth agenesis and alterations in shape of the dental crowns but no other obvious tooth abnormalities. This combination of features suggests that *WNT10A* is important at the early initiation stage of odontogenesis as well as in the later stages of crown and root morphogenesis, but not in hard tissue formation (Yang et al., 2015).

## Short Root Anomaly

Short root anomaly (SRA) has first been described by Lind (1972) and recently reviewed by Valladares Neto et al. (2013). Its overall prevalence is about 0.6–2.4%, but it occurs about 2.5–3 times

[1]OMIM: Online Mendelian Inheritance in Man®; http://omim.org/

more often in females than males. By far the most frequently affected teeth are the permanent maxillary central incisors, while other teeth, mainly premolars, are more rarely involved. The precise etiology of SRA is unknown, although clear familial clustering suggests that a genetic component at least plays a role (Lind, 1972). Since the crowns of affected teeth are perfectly normal, the anomaly is detected incidentally on radiographs. It is characterized by plump, short (only little longer or even shorter than the crowns) roots of inconspicuous radiodensity, which lack any signs of antecedent hard tissue resorption. This suggests that the basic processes of root morphogenesis progress normally, but root growth in length, i.e., the apical growth of HERS, is deficient.

## DISORDERS OF ROOT DEVELOPMENT ASSOCIATED WITH A GENERAL TOOTH DYSPLASIA

### Double Teeth

Double teeth result from the union of two adjacent teeth during odontogenesis. The etiology is unknown; presumed contributing factors are an evolutionary trend, trauma, environmental factors, and a hereditary component (Schuurs and van Loveren, 2000; Shashirekha and Jena, 2013; Hattab, 2014). Double teeth occur as two distinct entities which are referred to as gemination (with a prevalence of about 0.08–2.5%) and fusion (with a frequency of 0.1–0.85%; Shashirekha and Jena, 2013; Hattab, 2014). Gemination denotes a form of double teeth originating from the union of a regular and a supernumerary tooth, i.e., it reflects the incomplete splitting of one tooth germ. Fusion occurs when two regular tooth germs conjoin. Depending on the stage of development at which the union takes place, double teeth exhibit a broad crown with only an incisal/occlusal notch or labial/buccal groove and a single broad root (**Figures 4A–C**) or a partially divided crown and partially or completely separated roots (Schuurs and van Loveren, 2000; Hattab, 2014). Although, their validity has been doubted by Schuurs and van Loveren (2000), the classical criteria for discriminating gemination and fusion are a tooth count and the pulp anatomy of the conjoined teeth. When the oversized tooth is counted as one, the number of teeth is normal in cases of gemination and reduced in cases of fusion. Geminated teeth usually exhibit a partially or completely united pulp cavity (**Figure 4D**), while the pulp is completely divided in fused teeth. In cases of gemination the roots commonly are straight and broad and exhibit only a shallow groove in the area of the union (**Figures 4B,C**), whereas in cases of fusion the roots can be distorted because the germs of the conjoined teeth are not perfectly aligned (Schuurs and van Loveren, 2000). However, there are no indications that any component of the misshapen roots is defective. Thus, a normal HERS appears to develop from the cervical loop of the united enamel organs and to control all subsequent steps of radicular morphogenesis.

A condition related to but distinct from double teeth is an entity referred to as concrescence (Romito, 2004). Concrescence denotes a union of adjacent teeth by means of only radicular cementum. The etiology of such a union is unknown; trauma and a tight relationship of the neighboring tooth roots have been considered possible causative factors. Since concrescence can arise during or after root development (Romito, 2004), it is not always a true root malformation.

### Regional Odontodysplasia

Regional odontodysplasia (RO) is so uncommon that it mostly has been characterized in reports of isolated cases (Gardner and Sapp, 1973, 1977; Gibbard et al., 1973; Sapp and Gardner, 1973; Kerebel and Kerebel, 1983; Fearne et al., 1986; Gerlach et al., 1998), although several reviews cover the literature from successive time periods (Crawford and Aldred, 1989; Hamdan et al., 2004; Tervonen et al., 2004; Al-Tuwirqi et al., 2014). RO is an apparently non-hereditary disorder of enamel and dentin mostly affecting all or part of a quadrant, sometimes also two or more quadrants, and more often the maxilla than the mandible. The etiology is unclear; local circulatory disorders, viral infections, or a neural disturbance have been considered the most likely causes. Patients usually seek medical help at an early age because of a delay or failure in tooth eruption or because of pain resulting from pulp infections. Affected teeth exhibit a rough, discolored crown surface (**Figures 5A,D**)

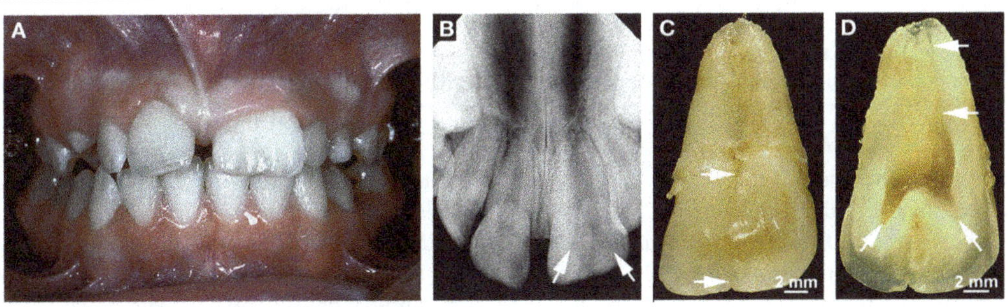


**FIGURE 4 | Clinical, radiographic, and macroscopic appearance of gemination. (A)** An intraoral view of a geminated permanent maxillary left central incisor shows the size of the double tooth in comparison with that of the normal right central incisor. Note that the tooth count is correct if the oversized incisor is counted as one. **(B)** The apical radiograph from the same incisor reveals two faintly visible separate pulp horns (arrows). **(C)** A lingual macroscopic view of the double tooth shows a small notch in the incisal edge and a groove in the cervical tubercle (arrows) which continues as a shallow groove on the root. **(D)** A macroscopic view of the mesio-distally cut incisor demonstrates the partially divided coronal pulp and the single root canal (arrows). Original magnifications **(C,D)** 4x.

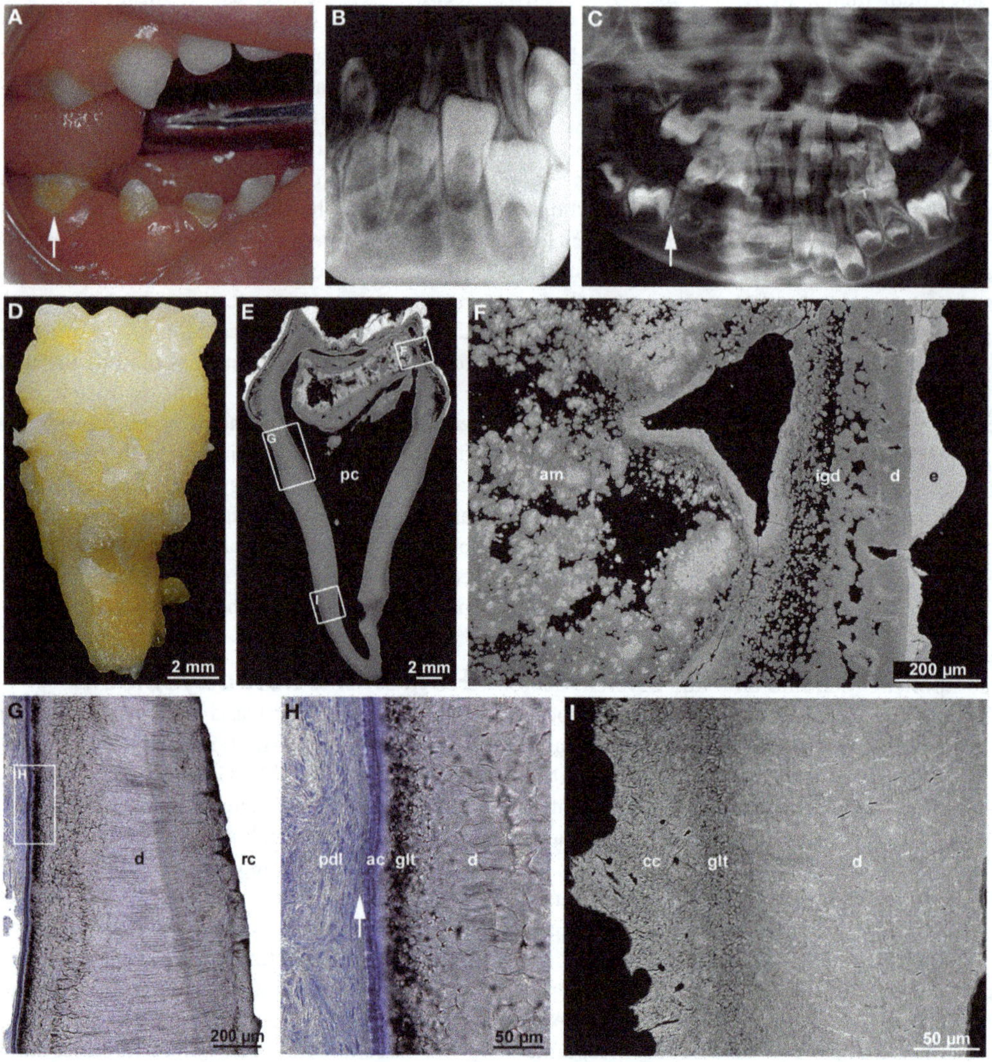


**FIGURE 5 | Clinical, radiographic, and microscopic features of regional odontodysplasia. (A)** An intraoral view of the affected mandibular right quadrant taken from a boy at the age of 2 years 8 months shows the primary second molar (arrow) which was later examined microscopically. **(B)** Apical radiograph of the mandibular front at the age of 4 years 7 months illustrating the ghost-like appearance of the permanent incisors. **(C)** A panoramic radiograph at the age of 5 years reveals a single root in the primary mandibular right second molar (arrow) as compared to the normally spread roots in the contralateral tooth. **(D)** Macroscopic buccal view of the single-rooted primary mandibular second molar extracted at the age of 5 years 4 months. **(E,F)** An overview **(E)** and detail **(F)** backscattered electron micrograph of a bucco-lingual ground section show hypoplastic enamel (e), tubular dentin containing clefts (d), interglobular dentin (igd), and amorphous masses (am) consisting of densely calcified globules and cellular dentin. **(G,H)** An overview **(G)** and detail **(H)** light micrograph of the cerviacl root surface stained with toluidine blue depict the root canal (rc), normal dentin (d), the granular layer of Tomes (glt), acellular cementum (ac), and Sharpey's fibers (arrow) attaching the periodontal ligament (pdl) to the root. **(I)** Backscattered electron micrograph of the apical root region revealing normal dentin (d), the granular layer of Tomes (glt), and cellular cementum (cc) with signs of hard tissue resorption. Original magnification **(D,E)** 5x, **(F)** 75x, **(G)** 50x, **(H)** 200x, **(I)** 220x.

and radiographically a characteristic "ghost-like" appearance (**Figures 5B,C**). Microscopically, dental enamel is hypoplastic and hypomineralized (**Figures 5E,F**). The hard tissue subjacent to the dentin-enamel junction often comprises thin layers of more or less regular tubular mantle dentin and interglobular dentin. Most of the space normally occupied by circumpulpal dentin and the pulp contains large voids as well as so-called amorphous masses of densely mineralized globules and less densely mineralized hard tissue which has been classified as cellular dentin (**Figures 5E,F**; Crawford and Aldred, 1989). No dentinal tubules exist in the dysplastic core of the crown, suggesting that the abnormal deposits do not constitute a mechanical obstacle for dentinogenesis. Rather odontoblasts must be assumed to have died for unknown reasons, after some circumpulpal dentin had been laid down.

The microscopic features probably account for the ghost-like radiographic appearance and the susceptibility to pulp infection in the absence of caries. Loss of pulp vitality might also be the reason why root formation often ends prematurely, leaving wide open apices (Gibbard et al., 1973; Fearne et al., 1986;

Crawford and Aldred, 1989; Hamdan et al., 2004). However, if the pulp remains vital long enough, radicular morphogenesis although somewhat delayed can be completed and result in a closed apex (Gardner and Sapp, 1973; Gibbard et al., 1973; Gerlach et al., 1998; Spini et al., 2007). This was also true for the primary mandibular right second molar of the case shown in **Figure 5**. In agreement with previous reports (Crawford and Aldred, 1989; Gerlach et al., 1998; Hamdan et al., 2004; Carlos et al., 2008), radicular dentin was much closer to normal than coronal dentin and in particular did not contain amorphous masses (**Figures 5E,G–I**). In the periphery, a granular layer of Tomes could be identified, and dentinal tubules traversed the entire wall of the root canal which, however, was abnormally wide and contained some scattered denticles. As in the crown, dentinogenesis obviously ended before the normal thickness of radicular dentin was attained. Whether, this occurred because the pulp died due to an infection or was caused by something else remains obscure. Irrespective of the premature termination of dentinogenesis, both accellular (**Figures 5G,H**) and cellular (**Figure 5I**) cementum were normal in appearance. This agrees with earlier reports (Gardner and Sapp, 1973; Gibbard et al., 1973) although there are also studies indicating that cementum is thin (Carlos et al., 2008) or even absent in places (Crawford and Aldred, 1989). Thus, even if possibly delayed, the transition from crown to root morphogenesis, apical growth of HERS and root elongation as well as the induction of radicular dentinogenesis and cementogenesis seem to progress properly in RO. Strikingly, however, a bifurcation dividing the root trunk into normally spread mesial and distal roots failed to form in the presented primary mandibular second molar (**Figures 5C,D**). Obviously, the epithelial projections of HERS did not unite and a furcation failed to form. This can also occur in the absence of other dental abnormalities although single-rooted primary molars are rare (Haridoss et al., 2014).

## Hypophosphatasia

Hypophosphatasia (HPP) is caused by homozygous, compound heterozygous, or heterozygous loss-of-function mutations in the *ALPL* gene encoding tissue-nonspecific alkaline phosphatase (TNALP). This enzyme controls biomineralization of organic matrices in bones and teeth by cleaving inorganic pyrophosphate which acts as a strong inhibitor of mineral crystal deposition (McKee et al., 2011, 2013). Based on the age at onset, HPP is classified into a perinatal, infantile (OMIM#241500), childhood (OMIM#241510), and adult (OMIM#146300) form. Clinical features include mineralization disorders of bones and teeth, which manifest themselves as rickets and early loss of teeth. These manifestations vary tremendously from severe (lethal) in the perinatal/infantile form to mild in the adult form of the disease. An additional form lacking any signs of skeletal involvement and showing only the dental features is referred to as odontohypophosphatasia.

The case illustrated in **Figure 6** is an example of odontohypophosphatasia which exhibits most of the typical dental features described in previous case reports (Baer et al., 1964; El-Labban et al., 1991; Lundgren et al., 1991; Chapple, 1993; Olsson et al., 1996; Lepe et al., 1997; Hu et al., 2000; Van den Bos et al., 2005). At the age of 3 years the boy was referred to a pediatric dentist because several primary front teeth had spontaneously exfoliated, before their roots were fully formed (**Figures 6C,D**). No radiographic signs of rickets could be detected. Only after a histological examination of the exfoliated primary teeth had revealed complete absence of acellular cementum (**Figures 6F,G**), laboratory tests were made which revealed markedly lowered serum concentrations of TNALP (32 U/l) and markedly elevated concentrations of pyridoxal-5-phosphate (317.1 $\mu$g/l). Also urinary levels of phosphoethanolamine, i.e., a hallmark of HPP (Lundgren et al., 1991), were increased. Complete aplasia of cementum has also been observed in earlier investigations (Hu et al., 2000), but a majority of authors described cementum as thin and only partially missing (Baer et al., 1964; El-Labban et al., 1991; Lundgren et al., 1991; Olsson et al., 1996). Notably, cellular cementum seems to be less severely affected than acellular cementum (McKee et al., 2013), possibly because formation of the cellular variety is rather insensitive to alterations in pyrophosphate (Zweifler et al., 2015). Instead of cementum, a thick subgingival dental plaque covered the root surface of the primary teeth in the presented patient (**Figure 6G**). Bacterial plaque on the roots of affected teeth has also been observed previously and was even considered responsible for the lack of periodontal support (El-Labban et al., 1991), but this inference was disputed by Olsson et al. (1996). Likewise in agreement with previous reports (Baer et al., 1964; Lundgren et al., 1991; Hu et al., 2000; Van den Bos et al., 2005), the radicular dentin of the exfoliated teeth was regularly tubular (**Figures 6F,G**) and the size of the pulp chamber corresponded fairly well to the stage of dental development (**Figures 6A,D,E**). Thus, it would appear that cementogenesis is particularly sensitive to a deficiency in TNALP, while dentinogenesis and root growth are less vulnerable (McKee et al., 2011). However, as suggested by a radiograph taken from the presented boy at the age of 10 years 8 months (**Figure 6B**), this may vary between primary and permanent teeth. While no permanent teeth had been lost by then and, hence, their periodontal support was obviously sufficient, both crowns and roots of the canines, premolars, and molars were malformed. This raises the question, whether TNALP in addition to mineralization of dental hard tissues directly or indirectly also affects tooth morphogenesis.

## Dentin Dysplasia Type I

Dentin dysplasia type I (DDI; OMIM#125400) is a heritable dentin disorder transmitted as an autosomal dominant trait (O Carroll and Duncan, 1994). However, the causative genetic defect has not been elucidated so far. The frequency of DDI is about 1 in 100,000 (Kim and Simmer, 2007). For this reason, knowledge on this disorder mainly originates from reports of isolated cases (Wesley et al., 1976; Kalk et al., 1998; Vieira et al., 1998; Neumann et al., 1999; Shankly et al., 1999; Özer et al., 2004; Da Rós Gonçalves et al., 2008; Rocha et al., 2011), although a few reviews (O Carroll et al., 1991; Ansari and Reid, 1997; Toomarian et al., 2010) are also available. The case shown in **Figure 7** illustrates the typical findings. Clinically, the crowns of affected teeth are usually normal in shape and color, but sometimes also slightly

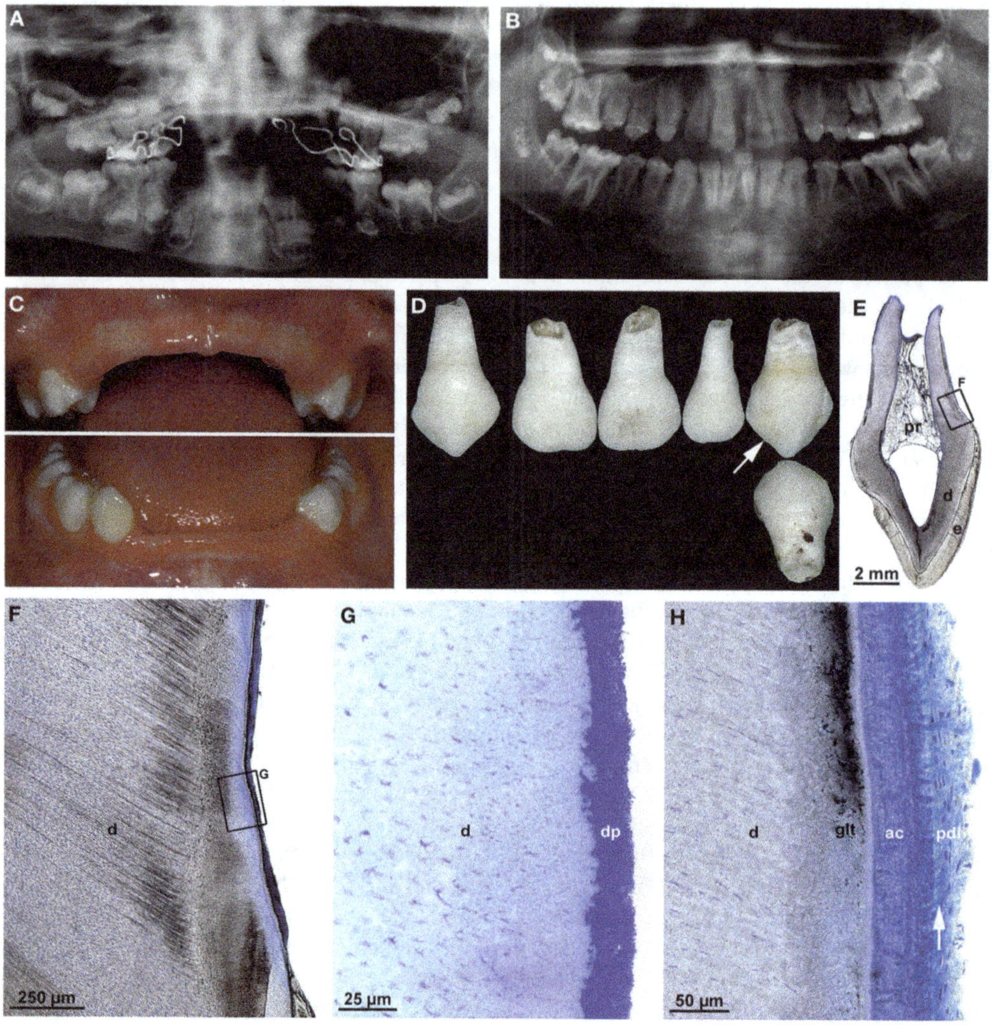


**FIGURE 6 | Clinical, radiographic, and microscopic features of hypophosphatasia. (A,B)** Panoramic radiographs taken from a boy at the ages of 5 years 6 months **(A)** and 10 years 8 months **(B)**; the early radiograph **(A)** shows the remaining primary molars as well as the germs of the permanent teeth, metal-dense structures in the maxilla originate from clasps of a prosthesis. The later radiograph **(B)** reveals aberrant shapes of the crowns and roots of the permanent teeth. **(C)** Intraoral view at the age of 3 years following the premature exfoliation of 11 of 12 primary front teeth. **(D)** Recovered exfoliated primary teeth, of which the maxillary left canine (arrow) was used for the microscopic investigation. **(E–G)** Overview **(E)** and detail **(F,G)** light micrographs from a bucco-lingual ground section stained with toluidine blue show normal enamel (e) and dentin (d), remnants of the pulp (pr), and dental plaque (dp). **(H)** A comparable detail micrograph from the root surface of a healthy primary canine reveals normal dentin (d), the granular layer of Tomes (glt), acellular cementum (ac), and Sharpey's fibers (arrow) attaching the periodontal ligament (pdl) to the root. Original magnifications **(E)** 5x, **(F)** 50x, **(G)** 400x, **(H)** 200x.

opalescent (**Figure 7A**). Radiographs reveal largely or completely obliterated pulp chambers and short, often pointed roots with apical radiolucencies in the absence of caries (**Figure 7B**). Based on these radiographic features, O Carroll et al. (1991) proposed a subdivision into four forms. However, this classification does not allow an unambiguous assignment of the presented case. Microscopic examination shows that in the crown, the enamel and a thin layer of dentin subjacent to the dentin-enamel junction is completely normal. Further inside, hard tissue comprises some still tubular interglobular dentin, but the bulk of the space normally occupied by the innermost circumpulpal dentin and pulp cavity is filled with roundish calcified bodies partially separated by crescent-shaped soft tissue spaces (**Figures 7C–E**). These calcified bodies are variably referred to as whorls (Wesley et al., 1976; O Carroll and Duncan, 1994) or denticles (Ranta et al., 1993). Shields et al. (1973) even considered them true denticles, which entailed the conclusion that their formation was induced by displaced fragments of a disintegrated HERS (Ranta et al., 1993). However, a close look at the denticle-like structures (**Figure 7E**) reveals that they lack the typical features of true denticles such as an epithelial core and tubules. Dentinal tubules rather appear to arise from the peripheral normal dentin and to curve around the calcified bodies. This suggests that normal odontoblasts attempt to lay down dentin, but on their way back from the advancing formation front are blocked and shunted by the preexisting ectopic obstacles in the dental papilla.

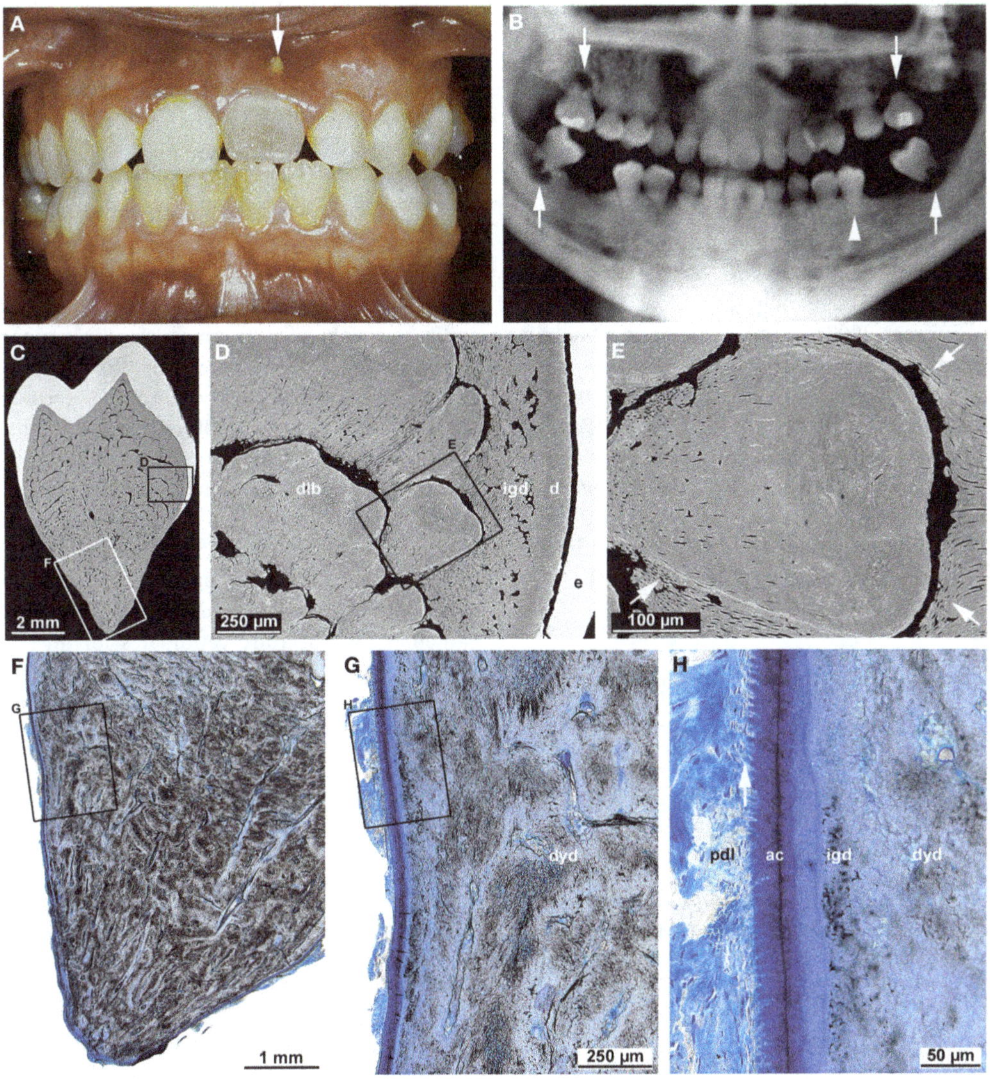


**FIGURE 7 | Clinical, radiographic, and microscopic characteristics of dentin dysplasia type I. (A)** An intraoral view of a female patient at the age of 16 years 3 months shows a slightly opalescent permanent maxillary central incisor with a fistula (arrow). **(B)** A panoramic radiograph taken at the same age reveals short roots in all permanent teeth as well as only rudimentary furcations and apical radiolucencies in the second molars (arrows); the mandibular left second premolar (arrow-head) served for the microscopic investigation. **(C–E)** Overview **(C)** and detail **(D,E)** backscattered electron micrographs from a bucco-lingual ground section of the premolar depict normal enamel (e) and dentin (d), interglobular dentin (igd), and denticle-like bodies (dlb). In the detail **(E)**, note the dentinal tubules (arrows) arising from the periphery and curving around the denticle-like body. **(F–H)** An overview **(F)** and details **(G,H)** of the root surface from the same ground section stained with toluidine blue reveal dysplastic dentin (dyd), interglobular dentin (igd), acellular cementum (ac), and Sharpey's fibers (arrow) attaching the periodontal ligament (pdl) to the root. Original magnifications **(C)** 10x, **(D)** 100x, **(E)** 350x, **(F)** 12.5x, **(G)** 50x, **(H)** 200x.

Nevertheless, the cause of the ectopic hard tissue formation in the dental papilla remains obscure.

In the root, individual denticle-like structures cannot be identified. Rather a mass of dysplastic hard tissue and interspersed small soft tissue canals fill the entire core of the root. In the periphery, however, thin layers of regular and interglobular dentin as well as acellular cementum with inserting periodontal Sharpey's fibers are still present (**Figure 7H**). Thus, it seems that the transition from crown to root formation is unaffected and the apical growth of HERS as well as the induction of radicular dentinogenesis and cementogenesis start normally, but are prematurely halted by the ectopic hard tissue formed in the dental papilla. In the permanent second molars of the presented case, this apparently occurred shortly after a futile attempt to build a furcation (**Figure 7B**).

## Dentinogenesis Imperfecta Types I, II, and III, X-linked Hypophosphatemia

Except for RO and DDI, dentin disorders do not appear to entail radicular malformations characterized by deviations in root length or shape, but rather alterations in pulp cavity dimensions. Dentinogenesis imperfecta type I associated with osteogenesis imperfecta (OMIM#166200) is caused by genetic defects of *COL1A1* and *COL1A2*, i.e., the two genes encoding the α1 and α2 chains of type I collagen. Dentinogenesis imperfecta type II (OMIM#125490) results from mutations in the *DSPP* gene which encodes dentin sialophosphoprotein, i.e., a non-collagenous component of the dentin matrix. Both forms of dentinogenesis imperfecta are characterized by early complete obliteration of the pulp cavity including the root canals. In contrast so-called shell teeth affected by dentinogenesis imperfecta type III (OMIM#125500) which is also caused by genetic defects of *DSPP*, exhibit excessively large pulp cavities (MacDougall et al., 2006; Kim and Simmer, 2007). X-linked hypophosphatemia (OMIM#307800) is due to mutations in the *PHEX* (phosphate-regulating gene with homologies to endopeptidases on the X chromosome) gene. Affected teeth exhibit hypomineralized dentin characterized by large amounts of so-called interglobular dentin (partly confluent globules of mineralized dentin separated by interstices of unmineralized matrix) and enlarged pulp cavities. These are sometimes mistaken as taurodontism although the furcation is not displaced apically (McKee et al., 2013).

## DISCUSSION

A summarizing comparison of the described most common human root dysplasias and the basic processes of root formation (**Table 1**) shows that the development of HERS at the transition from crown to root morphogenesis constitutes a particularly robust process, whereas apical growth of HERS associated with root elongation as well as the formation of the furcation in multirooted teeth seem to be rather susceptible to various intrinsic and extrinsic adverse effects.

The transition from crown to root formation and the concomitant development of HERS do not appear to be disrupted in any of the described radicular dysplasias. Thus, truly rootless teeth seem to be extremely rare in humans. Among the impacts affecting the apical proliferation of HERS, direct mechanical traumas to erupted immature teeth occur too late to exert influence on crown-root transition. On the other hand as revealed by the cases of root dilaceration, the effect of earlier indirect mechanical traumas via the primary predecessor do not appear to be harsh enough to completely disrupt HERS development, probably because the germ of the permanent tooth is rather well protected by the cushion of follicular soft tissues. Conceivably, early childhood cancer treatment using radiotherapy or chemotherapy could affect crown-root transition, but to the best of my knowledge no examples seem to exist in the literature. Considering that defects of the *Nfic* gene in mice completely prevent root formation (Steele-Perkins et al., 2003), human hereditary abnormalities associated with a radicular dysplasia are candidates for an effect on crown-root transition. In fact O Carroll et al. (1991) and O Carroll and Duncan (1994) displayed a graphical sketch of a tooth affected by DDI which virtually lacks roots. However, radiographs from real cases reveal at least small root stumps, suggesting that the designation "rootless teeth" in cases of DDI is not quite appropriate.

**TABLE 1 | Summary of the most common human root malformations as against potentially affected processes of root development.**

| Root malformation | Processes of root formation | | | | | | |
|---|---|---|---|---|---|---|---|
| | Hertwig's epithelial root sheath | | | | Dentinogenesis | Formation of furcation | |
| | Formation (crown-root transition) | Apical proliferation (root elongation) | Induction of odontoblast differentiation | Disintegration, cementogenesis | | Epithelial bridge formation | Interradicular dentinogenesis, cementogenesis |
| Short roots due to | | | | | | | |
| direct trauma | Unaffected | Disrupted | Disrupted | Continues | Disrupted | n.a.[a] | n.a.[a] |
| radiotherapy | Unaffected | Disrupted | Disrupted | Continues | Continues | Delayed | Unaffected (?) |
| chemotherapy | Unaffected | Disrupted | Disrupted | Continues | Continues | Delayed (?) | Unaffected (?) |
| Root dilaceration | Delayed (?) | In wrong direction | Unaffected | Unaffected | Unaffected | Unaffected (?) | Unaffected (?) |
| Taurodontism | Unaffected | Unaffected | Unaffected | Unaffected | Unaffected | Delayed | Unaffected |
| Short root anomaly | Unaffected | Impaired | Unaffected | Unaffected | Unaffected | n.a.[a] | n.a.[a] |
| Root malformation with CMD | Unaffected | Impaired | Unaffected | Unaffected | Mechanically impaired | Disturbed | d[b]: disrupted c[c]: excessive |
| Double teeth | Unaffected | Unaffected | Unaffected | Unaffected | Unaffected | n.a.[a] | n.a.[a] |
| Regional odontodysplasia | Unaffected | Impaired | Unaffected (?) | Unaffected | Impaired | Impaired | Impaired (?) |
| Hypophosphatasia | Unaffected | Unaffected | Unaffected | Dis[d]: unaffected (?) ac[e]: impaired cc[f]: unaffected (?) | Impaired (?) | Unaffected | Impaired (?) |
| Dentin dysplasia type I | Unaffected | Impaired | Unaffected | Unaffected | Mechanically Impaired | Impaired (?) | d[b]: mechanically impaired |

*[a]not applicable, because malformation largely occurs in single rooted teeth; [b]d, dentinogenesis; [c]c, cementogenesis; [d]dis, disintegration; [e]ac, acellular cementum formation; [f]cc, cellular cementum formation.*

Apical growth of HERS and the associated root elongation turn out to be one of the most susceptible processes of radicular morphogenesis (**Table 1**). Hence shortened roots would be the most prevalent malformation in humans, which agrees with clinical experience. However, the undisputable success of attempts at revascularization of necrotic teeth after dental injuries (Kottoor and Velmurugan, 2013) suggests that even the premature arrest of root growth is not necessarily as irreversible as previously thought. Intimately related to the apical proliferation of HERS are the induction of odontoblast differentiation and the subsequent radicular dentinogenesis. Therefore, the development of new odontoblasts from the ectomesenchymal cells of the dental papilla inevitably comes to a halt when root elongation is disrupted. However, further dentinogenesis also depends on the vitality of the pulp. If this is not challenged as in the case of radiotherapy or chemotherapy, dentinogenesis can continue even if root growth is arrested. Conversely, in cases of radicular dysplasias associated with enlarged root canals such as RO, it is often unclear whether the enlargement of the pulp cavity is due to impairment of dentinogenesis or the devitalization of the pulp, for example as a result of an infection. A remarkable observation in cases of severe dentinal disorders such as RO and DDI was that at least a thin peripheral layer of coronal and radicular dentin was normal. This suggests that the differentiation of odontoblasts is unaffected and dentinogenesis starts normally, until it encounters a mechanical obstacle (as in DDI) or is arrested for some unknown reason (as in RO).

Among the described human root malformations, HPP is the only one affecting cementogenesis, in particular the development of acellular cementum (**Table 1**). HPP is caused by mutations in the *ALPL* gene encoding tissue-nonspecific alkaline phosphatase (TNALPL) and the effect on cementogenesis seems to be due to defective mineralization resulting from a disrupted regulation of extracellular pyrophosphate cleavage (McKee et al., 2013). Although, a deficiency in TNALP can also entail consequences in dentin, the impact on cementum formation seems to be independent of that on dentinogenesis, as hypoplasia or even aplasia of cementum can occur in combination with completely normal radicular dentin. However, it remains mysterious how a disturbance of mineralization due to excessive concentrations of inorganic pyrophosphate can lead to complete absence of acellular cementum.

The processes involved in formation of the bi- or trifurcation in multirooted teeth appear to be particularly susceptible to extrinsic as well as genetic and other intrinsic influences (**Table 1**). In most conditions the formation of the epithelial bridges in the area of the future furcation is delayed, probably because epithelial proliferation is impaired. However, once the bridges are completed, the subsequent interradicular dentinogenesis and cementogenesis apparently can progress unaffected. Such a combination of a delay in furcation formation and normally progressing other processes of root development results in taurodontism which occurs as an isolated trait (Haskova et al., 2009), as part of hereditary syndromes (Wright et al., 1997; Yang et al., 2015), or as a feature accompanying consequences of radiotherapy and chemotherapy (Barbería et al., 2008). In RM-CMD/MIM the situation is exactly reversed: The roots of affected permanent first molars separate in an abnormally coronal position. Based on the microscopic structure of the misshapen furcation it is impossible to unambiguously derive whether epithelial bridges ever develop. Irrespectively the induction of odontoblast differentiation and dentinogenesis at the roof of the furcation and in the interradicular area are completely suppressed and no regular root trunk is formed. The most drastic disruption of furcation development leading to single-rooted posterior teeth apparently can occur in RO and most likely also in DDI. Whereas in RO the cause of the absent furcation formation is obscure, the masses of dysplastic hard tissue occupying the entire core of teeth affected by DDI conceivably interfere with the development of the epithelial bridges.

Thus, while many characteristics of the described most common human root dysplasias can be assigned to defects in specific processes of root development, the many question marks contained in **Table 1** indicate that inferences as to the precise pathogenesis of root malformations are rather speculative, because the processes involved in radicular morphogenesis and particularly in furcation development are incompletely understood.

## AUTHOR'S CONTRIBUTION TO FIGURES AND ETHICAL FRAMEWORK

All radiographs except the one shown in **Figure 2A** (**Figures 1A, 3A,B, 4B, 5B,C, 6A,B, 7B**) and intraoral photographs (**Figures 4A, 5A, 6C, 7A**) have been taken by dental technicians at the Center of Dental Medicine, University of Zurich. The radiograph shown in **Figure 2A** has been supplied by a private dental practice in Germany. All macroscopic photographs (**Figures 1B, 2D, 3C, 4C,D, 5D, 6D**), microCT reconstructions (**Figures 2B,C**), and micrographs (**Figures 1C,D, 2E–I, 3D–F, 5E–I, 6E–H, 7C–H**) have been made by the author.

Written informed consent regarding the usage of the clinical documentation and processing of extracted teeth for teaching and scientific research purposes was obtained from the patients or their parents upon admission to the Center of Dental Medicine, University of Zurich. This procedure was approved by the institutional ethics committee (Ethics Committee of the Canton of Zurich, Switzerland) provided that no identification of patients was possible. Therefore, all case evaluations were performed in an anonymized way.

## ACKNOWLEDGMENTS

I am grateful to my colleagues of the clinical departments for supplying case documentations as well as to Margrit Amstad-Jossi, Jinan Fierz, and Jacqueline Hofmann-Lobsiger for the skillful preparation of the microscopic specimens. This work was supported by institutional funds from the Center of Dental Medicine, University of Zurich.

## REFERENCES


Al-Tuwirqi, A., Lambie, D., and Seow, W. K. (2014). Regional odontodysplasia: literature review and report of an unusual case located in the mandible. *Pediatr. Dent.* 36, 62–67.

Andreasen, F. M., and Kahler, B. (2015). Pulpal response after acute dental injury in the permanent dentition: clinical implications - a review. *J. Endod.* 41, 299–308. doi: 10.1016/j.joen.2014.11.015

Andreasen, J. O. (1985). External root resorption: its implication in dental traumatology, paedodontics, periodontics, orthodontics and endodontics. *Int. Endod. J.* 18, 109–118. doi: 10.1111/j.1365-2591.1985.tb00427.x

Andreasen, J. O., and Flores, M. T. (2007). "Injuries to developing teeth," in *Textbook and Color Atlas of Traumatic Injuries to the Teeth*, ed J. O. Andreasen, F. M. Andreasen, and L. Andersson (Oxford: Blackwell Munksgaard), 542–576.

Andreasen, J. O., Sundström, B., and Ravn, J. J. (1971). The effect of traumatic injuries to primary teeth on their permanent successors. I. A clinical and histologic study of 117 injured permanent teeth. *Scand. J. Dent. Res.* 79, 219–283.

Ansari, G., and Reid, J. S. (1997). Dentinal dysplasia type I: review of the literature and report of a family. *J. Dent. Child.* 64, 429–434.

Bae, C. H., Kim, T. H., Ko, S. O., Lee, J. C., Yang, X., and Cho, E. S. (2015). Wntless regulates dentin apposition and root elongation in the mandibular molar. *J. Dent. Res.* 94, 439–445. doi: 10.1177/0022034514567198

Baer, P. N., Brown, N. C., and Hamner, J. E. (1964). Hypophosphatasia: report of two cases with dental findings. *Periodontics* 2, 209–215.

Bafna, Y., Kambalimath, H. V., Khandelwal, V., and Nayak, P. (2013). Taurodontism in deciduous molars. *BMJ Case Rep.* 2013:bcr2013010079. doi: 10.1136/bcr-2013-010079

Barbería, E., Hernandez, C., Miralles, V., and Maroto, M. (2008). Paediatric patients receiving oncology therapy: review of the literature and oral management guidelines. *Eur. J. Paediatr. Dent.* 9, 188–194.

Bosshardt, D. D., Stadlinger, B., and Terheyden, H. (2015). Cell-to-cell communication - periodontal regeneration. *Clin. Oral Implants Res.* 26, 229–239. doi: 10.1111/clr.12543

Carlos, R., Contreras-Vidaurre, E., de Almeida, O. P., Silva, K. R., Abrahão, P. G., Miranda, A. M. M. A., et al. (2008). Regional odontodysplasia: morphological, ultrastructural, and immunohistochemical features of the affected teeth, connective tissue, and odontogenic remnants. *J. Dent. Child.* 75, 144–150.

Chapple, I. L. C. (1993). Hypophosphatasia: dental aspects and mode of inheritance. *J. Clin. Periodontol.* 20, 615–622. doi: 10.1111/j.1600-051X.1993.tb00705.x

Crawford, P. J., and Aldred, M. J. (1989). Regional odontodysplasia: a bibliography. *J. Oral Pathol. Med.* 18, 251–263. doi: 10.1111/j.1600-0714.1989.tb00394.x

Da Rós Gonçalves, L., Oliveira, C. A. G. R., Holanda, R., Silva-Boghossian, C. M., Vieira Colombo, A. P., Maia, L. C., et al. (2008). Periodontal status of patients with dentin dysplasia type I: report of three cases within a family. *J. Periodontol.* 79, 1304–1311. doi: 10.1902/jop.2008.070426

Diekwisch, T. G. H. (2001). Developmental biology of cementum. *Int. J. Dev. Biol.* 45, 695–706.

Dineshshankar, J., Sivakumar, M., Balasubramanium, A. M., Kesavan, G., Karthikeyan, M., and Prasad, V. S. (2014). Taurodontism. *J. Pharm. Bioallied. Sci.* 6, S13–S15. doi: 10.4103/0975-7406.137252

Dong, J., Amor, D., Aldred, M. J., Gu, T., Escamilla, M., and MacDougall, M. (2005). DLX3 mutation associated with autosomal dominant amelogenesis imperfecta with taurodontism. *Am. J. Med. Genet.* 133A, 138–141. doi: 10.1002/ajmg.a.30521

Duverger, O., Zah, A., Isaac, J., Sun, H.-W., Bartels, A. K., Lian, J. B., et al. (2012). Neural crest deletion of Dlx3 leads to major dentin defects through down-regulation of Dspp. *J. Biol. Chem.* 287, 12230–12240. doi: 10.1074/jbc.M111.326900

El-Labban, N. G., Lee, K. W., and Rule, D. (1991). Permanent teeth in hypophosphatasia: light and electron microscopic study. *J. Oral Pathol. Med.* 20, 352–360. doi: 10.1111/j.1600-0714.1991.tb00944.x

Fearne, J., Williams, D. M., and Brook, A. H. (1986). Regional odontodysplasia: a clinical and histological evaluation. *J. Int. Assoc. Dent. Child.* 17, 21–25.

Fujiwara, N., Akimoto, T., Otsu, K., Kagiya, T., Ishizeki, K., and Harada, H. (2009). Reduction of Egf signaling decides transition from crown to root in the development of mouse molars. *J. Exp. Zool. B Mol. Dev. Evol.* 312B, 486–494. doi: 10.1002/jez.b.21268

Gardner, D. G., and Sapp, J. P. (1973). Regional odontodysplasia. *Oral Surg. Oral Med. Oral Pathol.* 35, 351–365. doi: 10.1016/0030-4220(73)90073-X

Gardner, D. G., and Sapp, J. P. (1977). Ultrastructural, electron-probe, and microhardness studies of the controversial amorphous areas in the dentin of regional odontodysplasia. *Oral Surg. Oral Med. Oral Pathol.* 44, 549–559. doi: 10.1016/0030-4220(77)90298-5

Gerlach, R. F., Jorge, J., de Almeida, O. P., Della Coletta, R., and Zaia, A. A. (1998). Regional odontodysplasia. Report of two cases. *Oral Surg. Oral Med. Oral Pathol.* 85, 308–313. doi: 10.1016/S1079-2104(98)90014-2

Gibbard, P. D., Lee, K. W., and Winter, G. B. (1973). Odontodysplasia. *Br. Dent. J.* 135, 525–532. doi: 10.1038/sj.bdj.4803111

Hamdan, M. A., Sawair, F. A., Rajab, L. D., Hamdan, A. M., and Al-Omari, I. K. H. (2004). Regional odontodysplasia: a review of the literature and report of a case. *Int. J. Paediatr. Dent.* 14, 363–370. doi: 10.1111/j.1365-263X.2004.00548.x

Han, X. L., Liu, M., Voisey, A., Ren, Y. S., Kurimoto, P., Gao, T., et al. (2011). Postnatal effect of overexpressed DKK1 on mandibular molar formation. *J. Dent. Res.* 90, 1312–1317. doi: 10.1177/0022034511421926

Haridoss, S. K., Swaminathan, K., Rajendran, V., and Rajendran, B. (2014). Single-rooted primary first mandibular molar. *BMJ Case Rep.* 2014:bcr2014206347. doi: 10.1136/bcr-2014-206347

Haskova, J. E., Gill, D. S., Figueiredo, J. A. P., Tredwin, C. J., and Naini, F. B. (2009). Taurodontism - a review. *Dent. Update* 36, 235–243.

Hattab, F. N. (2014). Double talon cusps on supernumerary tooth fused to maxillary central incisor: review of literature and report of case. *J. Clin. Exp. Dent.* 6, e400–e407. doi: 10.4317/jced.51428

Hu, J. C. C., Plaetke, R., Mornet, E., Zhang, C., Sun, X., Thomas, H. F., et al. (2000). Characterization of a family with dominant hypophosphatasia. *Eur. J. Oral Sci.* 108, 189–194. doi: 10.1034/j.1600-0722.2000.108003189.x

Huang, X., Bringas, P. Jr., Slavkin, H. C., and Chai, Y. (2009). Fate of HERS during tooth root development. *Dev. Biol.* 334, 22–30. doi: 10.1016/j.ydbio.2009.06.034

Huang, X. F., and Chai, Y. (2012). Molecular regulatory mechanism of tooth root development. *Int. J. Oral Sci.* 4, 177–181. doi: 10.1038/ijos.2012.61

Jafarzadeh, H., and Abbott, P. V. (2007). Dilaceration: review of an endodontic challenge. *J. Endod.* 33, 1025–1030. doi: 10.1016/j.joen.2007.04.013

Jaffe, N., Toth, B. B., Hoar, R. E., Ried, H. L., Sullivan, M. P., and McNeese, M. D. (1984). Dental and maxillofacial abnormalities in long-term survivors of childhood cancer: effects of treatment with chemotherapy and radiation to the head and neck. *Pediatrics* 73, 816–823.

Kalk, W. W. I., Batenburg, R. H. K., and Vissink, A. (1998). Dentin dysplasia type I. Five cases within one family. *Oral Surg. Oral Med. Oral Pathol.* 86, 175–178. doi: 10.1016/S1079-2104(98)90121-4

Kerebel, L.-M., and Kerebel, B. (1983). Soft-tissue calcifications of the dental follicle in regional odontodysplasia: a structural and ultrastructural study. *Oral Surg. Oral Med. Oral Pathol.* 56, 396–404. doi: 10.1016/0030-4220(83)90350-X

Kim, J.-W., and Simmer, J. P. (2007). Hereditary dentin defects. *J. Dent. Res.* 86, 392–399. doi: 10.1177/154405910708600502

Kim, T. H., Bae, C. H., Lee, J. C., Kim, J. E., Yang, X., de Crombrugghe, B., et al. (2015). Osterix regulates tooth root formation in a site-specific manner. *J. Dent. Res.* 94, 430–438. doi: 10.1177/0022034514565647

Kottoor, J., and Velmurugan, N. (2013). Revascularization for a necrotic immature permanent lateral incisor: a case report and literature review. *Int. J. Paediatr. Dent.* 23, 310–316. doi: 10.1111/ipd.12000

Kupczik, K., and Hublin, J.-J. (2010). Mandibular molar root morphology in Neanderthals and Late Pleistocene and recent *Homo sapiens*. *J. Hum. Evol.* 59, 525–541. doi: 10.1016/j.jhevol.2010.05.009

Larson, E. K., Cahill, D. R., Gorski, J. P., and Marks, S. C. Jr. (1994). The effect of removing the true dental follicle on premolar eruption in the dog. *Arch. Oral Biol.* 39, 271–275. doi: 10.1016/0003-9969(94)90116-3

Lee, H.-S., Kim, S.-H., Kim, S.-O., Choi, B.-J., Cho, S.-W., Park, W., et al. (2015). Microscopic analysis of molar-incisor malformation. *Oral Surg. Oral Med. Oral Pathol. Oral Radiol.* 119, 544–552. doi: 10.1016/j.oooo.2014.10.013

Lee, H.-S., Kim, S.-H., Kim, S.-O., Lee, J.-H., Choi, H.-J., Jung, H.-S., et al. (2014). A new type of dental anomaly: molar-incisor malformation (MIM). *Oral Surg. Oral Med. Oral Pathol. Oral Radiol.* 118, 101–109. doi: 10.1016/j.oooo.2014.03.014

Lepe, X., Rothwell, B. R., Banich, S., and Page, R. C. (1997). Absence of adult dental anomalies in familial hypophosphatasia. *J. Periodontal Res.* 32, 375–380. doi: 10.1111/j.1600-0765.1997.tb00547.x

Lind, V. (1972). Short root anomaly. *Scand. J. Dent. Res.* 80, 85–93. doi: 10.1111/j.1600-0722.1972.tb00268.x

Özer, L., Karasu, H., Aras, K., Tokman, B., and Ersoy, E. (2004). Dentin dysplasia type I: report of atypical cases in the permanent and mixed dentitions. *Oral Surg. Oral Med. Oral Pathol. Oral Radiol. Endod.* 98, 85–90. doi: 10.1016/j.tripleo.2004.01.005

Luan, X., Ito, Y., and Diekwisch, T. G. H. (2006). Evolution and development of Hertwig's epithelial root sheath. *Dev. Dyn.* 235, 1167–1180. doi: 10.1002/dvdy.20674

Lundgren, T., Westphal, O., Bolme, P., Modéer, T., and Norén, J. G. (1991). Retrospective study of children with hypophosphatasia with reference to dental changes. *Scand. J. Dent. Res.* 99, 357–364. doi: 10.1111/j.1600-0722.1991.tb01041.x

MacDougall, M., Dong, J., and Acevedo, A. C. (2006). Molecular basis of human dentin diseases. *Am. J. Med. Genet.* 140A, 2536–2546. doi: 10.1002/ajmg.a.31359

Marks, S. C. Jr., and Cahill, D. R. (1984). Experimental study in the dog of the non-active role of the tooth in the eruptive process. *Arch. Oral Biol.* 29, 311–322. doi: 10.1016/0003-9969(84)90105-5

McKee, M. D., Hoac, B., Addison, W. N., Barros, N. M. T., Millán, J. L., and Chaussain, C. (2013). Extracellular matrix mineralization in periodontal tissues: noncollagenous matrix proteins, enzymes, and relationship to hypophosphatasia and X-linked hypophosphatemia. *Periodontol. 2000* 63, 102–122. doi: 10.1111/prd.12029

McKee, M. D., Nakano, Y., Masica, D. L., Gray, J. J., Lemire, I., Heft, R., et al. (2011). Enzyme replacement therapy prevents dental defects in a model of hypophosphatasia. *J. Dent. Res.* 90, 470–476. doi: 10.1177/00220345103 93517

Minicucci, E. M., Lopes, L. F., and Crocci, A. J. (2003). Dental abnormalities in children after chemotherapy treatment for acute lymphoid leukemia. *Leuk. Res.* 27, 45–50. doi: 10.1016/S0145-2126(02)00080-2

Nakatomi, M., Morita, I., Eto, K., and Ota, M. S. (2006). Sonic hedgehog signaling is important in tooth root development. *J. Dent. Res.* 85, 427–431. doi: 10.1177/154405910608500506

Neumann, F., Würfel, F., and Mundt, T. (1999). Dentin dysplasia type I. A case report. *Ann. Anat.*, 181, 138–140. doi: 10.1016/S0940-9602(99)80120-4

O Carroll, M. K., and Duncan, W. K. (1994). Dentin dysplasia type I. Radiologic and genetic perspectives in a six-generation family. *Oral Surg. Oral Med. Oral Pathol.* 78, 375–381.

O Carroll, M. K., Duncan, W. K., and Perkins, T. M. (1991). Dentin dysplasia: review of the literature and a proposed subclassification based on radiographic findings. *Oral Surg. Oral Med. Oral Pathol.* 72, 119–125. doi: 10.1016/0030-4220(91)90202-N

Olsson, A., Matsson, L., Blomquist, H. K., Larsson, Å., and Sjödin, B. (1996). Hypophosphatasia affecting the permanent dentition. *J. Oral Pathol. Med.* 25, 343–347. doi: 10.1111/j.1600-0714.1996.tb00274.x

Palit, M. C., Hegde, K. S., Bhat, S. S., Sargod, S. S., Mantha, S., and Chattopadhyay, S. (2014). Tissue engineering in endodontics: root canal revascularization. *J. Clin. Pediatr. Dent.* 38, 291–297. doi: 10.17796/jcpd.38.4.j5285857278 615r1

Park, J.-C., Herr, Y., Kim, H.-J., Gronostajski, R. M., and Cho, M.-I. (2007). *Nfic* gene disruption inhibits differentiation of odontoblasts responsible for root formation and results in formation of short and abnormal roots in mice. *J. Periodontol.* 78, 1795–1802. doi: 10.1902/jop.2007.060363

Pedersen, L. B., Clausen, N., Schrøder, H., Schmidt, M., and Poulsen, S. (2012). Microdontia and hypodontia of premolars and permanent molars in childhood cancer survivors after chemotherapy. *Int. J. Paediatr. Dent.* 22, 239–243. doi: 10.1111/j.1365-263X.2011.01199.x

Price, J. A., Bowden, D. W., Wright, J. T., Pettenati, M. J., and Hart, T. C. (1998). Identification of a mutation in *DLX3* associated with tricho-dento-osseous (TDO) syndrome. *Hum. Mol. Genet.* 7, 563–569. doi: 10.1093/hmg/7.3.563

Price, J. A., Wright, J. T., Walker, S. J., Crawford, P. J. M., Aldred, M. J., and Hart, T. C. (1999). Tricho-dento-osseous syndrome and amelogenesis imperfecta with taurodontism are genetically distinct conditions. *Clin. Genet.* 56, 35–40. doi: 10.1034/j.1399-0004.1999.550105.x

Ranta, H., Lukinmaa, P.-L., and Waltimo, J. (1993). Heritable dentin defects: nosology, pathology, and treatment. *Am. J. Med. Genet.* 45, 193–200. doi: 10.1002/ajmg.1320450209

Rocha, C. T., Nelson-Filho, P., da Silva, L. A. B., Assed, S., and de Queiroz, A. M. (2011). Variation of dentin dysplasia type I: report of atypical findings in the permanent dentition. *Braz. Dent. J.* 22, 74–78.

Romito, L. M. (2004). Concrescence: report of a rare case. *Oral Surg. Oral Med. Oral Pathol. Oral Radiol. Endod.* 97, 325–327. doi: 10.1016/j.tripleo.2003.10.015

Sapp, J. P., and Gardner, D. G. (1973). Regional odontodysplasia: an ultrastructural and histochemical study of the soft-tissue calcifications. *Oral Surg. Oral Med. Oral Pathol.* 36, 383–392. doi: 10.1016/0030-4220(73)90216-8

Schroeder, H. E. (1991). *Oral Structural Biology*. Stuttgart; New York, NY: Thieme Medical Publishers.

Schuurs, A. H. B., and van Loveren, C. (2000). Double teeth: review of the literature. *J. Dent. Child.* 67, 313–325.

Shabahang, S. (2013). Treatment options: apexogenesis and apexification. *Pediatr. Dent.* 35, 125–128. doi: 10.1016/j.joen.2012.11.046

Shankly, P. E., Mackie, I. C., and Sloan, P. (1999). Dentinal dysplasia type I: report of a case. *Int. J. Paediatr. Dent.* 9, 37–42. doi: 10.1046/j.1365-263x.1999.00106.x

Shashirekha, G., and Jena, A. (2013). Prevalence and incidence of gemination and fusion in maxillary lateral incisors in Odisha population and related case report. *J. Clin. Diagn. Res.* 7, 2326–2329.

Shields, E. D., Bixler, D., and el-Kafrawy, A. M. (1973). A proposed classification for heritable human dentine defects with a description of a new entitiy. *Arch. Oral Biol.* 18, 543–553. doi: 10.1016/0003-9969(73)90075-7

Sonis, A. L., Tarbell, N., Valachovic, R. W., Gelber, R., Schwenn, M., and Sallan, S. (1990). Dentofacial development in long-term survivors of acute lymphoblastic leukemia. A comparison of three treatment modalities. *Cancer* 66, 2645–2652.

Spini, T. H., Sargenti-Neto, S., Cardoso, S. V., Souza, K. C. N., de Souza, S. O. M., de Faria, P. R., et al. (2007). Progressive dental development in regional odontodysplasia. *Oral Surg. Oral Med. Oral Pathol. Oral Radiol. Endod.* 104, e40–e45. doi: 10.1016/j.tripleo.2007.02.027

Steele-Perkins, G., Butz, K. G., Lyons, G. E., Zeichner-David, M., Kim, H.-J., Cho, M.-I., et al. (2003). Essential role for NFI-C/CTF transcription-replication factor in tooth root development. *Mol. Cell. Biol.* 23, 1075–1084. doi: 10.1128/MCB.23.3.1075-1084.2003

Tananuvat, N., Charoenkwan, P., Ohazama, A., Ketuda Cairns, J. R., Kaewgahya, M., and Kantaputra, P. N. (2014). Root dentin anomaly and a PLG mutation. *Eur. J. Med. Genet.* 57, 630–635. doi: 10.1016/j.ejmg.2014.09.006

Tervonen, S. A., Stratmann, U., Mokrys, K., and Reichart, P. A. (2004). Regional odontodysplasia: a review of the literature and report of four cases. *Clin. Oral Investig.* 8, 45–51. doi: 10.1007/s00784-003-0245-0

Toomarian, L., Mashhadiabbas, F., Mirkarimi, M., and Mehrdad, L. (2010). Dentin dysplasia type I: a case report and review of the literature. *J. Med. Case. Rep.* 4, 1. doi: 10.1186/1752-1947-4-1

Topouzelis, N., Tsaousoglou, P., Pisoka, V., and Zouloumis, L. (2010). Dilaceration of maxillary central incisor: a literature review. *Dent. Traumatol.* 26, 335–341. doi: 10.1111/j.1600-9657.2010.00915.x

Tronstad, L. (1988). Root resorption - etiology, terminology and clinical manifestations. *Endod. Dent. Traumatol.* 4, 241–252. doi: 10.1111/j.1600-9657.1988.tb00642.x

Tummers, M., and Thesleff, I. (2003). Root or crown: a developmental choice orchestrated by the differential regulation of the epithelial stem cell niche in the tooth of two rodent species. *Development* 130, 1049–1057. doi: 10.1242/dev.00332

Valladares Neto, J., Rino Neto, J., and de Paiva, J. B. (2013). Orthodontic movement of teeth with short root anomaly: should it be avoided, faced or ignored? *Dental Press, J. Orthod.* 18, 72–85. doi: 10.1590/S2176-94512013000600012

Van den Bos, T., Handoko, G., Niehof, A., Ryan, L. M., Coburn, S. P., Whyte, M. P., et al. (2005). Cementum and dentin in hypophosphatasia. *J. Dent. Res.* 84, 1021–1025. doi: 10.1177/154405910508401110

Vieira, A. R., Modesto, A., and Cabral, M. G. (1998). Dentinal dysplasia type I: report of an atypical case in the primary dentition. *J. Dent. Child.* 65, 141–144.

Wesley, R. K., Wysocki, G. P., Mintz, S. M., and Jackson, J. (1976). Dentin dysplasia type I. *Oral Surg. Oral Med. Oral Pathol.* 41, 516–524. doi: 10.1016/0030-4220(76)90279-6

Wigler, R., Kaufman, A. Y., Lin, S., Steinbock, N., Hazan-Molina, H., and Torneck, C. D. (2013). Revascularization: a treatment for permanent teeth with necrotic pulp and incomplete root development. *J. Endod.* 39, 319–326. doi: 10.1016/j.joen.2012.11.014

Witt, C. V., Hirt, T., Rutz, G., and Luder, H. U. (2014). Root malformation associated with a cervical mineralized diaphragm - a distinct form of tooth abnormality? *Oral Surg. Oral Med. Oral Pathol. Oral Radiol.* 117, e311–e319. doi: 10.1016/j.oooo.2013.06.030

Wright, J. T., Hong, S. P., Simmons, D., Daly, B., Uebelhart, D., and Luder, H. U. (2008). *DLX3* c.561_562delCT mutation causes attenuated phenotype of tricho-dento-osseous syndrome. *Am. J. Med. Genet.* 146A, 343–349. doi: 10.1002/ajmg.a.32132

Wright, J. T., Kula, K., Hall, K., Simmons, J. H., and Hart, T. C. (1997). Analysis of the tricho-dento-osseous syndrome genotype and phenotype. *Am. J. Med. Genet.* 72, 197–204.

Xiong, J., Gronthos, S., and Bartold, P. M. (2013). Role of the epithelial cell rests of Malassez in the development, maintenance and regeneration of periodontal ligament tissues. *Periodontol. 2000* 63, 217–233. doi: 10.1111/prd.12023

Xue, Y., Wang, W., Mao, T., and Duan, X. (2012). Report of two Chinese patients suffering from *CLCN7*-related osteopetrosis and root dysplasia. *J. Craniomaxillofac. Surg.* 40, 416–420. doi: 10.1016/j.jcms.2011.07.014

Yang, J., Wang, S.-K., Choi, M., Reid, B. M., Hu, Y., Lee, Y.-L., et al. (2015). Taurodontism, variations in tooth number, and misshapened crowns in Wnt10a null mice and human kindreds. *Mol. Genet. Genomic Med.* 3, 40–58. doi: 10.1002/mgg3.111

Yokohama-Tamaki, T., Ohshima, H., Fujiwara, N., Takada, Y., Ichimori, Y., Wakisaka, S., et al. (2006). Cessation of Fgf10 signaling, resulting in a defective dental epithelial stem cell compartment, leads to the transition from crown to root formation. *Development* 133, 1359–1366. doi: 10.1242/dev.02307

Zarina, R. S. R., and Nik-Hussein, N. N. (2005). Dental abnormalities of a long-term survivor of a childhood hematological malignancy: literature review and report of a case. *J. Clin. Pediatr. Dent.* 29, 167–174. doi: 10.17796/jcpd.29.2.hq7307703428nt3v

Zweifler, L. E., Patel, M. K., Nociti, F. H. Jr., Wimer, H. F., Millán, J. L., Somerman, M. J., et al. (2015). Counter-regulatory phosphatases TNAP and NPP1 temporally regulate tooth root cementogenesis. *Int. J. Oral Sci.* 7, 27–41. doi: 10.1038/ijos.2014.62

# 15

# Orthodontic Forces Induce the Cytoprotective Enzyme Heme Oxygenase-1 in Rats

**Edited by:**
Giovanna Orsini,
Polytechnic University of Marche, Italy

***Correspondence:**
Frank A. D. T. G. Wagener
frank.wagener@radboudumc.nl

*Christiaan M. Suttorp, Rui Xie, Ditte M. S. Lundvig, Anne Marie Kuijpers-Jagtman, Jasper Tom Uijttenboogaart, René Van Rheden, Jaap C. Maltha and Frank A. D. T. G. Wagener**

*Department of Orthodontics and Craniofacial Biology, Radboud university medical centre, Radboud Institute for Molecular Life Sciences, Nijmegen, Netherlands*

Orthodontic forces disturb the microenvironment of the periodontal ligament (PDL), and induce craniofacial bone remodeling which is necessary for tooth movement. Unfortunately, orthodontic tooth movement is often hampered by ischemic injury and cell death within the PDL (hyalinization) and root resorption. Large inter-individual differences in hyalinization and root resorption have been observed, and may be explained by differential protection against hyalinization. Heme oxygenase-1 (HO-1) forms an important protective mechanism by breaking down heme into the strong anti-oxidants biliverdin/bilirubin and the signaling molecule carbon monoxide. These versatile HO-1 products protect against ischemic and inflammatory injury. We postulate that orthodontic forces induce HO-1 expression in the PDL during experimental tooth movement. Twenty-five 6-week-old male Wistar rats were used in this study. The upper three molars at one side were moved mesially using a Nickel-Titanium coil spring, providing a continuous orthodontic force of 10 cN. The contralateral side served as control. After 6, 12, 72, 96, and 120 h groups of rats were killed. On parasagittal sections immunohistochemical staining was performed for analysis of HO-1 expression and quantification of osteoclasts. Orthodontic force induced a significant time-dependent HO-1 expression in mononuclear cells within the PDL at both the apposition- and resorption side. Shortly after placement of the orthodontic appliance HO-1 expression was highly induced in PDL cells but dropped to control levels within 72 h. Some osteoclasts were also HO-1 positive but this induction was shown to be independent of time- and mechanical stress. It is tempting to speculate that differential induction of tissue protecting- and osteoclast activating genes in the PDL determine the level of bone resorption and hyalinization and, subsequently, "fast" and "slow" tooth movers during orthodontic treatment.

**Keywords: orthodontic tooth movement, alveolar bone remodeling, cytoprotective enzymes, hyalinization, root resorption**

## INTRODUCTION

Although orthodontic tooth movement has been described in multiple studies the exact biological mechanisms are still not elucidated. Large differences in the rate of orthodontic tooth movement are found between individuals in identical experimental settings and are largely independent of the magnitude of the orthodontic force (Pilon et al., 1996; Iwasaki et al., 2006; Van Leeuwen et al., 2010).

The PDL contains a variety of cells, blood vessels, nerves, and extracellular matrix (ECM) molecules. Forces applied to a tooth compress the blood vessels at the resorption side, while dilating them at the apposition side leading to inflammation and subsequent remodeling of periodontal tissues. At the resorption side, recruited osteoclasts will degrade the alveolar bone allowing tooth movement (Krishnan and Davidovitch, 2009; Sanuki et al., 2010; Kook et al., 2011), whereas at the apposition side signaling pathways are activated to stimulate precursor cells in the PDL to differentiate into osteoblasts (Park et al., 2010; Tamura et al., 2010).

Unfortunately, at the resorption side, ischemic injury can result in cell death in a process called hyalinization. At these hyalinized regions of the PDL no living osteoclasts are present to facilitate alveolar bone resorption. The necrotic tissue needs to be removed by macrophages and multinucleated giant cells, and to be replaced by newly formed connective tissue. However, these multinucleated giant cells and macrophages can also initiate root resorption, one of the most important challenges in orthodontics (Brudvik and Rygh, 1994; von Bohl and Kuijpers-Jagtman, 2009). Orthodontic patients can be classified as "fast" or "slow" tooth movers, indicating variance in response of the periodontal ligament (PDL) to hyalinization formation (van Leeuwen et al., 1999).

Protection against inflammatory, mechanical, and ischemic stresses, as present during hyalinization, may determine the efficacy of individual orthodontic tooth movement. Interestingly, it was recently observed that differential levels of the osteoclast activating cytokine IL-1β also modulate orthodontic tooth movement (Iwasaki et al., 2006; Cao et al., 2016). "Fast tooth movers" may have decreased levels of hyalinization via higher induction of cytoprotective genes and/or increased levels of osteoclast activating genes. Heme oxygenase-1 (HO-1) is one of the most important examples of cytoprotective genes against ischemia reperfusion injury (Katori et al., 2002; Wagener et al., 2003). Protection against ischemic injury and cell death by HO-1 overexpression is demonstrated for example in liver and heart transplantations (Exner et al., 2004). HO-1 degrades heme into free iron, carbon monoxide (CO) and biliverdin (Grochot-Przeczek et al., 2012). Biliverdin is then directly converted into bilirubin by biliverdin reductase. CO is a signaling molecule that regulates inflammation, angiogenesis, and apoptotic signaling. Biliverdin and bilirubin are both potent antioxidants, while free iron is scavenged by co-induced ferritin (Babusikova et al., 2008). The level of HO-1 induction following a stimulus varies within the human population because of its highly polymorphic promoter (Wagener et al., 2008).

HO-1 is induced by a wide array of stresses (Wagener et al., 2003). In an *in vitro* study, HO-1 induction by mechanical stress in PDL cells was previously demonstrated (Cho et al., 2010). In the present study we aim to translate this *in vitro* finding of HO-1 induction in the PDL cells to an *in vivo* experimental setting in rats using orthodontic forces. We postulate that HO-1 will be induced by orthodontic forces and subsequently reduces or prevents hyalinization formation and root resorption. Protection against those unwanted side effects may ameliorate orthodontic tooth movement.

## MATERIALS AND METHODS

### Experimental Animals

Twenty-five 6-week-old male Wistar rats were used in this study. The animals were housed under normal laboratory conditions with *ad libitum* access to water and powdered rodent chow (Sniff, Soest, The Netherlands). The animals were allowed to acclimatize for at least 1 week before the start of the experiment. Ethical permission for the study was obtained according to the guidelines of the Board for Animal Experiments of the Radboud University Nijmegen (Reference number: RU-DEC-2006-160).

### Force Application

The rats were at random divided into 5 groups, with 5 animals per group. A split-mouth design was used to control for individual variances. The three maxillary molars on one randomly chosen side were moved mesially as one unit by means of a coil spring as described previously (Ren et al., 2003; Xie et al., 2009). The contralateral maxillary molars served as controls. A Nickel-Titanium (Ni-Ti) 10 cN Santalloy® closing coil spring (GAC, New York, NY, USA) was attached to the molar block via incisor anchorage to deliver a constant mesially directed force. An important advantage of this biomechanical design is that a constant low force per molar was applied preventing tipping of the molars. The effect could be estimated as a force of 170 cN per human molar which is within the range used in the clinic. This design has been proved to be functional and caused tooth movement during an period of 12 weeks (Ren et al., 2004).

After 6, 12, 72, 96, and 120 h of force application, groups of rats were killed and perfused with 4% paraformaldehyde (PFA) in phosphate-buffered saline (PBS). The maxillae were removed, post-fixed for 24 h in 4% PFA, decalcified in 10% EDTA, and embedded in paraffin.

### Haematoxylin-Eosin Staining of Maxillary Parasagittal Sections

Serial parasagittal sections (5 μm) mounted on Superfrost Plus slides (Menzel-Gläser, Braunschweig, Germany) were routinely stained with haematoxylin and eosin (HE) for general tissue survey. For immunohistochemical evaluation, sections containing at least the radicular pulp of three roots of the maxillary molars were selected.

### Immunohistochemical Staining

Immunostaining for HO-1 and CD68 was done essentially as previously described (Tan et al., 2009). CD68 is a marker for cells of the macrophage lineage, including monocytes, giant cells and osteoclasts and is recognized by the ED1 antibody (Sminia and Dijkstra, 1986). Cells within the PDL were counted as osteoclasts when they were ED1-positive, multinuclear, and located at the alveolar bone outline.

In brief, tissue sections were deparaffinized and rehydrated, followed by quenching of endogenous peroxidase activity using 3% $H_2O_2$ in methanol. After post-fixation in 4% PFA, antigen retrieval was performed by heating sections in 10 mM citrate pH 6 at 70°C for 10 min, followed by incubation in 1% trypsin (Difco Laboratories, Detroit, MI) at 37°C for 7 min.

Sections were subsequently blocked in 10% normal donkey serum (NDS; Chemicon, Temecula, CA) before overnight incubation at 4°C with primary antibody diluted in 2% NDS. The primary antibodies were polyclonal rabbit anti-HO-1 antibody (1:600; SPA-895, Stressgen, Ann Arbor, MI) and monoclonal mouse anti-CD68 ED1 antibody (1:200; MCA341R, Serotec, Breda, The Netherlands). Then sections were incubated with biotin-conjugated donkey anti-rabbit or anti-mouse secondary antibodies (1:3000–1:5000; Jackson Labs, West Grove, PA) for 1 h, followed by 45 min incubation with Vectastain ABC-Elite kit (Vector Laboratories, Burlingame, CA). Immunostaining was visualized by incubating the sections for 10 min with 3′3′-diaminobenzidine tetrahydrochloride (DAB; Sigma, St. Louis, MO). Staining was intensified with 0.5% $CuSO_4$, and counterstained with haematoxylin. Photographs were taken on a Carl Zeiss Imager Z.1 system (Carl Zeiss Microimaging Gmbh, Jena, Germany) under bright field conditions.

## Analysis of Immunohistochemical Data

The PDL region containing the roots of first and second molars was selected for quantitative measurement of HO-1 positive cells. Roots fulfilling the following criteria were included in the study: (1) The root structure is present from the cementoenamel junction to the apex, (2) the radicular pulp is present in the root structure, (3) no artifacts are present in the PDL structure. Almost all third molars were excluded because the root structure was not present over the whole length of the root in most sections. For standardization, root length was measured from apex to the top of the alveolar crest at the line through the middle of the root by using an ocular graticule (**Figure 1**). This allowed us to quantify the number of HO-1 and ED1 positive cells per mm of root length.

HO-1 positive mononuclear PDL cells and ED1 positive multinuclear osteoclasts were counted along the mesial and distal areas of the PDL in both experimental and control sides by blinded observers. Because the three maxillary molars were moved mesially as one unit, the mesial areas of all roots at the experimental sides were considered resorption sides, whereas the distal areas were considered apposition sides (**Supplementary Figure 1**). To determine the inter-examiner reliability, 10 sections were measured by the two observers and acceptable $R^2 > 0.80$ were obtained for cell counting and root length measurements. For positively stained mononuclear and osteoclast cells, data was presented as the number of positive cells per mm of root length.

## Statistical Analysis

The data from HO-1 positive mononuclear cells for control samples showed a normal distribution as measured by the Kolmogorov-Smirnov test (KS-test). No time dependency throughout the experimental period and no side dependency by one-way analysis of variance (ANOVA) was found. Therefore, these data were pooled and used as baseline HO-1 expression in PDL.

The data from both HO-1 positive mononuclear PDL cells for experimental samples and the control and experimental osteoclasts (HO-1 and ED1) showed a non-normal distribution and was analyzed using non-parametric Kruskal-Wallis ANOVA on ranks and Mann-Whitney tests.

The data for the HO-1 positive osteoclasts at the distal area of the control samples was normally distributed. Therefore, ANOVA and Tukey's multiple comparison *post-hoc* test were used to analyze the time dependency.

Independent-Samples *T*-test was performed to compare differences between osteoclasts for each marker (HO-1 and ED1) at the distal areas. Differences were assumed to be significant if $p < 0.05$.

# RESULTS

## Effects of Orthodontic Force on HO-1 Expression in PDL Cells

Histological evaluation of HE-stained sections demonstrated that application of mechanical stress significantly reduced the width of the PDL at the resorption side, whereas the width at the apposition site was increased (**Supplementary Figure 1**). This confirms that the Ni-Ti coil spring appliance produced a mesially-orientated force acting on the PDL and the molar block. Hyalinized regions in the PDL were only observed at the

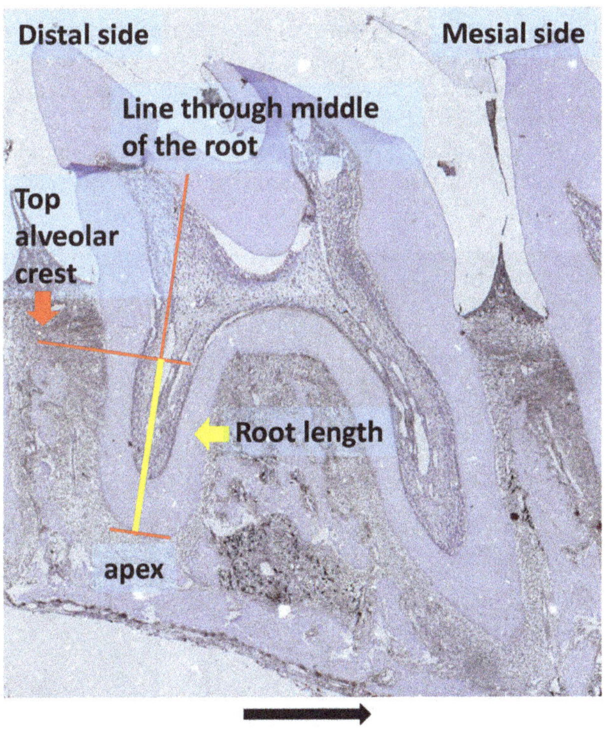


**FIGURE 1 | Root length measurement (yellow line) as used for determining the number of cells/mm root explained in detail: root length was measured from apex to the top of the alveolar crest at the line through the middle of the root (HO-1 immunostaining, magnification: x25, experimental group 120 h, black arrow indicated the direction of the tooth movement).**

resorption side in the experimental group (**Figure 5**), but not in the control group.

First we investigated the HO-1 expression in parasagittal sections at the control (no force) side. In these sections, HO-1 positive cells were strongly present in the bone marrow and only few HO-1 expressing cells were found in the PDL. The large number of cells expressing high levels of HO-1 in the bone marrow was used as an internal control for the staining procedure. Hardly any HO-1 positive cells were found in sections from pulp tissue, whereas interdental papillae were positive for HO-1 expressing cells (**Figure 2**).

Next, we compared the effect of orthodontic force on HO-1 expression. We observed no change in the levels of HO-1 staining for the bone marrow, pulp and interdental papilla following mechanical stress at the measured time points. However, we detected a strong increase in the number of HO-1 positive mononuclear cells in the PDL after force application (**Figure 3B**) compared to the contralateral control side (**Figure 3A**). This was especially evident in the vicinity of blood vessels.

In order to quantify HO-1 protein in PDL tissue during orthodontic tooth movement experimental sections were examined and compared to controls. In general there were low numbers of cells strongly expressing HO-1 (<10 cells/mm root) observed in the PDL at the control side. At the control side no statistically significant differences were detected between the number of HO-1 positive mononuclear PDL cells at the distal- and mesial side at any of the investigated time points nor between the different time points ($p = 0.110$). These data were therefore pooled, considered as base-line HO-1 expression in PDL (**Figure 3C**, red horizontal line).

At the experimental side there was a statistically significant time-dependent increase in the number of HO-1 positive cells per mm of root length and the data was therefore separated for the different time points and for both the resorption- and apposition side. Both for the resorption- and apposition side the number of HO-1 positively stained mononuclear PDL cells was significantly increased for the time points 6 and 12 h compared to no force application ($p < 0.001$, **Figure 3C**). Although the number of HO-1 positive stained mononuclear cells was higher at the resorption side after 12 h compared to the apposition side, this did not reach statistical significance ($p = 0.083$).

Summarizing, following orthodontic treatment, the PDL tissue showed a strong increase in the number of HO-1 positive cells at both the apposition- and resorption side compared to the contralateral control side, but returned within 72 h to baseline levels.

## HO-1 Expression in Osteoclasts

When no force was applied, osteoclasts were mainly observed in the bone marrow and in the PDL at the distal side (molar distal drift in rats, **Supplementary Figure 1**). However, upon mechanical stress, the number of osteoclasts within the PDL decreased at the distal side (apposition side), whereas at the resorption side the osteoclast numbers increased. A portion of the observed osteoclasts were also positively stained for HO-1 (**Figure 4A**). In control sections, HO-1 positively stained osteoclasts were observed in both the PDL and the bone marrow. The HO-1 expression levels in osteoclasts were, however, less intense compared to those in the HO-1 positive mononuclear PDL cells and bone marrow cells (**Figures 2–4A**).

In control sections the number of HO-1 and ED1 positive osteoclasts per mm of root length was significantly higher at the distal side compared to the mesial side (**Figure 4B**). The data were therefore separated for both areas.

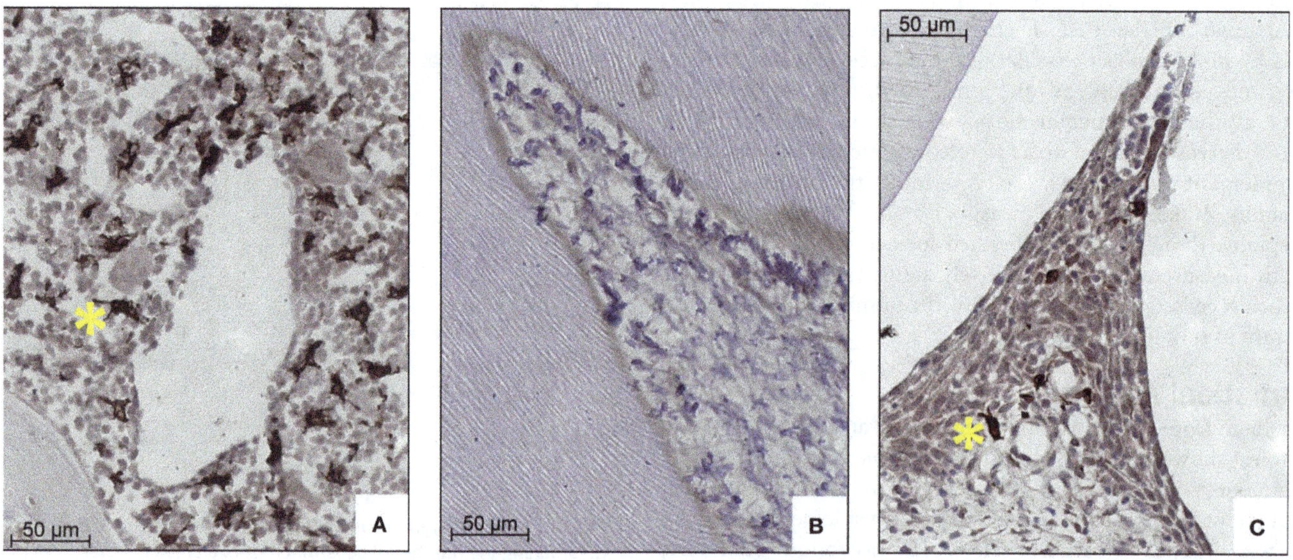


**FIGURE 2 | HO-1 expression in bone marrow, pulp tissue and interdental papilla tissue representative for both control and experimental group (HO-1 immunostaining, magnification: x400, yellow asterisk indicates a HO-1 overexpressing cell). (A)** Large numbers of HO-1 overexpressing cells in bone marrow (control group 120 h). **(B)** Negligible numbers of HO-1 positive cells were present in pulp tissue (experimental group 12 h). **(C)** Few HO-1 positive cells in interdental papilla tissue (control group 120 h).

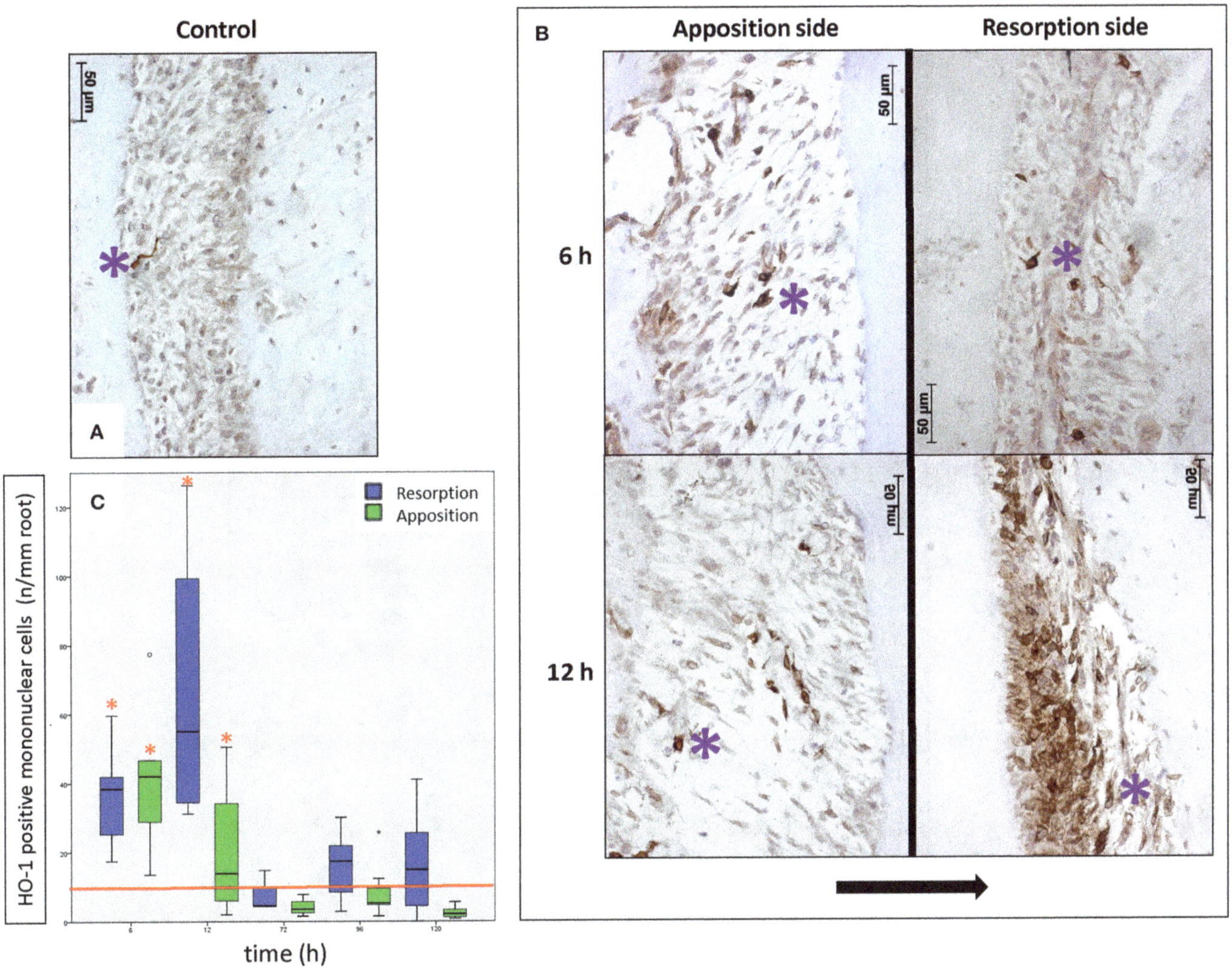


**FIGURE 3 | Effects of orthodontic force on HO-1 expression in the PDL (HO-1 immunostaining, magnification: x400, purple asterisk indicates a HO-1 overexpressing cell, black arrow indicates the direction of the tooth movement). (A)** Only few strong HO-1 positive cells are observed in PDL tissue in control sections (control group 6 h). **(B)** Many HO-1 overexpressing cells were present in PDL tissue at both the apposition- and resorption side in experimental sections of experimental time 6 and 12 h. This was especially evident in the vicinity of blood vessels. **(C)** Box-plot of mononuclear PDL cells at the experimental sides compared to control. The number of HO-1 positive mononuclear PDL cells is significantly higher at 6 and 12 h of force application compared to the control group (base-line HO-1 expression in PDL, red horizontal line), for both the apposition- and resorption side (Kruskal-Wallis ANOVA on ranks tests, $p < 0.001$). *Significantly different from base-line HO-1 expression in PDL, $p < 0.05$.

When applying the mesially directed force, changes in the numbers of osteoclasts were observed at both sides (**Figure 4B**). After 120 h the numbers of HO-1 positive ($p = 0.349$) and ED1 positive ($p = 0.065$) osteoclasts found at the mesial side (resorption side) were similar to the distal side in control sections, and with a similar HO-1/ED1 ratio. In conclusion, expression of HO-1 in osteoclasts was demonstrated to be independent of time- and mechanical stress.

## DISCUSSION

We demonstrated here for the first time that applying an orthodontic force strongly induces expression of the cytoprotective enzyme HO-1 in PDL cells at both the resorption- and apposition side in rats. Morphological changes within the PDL as a result of ischemic stress at the resorption side (compression of blood vessels, hyalinization areas) and mechanical stress at the apposition side (stretched blood vessels and increased PDL width) were observed (Supplemental Figure 1). In general the control side demonstrated relatively low numbers of HO-1 positive cells. Only bone marrow cells showed constitutively high expression levels of HO-1. Orthodontic force strongly induced HO-1 expression in cells situated closely around blood vessels, suggesting that these cells may be pericytes or infiltrated leukocytes (Zeng et al., 2015). A major part of the HO-1 positive PDL cells are fibroblasts, while only a minor part of osteoblasts and cementoblasts are HO-1 positive. In PDL cells HO-1 induction occurred shortly after placing the orthodontic

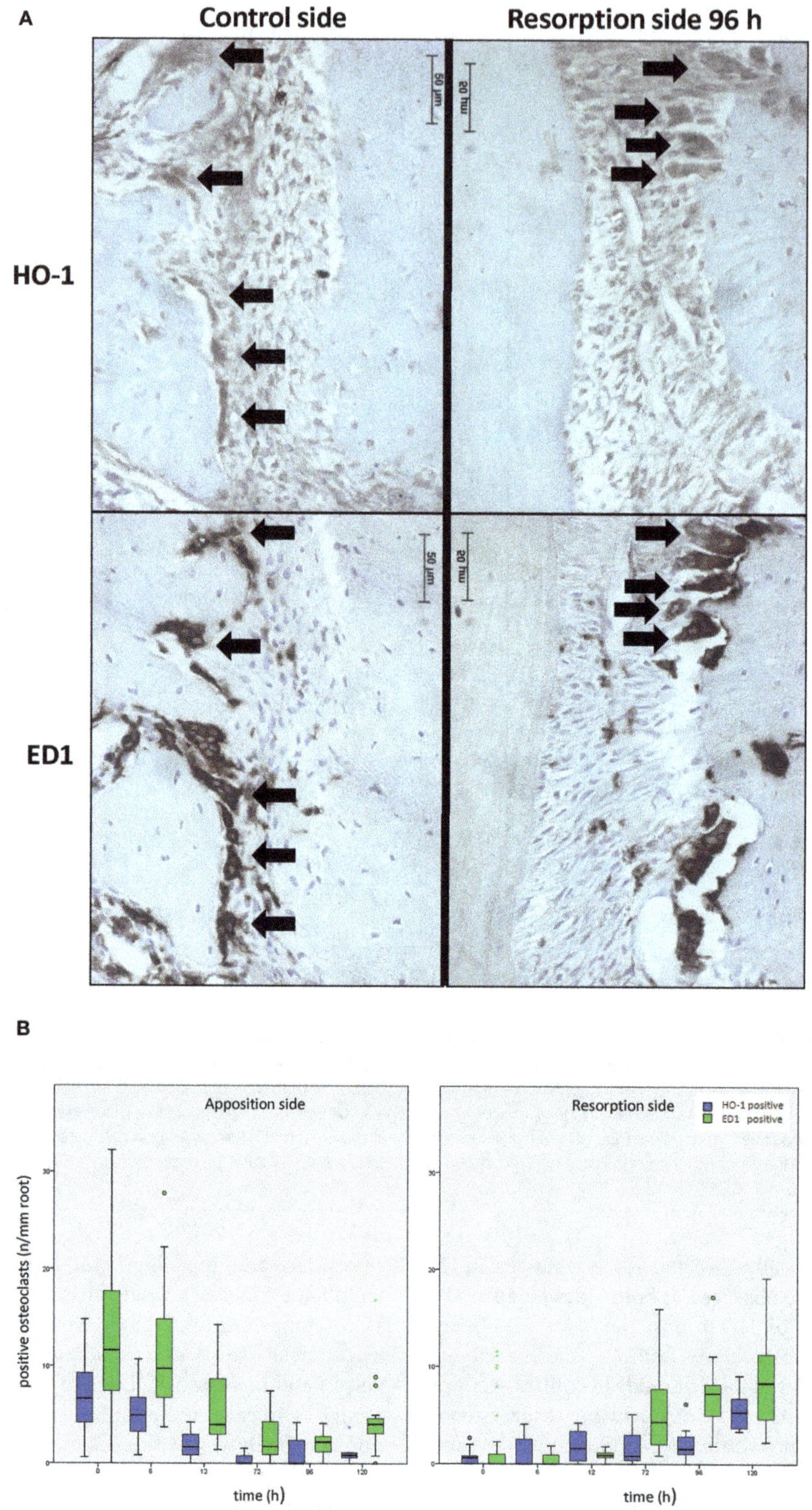


**FIGURE 4 | Effects of orthodontic force on HO-1 and ED1 positive osteoclasts. (A)** HO-1 (upper lane) and ED1 (lower lane) positive osteoclasts are found both before [control group, distal side (left panel)] and after [experimental group 96 h, resorption side (right panel)] force application as shown by immunohistochemistry. (magnification: x400, black arrows indicating an HO-1 and ED1 positive osteoclast, cells that were multinuclear and located at the alveolar bone outline were marked as osteoclasts). **(B)** When no force is present osteoclasts are mainly present at the distal site. Upon mechanical stress, ED1 or HO-1 positive osteoclast numbers decrease at the distal side, what is now called the apposition side (left panel), whereas the amount of osteoclasts at the resorption side increase (right panel). HO-1 expression levels in the osteoclasts and the HO-1/ED1 ratio remain similar following mechanical stress (Independent-Samples $T$-tests, $p > 0.05$).

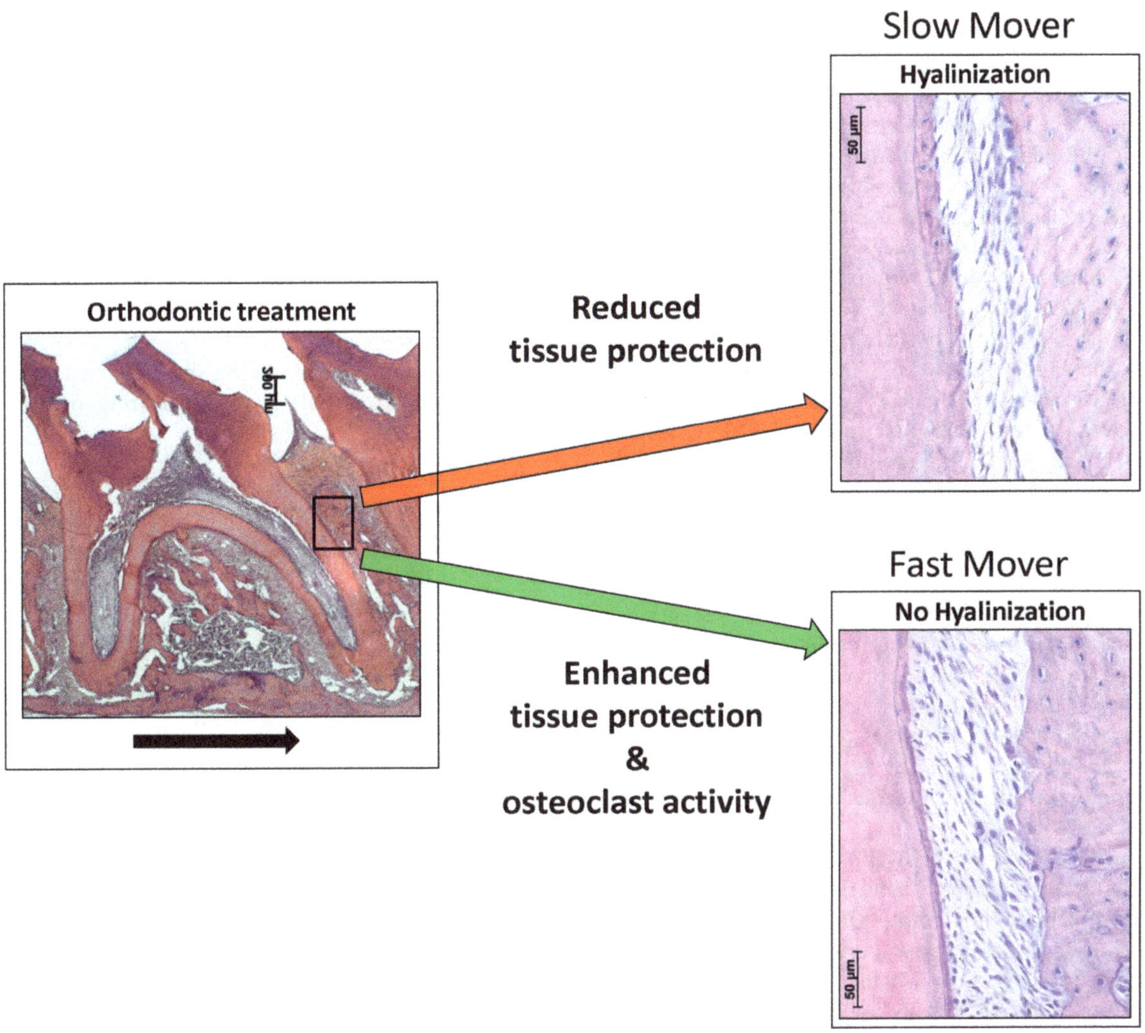


**FIGURE 5 | Orthodontic force can result in hyalinization- or no hyalinization formation in the PDL, resulting in "slow" or "fast" tooth movers.** In this hypothetical model we postulate that differential expression of tissue protective genes determine, in concert with osteoclast activating genes, the tooth movement. Applied orthodontic force results in mechanical stress within the PDL. This mechanical stress induces expression of HO-1 in PDL cells. Reduced HO-1 expression levels may lead to increased levels of ischemic injury and cell death (hyalinization), resulting in a hampered orthodontic tooth movement rate. Expression of cytoprotective enzymes, as HO-1, likely reduces ischemic injury and cell death. We hypothesize that differential expression of osteoclast activating genes (e.g., IL-1 β) and tissue protecting genes (e.g., HO-1) determines the remodeling of the PDL, or alveolar bone and therefore the orthodontic tooth movement rate. Differences in gene expression levels (e.g., as a result of polymorphisms) levels possibly explain the "slow" and "fast" tooth movers following orthodontic treatment. "Fast" tooth movers have enhanced osteoclastic activity (e.g., high IL-1 β) and protection against hyalinization (e.g., high HO-1), whereas "slow" tooth movers show hyalinization hampering osteoclast activity (black arrow indicates the direction of the tooth movement).

appliance but dropped within 72 h to control values. Thus, although the orthodontic force was applied continuously HO-1 induction within the PDL cells was only temporary. Induction of HO-1 by mechanical stress was previously demonstrated in several *in vivo* (Rawlinson et al., 1998) and *in vitro* (Cho et al., 2010) experimental settings but not yet during orthodontic tooth movement.

Osteoclasts are bone-specific, indicating the existence of different subsets of osteoclasts at different bone-sites (Everts et al., 2009; Henriksen et al., 2011). Induction of HO-1 inhibited osteoclastogenesis *in vitro* and *in vivo* in arthritis models (Zwerina et al., 2005). It was demonstrated that induction of HO-1 in osteoclast precursors resulted in reduced osteoclast differentiation and subsequently decreased bone resorption. It was also shown that the majority of osteoclasts attached to bone erosions in human joints from patients with rheumatoid arthritis were negative for HO-1 (Zwerina et al., 2005). If these findings of osteoclasts in an arthritic setting could be seen in the oral setting as well, this could have major impact on our understanding of both tooth movement and root resorption. Effects of orthodontic force on HO-1 expression in osteoclasts was therefore studied in more detail.

As demonstrated previously, after application of a mesially-directed force with a Ni-Ti coil spring almost all osteoclasts had disappeared from the distal side within 12 h, while at the mesial side (new resorption side) the number of osteoclasts increased and after 120 h the numbers were similar to the distal side in the control group (Xie et al., 2009). There giant cells are also multinuclear and ED1 positive, we cannot exclude that giant cells entering the PDL and accidentally located at the alveolar bone outline were marked as osteoclasts. However, we remain confident that the large majority of the observed multinuclear, ED1 positive alveolar bone lining cells were osteoclasts.

Both experimental- and control sides demonstrated comparable proportions of HO-1 positive osteoclasts. The proportions of HO-1/ED1 positive cells had not changed significantly, indicating that the basal levels of HO-1 expression in osteoclasts was independent of time and mechanical strain. Thus, mechanical stress did not induce HO-1 expression in osteoclasts. This was also true for the dental pulp cells, interdental papilla tissue, and bone marrow cells. Since large numbers of HO-1 positive osteoclasts are present in the bone marrow, where normal osteoclast differentiation occurs it is unlikely that osteoclastogenesis is hampered following force induction. In rheumatoid arthritis bone resorption is mainly a pathological process (Wagener et al., 2008), whereas alveolar bone resorption is a normal physiological adaptive process. Functional differences were indeed described between osteoclasts located at long flat bones (craniofacial region) and long bones (axial skeleton) with respect to their acid- and protease secretion during bone degradation (Everts et al., 2009; Henriksen et al., 2011).

Reduction or prevention of hyalinized tissue formation is thought to facilitate orthodontic tooth movement and to decrease undermining resorption. It is tempting to speculate that the levels of cytoprotective genes that are activated during orthodontic tooth movement determine whether tooth movement or hyalinization take place. HO-1 has been demonstrated to attenuate inflammation and to prevent tissue injury and apoptosis following ischemic injury (Zarjou et al., 2011; Kumar et al., 2013). Expression of this cytoprotective HO-1 within the PDL likely generates a protecting environment and subsequently inhibits ischemic injury (von Bohl and Kuijpers-Jagtman, 2009).

In humans the levels of HO-1 induction are largely controlled by a promoter polymorphism, that has been shown to have strong clinically significance (Exner et al., 2004; Wagener et al., 2008). The existence of "slow" and "fast" tooth movers (van Leeuwen et al., 1999) could thus possibly be explained by differences in individual expression of HO-1. The HO-1 promoter polymorphism in humans, determining the levels of HO-1 induction, are not present at the equivalent positions in the rat and mouse ho-1 genes (Shibahara et al., 2002). The influence of gene polymorphism of IL-1β at the tooth movement rate has been demonstrated previously in orthodontic patients (Iwasaki et al., 2006). Therefore, we hypothesize that remodeling of the PDL and alveolar bone is determined by the sum of the expression of osteoclast activating- and tissue protecting genes in the PDL microenvironment. Differences found in tooth movement rate could be explained by differential expression of these genes (**Figure 5**). Interestingly, HO-1 induction is attenuated at higher age (Abraham and Kappas, 2008), which may further explain the increased levels of root resorption and hyalinization after orthodontic treatment at older age.

Since HO-1 was only shortly induced during the application of the continuous orthodontic force, this suggests that accommodation to the mechanical and ischemic stress takes place. Interestingly, when orthodontic forces are interrupted with inactive periods strongly reduced root resorption has been observed in rats and dogs (Kameyama et al., 2003). The mechanism of this protection remains unknown. Possibly, renewal of HO-1 induction occurs during intermittent force application, contributing to decreased root resorption and hyalinization formation. Further research to tooth displacement and hyalinization by modulating the HO-1 system is warranted to reveal the exact role of HO-1 during orthodontic tooth movement.

## CONCLUSION

Summarizing, the present study showed that orthodontic forces induced HO-1 expression in the PDL in rats in the mononuclear cell population. Although the force was applied continuously, the HO-1 expression was only temporarily. HO-1 positive osteoclasts are present but this expression was shown to be independent of time- and mechanical stress. HO-1 induction may be a novel target for reducing unwanted side effects of orthodontic force application in the future.

## AUTHOR CONTRIBUTIONS

CS: analyzed data, wrote manuscript. RX: performed experiments, edited manuscript. DL: analyzed data, wrote manuscript. AK: analyzed data, wrote manuscript. JU: performed experiments. RV: performed experiments, edited manuscript. JM: analyzed data, designed experiments, wrote manuscript. FW: analyzed data, designed experiments, wrote manuscript.

## ACKNOWLEDGMENTS

This study was supported by the Radboud university medical center, Nijmegen, The Netherlands. The authors declare that they have no conflict of interest in the research.

## REFERENCES

Abraham, N. G., and Kappas, A. (2008). Pharmacological and clinical aspects of heme oxygenase. *Pharmacol. Rev.* 60, 79–127. doi: 10.1124/pr.107.07104

Babusikova, E., Jesenak, M., Durdik, P., Dobrota, D., and Banovcin, P. (2008). Exhaled carbon monoxide as a new marker of respiratory diseases in children. *J. Physiol. Pharmacol.* 59, 9–17.

Brudvik, P., and Rygh, P. (1994). Multi-nucleated cells remove the main hyalinized tissue and start resorption of adjacent root surfaces. *Eur. J. Orthod.* 16, 265–273. doi: 10.1093/ejo/16.4.265

Cao, Y., Jansen, I. D., Sprangers, S., Stap, J., Leenen, P. J., Everts, V., et al. (2016). IL-1beta differently stimulates proliferation and multinucleation of distinct mouse bone marrow osteoclast precursor subsets. *J. Leukoc. Biol.* doi: 10.1189/jlb.1A1215-543R. [Epub ahead of print].

Cho, J. H., Lee, S. K., Lee, J. W., and Kim, E. C. (2010). The role of heme oxygenase-1 in mechanical stress- and lipopolysaccharide-induced osteogenic differentiation in human periodontal ligament cells. *Angle Orthod.* 80, 552–559. doi: 10.2319/091509-520.1

Everts, V., de Vries, T. J., and Helfrich, M. H. (2009). Osteoclast heterogeneity: lessons from osteopetrosis and inflammatory conditions. *Biochim. Biophys. Acta* 1792, 757–765. doi: 10.1016/j.bbadis.2009.05.004

Exner, M., Minar, E., Wagner, O., and Schillinger, M. (2004). The role of heme oxygenase-1 promoter polymorphisms in human disease. *Free Radic. Biol. Med.* 37, 1097–1104. doi: 10.1016/j.freeradbiomed.2004.07.008

Grochot-Przeczek, A., Dulak, J., and Jozkowicz, A. (2012). Haem oxygenase-1: non-canonical roles in physiology and pathology. *Clin. Sci.* 122, 93–103. doi: 10.1042/CS20110147

Henriksen, K., Bollerslev, J., Everts, V., and Karsdal, M. A. (2011). Osteoclast activity and subtypes as a function of physiology and pathology–implications for future treatments of osteoporosis. *Endocr. Rev.* 32, 31–63. doi: 10.1210/er.2010-0006

Iwasaki, L. R., Gibson, C. S., Crouch, L. D., Marx, D. B., Pandey, J. P., and Nickel, J. C. (2006). Speed of tooth movement is related to stress and IL-1 gene polymorphisms. *Am. J. Orthod. Dentofacial Orthop.* 130, 698.e1–9. doi: 10.1016/j.ajodo.2006.04.022

Kameyama, T., Matsumoto, Y., Warita, H., and Soma, K. (2003). Inactivated periods of constant orthodontic forces related to desirable tooth movement in rats. *J. Orthod.* 30, 31–37. discussion: 21–22. doi: 10.1093/ortho/30.1.31

Katori, M., Anselmo, D. M., Busuttil, R. W., and Kupiec-Weglinski, J. W. (2002). A novel strategy against ischemia and reperfusion injury: cytoprotection with heme oxygenase system. *Transpl. Immunol.* 9, 227–233. doi: 10.1016/S0966-3274(02)00043-6

Kook, S. H., Jang, Y. S., and Lee, J. C. (2011). Human periodontal ligament fibroblasts stimulate osteoclastogenesis in response to compression force through TNF-alpha-mediated activation of CD4+ T cells. *J. Cell. Biochem.* 112, 2891–2901. doi: 10.1002/jcb.23205

Krishnan, V., and Davidovitch, Z. (2009). On a path to unfolding the biological mechanisms of orthodontic tooth movement. *J. Dent. Res.* 88, 597–608. doi: 10.1177/0022034509338914

Kumar, K. J., Yang, H. L., Tsai, Y. C., Hung, P. C., Chang, S. H., Lo, H. W., et al. (2013). Lucidone protects human skin keratinocytes against free radical-induced oxidative damage and inflammation through the up-regulation of HO-1/Nrf2 antioxidant genes and down-regulation of NF-kappaB signaling pathway. *Food Chem. Toxicol.* 59, 55–66. doi: 10.1016/j.fct.2013.04.055

Park, K. H., Han, D. I., Rhee, Y. H., Jeong, S. J., Kim, S. H., and Park, Y. G. (2010). Protein kinase C betaII and delta/theta play critical roles in bone morphogenic protein-4-stimulated osteoblastic differentiation of MC3T3-E1 cells. *Biochem. Biophys. Res. Commun.* 403, 7–12. doi: 10.1016/j.bbrc.2010.10.074

Pilon, J. J., Kuijpers-Jagtman, A. M., and Maltha, J. C. (1996). Magnitude of orthodontic forces and rate of bodily tooth movement. An experimental study. *Am. J. Orthod. Dentofacial Orthop.* 110, 16–23. doi: 10.1016/S0889-5406(96)70082-3

Rawlinson, S. C., Zaman, G., Mosley, J. R., Pitsillides, A. A., and Lanyon, L. E. (1998). Heme oxygenase isozymes in bone: induction of HO-1 mRNA following physiological levels of mechanical loading *in vivo*. *Bone* 23, 433–436. doi: 10.1016/S8756-3282(98)00125-2

Ren, Y., Maltha, J. C., and Kuijpers-Jagtman, A. M. (2004). The rat as a model for orthodontic tooth movement–a critical review and a proposed solution. *Eur. J. Orthod.* 26, 483–490. doi: 10.1093/ejo/26.5.483

Ren, Y., Maltha, J. C., Van 't Hof, M. A., and Kuijpers-Jagtman, A. M. (2003). Age effect on orthodontic tooth movement in rats. *J. Dent. Res.* 82, 38–42. doi: 10.1177/154405910308200109

Sanuki, R., Shionome, C., Kuwabara, A., Mitsui, N., Koyama, Y., Suzuki, N., et al. (2010). Compressive force induces osteoclast differentiation via prostaglandin E(2) production in MC3T3-E1 cells. *Connect. Tissue Res.* 51, 150–158. doi: 10.3109/03008200903168484

Shibahara, S., Kitamuro, T., and Takahashi, K. (2002). Heme degradation and human disease: diversity is the soul of life. *Antioxid. Redox Signal.* 4, 593–602. doi: 10.1089/15230860260220094

Sminia, T., and Dijkstra, C. D. (1986). The origin of osteoclasts: an immunohistochemical study on macrophages and osteoclasts in embryonic rat bone. *Calcif. Tissue Int.* 39, 263–266. doi: 10.1007/BF02555216

Tamura, M., Nemoto, E., Sato, M. M., Nakashima, A., and Shimauchi, H. (2010). Role of the Wnt signaling pathway in bone and tooth. *Front. Biosci.* 2, 1405–1413. doi: 10.2741/e201

Tan, S. D., Xie, R., Klein-Nulend, J., van Rheden, R. E., Bronckers, A. L., Kuijpers-Jagtman, A. M., et al. (2009). Orthodontic force stimulates eNOS and iNOS in rat osteocytes. *J. Dent. Res.* 88, 255–260. doi: 10.1177/00220345083 30861

Van Leeuwen, E. J., Kuijpers-Jagtman, A. M., Von den Hoff, J. W., Wagener, F. A., and Maltha, J. C. (2010). Rate of orthodontic tooth movement after changing the force magnitude: an experimental study in beagle dogs. *Orthod. Craniofac. Res.* 13, 238–245. doi: 10.1111/j.1601-6343.2010.01500.x

van Leeuwen, E. J., Maltha, J. C., and Kuijpers-Jagtman, A. M. (1999). Tooth movement with light continuous and discontinuous forces in beagle dogs. *Eur. J. Oral Sci.* 107, 468–474. doi: 10.1046/j.0909-8836.1999.eos107608.x

von Bohl, M., and Kuijpers-Jagtman, A. M. (2009). Hyalinization during orthodontic tooth movement: a systematic review on tissue reactions. *Eur. J. Orthod.* 31, 30–36. doi: 10.1093/ejo/cjn080

Wagener, F. A., Toonen, E. J., Wigman, L., Fransen, J., Creemers, M. C., Radstake, T. R., et al. (2008). HMOX1 promoter polymorphism modulates the relationship between disease activity and joint damage in rheumatoid arthritis. *Arthritis Rheum.* 58, 3388–3393. doi: 10.1002/art.23970

Wagener, F. A., Volk, H. D., Willis, D., Abraham, N. G., Soares, M. P., Adema, G. J., et al. (2003). Different faces of the heme-heme oxygenase system in inflammation. *Pharmacol. Rev.* 55, 551–571. doi: 10.1124/pr.55.3.5

Xie, R., Kuijpers-Jagtman, A. M., and Maltha, J. C. (2009). Osteoclast differentiation and recruitment during early stages of experimental tooth movement in rats. *Eur. J. Oral Sci.* 117, 43–50. doi: 10.1111/j.1600-0722.2008.00588.x

Zarjou, A., Kim, J., Traylor, A. M., Sanders, P. W., Balla, J., Agarwal, A., et al. (2011). Paracrine effects of mesenchymal stem cells in cisplatin-induced renal injury require heme oxygenase-1. American journal of physiology. *Ren. Physiol.* 300, F254–F262. doi: 10.1152/ajprenal.00594.2010

Zeng, M., Kou, X., Yang, R., Liu, D., Wang, X., Song, Y., et al. (2015). Orthodontic force induces systemic inflammatory monocyte responses. *J. Dent. Res.* 94, 1295–1302. doi: 10.1177/0022034515592868

16

# Varanoid Tooth Eruption and Implantation Modes in a Late Cretaceous Mosasaur

**Edited by:**
Giovanna Orsini,
Polytechnic University of Marche, Italy

***Correspondence:**
Thomas G. H. Diekwisch
diekwisch@bcd.tamhsc.edu

[†] These authors have contributed equally to this work.

*Min Liu[1†], David A. Reed[2†], Giancarlo M. Cecchini[3], Xuanyu Lu[2], Karan Ganjawalla[4], Carol S. Gonzales[5], Richard Monahan[5], Xianghong Luan[2] and Thomas G. H. Diekwisch[2,6*]*

*[1] Department of Periodontology, Stomatological Hospital, Jilin University, Changchun, China, [2] Department of Oral Biology, University of Illinois, Chicago, IL, USA, [3] College of Dentistry, Midwestern University, Downers Grove, IL, USA, [4] School of Dental Medicine, Harvard University, Boston, MA, USA, [5] Department of Oral Diagnosis, University of Illinois College of Dentistry, Chicago, IL, USA, [6] Center for Craniofacial Research and Diagnosis and Department of Periodontics, Texas A&M University Baylor College of Dentistry, Dallas, TX, USA*

Erupting teeth are some of the oldest witnesses of developmental processes in the vertebrate fossil record and provide an important resource for vertebrate cladistics. Here, we have examined a mosasaur jaw fragment from central Texas using ultrathin ground section histology and 3D tomographic imaging to assess features critical for the cladistic placement of mosasaurs among varanoids vs. snakes: (i) the orientation of replacement teeth compared to the major tooth axis, (ii) the occurrence of resorption pits, and (iii) the mode of tooth implantation/attachment to the tooth bearing element (TBE). The replacement tooth studied here developed in an inclined position slightly distal of the deciduous parent tooth, similar to another varanoid squamate, the Gila monster *Heloderma suspectum*. Ground sections and tomographs also demonstrated that the replacement tooth attachment apparatus was entirely intact and that there was no evidence of mechanical deformation. Sections and tomographs further illustrated that the replacement tooth was located within a bony crypt and the inclination of the crypt matched the inclination of the replacement tooth. These preparations also revealed the presence of a resorption pit within the boundaries of the deciduous tooth that surrounded the developing replacement tooth. This finding suggests that developing mosasaur teeth developed within the walls of resorption pits similar to varanoid tooth germs and unlike developing snake teeth which are surrounded by fibrous connective tissue integuments. Finally, mosasaurs featured pseudo-thecodont tooth implantation with teeth anchored within a socket of mineralized tissue by means of a mineralized periodontal ligament. Together, these data indicate that the moderate inclination of the erupting mosasaur tooth studied here is neither a result of postmortem displacement nor a character representative of snakes, but rather a shared character between Mosasaurs and other varanoids such as *Heloderma*. In conjunction with the presence of resorption pits and the evidence for pseudothecodont tooth implantation, the tooth eruption and implantation characters described in the present study either place mosasaurs among the varanoids or suggest convergent evolution mechanisms between both clades, with mosasaurs evolving somewhat independently from a common varanoid ancestor.

**Keywords: tooth eruption, tooth replacement, resorption pits, reptilian phylogeny, mosasaurs**

## INTRODUCTION

Mosasaurs are an extinct group of large marine squamates that dominated mid- and late- Cretaceous oceans some 65–100 million years ago (MYA, *Clidastes*, Luan et al., 2009a). The phylogenetic classification of these large marine predators has been the subject of an animated scientific debate for centuries. The majority of scholars consider mosasaurs to belong to an evolved superfamily of squamates, the Varanoidea, which includes besides the Mosasauridae also a number of extant lizards such as the Komodo dragon (*Varanus komodoensis*) and the Gila monsters (*Heloderma*; Carroll, 1988). Most recent integrated analyses place mosasaurs within Toxicofera as a sister group of snakes (Reeder et al., 2015). Mosasaur-snake affinities go back to earlier theories based on a number of properties of the mosasaur dentition, including tooth attachment and tooth replacement (Cope, 1869, 1872; Owen, 1877, 1878; Caldwell and Lee, 1997; Lee, 1997a,b; Zaher and Rieppel, 1999; Tchernov et al., 2000; reviewed in Greene and Cundall, 2000; Rieppel et al., 2003), re-awakening a century-old concept of an aquatic origin of snakes first introduced by Cope (1872). Cope noted certain similarities in the feeding apparatus between mosasaurs and macrostomatan snakes, including a separation between the mandibular rami allowing for feeding on large prey (Luan et al., 2009b). Lee (1997a,b) returned to Cope's original hypothesis, largely based on similarities in tooth eruption patterns between mosasaurs and snakes, suggesting that snakes and mosasaurs are derived from a common ancestor characterized by recumbent replacement teeth, which he thought of as the most important character (Lee, 1997a). He believed that these characters were in favor of an aquatic origin of snakes, when compared to the classic terrestrial burrowing theory (Lee, 1997b; Caldwell and Lee, 1997). However, most recent fossil discoveries and analyses do not support a marine origin of snakes based on the placement of the borrowing scolecophidians and the discovery of the four-legged *Tetrapodophis* as the earliest snake lineages (Martill et al., 2015, Reeder et al., 2015). The purpose of the present study is to investigate a well preserved fossil of a mosasaur replacement tooth for three characters thought to be crucial for the distinction between ophidian and varanoid dentitions (Zaher and Rieppel, 1999): (i) the recumbent or axial position of replacement teeth, (ii) the occurrence of resorption pits, and (iii) the presence of sockets or bony pedicels that anchor the tooth apex to the jaw. The direction of tooth eruption is one of the characters important for the varanoid/snake distinction of mosasaur dentitions. Replacement teeth in most squamates and crocodilians develop apical of the deciduous tooth, and teeth erupt in vertical direction and displace the erupted tooth, while snake replacement teeth are commonly found in an inclined or recumbent position. The mosasaur condition differs from the classic varanoid mode of tooth attachment because replacement teeth in some mosasaur fossils are preserved in an inclined position (Zaher and Rieppel, 1999, Rieppel and Kearney, 2005). These observations have prompted some authors to seek parallels between the inclined replacement teeth and pseudothecodont tooth implantation in mosasaurs with the recumbent replacement teeth and their synostotic mode of attachment in ophidians such as snakes as a morphological argument for the aquatic origin or snakes (Caldwell and Lee, 1997; Lee, 1997b).

The second character crucial to classify mosasaur dentitions among varanoids and snakes is the presence of resorption pits. In squamates, the resorption pit is a structure-less condensate that grows at the apex of a deciduous tooth through mineralized bone and dentin resorption to facilitate the growth of a new tooth within its boundaries. The terminology "resorption pit" is confusing as also the Howship's lacunae of cellular level osteoclast bone resorption are called resorption pits (Hefti et al., 2010). Replacement teeth in most squamates and in crocodilian archosaurs develop within resorption pits of deciduous teeth (Edmund, 1960; Martin et al., 1980; Zaher and Rieppel, 1999), while snake teeth develop in the free connective tissue between tooth bearing elements and oral mucosa without any bony encasement (Lee, 1997b; Rieppel, 1980; Vonk et al., 2008). From a functional perspective, the formation of resorption pits in squamates ensures removal of the deciduous tooth anchorage and also provides protection of the successional tooth within the already existing theca of the previous generation tooth.

The third feature important for the standing of mosasaurs in the varanoid/snake origin debate is the type of tooth implantation. Tooth implantation in most non-mosasauroid varanoids has been characterized as classical pleurodont while in snakes, tooth implantation is acrodont and teeth are ankylosed to the rim of the socket by means of a cementoid synostosis between the tooth apex and the tooth bearing element (TBE; Zaher and Rieppel, 1999). In contrast, tooth attachment in mosasaurs is lacking the non-mineralized periodontal ligament of mammalian and crocodilian teeth and instead features a mineralized ligamentous interface between cementum (bone of attachment) and interdental ridge (McIntosh et al., 2002; Luan et al., 2009b). Moreover, the interdental ridges between individual mosasaur teeth are relatively thinner and cover only a portion of the mosasaur root surface compared to the alveolar theca that surrounds most of the mammalian tooth root surface (Luan et al., 2009b). Thus, it makes sense to classify the mosasauroid mode of tooth implantation as pseudothecodont or subthecodont (Zaher and Rieppel, 1999).

The debate on Mosasaur-snake origins focuses on three features related to the dentition, the recumbent position of replacement teeth, the lack or presence of resorption pits, and the type of tooth implantation. To address key questions of tooth eruption and implantation in mosasaurs, we have analyzed a newly discovered and well-preserved specimen from the Texas shore of the Western Interior Seaway using ground sections as well as cone beam and microcomputer tomography. Our data provide novel insights into mosasaur tooth implantation and their phylogenetic implications.

## MATERIALS AND METHODS

### Samples Used for Comparative Analysis

A jaw fragment of a late Cretaceous mosasaur featuring erupted and replacement teeth was obtained from an unspecified central Texas excavation site. Five representative extant species were chosen to provide a frame of reference for the position of the mosasaur replacement tooth: a rodent (mouse, *Mus musculus*), a marsupial (opossum, *Monodelphis domestica*), a crocodilian (American alligator, *Alligator mississippiensis*), a snake (ball python, *Python regius*), and a squamate (Iguana, *Iguana iguana*). Mouse, opossum, alligator, snake and iguana were sacrificed according to UIC animal care regulations and studies were approved by the UIC animal care committee. The Gila monster skull was from a private collection.

## X-Ray Tomography of Calcified Tissues

The position of replacement teeth vs. the position of already erupted teeth was assessed in all six extant species using micro-CTs (Scanco Model 40) at 70 kV for optimal imaging of teeth. Tomographic data of the jaw fragment were obtained using an iCAT cone beam tomograph (Imaging Sciences International LLC, Hatfield, PA) at 120 kV, and individual images were segmented using Azivo (FEI Visualization) to visualize the orientation of the mosasaur replacement tooth relative to the erupted tooth.

## Ultrathin Ground Sections of Mosasaur Jaw Fragments

The fossil mandible and teeth were sectioned using an EXAKT diamond band saw. Sections were mounted and polished to 40 μm thickness using an EXAKT ultrathin grinding system to assess the histological context of the replacement tooth in our mosasaur jaw fragment.

## Skull Preparation, Whole Mount Stains, and Paraffin Sections

Mature skulls from mouse, opossum, alligator, snake, and iguana were photographed in lateral position. For whole mount and paraffin preparations, animals were sacrificed according to UIC animal regulations and either fixed in 70% ethanol (whole mount stains) or 10% formalin (paraffin sections). For whole mount stains, jaws were fixed and dehydrated with ethanol and acetone, stained with alcian blue and alizarin red S for 2 days, immersed in 0.5% potassium hydroxide solution, and stored in 80% glycerol. For paraffin sections, tissues were fixed in formalin, dehydrated using a graded series of ethanols, embedded in paraffin, and cut in 5 μm thick sections. Sections were stained using Mallory's trichrome stain.

# RESULTS

## The Sampled Mosasaur Replacement Tooth Was Inclined at a 28° Angle in Distal Direction, Surrounded by an Undistorted Bony Crypt, and Located Within a Deciduous Resorption Pit

To conduct a detailed analysis of mosasaur tooth eruption and implantation, a well-preserved specimen from North Texas was analyzed using ground sections and micro-computed tomography. Macroscopic analysis identified the replacement tooth as a black-colored conical object protruding between the apex of the adjacent sand-colored erupted tooth and the dark brown-colored tooth-bearing element (**Figures 1A,D**). Ground sections prepared in a plane labial from the replacement tooth reveal an intact interdental ridge and tooth attachment apparatus (**Figures 1B,C**). The erupting tooth was surrounded by its own bony crypt and associated pedicel (a mineralized periodontium, **Figures 1E,F**). The inclined direction of the replacement tooth axis pointed toward the opening of the bony crypt (**Figure 1E**), indicating that the tooth had not rotated within the crypt. There was no tissue compression or distortion visible (**Figures 1B,C,E,F**), suggesting that the inclination of the replacement tooth was not a result of postmortem mechanical distortion or deformation.

Large scale cone beam tomographs of the 8 cm long mosasaur jaw fragment illustrated the position of the replacement tooth adjacent to the apex of the deciduous tooth (**Figure 1H** vs. **Figure 1G**). Individual cone beam tomographs were used to calculate the 28° distal inclination angle of the replacement tooth when measured against the vertical axis of the deciduous tooth (**Figure 1K**) and to visualize the spatial relationship between both teeth from various angles when rotated in horizontal direction (**Figures 1I–L**). The individual tomographs also illustrated the location of the replacement tooth within an electron lucent resorption pit. In this tomograph, both replacement tooth and deciduous tooth were positioned within the same pseudotheca formed by the electron dense interdental ridges (**Figure 1J**).

## On-Axis and Recumbent Modes of Tooth Replacement in Amniotes

To ask how mosasaur tooth replacement relates to tooth replacement mechanisms in various amniotes, tooth eruption and implantation were examined in five distinct amniote species on a macroscale and microscale level, including a squamate (Iguana, *I. iguana*), a snake (ball python, *P. regius*), a crocodilian (American alligator, *A. mississippiensis*), a marsupial (opossum, *M. domestica*), and a rodent (mouse, *M. musculus*)(**Figure 2**). For macroscopic comparison, skulls of all five species were photographed (**Figures 2A–E**). Individual tooth rows including replacement teeth and their relationship to the jaw bone were visualized using whole mount stains (**Figures 2F–J**). Histological preparations of tooth replacement or individual teeth in mammalian dentitions were illustrated using Mallory stains (**Figures 2K–O**). The replacement dentition in the *Iguana* was positioned immediately apical of the deciduous erupted tooth, suggesting eruption of the replacement tooth in vertical direction (**Figures 2F,K**). Replacement teeth in the python were positioned at a ~15° inclination when compared to the horizontal jaw bone axis, while erupted teeth were inclined at an angle between ~35 and 60° in distal direction (**Figure 2G**). The histological section of a *P. regius* replacement dentition showed numerous replacement teeth prior to eruption and implantation (**Figure 2L**). None of these teeth demonstrated evidence of a mineralized pseudotheca surrounding the apical portion of the developing tooth (**Figure 2L**). In contrast, alligator (*A. mississippiensis*) tooth roots were surrounded by bony sockets

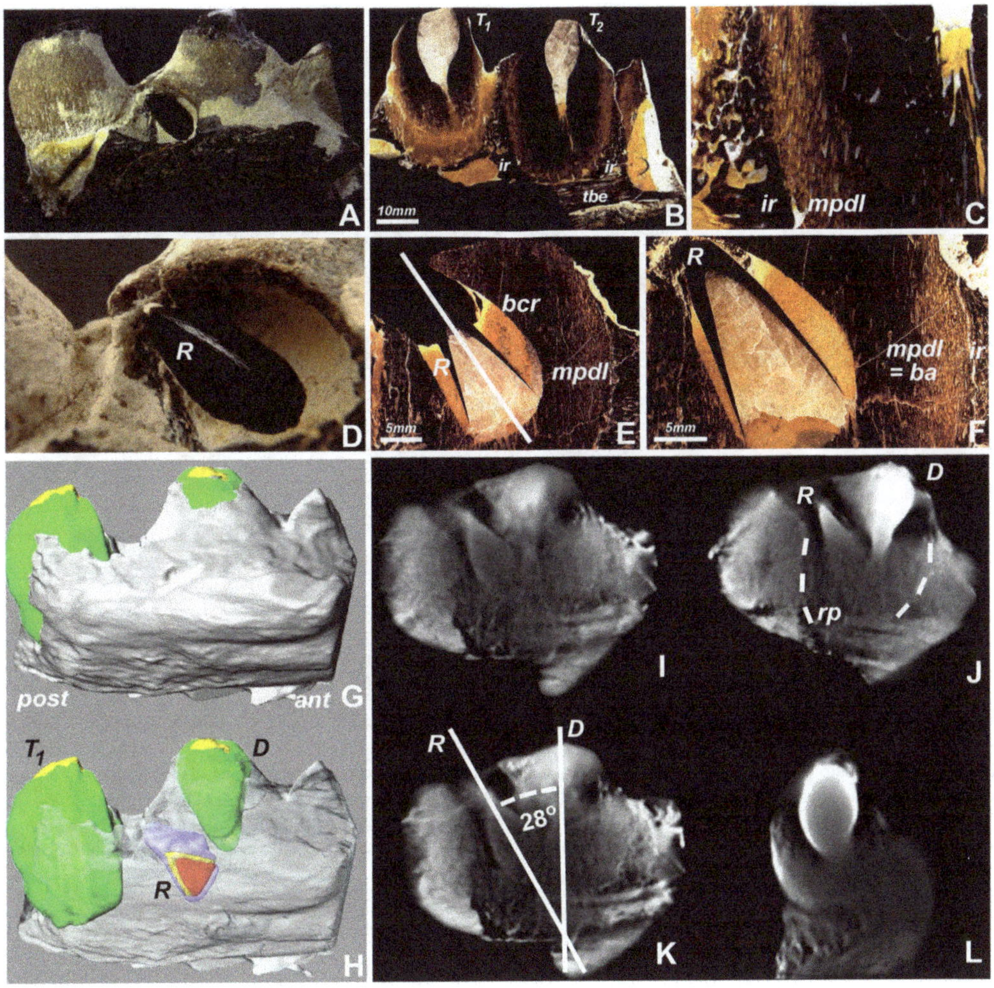


**FIGURE 1 | Replacement tooth position in a fossil Mosasaur jaw fragment from central Texas. (A,D)** are macrographic images of the intact fragment, **(B,C,E,F)** are ultrathin ground sections, **(G,H)** are 3D-reconstructions of stacked tomographs highlighting individual tooth positions, and **(I–L)** are individual tomographs illustrating the relationship between the center tooth, its replacement tooth, and surrounding socket. **(H)** was generated by digitally removing the superficial set of tomographs and coloring the replacement tooth (R), and **(I–L)** are individual cone beam tomographs generated while rotating the individual jaw fragment during the 3D tomography rendering process. The interrupted lines in **(J)** indicate the boundaries between the tooth-pedicel complex and the pseudotheca formed by the adjacent interdental ridges. Abbreviations: $T_1$ and $T_2$, neighboring teeth; ir, interdental ridge; tbe, tooth bearing element; mpdl, mineralized periodontal ligament; pedicel, or ba, bone of attachment; R, replacement tooth; E, Deciduous tooth; bcr, bony crypt of the replacement tooth R; rp, resorption pit; ant, anterior (mesial); post, posterior (distal). The mpdl descriptor in **(E,F)** refers to the pedicel of the replacement tooth, while the mpdl in **(C)** represents the pedicel of the exfoliating tooth $T_2$.

(**Figures 2H,M**), and replacement teeth developed in tandem with partial resorption of the apical dentin/pulp complex of the deciduous tooth (**Figure 2M**). The two mammals employed in the present study were characterized by monophyodont dentitions, and there was no evidence of tooth replacement *per-se*. However, the frontal incisors of the *Monodelphis* were inclined at a 30–60° angle (**Figure 2I**), and the continuously erupting mouse incisor was positioned at a 60° angle (**Figure 2J**) illustrating that modes of tooth replacement and individual tooth inclination vary greatly among vertebrate species.

The Gila monster *Heloderma suspectum* employs a combination of drift and rotation to position the replacement tooth in alignment with the deciduous tooth.

One of the key arguments for mosasaur-snake affinities is the inclined orientation frequently observed in mosasaur replacement teeth, which at least in terms of its angular position resembles the recumbent position of replacement teeth in snakes. In contrast, most squamates other than snakes feature on-axis vertical tooth replacement modes. To ask the question whether off-axis tooth replacement also occurs in other varanoids, the skull of a Gila monster, *H. suspectum*, was subjected to 3D microtomography and X-ray analysis (**Figure 3**). X-ray images and micro-CTs revealed a replacement tooth in the lower jaw located slightly distal (posterior) of the deciduous tooth (**Figures 3A–C**). As demonstrated by X-ray analysis, radiolucent areas of the newly formed tooth overlapped with those of the

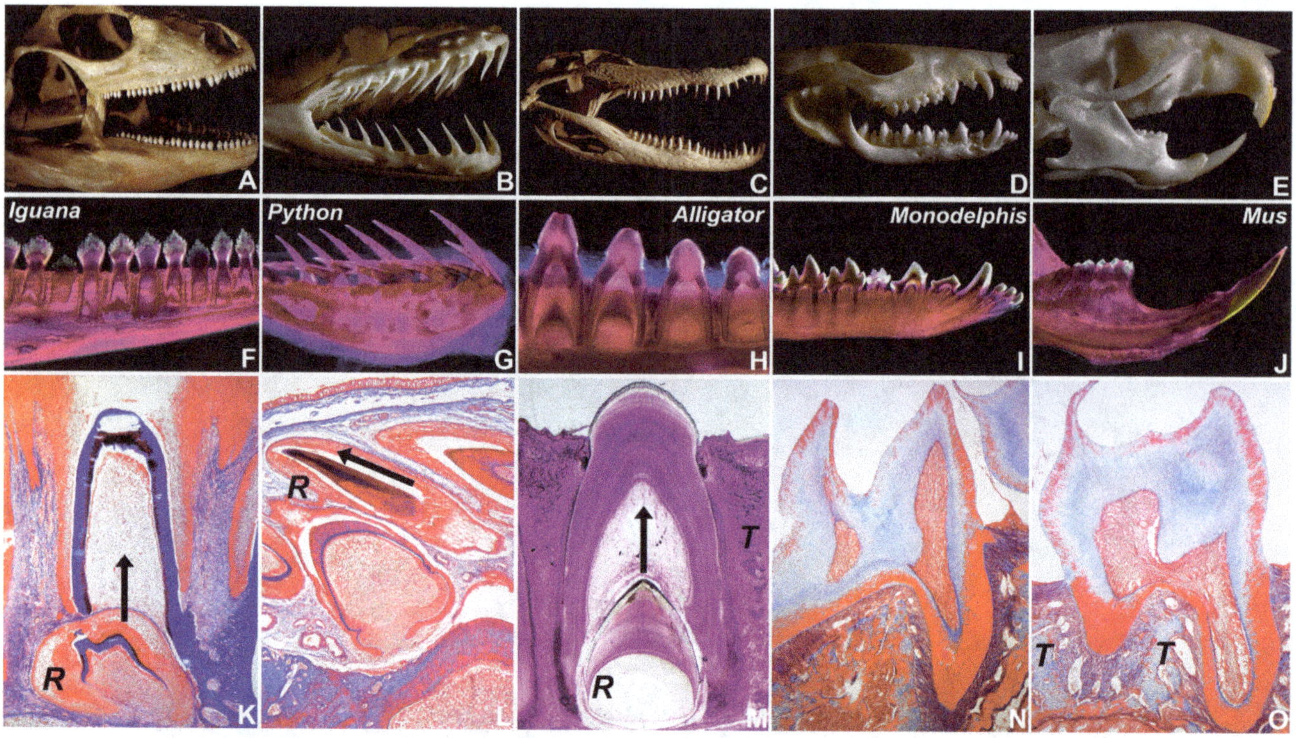


**FIGURE 2 | Tooth shape and succession in select amniotes. (A–E)** are skull photographs, **(F–J)** are macrographs of whole mount stains, and **(K–O)** are micrographs of histological preparations based on the following specimen: **(A,F,K)** Green iguana (*Iguana iguana*), **(B,G,L)** Ball python (*Python regius*), **(C,H,M)** American alligator (*Alligator mississippiensis*), **(D,I,N)** Short-tailed opossum (*Monodelphis domestica*), and **(E,J,O)** house mouse (*Mus musculus*). (R) indicates the position of the replacement tooth **(K–M)**, (T) labels the alveolar bone theca in alligator and mouse **(M,O)**, and the arrows represent the direction of tooth eruption **(K–M)**.

deciduous tooth, suggesting that the replacement tooth formed inside of a resorption pit within the deciduous tooth (**Figure 3C**).

## The Relationship between Vertical Tooth Axis Orientation and Replacement Tooth Position Varies among Amniotes

In the present study we asked the question whether mosasaur tooth replacement and successional tooth implantation mechanisms are identifying characters that establish mosasaurs as a family unequivocally positioned within squamates and define its relationship with other squamates such as snakes and varanoids (**Figure 4**). For this purpose, fossil mosasaur jaw fragment preparations were compared against skeletal and histological preparations of extant amniotes, representing various groups, including varanoids, snakes, crocodilians, marsupials, and rodents. Vertebrate systematics place Mosasaurs together with other varanoids (e.g., the iguana and the Gila monster used in the present study) and snakes (e.g., the python used in the present study) within the order of squamates (Squamata), which in turn belongs to the superorder lepidosaurs. Together with the archosaurs (represented here by the alligator), lepidosaurs are part of the diapsid clade, while the two mammals studied here, the Monodelphis (a marsupial) and the mouse (a rodent), belong to the synapsid clade. Both diapsids and synapsids are amniotes.

Three-dimensional micro-CT reconstructions of tooth bearing jaw fragments of all six species illustrate the orientation of tooth axis and replacement teeth in relationship to the jaw bone (**Figure 4**, right panel). These reconstructions illustrate that the replacement teeth in iguana and alligator were oriented in vertical direction, while the python replacement teeth were positioned at a 60° distal inclination to the erupted teeth. In another varanoid studied here, the Gila monster *Heloderma*, tooth crowns were slightly (~10–20°) inclined in distal direction when compared to the horizontal jaw axis, and replacement teeth were located posterior (distal) of the fully erupted tooth (**Figure 4**). In contrast to the four diapsids studied here, the dentition of the two mammals investigated (*Monodelphis* and *Mus*) lacked classic replacement teeth (monophyodont dentition), and only the mouse incisor featured permanent eruption and was inclined at a 60° angle when compared to the erupted molars (**Figure 4**).

The rotational drift employed during mosasaur tooth eruption and implantation resembles tooth eruption/implantation mechanisms found in Heloderma, while other varanoids such as the Iguana feature on-axis tooth eruption/replacement, and snakes such as the Python develop recumbent replacement teeth.

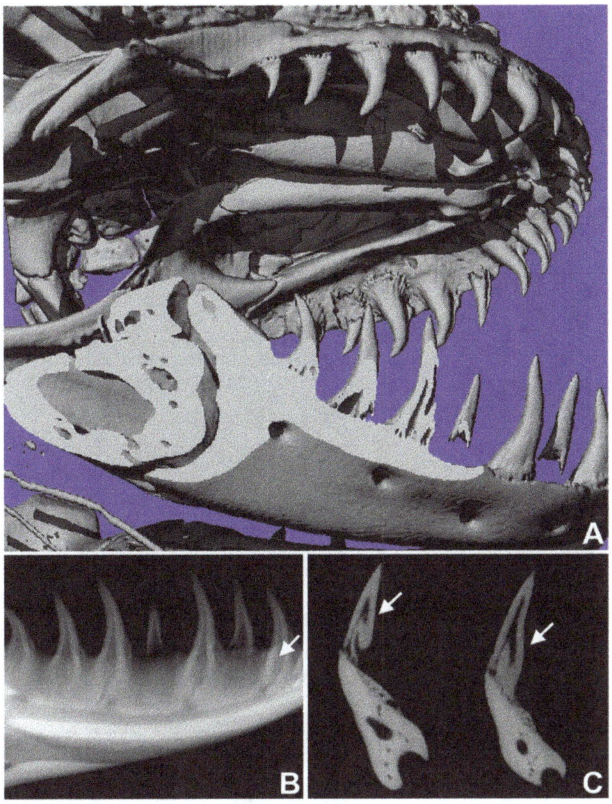


**FIGURE 3 | Replacement tooth position in the Gila monster (*Heloderma suspectum*). (A)** is a microCT image of the entire skull, **(B,C)** are radiographs in sagittal **(B)** and transverse **(C)** orientation, revealing the position of the replacement tooth (arrows).

In the present study, we distinguish between three different modes of tooth eruption and implantation in diapsid amniotes (**Figure 5**). Squamates and crocodilia favor on axis tooth replacement with the replacement tooth germ developing within a resorption pit at the apical portion of the deciduous tooth (**Figures 5A,D**). In most squamates, replacement teeth are then implanted in a pleurodont fashion, while crocodilian archosaur teeth are implanted into a *theca*. We propose that the replacement teeth in evolved varanoids such as *Mosasauridae* and *Helodermitidae* develop within resorption pits and then move into the position of the deciduous teeth through distal drift and a rotational movement (**Figure 5B**). Finally, ophidian tooth development differs from mosasaurian and varanoid tooth development as snake teeth develop within the supramandibular odontogenic connective tissue and only after completion of crown formation attach to the tooth bearing element through synostosis (ankylosis; **Figure 5C**).

## DISCUSSION

In the present study a fossil mosasaur jaw fragment containing an erupting tooth was analyzed using ultrathin ground sections and cone beam 3D computer tomography to compare mosasaur tooth eruption and implantation with tooth replacement mechanisms in extant amniotes, including an iguana, a python, a Gila monster, an alligator, a *Monodelphis* marsupial, and a mouse. In the fossil Mosasaur jaw fragment studied here, the replacement tooth was inclined, and there was no evidence of postmortem displacement as the surrounding bone microstructure was intact. Cone beam-CT analysis revealed the presence of a resorption pit and indicated that both the deciduous tooth and its replacement tooth were positioned within the same pseudo-theca. Ultrathin ground sections confirmed the presence of a pedicel formed by a mineralized periodontal ligament, connecting the mosasaur tooth root with the adjacent interdental ridge to provide a pseudo-thecodont attachment. The combination of drift and rotation as the proposed mode of Mosasaur tooth replacement resembled similar tooth replacement/implantation movements in the extant Gila monster *H. suspectum*. In contrast, other amniotes studied here featured vertical on-axis tooth replacement, while recumbent replacement teeth were only detected in our python sample, and mammals exhibited a variety of tooth axis orientations.

### Replacement Tooth Rotation: Artifact, Ophidian, or Varanoid Character?

The mosasaur replacement tooth examined in the present study was observed in an inclined position similar to replacement teeth previously described in a number of mosasaurs including *Leiodon*, *Platecarpus*, *Tylosaurus*, and *Clidastes* (Lee, 1997a). Moreover, our ultrathin ground sections and 3D cone beam tomographs demonstrated that the position and shape of the bony crypt opening matched the inclination angle of the replacement tooth. These ground sections and tomographs did not provide any evidence of postmortem displacement or deformation, but rather demonstrated that inclined replacement teeth and their integument were fairly well-preserved. Thus, our evidence suggests that the inclined position of our mosasaur replacement tooth is representative of the actual position of these teeth in at least some Cretaceous mosasaur species.

However, not only snakes and mosasaurs have off-axis and lingual replacement teeth that are often inclined or recumbent, but also closely related extant varanoids such as the Gila monster *Heloderma* are characterized by similar rotational and off-axis replacement teeth as demonstrated in the present study and as previously described by Smith (1958, note Figure 6). Moreover, inclined or recumbent tooth positions are prominent in a broad range of amniotes including some mammals (rodents, marsupials). Thus, a recumbent tooth position is not necessarily a defining character for synaptomorphic mosasaur-snake affinities, but rather a homoplastic character that occurs in a number of amniotes. From a morphological position alone, which is the basis of Lee's argument (Lee, 2005), Mosasaur-Heloderma tooth eruption/implantation synaptomorphies are more plausible than those between mosasaurs and snakes, suggesting that mosasaurs and Helodermatidae may safely be grouped among the varanoids, as suggested by Zaher and Rieppel (1999). A possible relationship between mosasaurs and Helodermatidae is also supported by earlier studies on tongue morphologies (Schulp et al., 2005)

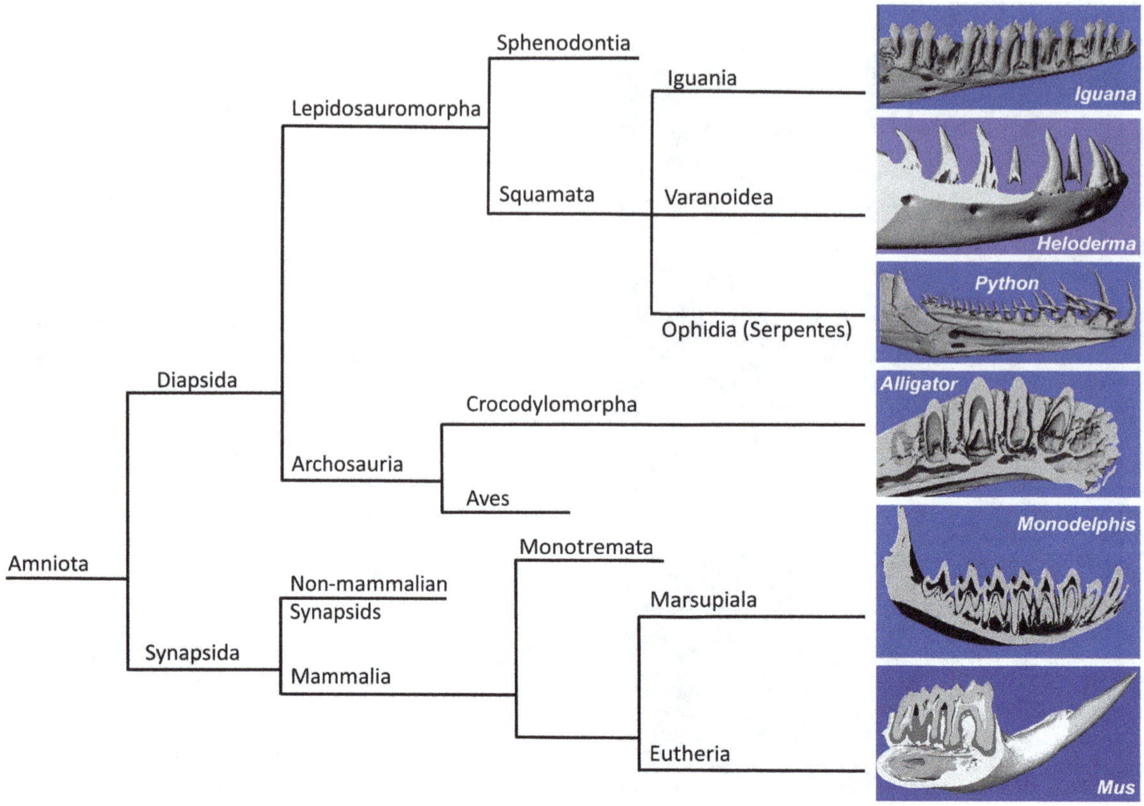


**FIGURE 4 | Consensus phylogeny illustrating the relationships of the species included in the present analysis.** The left side of the diagram illustrates the phylogenetic relationship between the species studies in the present analysis, including green iguana (*Iguana iguana*), ball python (*Python regius*), Gila monster (*Heloderma suspectum*), American alligator (*Alligator mississippiensis*), short-tailed opossum (*Monodelphis domestica*), and house mouse (*Mus musculus*). Three-dimensional micro-CT reconstructions of the tooth rows are presented on the right side of the illustration.

and by the posterolingual (distal) replacement tooth position described in the present study in both the *Heloderma* specimen and the mosasaur fragment. One benefit of an inclined or somewhat recumbent position would be a longer period of protected development for the replacement tooth, which might provide an important advantage for mosasaurs when it comes to the preservation of a fairly complete tooth row as a prerequisite for preying on large organisms with calcareous shells.

## The Resorption Pit: Unprotected *De novo* Tooth Formation or Protected Replacement of Existing Teeth?

Our study indicated that the developing mosasaur replacement tooth was surrounded by a resorption pit within the boundaries of the deciduous tooth. Replacement tooth and deciduous tooth were located within the same pseudotheca formed by the interdental ridges between adjacent teeth. As demonstrated in the present study, mosasaurian, iguanid, and crocodilian replacement teeth developed within resorption pits generated at the apex of the previous generation tooth and at the expense of the deciduous tooth mineral substance, while the python snake teeth studied here do not. Specifically, developing python tooth germs were not surrounded by any mineralized tissue as demonstrated in the present study, making it impossible for resorption pits to form. In terms of the mosasaur-sake debate, Lee was aware that mosasaurs and many other squamates form resorption pits for tooth replacement, while there are no resorption pits in snake teeth and replacement teeth lie outside the jawbone throughout their entire development (Lee, 1997a). It is thus surprising that he gave mosasaur-snake synaptomorphies serious consideration. The presence of resorption pits in mosasaurs and varanoids vs. their absence in snakes as documented in the present study certainly argues in favor of mosasaur-varanoid homologies.

## Tooth Implantation: Pseudotheca or Synostosis?

In terms of tooth implantation, our specimen demonstrated anchorage of the bulbous mosasaur root cementum by means of a mineralized periodontal ligament in a bowl-shaped groove between interdental ridges as described earlier (Luan et al., 2009b). This mode of attachment resembled thecoid forms of tooth attachment but fell short of true thecodont attachment because of the mineralized state of the ligament and because of the shallow interdental ridges that only provided incomplete anchorage for the protruding tooth. As such, we

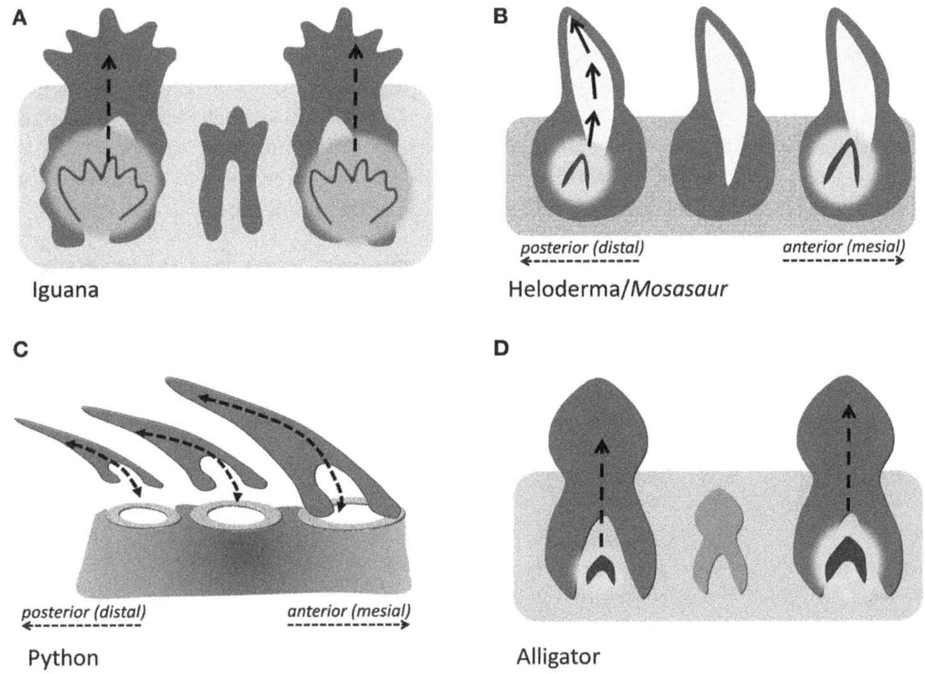


**FIGURE 5 | Direction of tooth eruption in select amniotes.** Sketch illustrating the common straight upright eruption pattern in iguana and alligator **(A,D)**, the recumbent position of replacement teeth in snakes **(C)**, and the rotational shift that the replacement tooth undergoes when erupting to replace its predecessor tooth **(B)**, as a proposed mechanism in Helodermitidae and Mosasaurs.

have chosen the term pseudothecodont to define the mode of mosasauroid tooth attachment as an intermediary between ankylosis and ligamentous thecodont attachment. Our term pseudothecodont is based on the ligamentous structure and mineralized composition of the mosasaur attachment tissue that interfaces between interdental ridges and the bulbous root cementum (Luan et al., 2009b), and describes similar forms of implantation as identified by the earlier terms "subthecodont" or "ankylosed thecodont" (Zaher and Rieppel, 1999). Thus, our data indicate that mosasaur teeth are truly unique and can neither be compared with the cementoid ankylosis to the socket rim as it occurs in snakes nor with the pleurodont ankylosis that is typical for most extant varanoids.

## The Origin of Snakes—A Flashback from the Bone Wars?

In the present study we have demonstrated (i) that the presence of inclined replacement teeth is not unique to mosasauroid varanoids but also occurs in helodermatoid squamates and is therefore is not a synaptomorphic character exclusive for mosasaurs and snakes, (ii) that the occurrence of resorption pits as structural basis for replacement tooth formation within the deciduous precursor theca is a character found both in mosasaurs and varanoids, but not in snakes, supporting mosasaur-varanoid affinities, and (iii) that the pseudothecodont mode of tooth implantation in mosasaurs is different from the pleurodont type of tooth attachment as it occurs in many varanoids and from the ankylotic synostosis on the rim of the TBE as it is representative of most snakes, suggesting that mosasaurian pseudothecodont tooth implantation is an autopomorphic character for mosasaurs alone. Together, our study suggests that the mosasaur tooth apparatus is distinct from varanoids and snakes and shares common features with both groups, while the pseudothecodont implantation of mosasaurs does not occur in either of the other two groups.

The original concept of mosasaur-snake affinities goes back to Edward D. Cope (1840–1897), who together with Othniel Charles Marsh (1831–1899) was known for his fossil-finding expeditions during the Bone Wars. Cope argued for a systematic relationship between mosasaurs and snakes based on common traits in their lower jaws, including a free mandibular symphysis and a straight vertical splenial-angular joint, allowing for a large gape to facilitate feeding on large prey (Cope, 1869, 1872; Lee, 1997b; Luan et al., 2009b). Cope's account was originally disputed by Owen (1877, 1878), but later adopted by Lee (1997a,b) based on two derived traits, (i) the presence of recumbent replacement teeth and (ii) the establishment of a discrete socket under each tooth (Lee, 1997a). For Cope, the transformation of marine mosasaurs into modern snakes was just one example for his Neo-Lamarckian school of thought, according to which organisms slowly evolve over time and pass on their fittest traits toward their offspring (Cope, 1889).

Proponents of the snake-mosasaur common ancestor school of thought have invoked the discovery of fossil marine snakes with limbs as supportive of mosasaur-snake origins (Caldwell and Lee, 1997). However, a close relationship between snakes and monitor lizards has been refuted by recent DNA evidence (Vidal and Hedges, 2004), and an extensive study including

161 squamate species and up to 44 nuclear genes reported a paraphyletic relationship between scolecophidians and other snakes, supporting the burrowing hypothesis of snake origins and at the same time rejecting the hypothesis of marine origins of snakes (Wiens et al., 2012).

It appears as if the mosasaur feeding apparatus was uniquely specialized to anchor large-sized teeth within powerful jaws (TBEs) and to provide optimum protection for replacement teeth within a bony crypt that develops within a resorption pit at the apex of its predecessor. While the recumbent orientation of snake dentitions facilitates retention of prey and prevents a possible escape of captured organisms, mosasaur dentitions appear to be adept at feeding on a broad range of food, including a diet of large fish, ammonites, sea turtles, and crustaceans (Polcyn et al., 2014). Crushing the bones and mineralized shells of such prey would be traumatic for developing teeth, unless they were protected by bony crypts or the covers of already erupted teeth with a rigid yet flexible attachment apparatus (Luan et al., 2009b). It seems as if Cope was captivated by the morphological similarities between large angioform animals such as mosasaurs and snakes, and the skeletal similarities that supported his Neo-Lamarckian views, while he appeared to have overlooked the selective pressures in late Cretaceous oceans.

## AUTHOR CONTRIBUTIONS

ML, GC, XL, KG, CG prepared samples and conducted experiments; XL analyzed data and generated images; DR, RM, XL, and TD analyzed data and wrote the manuscript.

## REFERENCES


Caldwell, M. W., and Lee, M. S. (1997). A snake with legs from the marine Cretaceous of the Middle East. *Nature* 386, 705-709. doi:10.1038/386 705a0

Carroll, R. L. (1988). *Vertebrate Paleontology and Evolution.* New York, NY: WH Freeman and Company.

Cope, E. D. (1869). On the reptilian orders, Pythonomorpha and Streptosauria. *Proc. Boston Soc. Nat. Hist.* 12, 250–266.

Cope, E. D. (1872). On the geology and paleontology of the Cretaceous strata of Kansas. *US Geol. Sur.* 5, 318–349.

Cope, E. D. (1889). Lamarck *versus* Weismann. *Nature* 41, 79.

Edmund, A. G. (1960). Tooth replacement phenomena in the lower vertebrates. *R. Ont. Mus. Life Sci. Div. Contrib.* 52, 1–190.

Greene, H. W., and Cundall, D. (2000). Limbless tetrapods and snakes with legs. *Science* 287, 1939–1941. doi: 10.1126/science.287.5460.1939

Hefti, T., Frischherz, M., Spencer, N. D., Hall, H., and Schlottig, F. (2010). A comparison of osteoclast resorption pits on bone with titanium and zirconia surfaces. *Biomaterials* 31, 7321–7331. doi: 10.1016/j.biomaterials.2010.06.009

Lee, M. S. (1997a). On snake-like dentition in mosasaurian lizards. *J. Nat. Hist.* 31, 303–314.

Lee, M. S. (1997b). The phylogeny of varanoid lizards and the affinities of snakes. *Philos. Trans. R. Soc. Lond. Biol.* 352, 53–91.

Lee, M. S. (2005). Molecular evidence and marine snake origins. *Biol. Lett.* 1, 227-230. doi: 10.1098/rsbl.2004.0282

Luan, X., Dangaria, S., Ito, Y., Walker, C., Jin, T., Schmidt, M., et al. (2009a). Neural crest lineage segregation: a blueprint for periodontal regeneration. *J. Dent. Res.* 88, 781–791. doi: 10.1177/0022034509340641

Luan, X., Walker, C., Dangaria, S., Ito, Y., Druzinsky, R., Jarosius, K., et al. (2009b). The mosasaur tooth attachment apparatus as paradigm for the evolution of the gnathostome periodontium. *Evol. Dev.* 11, 247–259. doi: 10.1111/j.1525-142X.2009.00327.x

Martill, D. M., Tischlinger, H., and Longrich, N. R. (2015). A four-legged snake from the early Cretaceous of Gondwana. *Science* 349, 416–419. doi: 10.1126/science.aaa9208

Martin, L., Stewart, J., and Whetstone, K. (1980). The origin of birds: structure of the tarsus and teeth. *Auk* 97, 86–93.

McIntosh, J. E., Anderson, X., Flores-de-jacoby, L., Carlson, D., Shuler, C., and Diekwisch, T. (2002). Caiman periodontium as an intermediate between basal vertebrate ankylosis-type attachment and mammalian "true" periodontium. *Microsc. Res. Tech.* 59, 449–459. doi: 10.1002/jemt.10222

Owen, R. (1877). *On the Rank and Affinities in the Reptilian Class of Mosasauridae.* London: Quarterly Journal of the Geological Society.

Owen, R. (1878). On the affinities of the Mosasauridae Gervais, as exemplified in the bony structure of the fore fin. *Q. J. Geol. Soc. Lond.* 34, 784–753.

Polcyn, M. J., Jacobs, L. L., Araújo, R., Schulp, A. S., and Mateus, O. (2014). Physical drivers of mosasaur evolution. *Palaeogeog. palaeoclim. palaeoecol.* 400, 17–27. doi: 10.1016/j.palaeo.2013.05.018

Reeder, T. W., Townsend, T. M., Mulcahy, D. G., Noonan, B. P., Wood, P. L., Sites, J. W., et al. (2015). Integrated analyses resolve conflicts over squamate reptile phylogeny and reveal unexpected placements for fossil taxa. *PLoS ONE* 10:e0118199. doi: 10.1371/journal.pone.0118199

Rieppel, O. (1980). The trigeminal jaw adductors of primitive snakes and their homologies with the lacertilian jaw adductors. *J. Zool.* 190, 447–471.

Rieppel, O., and Kearney, M. (2005). Tooth replacement in the Late Cretaceous mosasaur Clidastes. *J. Herpetol.* 39, 688–692. doi: 10.1670/119-05A.1

Rieppel, O., Kluge, A. G., and Zaher, H. (2003). Testing the phylogenetic relationships of the Pleistocene snake Wonambi naracoortensis Smith. *J. Vertebr. Paleontol.* 22, 812–829. doi: 10.1671/0272-4634(2002)022[0812:TTPROT]2.0.CO;2

Schulp, A., Molder, E., and Schwenk, K. (2005). Did mosasaurs have forked tongues? *Neth. J. Surg. Geosci.* 84, 359–371. doi: 10.1017/S0016774600021144

Smith, H. M. (1958). Evolutionary lines in tooth attachment and replacement in reptiles: their possible significance in mammalian dentition. *Trans. Kan. Acad. Sci. (1903)*, 61, 216–225.

Tchernov, E., Rieppel, O., Zaher, H., Polcyn, M. J., and Jacobs, L. L. (2000). A fossil snake with limbs. *Science* 287, 2010–2012. doi: 10.1126/science.287.5460.2010

Vidal, N., and Hedges, S. B. (2004). Molecular evidence for a terrestrial origin of snakes. *Proc. R. Soc. Lond. Biol.* 271(Suppl. 4), S226–S229. doi: 10.1098/rsbl.2003.0151

Vonk, F. J., Admiraal, J. F., Jackson, K., Reshef, R., de Bakker, M. A., Vanderschoot, K., et al. (2008). Evolutionary origin and development of snake fangs. *Nature* 454, 630–633. doi: 10.1038/nature07178

Wiens, J. J., Hutter, C. R., Mulcahy, D. G., Noonan, B. P., Townsend, T. M., Sites, J. W., et al. (2012). Resolving the phylogeny of lizards and snakes (Squamata) with extensive sampling of genes and species. *Biol. Lett.* 8, 1043–1046. doi: 10.1098/rsbl.2012.0703

Zaher, H., and Rieppel, O. (1999). Tooth implantation and replacement in squamates, with special reference to mosasaur lizards and snakes. *Am. Mus. Novit.* 3271, 1–19.

17

# Small-Scale Fabrication of Biomimetic Structures for Periodontal Regeneration


**Edited by:**
Thimios Mitsiadis,
University of Zurich, Switzerland

***Correspondence:**
Han-Sung Jung
hsjung@yuhs.ac

†Joint first authors.

*David W. Green* [1,2†], *Jung-Seok Lee* [3†] *and Han-Sung Jung* [1,2*]

[1] Division in Anatomy and Developmental Biology, Department of Oral Biology, Oral Science Research Center, BK21 PLUS Project, Yonsei University College of Dentistry, Seoul, South Korea, [2] Oral Biosciences, Faculty of Dentistry, The University of Hong Kong, Hong Kong, Hong Kong, [3] Department of Periodontology, Research Institute for Periodontal Regeneration, Yonsei University College of Dentistry, Seoul, South Korea



The periodontium is the supporting tissues for the tooth organ and is vulnerable to destruction, arising from overpopulating pathogenic bacteria and spirochaetes. The presence of microbes together with host responses can destroy large parts of the periodontium sometimes leading tooth loss. Permanent tissue replacements are made possible with tissue engineering techniques. However, existing periodontal biomaterials cannot promote proper tissue architectures, necessary tissue volumes within the periodontal pocket and a "water-tight" barrier, to become clinically acceptable. New kinds of small-scale engineered biomaterials, with increasing biological complexity are needed to guide proper biomimetic regeneration of periodontal tissues. So the ability to make compound structures with small modules, filled with tissue components, is a promising design strategy for simulating the anatomical complexity of the periodotium attachment complexes along the tooth root and the abutment with the tooth collar. Anatomical structures such as, intima, adventitia, and special compartments such as the epithelial cell rests of Malassez or a stellate reticulum niche need to be engineered from the start of regeneration to produce proper periodontium replacement. It is our contention that the positioning of tissue components at the origin is also necessary to promote self-organizing cell–cell connections, cell–matrix connections. This leads to accelerated, synchronized and well-formed tissue architectures and anatomies. This strategy is a highly effective preparation for tackling periodontitis, periodontium tissue resorption, and to ultimately prevent tooth loss. Furthermore, such biomimetic tissue replacements will tackle problems associated with dental implant support and perimimplantitis.



**Keywords: periodontium, tissue engineering, modular biomaterials, 3D bioprinting, cell sheet engineering**


## INTRODUCTION

The periodontium tissue complex is adapted to fixing and supporting the tooth into the mandibular and maxillary bone sockets and preserving its structure under extreme masticatory forces. Unfortunately, there are currently no permanent cures for chronic and advanced periodontal tissue degeneration. This situation has spurred efforts to grow new replacement patient-matched periodontal tissue for transplantation into the periodontal pocket. Arguably, this represents the only clear permanent solution for periodontal tissue degeneration.

To gain acceptance and to be relevant in the clinic, prospective engineered tissue replacements must display higher levels of tissue biomimicry, to promote coherent host integration. Biomimetic tissue systems can be engineered to program tissue morphogenesis and produce good clinical outcomes. How should tissue engineers design and produce structures that enable embedded tissue components to self-organize and spontaneously grow into proper tissues? Modular design of biomaterials may be a good starting point.

Modular biomaterials are a useful way of building tissue complexity in the laboratory. They are composites of limitless structural units. These units can have any type of size, composition, morphology, and topology. They can be fused together in any sort of position to make intricate patterns. When built-up in scale they can form hierarchies. The combination of structure and composition enables them to perform the numerous roles and behaviors of native tissue development and regeneration. This level of organization is not possible with conventional cell sheet engineering. Infact, tissue biology is highly modular itself. There are many delineations, partitionings, dissociations, associations, and complex organizations made between tissue components (cells, proteins, and matrices). By engineering in a modular fashion with assorted functional tissue units is to emulate native tissue organization. Assembling tissues in this manner will accelerate correct mimetic tissue morphogenesis and near normal tissue functioning. Once structure and function are synergized then tissues can remain permanent.

## ENGINEERING CRITERIA FOR PERIODONTAL REGENERATION

Conventional periodontal clinical therapy focuses on bacteria removal (plaque control), pocket depth reduction by surgical reattachment, reattachment to the root surfaces, forming a hermetic epithelial barrier, and tackling inflammation (**Figures 1A,B**). However, the grand prize for periodontal therapy is the total replacement of missing and degenerate tissue with healthy functional tissue originating from patient cells. This is only achieved by creating proper conditions for *de novo* tissue formation engineered in the laboratory or inside the periodontal pocket (**Figure 1C**). There are two dimensions to periodontium tissue regeneration. There is the attachment complex along the root of the tooth and the attachment complex that forms the epithelial seal against the neck of the tooth masticatory surface (**Figure 1A**; left side of tooth diagram). These union structures are partitioned into numerous anatomical compartments, (some well-delineated and some diffuse) each typified with its own specialized functional properties, ultrastructure, size and morphology.

To ensure fast, effective, and accurate biomimetic translation from concept to clinic, these compartments must be stacked together as layers (between 5 and 100 $\mu$m) in a specific functional sequence and fixed together with interconnecting embedded union structures made from regionally specialized collagen fibers (**Figure 1B**). Another compartment of significance to driving regeneration of cementum is the epithelial cell rests of Malassez. Modular design can incorporate this cellular assembly and other stem cell niche compartments as adjuncts. Ultimately, this must be a synchronized production from collective cellular programming and self-organization biological processes. These are the prime drivers, for producing final functional complexity. The proper positioning of compartments establishes a set of functional pre-arrangements of cells and matrix components that spontaneously and inevitably give rise to correct tissue ultrastructures, morphologies, and anatomies.

Strategies being developed for periodontal regeneration are embracing numerous tissue engineering techniques to recreate a living replacement that can spontaneously graft into the walls of periodontal pocket and so provide fresh, permanent replacement to re-support the compromised tooth organ. To generate high volumes of good quality biomimetic tissue the physical environment for growth and regeneration needs to emulate the physical (e.g., mechanical, patterning) and topological complexity of normal periodontium structures. Modular biomaterials can be a good beginning for representing this organizational complexity and an approach for translating biocomplexity into tissue engineered biosystems. For instance, modular biomaterials will be capable of mapping networks and relationships between cells and components that promote self-regeneration processes. In this short article, we focus exclusively on modular biomaterials to engineer the periodontium and speculate on how this can improve tissue engineered outcomes.

## FRAMEWORKS TO SUPPORT PERIODONTAL TISSUE REGENERATION

The engineering of periodontal tissue sets is at a crossroads of approaches: biomaterial-free tissue morphogenesis, tissue morphogenesis with biomaterial engagement of endogenous regeneration, and fully engaged biomaterials seeded with cells. Biomaterials with regeneration potential have nominally provided transient stop-gaps and bridges across the periodontal pocket.

An important contribution to the existing panel of engineered periodontal replacements has been essentially devoid of biomaterials involving cells assembled into sheets (Asakawa et al., 2010). Cell sheet engineering has been widely used to construct tissues with translation into stratified tissue types and simple anatomical cellular organizations such as, the skin, myocardium, corneal, and mucosal epithelium as well as, PDL, cementum, and the alveolar bone lining (Iwata et al., 2009). It is a relatively low-tech and effective fabrication method. There is a capacity with this technique to grow coherent, self-supporting monolayers of tissue-specific cells and then deploy them as stratified constructs into small tissue defects. Cell sheets and multiple sheets have also been used to encase implantable devices (not exceeding 3–6 layers or 80–100 $\mu$m). Cell sheets are reminiscent of the organization of periodontal tissues and have been used in reconstructions. There is an attempt to replicate the different layers using more rationally designed material frameworks to restore different tissue morphologies. In one

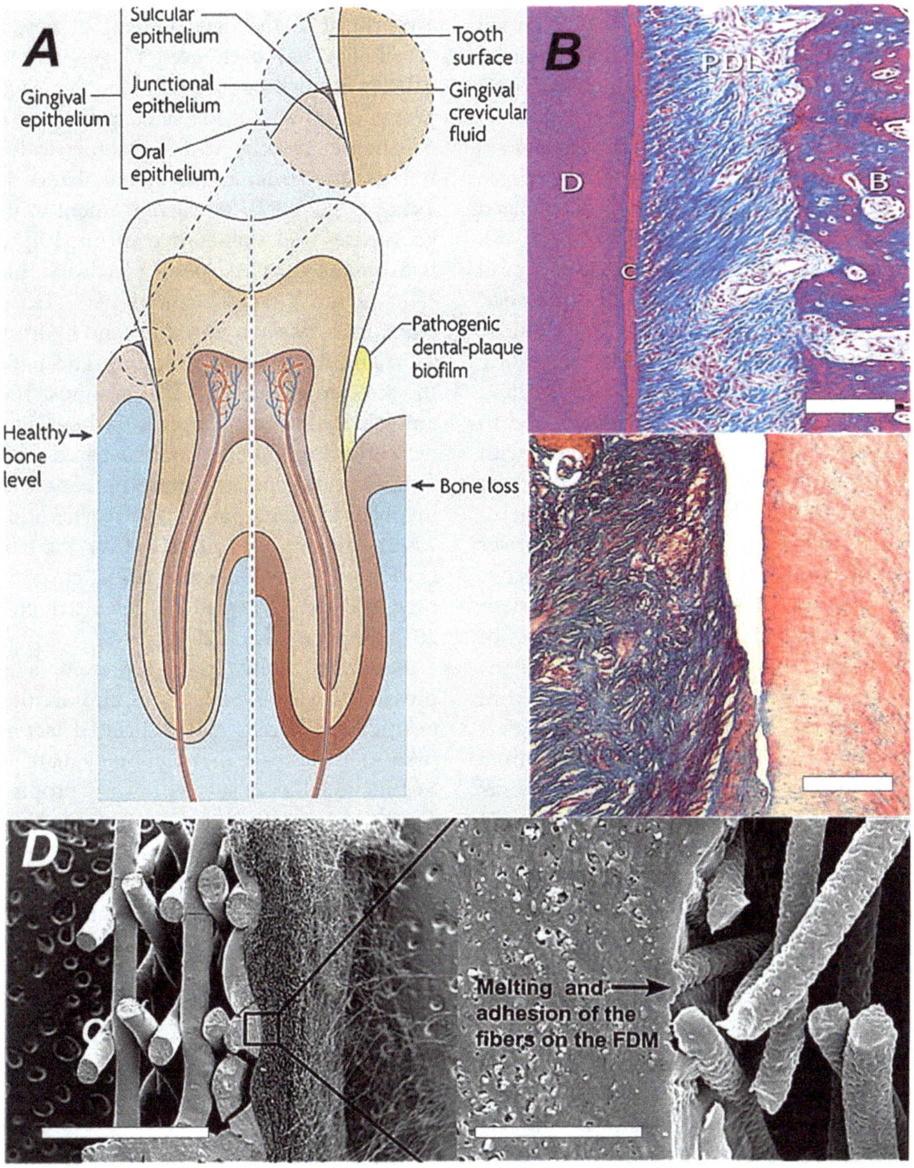


**FIGURE 1 | The comparative anatomy and histoarchitecture of healthy and diseased periodontal tissue and a typical biomaterial replacement for lost union structures. (A)** A diagram showing the difference in the tooth supporting structures between normal healthy periodontium and diseased periodontium. In particular, the "periodontal connective tissue" and bone are destroyed by growth of a dental plaque biofilm that attaches and develops first at the sulcus, progressing along the tooth root and then creating a deepening pocket (Darveau, 2010; Reproduced with kind permission from Macmillan). **(B)** The healthy periodontal ligament at the centre of the periodontium complex shown in polarized light at high magnification. In this view we can see the densified collagen fiber bundles arranged in very high order corresponding to strong birefringence. Along the tooth root the collagen fiber mass is anchored and suspended between the cementum (C)/dentine and alveolar bone (AB). This image depicts the histoarchitecture of the periodontium. It shows the complex nature of the tissue architecture. The periodontal "hinge" ligament tissue is filled with cell assemblies and blood vessels servicing its role in continual cycles of readjustment, repair and regeneration. (Reproduced with kind permission from John Wiley and Sons A/S; Bosshardt and Sculean, 2009). **(C)** Close-up histosection of an advanced gingival mucosa lesion at the tooth surface caused by the infiltration of periodontitis causing bacteria. The periodontal ligament has clearly separated and peeled away from the tooth surface (dentine) on the right. Cementum is lost and the junctional epithelium disappears from the tooth surface as the gingival pocket opens-up. Tissue engineering approaches involve infilling the space and regenerating a new periodontium in between pulling a whole new union "cable" structure of collagen fibers (Type I) from a *de novo* periodontal ligament into reconstituted *de novo* alveolar bone and Sharpeys collagen fiber tips from the periodontal ligament embedded into the cementum at the tooth surface (Type III; Hasegawa et al., 2005; Reproduced with kind permission from Mary Anne Liebert). **(D)** One conventional biomaterial led strategy is simpy to combine thin layers of material with tissue-specific architectures that mimic periodontal ligament and the cementum layer. Each structure provides contact guidance for the proper organization of cementum cells and the alignment of the peridontal ligament fibers. The seeded cells collectively organize themselves into a coherent functional unit. The SEM image shows an engineered bi-layered polymer structure that provides the appropriate physical framework for the periodontal ligament cells and the cementum. The PDL housing consists of an electrospun structure with fibrous mesh architecture, to align and guide the extension of PDL fibers. This meshwork was melted onto the porous solid layer with a technique called fused deposition modeling (FDM; Obregon et al., 2015; Reproduced with kind permission from Elsevier).

Periodontal related example, electrospinning (to create a fibrous network) and fused deposition modeling (FDM; to create a small porous solid membrane) recreated the PDL and mineralized layer of bone or cementum respectively (Obregon et al., 2015; **Figure 1D**).

Modular biomaterials are tissue engineering structures divided into a network of small segments containing tissue components tailored toward synergistic and synchronized function between neighboring segments (Zorlutuna et al., 2013). The cell-containing building blocks are arranged so as to mimic the organization of native tissue. Traditional cell-seeded frameworks are a scramble of tissue components. The modular approach is a way of ordering tissue components according to native anatomical organization, which is always diverse and complex (**Figure 2A**). These design principles when applied to the periodontium then translate into semi-permeable layers, with physical guides to direct the fiber alignments across different regions, for the PDL and cementum. They translate into spheres and rods to form a template for epithelialization and barrier formation and spherical outgrowths representing regional niches and crypts for epithelial cell rests of Malassez ERM's and stem cell phenotypes. Modular design facilitates the accumulation of cellular assemblies and other stem cell niche compartments. Ultimately, this must be a synchronized production from collective cellular programming and self-organization biological processes. These are the prime drivers, for producing the final functional complexity. The proper positioning of compartments establishes a set of functional pre-arrangements of cells and matrix components that spontaneously and inevitably give rise to correct tissue ultrastructures, morphologies, and anatomies.

Now there are some notable module structures designed to house assorted cell populations and phenotypes. There are various methods to assemble them in rational networks related to selected tissue architecture (Khademhosseini et al., 2006; Gauvin and Khademhosseini, 2011; Hansen et al., 2013; Kolesky et al., 2014). Bioprinting in three-dimensions (programmable positioning of building blocks) combined with microfluidic technology (programmable size and shape generator of droplets for building blocks) could propel the manufacture of more highly intricate and complex morphologies and the deep internal structures and architectures that more accurately replicate the exact anatomical organization of many complex tissue and including periodontal tissues with its multi-planar differences in composition and architecture (Erdman et al., 2014). A standardized microengineering method of producing regular modules is with polymer microdroplets. Changes in droplet size (in nanoliter and microliter volumes) (Gruene et al., 2011), composition and deposition leads to single modules and module networks with biologically acceptable complexity (Durmus et al., 2013). Three-dimensional bioprinting and aqueous droplet microfluidics and nanofluidics are the highest precision tools in generating and depositing mixtures of aqueous biomaterials into precisely defined shapes, structures (including internalized structures) and assemblies of droplets and beads with well-delineated architectures at micron scales and nanoscales with picoliter droplets (Erdman et al., 2014; Murphy and Atala, 2014). Contained within the droplets are mixtures of cells, tissue components, and biological molecules. Blood vessel networks are critical to the development of new tissues. Microprinting technology has been used to generate branched networks of tubules mimicking natural blood vessels (Kucukgul et al., 2015; Wang et al., 2015). Repeated gelling of hydrogels, one on top of another, placed within geometrically patterned templates was used to generate hexagonal shaped hepatic structures (Liu Tsang et al., 2007). The arrangement of modules into deliberate geometries and shapes is controlled by deposition of aqueous hydrophilic droplets, onto a hydrophobic oil receiver solution (Nichol and Khademhosseini, 2009; Du et al., 2011). Chemical reactions between hydrophilic and hydrophobic components are a driving force for organization and patterning of objects into the directed geometries. This is almost 100% controlled. As with any fabrication tool the sizes of the individual modules and the networks are limited. Modular-based architectures also provide temporal and spatial patterning capabilities for vital processes involved in development and regeneration. There are instances where this has been delivered for the controlled and regulated elution of growth factors using core-shell arrangements and bead-in-bead arrangements (Babister et al., 2008; Perez et al., 2014; Perez and Kim, 2015).

Modular biomaterials represent a potential solution to provide temporary structures and architectures for the precise positioning of cells and associated factors (to generate proper tissues) in 3D space that accurately match normal tissue and lead to functional associations toward proper regeneration. A one-to-one biomimetic matching between the smallest units present in natural tissue and the replicated modules is not necessary for function. Function is designed to emerge from the interplay between the well-placed tissue components inside the combined modules. The fusion of tissue modules into clusters and networks establishes a provisional tissue mimicking anatomical structure. These arrangements also facilitate the directional release of factors designed to stimulate different types of pre-existing endogenous tissues to grow and develop into the modular replacement.

## TISSUE BIOMIMICRY WITH MODULAR BIOMATERIALS

Tissues are essentially divided into compartments bounded by cell linings (intima, adventitia), membranes (vesicles and pouches), and boundaries made from structural biomaterials. The intricate complexity of form and architecture are strongly and directly associated with function. There is a growing interest in designing biomaterial devices and products that reflect this compartmentalization arrangement, which facilitates, partitioning, gradation, and division of tissue entities (Nichol and Khademhosseini, 2009; **Figures 2A,B**). Crucially, the building of compartments relies on chemical self-organization processes rather than biologically driven self-assembly and self-organization processes toward tissue complexity (Jakab et al., 2010; Athanasiou et al., 2013). These can also be directed in specified ways by manipulating the steps in synthesis. The most commonly used and versatile semi-autonomous

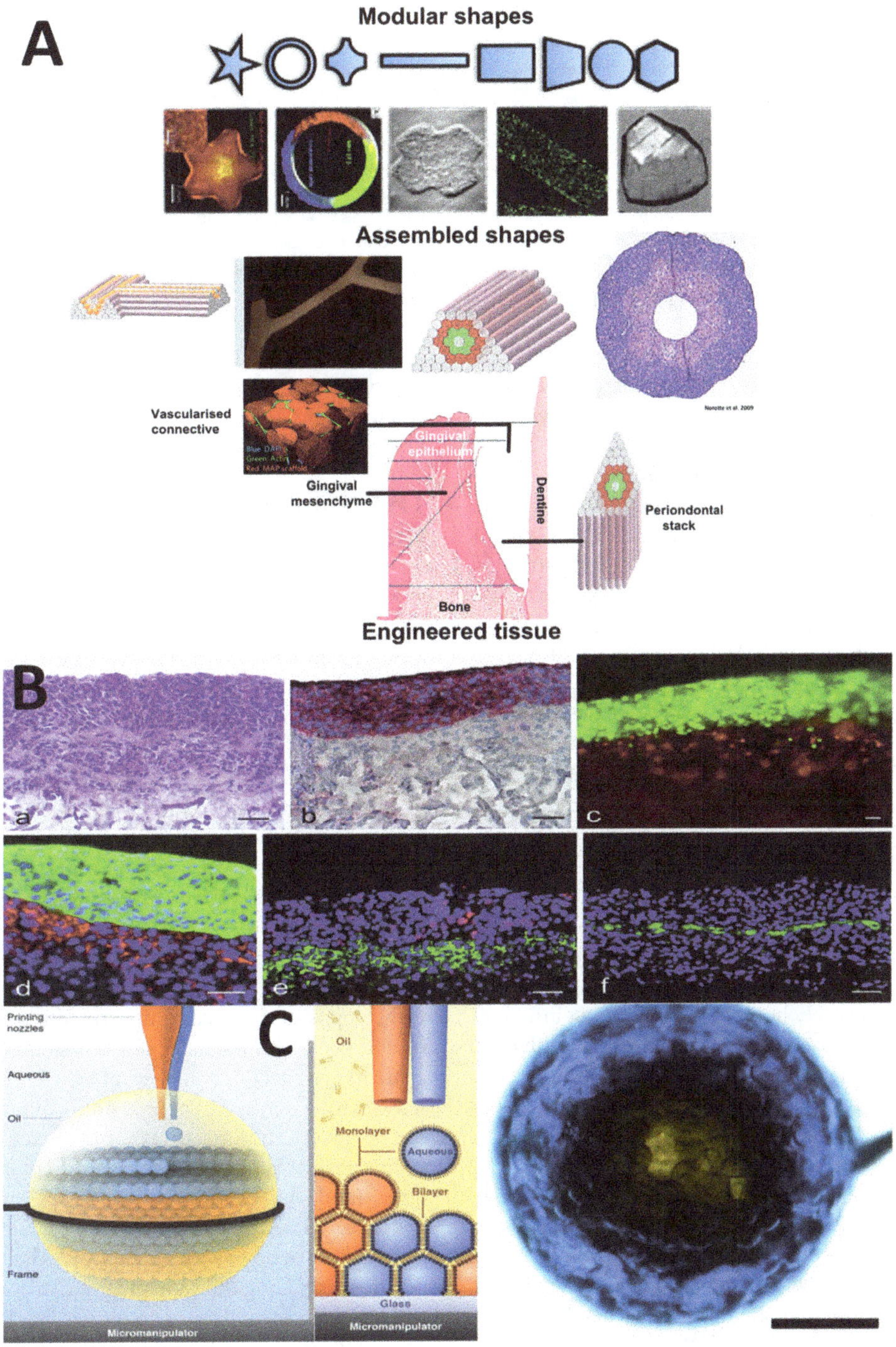


**FIGURE 2 | Selected Microfabricated modular biomaterials by laser printing, 3D microdroplet printing and microdroplet fluidics. (A)** (a) A diagram showing the basic concept for modular biomaterials design. Particular shaped blocks of material (mainly hydrogels) are created by one of the micro fabrication techniques listed. The assembly of those building blocks can be directed or allowed to randomly self-assemble. It is then possible to generate large blocks of material using combinations of the small modules. A range of different module shapes, that have been fabricated, is shown in (b). In (c) we present a diagram showing the different module structures and organization that could be used to represent the various periodontium tissues structurally and compositionally in a very basic representation to mimic the structural environments necessary for gingival epithelium development, subepithelial connective tissue formation and the stacked layers of cementum, ligament and the alveolar bone lining (McGuigan and Sefton, 2006; McGuigan et al., 2006, 2008; Nichol and Khademhosseini, 2009; Chamberlain et al., 2010; Reproduced with kind permission from PLoS, MacMillan Publishing, MYJoVE Corporation, American Association for the Advancement of Science, Royal Society of Chemistry). **(B)** (a) Showing the arrangement of printed cells in a distribution reminiscent of skin tissue; (b) Red staining to highlight the distinct keratinocyte cell region; (c) Fluorescently labeled red fibroblasts and green keratinocytes printed using the laser technique into tight and clear layers; (d) Phenotype related fluorescence tagging of fibroblasts (red) and keratinocytes for cytokeratin 14 expression. Note the densification of cells in this layer; (e) Fluorescent labeling of the printed cellular construct for proliferation using red Ki-67 and in (f) for presence of laminin basement membrane protein in green, which forms a distinct supporting layer

*(Continued)*

**FIGURE 2 | Continued**
(all scale bars = 50 microns). "Laser-Assisted BioPrinting" was used to manufacture a layered skin reproduction, which can easily be translated to other multi-layered tissues such as, the periodontium. In this microfabrication technique, a solution containing fibroblasts and keratinocytes were ejected from the solution as a continuous jet of droplets using laser force field. The droplets are collected into compound structures, onto a solid receiver substrate, where the solution is able to gel. New layers are stacked-up on the preceding layer using the same procedure. Different cell types of the skin were infused into the different layers representing the native cellular composition of human skin. This fast, automated type of layering procedure can be easily tailored to recreate the laminate "sandwich" of tissues in the periodontium (Koch et al., 2012; Reproduced with kind Permission from Wiley) **(C)** An ordered, aggregated array of droplets that can mimic certain forms of simple tissue structures. Three-dimensional printing is used to arrange assorted aqueous droplets (modules) into highly organized globular shaped microstructures. The water droplets are printed into "lipid-containing oil droplets" and coated in a lipid bi-layer. As well they are supported inside the macrodroplet. The lipid provides a soft substrate in which membrane proteins can be inserted. This provides channels between individual droplet-based mdules. The whole process is precisely controlled by the printer program settings so that diverse arrangements of architectures are conceived via computer-aided designs (Villar et al., 2013) (Reproduced with Kind permission of the American Association for the Advancement of Science).

system is hydrogel in oil at interfaces and with droplets, which enables well-delineated shapes to be generated (Gauvin and Khademhosseini, 2011). Another chemically driven system employs capillary forces to force microgel units into packing arrangements that can support themselves in tight ball and rod-like structures, for example (Fernandez and Khademhosseini, 2010). Using DNA links attached to their external surfaces, building blocks of microgel are instilled with a program for self-assembly or piecing together in precise ways coded for by the complementarity of the DNA molecules (Qi et al., 2013).

Modular biomaterial strategies have tended to employ small, single blocks of material in a thus-far limited selection of shapes (typically spheres and rods, the products of chemical laws used in their formation in aqueous solutions; **Figures 2A,C**) with variable dimensions. These small building blocks are constructed into high order architectures by three defined assembly routes: random assembly, which is governed by the chemical and physical properties of the chemical environment; stacking together layers of material; or by directed assembly in which the modules are purposefully pieced together by the action of external forces or by molecular "lock and key" decorations at the surfaces of modules (Nichol and Khademhosseini, 2009; Liu et al., 2010). However, the scale is limited to an individual function and encapsulating modules inside a bulk material. An early example was the construction of collagen microrods encased in endothelial cells (McGuigan et al., 2008). Microfluidic engineering is a powerful method for compartmentalizing many types of tissue-specific cells and microtissues for the regeneration of various tissues, production of organoids and synthesis of vascular-branched networks (Lu et al., 2015). Modular microtissues supported inside collagen-fibrin beads, up to 300 µm in diameter, grew internal vascular networks (vascularization). Embedded inside a gel, the networks extended beyond the original beads into vessel structures that formed networks, mimicking angiogenesis, after 14 days (Peterson et al., 2014). Modular biomaterials have gained popularity in drug delivery, targeting therapeutics and for immunotherapy. The increasingly complex shaping of modules is made possible by using complex fluids such as with mixtures of polyelectrolytes and surfactants (Lapitsky et al., 2008). Compartments built with biomaterials are referred to as modules. The ability to create modules small enough to mirror those in nature has profoundly increased due to advances in microfabrication strategies (Zorlutuna et al., 2012). Modules of different shapes and sizes can be printed with inkjets or molded using lithography (**Figures 2B,C**).

## TRANSFERRING MODULAR BIOMATERIALS INTO THE DENTAL CLINIC

We have described an idea about how to compartmentalize and arrange cells and their supporting components into arrangements that imitate the basic organization of the tissue units. We have provided examples of the first steps, where this has been used to mimic hepatic tissue, and structures with hexagonal packing such as, retinal pigment epithelium, corneal endothelium, and kidney papillary ducts. Layer-by-layer reconstructions with regional variations can be recreated with high aspect ratio compartments filled with nested modules, compounded too with modules representing folds and pouches containing regenerative progenitors (Nanci and Bosshardt, 2006). An important biomimetic property for the modules, housing specialized tissue, and cell specific microenvironments, is to have interfaces that permit physical and molecular exchanges with apposing tissue compartments so that growth factor receptors are bound and cell-to-cell and cell-matrix junction proteins connections are established. These are needed for self-organization (via cell fusion, differential cell adhesions and contact minimizations) and tissue morphogenesis. The positioning arrangements of the individual periodontium tissue types (and the anatomical sub-types) must be synchronized and coordinated to create the tight biological and mechanical interlocking of bone with ligamentous tissue, with cementum and with dentine along the root and gingiva epithelium, mesenchyme and epithelium at the enamel/dentine junction of the tooth. The positioning, integration, connectivity, and coordination of the anatomical and functional units of multiple tissues can be achieved using one of the various microfabrication technologies ranging between microfluidics to 3D printing techniques (**Figure 2**). Regional variations in tissue dimensionality and tissue component density, distributions, types of co-mixtures, and gradations can be engineered with modular approaches.

To improve the interplay between the components of distinct units, we anticipate constructing compartment boundaries that replicate the behavior of basement membranes and cell linings in which the cross-boundary throughput of biomolecules can be autonomously regulated by including membrane voltage-gated ion channels (out of 300), water channels (aquaporins), and cell integrins receptors (attachment and signal transduction), contact junctions, and cell-and matrix specific ligands. The design must also facilitate cell-to-cell connections and cross-migrations between compartments and networks of modules.

We have described numerous ways of building the individual microscale modules and microtissue units into larger macrostructures that can bridge the gap of the periodontal pocket. "Layer-by-layer" building designs suit the specific sandwich design (tooth–cementum–PDL–bone) of the natural human periodontium. Cell sheet engineering has created impressive reconstructions of the periodontal ligament, but the low initial mechanical properties, low blood supply through an interpenetrating vasculature and regulation of growth *in situ* are unresolved problems of cell sheets (Matsuda et al., 2007; Sawa and Miyagawa, 2013).

To achieve clinical relevance and acceptability, the modularization technique must incorporate specific tissue microenvironments that trigger and drive the development of each tissue type along its pre-programmed pathways and cascade. The individual tailoring of module microenvironments, so significant in delineating cell phenotype, proliferation, apoptosis and future fates, has already been demonstrated, as has the packing together of modules holding different environmental qualities (Guillame-Gentil et al., 2010). The partitioning and re-aggregation of such units will facilitate the programming of dynamic changes, in line with transitional phases in development and morphogenesis, as materials can be engineered with environmental responsiveness to external cues in regeneration. In addition, the modular approach allows for the integration of spaces for vasculature templating.

We have introduced a concept to biomaterials design that is not mainstream and has not been thoroughly explored as strategy for biomimetic translation of tissue organization from nature to the laboratory. The hardware is available to construct appropriate modules with sizes, shapes and attachments, which bring together tissue components and mimic tissue anatomical organization. One of the greatest unment challenges for modular tissue engineering is simulating structures for blood vessel networks without which the engineered tissue is unusable. Models for biomimicry include adult tissues as well as embryonic tooth development. Maps on how to arrange modules and their tissue components in biomimetic fashion will need to be drawn, trialed and tested for the best clinical outcomes in treating periodontitis and supporting failing and infected dental implants.

## FUNDING

This work was supported by the National Research Foundation of Korea (NRF) grant funded by the Korea government (MSIP) (No. 2014R1A2A1A11050764). This work was supported by the Korean Federation of Science and Technology Societies (KOFST) grant funded by the Korean government (MSIP: Ministry of Science, ICT and Future Planning).

## REFERENCES

Asakawa, N., Shimizu, T., Tsuda, Y., Sekiya, S., Sasagawa, T., Yamato, M., et al. (2010). Pre-vascularization of *in vitro* three-dimensional tissues created by cell sheet engineering. *Biomaterials* 14, 3903–3909. doi: 10.1016/j.biomaterials.2010.01.105

Athanasiou, K. A., Eswaramoorthy, R., Hadidi, P., and Hu, J. C. (2013). Self-organization and the self-assembling process in tissue engineering. *Annu. Rev. Biomed. Eng.* 15, 115–136. doi: 10.1146/annurev-bioeng-071812-152423

Babister, J. C., Tare, R. S., Green, D. W., Inglis, S., Mann, S., and Oreffo, R. O. (2008). Genetic manipulation of human mesenchymal progenitors to promote chondrogenesis using "bead-in-bead" polysaccharide capsules. *Biomaterials* 29, 58–65. doi: 10.1016/j.biomaterials.2007.09.006

Bosshardt, D. D., and Sculean, A. (2009). Does periodontal tissue regeneration really work? *Periodontol 2000* 51, 208–219. doi: 10.1111/j.1600-0757.2009.00317.x

Chamberlain, M. D., Butler, M. J., Ciucurel, E. C., Fitzpatrick, L. E., Khan, O. F., Leung, B. M., et al. (2010). Fabrication of micro-tissues using modules of collagen gel containing cells. *J. Vis. Exp.* 46:2177. doi: 10.3791/2177

Darveau, R. P. (2010). Periodontitis: a polymicrobial disruption of host homeostasis. *Nat. Rev. Microbiol.* 7, 481–490. doi: 10.1038/nrmicro2337

Du, Y., Ghodousi, M., Qi, H., Haas, N., Xiao, W., and Khademhosseini, A. (2011). Sequential assembly of cell-laden hydrogel constructs to engineer vascular-like microchannels. *Biotechnol. Bioeng.* 7, 1693–1703. doi: 10.1002/bit.23102

Durmus, N. G., Tasoglu, S., and Demirci, U. (2013). Bioprinting: functional droplet networks. *Nat. Mater.* 6, 478–479. doi: 10.1038/nmat3665

Erdman, N., Schmidt, L., Qin, W., Yang, X., Lin, Y., DeSilva, M. N., et al. (2014). Microfluidics-based laser cell-micropatterning system. *Biofabrication* 3:035025. doi: 10.1088/1758-5082/6/3/035025

Fernandez, J. G., and Khademhosseini, A. (2010). Micro-masonry: construction of 3D structures by microscale self-assembly. *Adv. Mater. Weinheim.* 22, 2538–2541. doi: 10.1002/adma.200903893

Gauvin, R., and Khademhosseini, A. (2011). Microscale technologies and modular approaches for tissue engineering: moving toward the fabrication of complex functional structures. *ACS Nano.* 5, 4258–4264. doi: 10.1021/nn201826d

Gruene, M., Unger, C., Koch, L., Deiwick, A., and Chichkov, B. (2011). Dispensing pico to nanolitre of a natural hydrogel by laser-assisted bioprinting. *Biomed. Eng.* 10:19. doi: 10.1186/1475-925X-10-19

Guillame-Gentil, O., Semenov, O., Roca, A. S., Groth, T., Zahn, R., Vörös, J., et al. (2010). Engineering the extracellular environment: strategies for building 2D and 3D cellular structures. *Adv. Mater. Weinheim.* 22, 5443–5462. doi: 10.1002/adma.201001747

Hansen, C. J., Aksena, R., Kolesky, D. B., Vericella, J. J., Kranz, S. J., Muldowney, G. P., et al. (2013). High-throughput printing via microvascular multinozzle arrays. *Adv. Mater. Weinheim.* 25, 96–102. doi: 10.1002/adma.201203321

Hasegawa, M., Yamato, M., Kikuchi, A., Okano, T., and Ishikawa, I. (2005). Human periodontal ligament cell sheets can regenerate periodontal ligament tissue in an athymic rat model. *Tissue Eng.* 11, 469–478. doi: 10.1089/ten.2005.11.469

Iwata, T., Yamato, M., Tsuchioka, H., Takagi, R., Mukobata, S., Washio, K., et al. (2009). Periodontal regeneration with multi-layered periodontal ligament-derived cell sheets in a canine model. *Biomaterials* 14, 2716–2723. doi: 10.1016/j.biomaterials.2009.01.032

Jakab, K., Norotte, C., Marga, F., Murphy, K., Vunjak-Novakovic, G., and Forgacs, G. (2010). Tissue engineering by self-assembly and bio-printing of living cells. *Biofabrication* 2:022001. doi: 10.1088/1758-5082/2/2/022001

Khademhosseini, A., Eng, G., Yeh, J., Fukuda, J., Blumling, J. III, and Langer, R., et al. (2006). Micromolding of photocrosslinkable hyaluronic acid for cell encapsulation and entrapment. *J. Biomed. Mater. Res. A.* 79, 522–532. doi: 10.1002/jbm.a.30821

Koch, L., Deiwick, A., Schlie, S., Michael, S., Gruene, M., Coger, V., et al. (2012). Skin tissue generation by laser cell printing. *Biotechnol. Bioeng.* 7, 1855–1863. doi: 10.1002/bit.24455

Kolesky, D. B., Truby, R. L., Gladman, A. S., Busbee, T. A., Homan, K. A., and Lewis, J. A. (2014). 3D bioprinting of vascularized, heterogeneous cell-laden tissue constructs. *Adv. Mater. Weinheim.* 26, 3124–3130. doi: 10.1002/adma.201305506

Kucukgul, C., Ozler, S. B., Inci, I., Karakas, E., Irmak, S., Gozuacik, D., et al. (2015). 3D bioprinting of biomimetic aortic vascular constructs with self-supporting cells. *Biotechnol. Bioeng.* 112, 811–821. doi: 10.1002/bit.25493

Lapitsky, Y., Zahir, T., and Shoichet, M. S. (2008). Modular biodegradable biomaterials from surfactant and polyelectrolyte mixtures. *Biomacromolecules* 1, 166–174. doi: 10.1021/bm7009416

Liu, B., Liu, Y., Lewis, A. K., and Shen, W. (2010). Modularly assembled porous cell-laden hydrogels. *Biomaterials* 31, 4918–4920. doi: 10.1016/j.biomaterials.2010.02.069

Liu Tsang, V., Chen, A. A., Cho, L. M., Jadin, K. D., Sah, R. L., DeLong, S., et al. (2007). Fabrication of 3D hepatic tissues by additive photopatterning of cellular hydrogels. *FASEB J.* 21, 790–801. doi: 10.1096/fj.06-7117com

Lu, Y.-C., Song, W., An, D., Kim, B. J., Scwartz, R., Wu, M., et al. (2015). Designing compartmentalized hydrogel microparticles for cell encapsulation and scalable 3D cell culture. *J. Mater. Chem. B.* 3, 353–360. doi: 10.1039/C4TB01735H

Matsuda, N., Shimizu, T., Yamato, M., and Okano, T. (2007). Tissue Engineering Based on Cell Sheet Technology. *Adv. Mater. Weinheim.* 19, 3089–3099. doi: 10.1002/adma.200701978

McGuigan, A. P., Bruzewicz, D. A., Glavan, A., Butte, M. J., and Whitesides, G. M. (2008). Cell encapsulation in sub-mm sized gel modules using replica molding. *PLoS ONE* 3:e2258. doi: 10.1371/journal.pone.0002258

McGuigan, A. P., Leung, B., and Sefton, M. V. (2006). Fabrication of cell-containing gel modules to assemble modular tissue-engineered constructs [corrected]. *Nat Protoc.* 1:2963–2969. doi: 10.1038/nprot.2006.443

McGuigan, A. P., and Sefton, M. V. (2006). Vascularized organoid engineered by modular assembly enables blood perfusion. *Proc. Natl. Acad. Sci. U.S.A.* 103, 11461–11466. doi: 10.1073/pnas.0602740103

Murphy, S. V., and Atala, A. (2014). 3D bioprinting of tissues and organs. *Nat. Biotechnol.* 32, 773–785. doi: 10.1038/nbt.2958

Nanci, A., and Bosshardt, D. D. (2006). Structure of periodontal tissues in health and disease. *Periodontology 2000* 40, 11–28. doi: 10.1111/j.1600-0757.2005.00141.x

Nichol, J. W., and Khademhosseini, A. (2009). Modular tissue engineering: engineering biological tissues from the bottom up. *Soft Matter.* 5, 1312–1319. doi: 10.1039/b814285h

Obregon, F., Vaquette, C., Ivanovski, S., Hutmacher, D. W., and Bertassoni, L. E. (2015). Three-dimensional bioprinting for regenerative dentistry and craniofacial tissue engineering. *J. Dent. Res.* 94, 143S–152S. doi: 10.1177/0022034515588885

Perez, R. A., and Kim, H. W. (2015). Core-shell designed scaffolds for drug delivery and tissue engineering. *Acta Biomater.* 21, 2–19. doi: 10.1016/j.actbio.2015.03.013

Perez, R. A., Kim, M., Kim, T. H., Kim, J. H., Lee, J. H., Park, J. H., et al. (2014). Utilizing core-shell fibrous collagen-alginate hydrogel cell delivery system for bone tissue engineering. *Tissue Eng. A* 20, 103–114. doi: 10.1089/ten.tea.2013.0198

Peterson, A. W., Caldwell, D. J., Rioja, A. Y., Rao, R. R., Putnam, A. J., and Stegemann, J. P. (2014). Vasculogenesis and angiogenesis in modular collagen-fibrin microtissues. *Biomater. Sci.* 2, 1497–1508. doi: 10.1039/C4BM00141A

Qi, H., Ghodousi, M., Du, Y., Grun, C., Bae, H., Yin, P., et al. (2013). DNA directed self-assembly of shape-controlled hydrogels. *Nat. commun.* 4:2275. doi: 10.1038/ncomms3275

Sawa, Y., and Miyagawa, S. (2013). Present and future perspectives on cell sheet-based myocardial regeneration therapy. *BioMed. Res. Int.* 2013:ID583912. doi: 10.1155/2013/583912

Villar, G., Graham, A. D., and Bayley, H. (2013). A tissue-like printed material. *Science* 340, 48–52. doi: 10.1126/science.1229495

Wang, M. O., Vorwald, C. E., Dreher, M. L., Mott, E. J., Cheng, M. H., Cinar, A., et al. (2015). Evaluating 3D-printed biomaterials as scaffolds for vascularized bone tissue engineering. *Adv. Mater. Weinheim.* 27, 138–144. doi: 10.1002/adma.201403943

Zorlutuna, P., Annabi, N., Camci-Unal, G., Nikkhah, M., Cha, J. M., Nichol, J. W., et al. (2012). Microfabricated biomaterials for engineering 3D tissues. *Adv. Mater. Weinheim.* 24, 1782–1804. doi: 10.1002/adma.201104631

Zorlutuna, P., Vrana, N. E., and Khademhosseini, A. (2013). The expanding world of tissue engineering: the building blocks and new applications of tissue engineered constructs. *IEEE Rev. Biomed. Eng.* 6, 47–62. doi: 10.1109/RBME.2012.2233468

# 18

# HEMA but not TEGDMA induces autophagy in human gingival fibroblasts

**Edited by:**
Gianpaolo Papaccio,
Second University of Naples, Italy

***Correspondence:**
Mirella Falconi,
Department of Biomedical and Neuromotor Sciences - Human Anatomy, University of Bologna, Via Imerio, 48, 40126 Bologna, Italy
mirella.falconi@unibo.it

*Gabriella Teti [1], Giovanna Orsini [2], Viviana Salvatore [1], Stefano Focaroli [1], Maria C. Mazzotti [3], Alessandra Ruggeri [1], Monica Mattioli-Belmonte [4] and Mirella Falconi [1]**

[1] Department of Biomedical and Neuromotor Sciences, University of Bologna, Italy, [2] Department of Clinical Sciences and Stomatology, Polytechnic University of Marche, Ancona, Italy, [3] Department of Medical and Surgical Sciences, University of Bologna, Italy, [4] Department of Clinical and Molecular Sciences, Polytechnic University of Marche, Ancona, Italy

Polymerized resin-based materials are successfully used in restorative dentistry. Despite their growing popularity, one drawback is the release of monomers from the polymerized matrix due to an incomplete polymerization or degradation processes. Released monomers are responsible for several adverse effects in the surrounding biological tissues, inducing high levels of oxidative stress. Reactive oxygen species are important signaling molecules that regulate many signal-trasduction pathways and play critical roles in cell survival, death, and immune defenses. Reactive oxygen species were recently shown to activate autophagy as a mechanism of cell survival and cell death. Although the toxicity induced by dental resin monomers is widely studied, the cellular mechanisms underlying these phenomena are still unknown. The aim of the study was to investigate the behavior of human gingival cells exposed to 2-hydroxy-ethyl methacrylate (HEMA) and triethylene glycol dimethacrylate (TEGDMA) to better elucidate the mechanisms of cell survival and cell death induced by resin monomers. Primary culture of human gingival cells were exposed to 3 mmol/L of HEMA or 3 mmol/L of TEGDMA for 24, 48, and 72 h. Morphological investigations were performed by transmission electron microscopy to analyze the ultrastructure of cells exposed to the monomers. The expression of protein markers for apoptosis (caspase – 3 and PARP) and autophagy (beclin – 1 and LC3B I/II) were analyzed by western blot to investigate the influence of dental resin monomers on mechanisms underlying cell death. Results showed that HEMA treatment clearly induced autophagy followed by apoptosis while the lack of any sign of autophagy activation is observed in HGFs exposed to TEGDMA. These data indicate that cells respond to monomer-induced stress by the differential induction of adaptive mechanisms to maintain cellular homeostasis.

**Keywords: dental resin monomers, autophagy, apoptosis, human gingival fibroblasts, adaptive cell response**

## Introduction

The development of new generations of resin-based dental restorative materials has allowed for the application of more conservative, esthetic, and long lasting restorative techniques. These adhesive techniques are extensively used in a wide variety of applications in dentistry, including restorative procedures, prosthodontics, orthodontics and preventive dentistry, making resin-based composites one of the most important groups of materials in dental practice (Bakopoulou et al., 2009). Most of these products consist of a mixture of various methacrylate monomers, such as BisGMA (2,2-bis[4-(2-hydroxy-3- metha cryloxypropoxy)phenyl]propane) and UDMA (urethane dimethacrylate) in combination with comonomers of lower viscosity, such as TEGDMA (triethyleneglycol dimethacrylate), EGDMA (ethyleneglycol dimethacrylate), or DEGDMA (diethyleneglycol dimethacrylate) (Peutzfeldt, 1997; Ilie and Hickel, 2011).

These methacrylate monomers are responsible for major clinical disadvantages, such as polymerization shrinkage of the composites leading to microleakage phenomena in the tooth-material interface (Braga et al., 2005), as well as adverse effects caused by substances released from the resinous matrix due to incomplete polymerization or resin degradation (Schweikl et al., 2006, 2007; Bakopoulou et al., 2009). Incomplete polymerization and the leaching of monomers not only decrease the mechanical properties of a restoration, but can also negatively impact the biocompatibility of the materials (Bakopoulou et al., 2009). Based on *in vitro* cell culture experiments of multiple target cells, resin monomers, such as 2-hydroxyethyl methacrylate (HEMA) and TEGDMA, were shown to specifically interfere with various vital cellular functions (Schweikl et al., 2006; Krifka et al., 2013). Dental resin monomers cause persistent inflammatory responses (Schmalz et al., 2011), down-regulate several extracellular matrix proteins (Falconi et al., 2007, 2010; Zago et al., 2008; Teti et al., 2009), disturb reparative dentinogenesis and reduce the expression of genes involved in biomineralization (About et al., 2002; Galler et al., 2011).

HEMA and TEGDMA are a likely cause of cellular stress via the formation of reactive oxygen species (ROS) (Stanislawski et al., 2003; Chang et al., 2005). Resin monomers deplete the amount of intracellular antioxidant glutathione (GSH), while in parallel increasing the formation of ROS (Chang et al., 2005) thereby inducing cell death via apoptosis, delayed cell proliferation and mineralization processes (Schweikl et al., 2007). The cellular mechanisms underlying these phenomena remain poorly understood.

Autophagy is a catabolic process aimed at recycling cellular components and damaged organelles in response to diverse conditions of stress, such as nutrient deprivation, viral infection and genotoxic stress. A growing amount of evidence in recent years argues for oxidative stress acting as the converging point of these stimuli, with ROS and reactive nitrogen species (RNS) being among the main intracellular signal transducers sustaining autophagy (Filomeni et al., 2015).

The autophagy pathway is based on distinct steps, including induction, vesicle nucleation, selective cargo recognition, autophagosome formation, autophagosome-lysosome fusion, cargo degradation, and nutrient recycling (Huang et al., 2011). More than 30 key components of the autophagy machinery encoded by autophagy-related genes (ATGs) function at different steps of this process. Beclin - 1 protein represents a primary cellular activator of autophagy involved in the autophagosome initiation and assembly (Huang et al., 2011), while microtubule associated protein light chain 3 (LC3) is mainly involved in the elongation of the autophagosome. Endogenous LC3 is detected as two bands following SDS-PAGE and immunoblotting: one represents LC3-I, which is cytosolic, and the other LC3-II, which is conjugated with autophagosomes (Parzych and Klionsky, 2014).

The aim of this study was to verify an involvement of autophagy in human gingival fibroblasts exposed to HEMA and TEGDMA. Cell viability data, transmission electron microscopy and western blotting were carried out to this aim. The main goal is to demonstrate a further adaptive cell response to oxidative stress caused by monomers, for a better understanding of the mechanisms involved in toxicity induced by resin dental materials.

## Materials and Methods

### Human Gingival Fibroblasts (HGFs)

HGFs were obtained from healthy patients subjected to gingivectomy of the molar region. Informed consent was obtained from each patient. Immediately after removal, the tissues were washed in phosphate buffer, cut in small pieces and placed in Dulbecco's Modified Eagles' Medium (DMEM) (Life Technologies, Milan, Italy), supplemented with 10% fetal calf serum (FCS), penicillin (50 UI $mL^{-1}$), and streptomycin (0.05 mg $mL^{-1}$), at 37°C in a 5% humidified $CO_2$ atmosphere. After the first passage, the HGFs were routinely cultured in DMEM supplemented with 10% FCS and were not used beyond the fifth passage.

### Cell Viability Assay

HGFs were seeded into 96-well plates ($2 \times 10^4$/well) for 24 h. Then, the medium was changed with a new one containing different concentrations of HEMA or TEGDMA and incubated for 24 h. Cell viability was established using the resazurin-based reagent cell viability reagent (PrestoBlue; Life Technologies, Grand Island, NY) diluted at 1:20 with the culture medium, allowing incubation of the reaction for 2 h at 37°C. The optical density in each well was immediately measured using a spectrophotometer Microplate Reader (Model 680, Biorad Lab Inc., CA, USA) at a wavelength of 570 nm. Each experiment was performed three times, and four replicate cell cultures were analyzed in each experiment. The optical density obtained from treated cell cultures was expressed as the percentage of untreated cells.

### HEMA and TEGDMA Treatment

HEMA and TEGDMA were previously dissolved in ethanol as solvent at a concentration of 1 mol/L (stock solution). Subsequently, HGFs were treated with 3 mmol/L HEMA or 3 mmol/L of TEGDMA for 24, 48, and 72 h.

For each concentration of HEMA and TEGDMA treatment, the final concentration of ethanol used for cell incubation was no more than 0.5%, which corresponds to a nontoxic concentration (Falconi et al., 2007). Controls consisted in untreated HGFs and HGFs exposed to the same concentration of solvent for the previously described periods of time.

### Transmission Electron Microscopy (TEM)

HGFs were initially collected after each experimental point, and fixed with 2.5% glutaraldehyde in 0.1 M cacodylate buffer for 2 h and post fixed with a solution of 1% osmium tetroxide in 0.1 M cacodylate buffer. The cells were then embedded in epoxy resins after a graded-ethanol serial dehydration step. The embedded cells were sectioned into ultrathin slices, stained by uranyl acetate solution and lead citrate, and then observed with transmission electron microscope CM10 Philips (FEI Company, Eindhoven, The Netherlands) at an accelerating voltage of 80 kV. Images were recorded by Megaview III digital camera (FEI Company, Eindhoven, The Netherlands).

### Protein Extraction and Western Blot Analysis

After each experimental point, HGFs were washed with PBS, collected and lysed in RIPA buffer (Pierce, Life technologies, Milan, Italy) containing protease inhibitor cocktail. Proteins (50μg/sample) were separated by 4-12% SDS/PAGE and transferred to a nitrocellulose membrane (GE Healthcare Europe GmbH, Milan, Italy). After being blocked with 5% skim milk powder diluted in TBS containing 5% Tween-20 for 30 min, the membrane was incubated with a primary antibody, anti-caspase - 3 (Cell Signaling Technology, Danvers, MA, USA), anti- beclin -1 (Cell Signaling Technology, Danvers, MA, USA), anti-LC3B I-II (Cell Signaling Technology, Danvers, MA, USA), anti-PARP (Santa Cruz Biotecnology, Inc, Santa Cruz, California), and anti β-tubulin (Sigma Aldrich, St. Louis, Missouri, USA) at 4°C overnight. Immunoreactive proteins were detected using an enhanced chemiluminescence light (ECL) detecting kit (GE Healthcare Europe GmbH, Milan, Italy). β-tubulin acted as a loading control. Images were obtained by Image Station 2000R (Kodak, New York, New York). The experiments were replicated at least three times, and representative results are shown.

### Statistical Analysis

Statistical differences were assessed by One-Way ANOVA ($P < 0.05$) and Dunnett multiple comparison test ($P < 0.05$). The statistical analysis was performed with GraphPad Prism 5.0 software.

## Results

### Cell Viability Assay

To establish the concentration of HEMA and TEGDMA to test in this study we firstly performed baseline dose–response curves to HEMA and TEGDMA for the human gingival cells. In HGFs exposed to HEMA for 24 h, a strong reduction in cell viability was observed at 4 and 8 mmol/L (**Figure 1A**) (IC50: 3.79 mmoL/L). A similar pattern was observed in HGFs exposed to different doses of TEGDMA where 4 and 8 mmol/L (IC50: 3.46 mmol/L) represented the concentrations to which the HGFs were extremely susceptible (**Figure 1B**). We decided to perform the following experiments testing the concentration of 3 mmoL/L for both resins, values below the respective IC50.

### TEM Analysis for HGFs exposed to HEMA

Ultrastructural analysis showed a preserved morphology in untreated HGFs, where nucleus and cytoplasmic organelles were easily detectable (**Figure 2A**). Control HGFs were characterized by several mitochondria scattered in the cytoplasm (**Figure 2E**). Cells exposed to 3 mmol/L of HEMA for 24 h showed a fibroblast like morphology, with the nucleus well preserved (**Figure 2B**). Some autophagic vesicles and empty vacuoles characterized the cytoplasm (**Figure 2F**). After 48 h of exposition, cells still showed a well preserved morphology, while in the cytoplasm a higher number of autophagic vesicles was detected (**Figures 2C,G**). Mitochondria were well preserved. At 72 h of HEMA exposition, cells showed a round or polygonal morphology (**Figure 2D**) with cytoplasm characterized by several autophagic vesicles. At higher magnification, condensed masses of chromatin were observed in the nucleus and the nuclear envelope was enlarged (**Figure 2H**). In the cytoplasm, several autophagic vesicles, swollen mitochondria and dilated rough endoplasmic reticulum (RER) were detectable (**Figure 2H**).

### Apoptosis and Autophagy in HGFs Exposed to 3 mmol/l of HEMA

To better evaluate the presence of apoptosis and autophagy in HGFs exposed to HEMA, the expression of protein markers for apoptosis (caspase – 3 and PARP) and autophagy (beclin – 1 and LC3B I/II) were analyzed by western blot. Results showed the activation of caspase – 3 (cleaved caspase -3) after 72 h of treatment, and no sign of PARP activation in all the experimental points (**Figure 3A**). On the contrary, Western blot analysis demonstrated an increase in the expression of both beclin-1 and the fast migrating form of LC3B (LC3B II, 14 kDa), while LCB I (16 kDa) decreased (**Figure 3B**), suggesting the activation of the autophagic pathway.

### TEM Analysis for HGFs Exposed to TEGDMA

TEM images showed untreated HGFs with a fibroblastic shape and a well preserved morphology. Regular cytoplasmic organelles were detected (**Figures 4A,E**). After 24 h of TEGDMA treatment, cells were slightly damaged (**Figure 4B**). The nucleus was still well preserved, while the cytoplasm was characterized by the presence of some damaged mitochondria and the lack of autophagic vesicles (**Figure 4F**). After 48 h of TEGMDA treatment, masses of condensed chromatin were observed (**Figure 4C**). Several damaged mitochondria and an enlarged Golgi apparatus were detected in the cytoplasm (**Figure 4G**). After 72 h of TEGDMA exposition, cells showed a clear morphological pattern of necrosis (**Figure 4D**). Cytoplasmic organelles were not distinguishable (**Figure 4H**).

### Apoptosis and Autophagy in HGFs Exposed to 3 mmol/l of TEGDMA

As previously described for HEMA, to better evaluate the presence of apoptosis and autophagy in HGFs exposed to TEGDMA, the expression of caspase – 3, PARP, beclin – 1 and LC3B I/II were analyzed by western blot. Results showed a light band corresponding to the cleaved fragment of caspase -3 in samples treated for 72 h, and no sign of PARP activation in all the experimental points (**Figure 5A**). Regarding autophagy, bands corresponding to the up-regulation of beclin-1 and of the fast migrating form of LC3B and LCB I were not observed (**Figure 5B**).

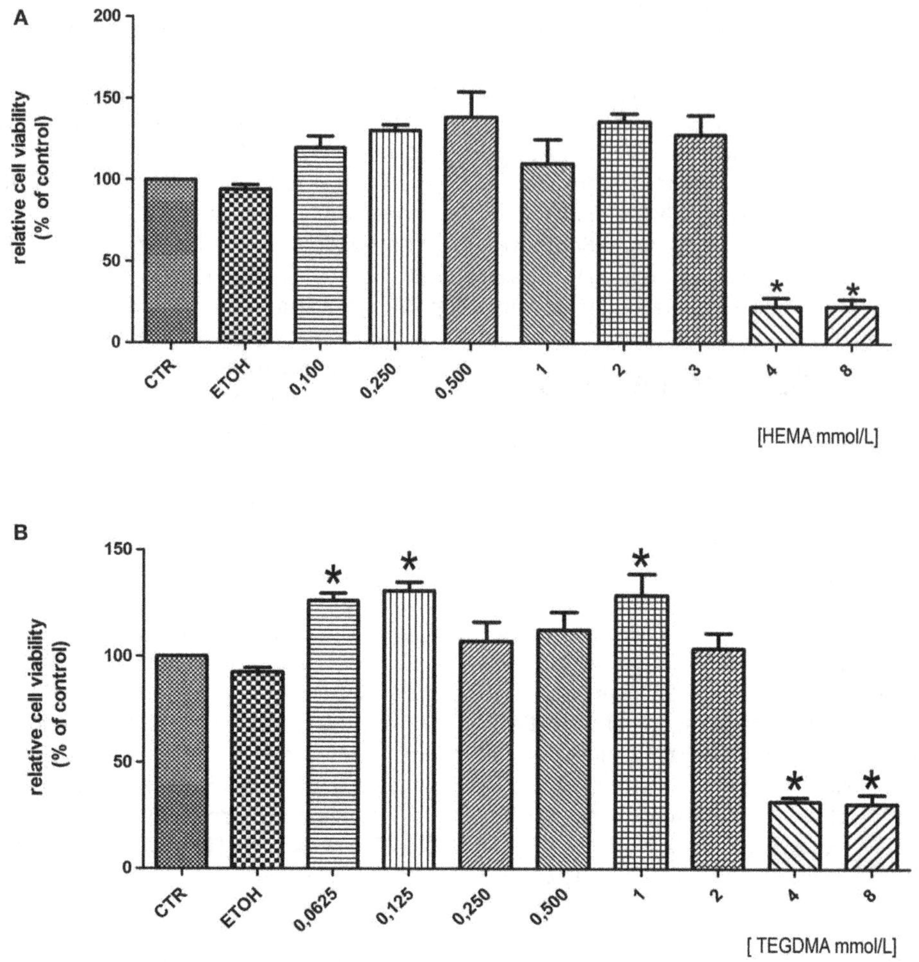


**FIGURE 1 | Cell viability assay of HGFs exposed to different concentration of HEMA (A) and TEGDMA (B) for 24 h.** Data were expressed as relative percentage ± SD compared to control HGFs (CTR). *Represents a significant difference compared to CTR HGFs, $P < 0.05$.

## Discussion

Dental resin composite are biomaterials commonly used to aesthetically restore the structure and function of teeth impaired by caries, erosion, or fracture (Krifka et al., 2013). Despite their growing popularity, there are concerns that resin-based materials may be toxic, based on the fact that they may release unpolymerized monomers, additives, and filler components in the oral environment (Van Landuyt et al., 2011; Reichl et al., 2012) responsible of adverse effects on cells and tissues nearby (Schweikl et al., 2006, 2007).

The cellular and molecular mechanisms underlying toxicity are still under discussion. Krifka et al. (2013) suggested the presence of multiple adaptive mechanisms in cell responses toward stress caused by dental resin monomers, but the role of autophagy induced by dental resin monomers as a mechanism of cell survival and/or cell death is not well understood.

The aim of the present study was to investigate the involvement of autophagy as a further adaptive mechanism against cell death in HGFs exposed to HEMA and TEGDMA.

The quantity of released dental monomers a patient may be exposed has yet to be determined.

Briefly, the rationale by which the authors have chosen the concentration of HEMA and TEGDMA is based on previous scientific reports, demonstrating that the direct contact of composite materials to dental pulp may induce local adverse effect to the dentin—pulp complex (Modena et al., 2009), even if the release of HEMA and TEGDMA has been estimated to be in micromolar and nanomolar concentrations, amounts far below levels required to cause systemic adverse effects (Van Landuyt et al., 2011; Michelsen et al., 2012). However, due to a great variety in analytical methodology employed in different studies, there is no agreement about the quantities detected in eluates of multiple composite filling materials (Nocca et al., 2011; Van Landuyt et al., 2011; Krifka et al., 2013; Botsali et al., 2014) and further studies are needed to quantify the exact amount of resin monomers release.

According to our previous works (Falconi et al., 2007; Zago et al., 2008; Teti et al., 2009) and cell viability results

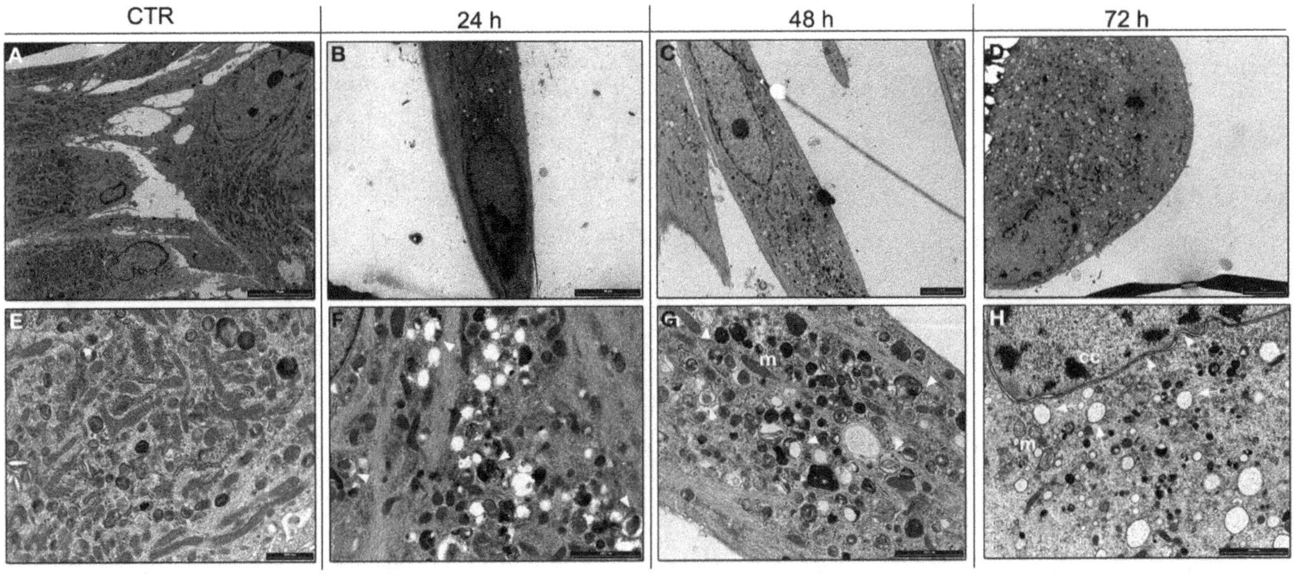


**FIGURE 2 | (A)** Control HGFs showing a well preserved morphology (bar: 10 um); **(E)** Detail of cytoplasm in control cells showing several mitochondria with a regular shape (bar: 1 um); **(B)** HGFs exposed to 3 mmol/L of HEMA for 24 h. Cells showed a preserved fibroblast morphology (bar: 10 um); **(F)** few autophagic vesicles (arrowhead) detected in the cytoplasm of HGFs treated for 24 h (bar: 2 um); **(C)** HGFs exposed to HEMA for 48 h. Nucleus is still well preserved (bar: 5 μm); **(G)** higher magnification of cytoplasm in HGFs exposed to HEMA for 48 h. Several autophagic vesicles (arrowhead) were detected. Mitochondria (m) still showed a regular shape (bar: 2.5 um); **(D)** HGFs exposed for 72 h. Cells appear round shaped and the nucleus showed masses of condensed chromatin (cc) (bar: 5 μm); **(H)** higher magnification of cytoplasm in HGFs exposed for 72 h. Dilated nucleus envelope (arrowhead) and enlarged RER (arrow) were detectable. Mitochondria (m) showed a degraded morphology (*) (bar: 2.5 um).

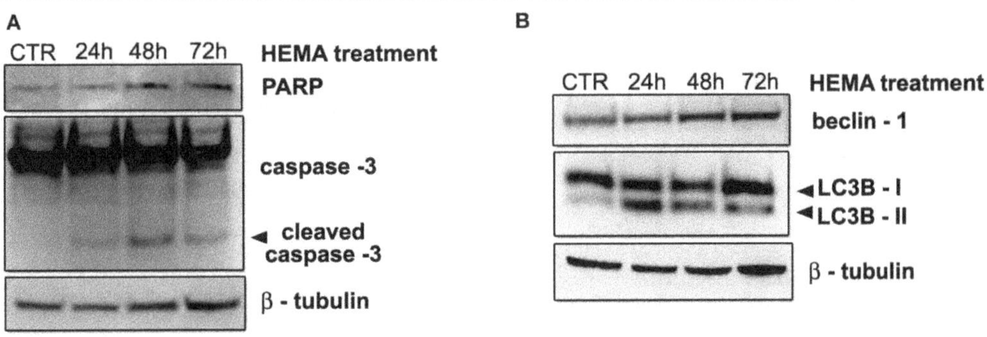


**FIGURE 3 | (A)** Western blot analysis of caspase -3 and PARP in HGFs treated with 3 mmol/L HEMA for 24, 48, 72 h. **(B)** Western blot analysis for Beclin-1 and LC3B I/II expression in HGFs exposed to 3 mmol/L HEMA for the indicated times. β—tubulin represents equal lane loading.

obtained in this study, we decided to perform all experiments at the concentration of 3 mmol/L for both monomers. These concentrations are just below the IC50 calculated for HEMA and TEGDMA.

Current findings strongly suggest that monomers enhance the formation of ROS, which is most likely the cause of cell death by apoptosis activated by dental composites and resin monomers (Stanislawski et al., 2003). Our data on ultrastructural analysis of HGFs exposed to HEMA up to 72 h demonstrated morphological features more connected with autophagy rather than apoptosis. Indeed, the presence of several intracellular double/multimembranus vesicles, called autophagosomes, which sequester cytoplasms, proteins and organelles are morphological hallmarks of autophagy (Edinger and Thompson, 2004). No ultrastructural features connected with apoptosis such as characteristic chromatin condensation and margination, as well as apoptotic bodies, (Saraste and Pulkki, 2000; Burattini et al., 2010) were detected. By the time of 72 h, damaged mitochondria, enlargement of RER and nuclear envelope suggested the presence of oxidative stress and endothelial reticulum stress (Burattini et al., 2010). The presence of autophagy in HGFs exposed to HEMA was confirmed by western blot data, in which the upregulation of beclin -1, LC3B-II and the down-regulation of LC3B-I were

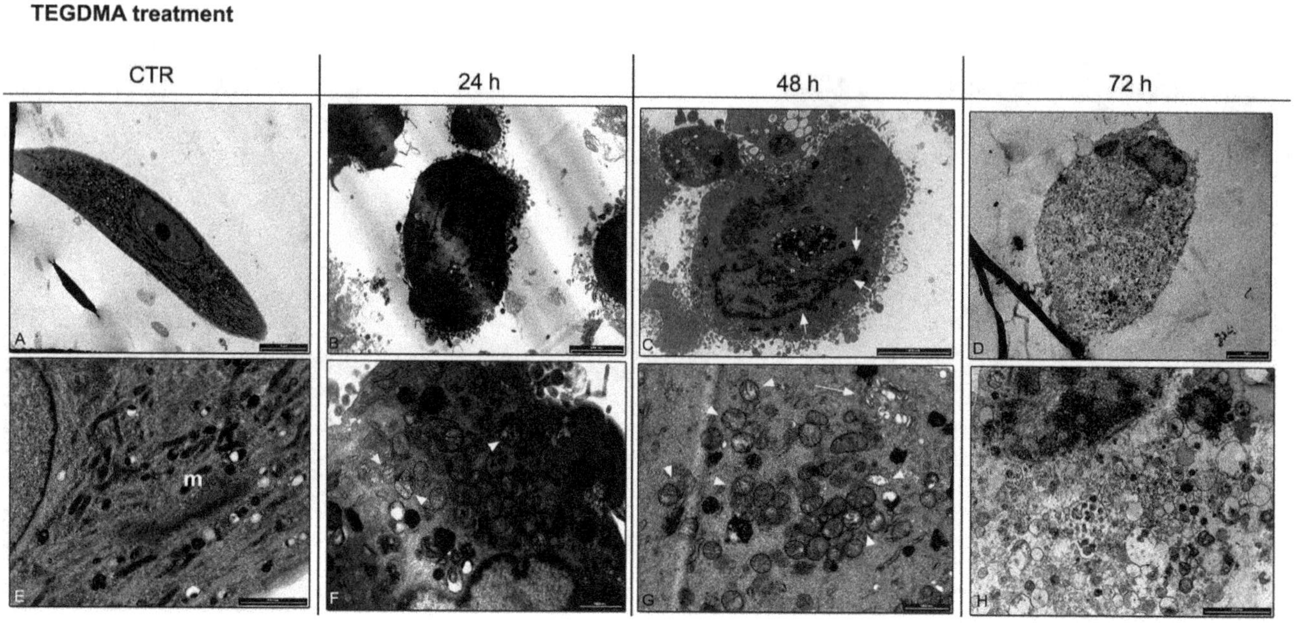


**FIGURE 4 | (A)** TEM image showing untreated HGFs with a well preserved morphology (bar: 10 um); **(E)** Detail of cytoplasm in control cells showing several mitochondria (m) with a regular shape (bar: 2 um); **(B)** HGFs exposed to 3 mmol/L of TEGDMA for 24 h. Cells showed a round shape morphology (bar: 5 um); **(F)** in the cytoplasm of HGFs treated for 24 h damage mitochondria (arrowhead) were detected (bar: 1 um). No autophagy vesicles were observed; **(C)** HGFs exposed to TEGDMA for 48 h. Chromatin condensation (arrow) was detected in the nucleus (bar: 5 um); **(G)** higher magnification of cytoplasm in HGFs exposed to TEGDMA for 48 h. Several damaged mitochondria (arrowhead) and an enlargement in Golgi apparatus (arrow) were observed (bar: 1 um); **(D)** Necrotic HGFs exposed for 72 h to 3 mmol/L of TEGDMA (bar: 10 um); **(H)** higher magnification of cytoplasm in HGFs exposed for 72 h. No cytoplasmic organelles were distinguishable (bar: 2 um).

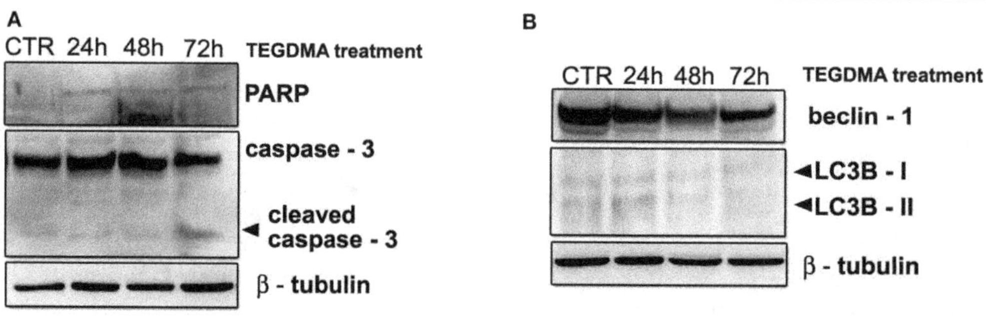


**FIGURE 5 | (A)** Western blot analysis of caspase -3 and PARP in HGFs treated with 3 mmol/L TEGDMA for 24, 48, 72 h. **(B)** Western blot analysis for Beclin-1 and LC3B I/II expression in HGFs exposed to 3 mmol/L TEGDMA for the indicated times. β—tubulin represents equal lane loading.

observed in all experimental conditions, while the activation of caspase -3 was detected only after 72 h of treatment. All these results suggest an early attempt of cells to survive by autophagy induction, followed by apoptosis after long term exposition (72 h).

Autophagy is foremost a survival mechanism that is activated in cells subjected to nutrient or obligate growth factor deprivation. When cellular stress continues, cell death may continue by autophagy alone, or else it often becomes associated with features of apoptotic or necrotic cell death (Edinger and Thompson, 2004; Krysko et al., 2008).

HGFs exposed to TEGDMA did not show a similar pattern. Electron microscopy images underlined morphological features connected with necrosis. A few morphological details connected with apoptosis, such as chromatin condensation, were observed just after 48 h of treatment (Burattini et al., 2010). Furthermore, a light band corresponding to the cleaved form of caspase – 3 was detected after 72 h of exposition. Regarding autophagy, there were no upregulation of beclin -1 protein and LC3B-II, suggesting the lack of this phenomena in cells treated with TEGDMA.

In recent years a growing amount of evidence suggests that reactive ROS and reactive nitrogen species (RNS) are among the main intracellular signal transducers sustaining autophagy (Filomeni et al., 2015). Oxidative stress induced by monomers as a result of elevated ROS generation apparently acts as a signal for the activation of pathways which control cell survival and death through the redox-sensitive activation of genes and antioxidant proteins (Krifka et al., 2013). In our experimental conditions, we believe elevated amounts of ROS induced by HEMA are responsible for the activation of autophagy as an adaptive mechanism for cells to survive. On the contrary, ROS do not activate autophagy in HGFs exposed to TEGDMA but exert cytotoxicity via apoptosis and more deeply via necrosis (Krysko et al., 2008).

In conclusion, our data indicate that cells actively respond to monomer-induced oxidative stress by the differential induction of cell death mechanism (autophagy, apoptosis and necrosis) to maintain cellular homeostasis and vital cell functions. Further experiments to investigate the exact molecular mechanisms involved in the induction of autophagy by HEMA treatment and the lack of such response in TEGDMA treated cells are in progress.

## Authorship

Each author substantially contributed to experimental procedure. In particular Dr. Teti, Prof. Falconi and Prof. Orsini planned the research and experiments. Dr. Focaroli and Dr. Mazzotti, were responsible for cell culture, dental monomers treatment and cell viability assay. Dr. Salvatore and Dr. Teti performed western blot analysis. Prof. Ruggeri and Dr. Mattioli Belmonte performed TEM analysis; Prof. Falconi and Prof. Orsini oversaw the whole research. All authors equally and competently contributed to the draft.

## Funding

This work was supported by Fondazione del Monte di Bologna e Ravenna.

## Ethical Statement

All patients provided their informed consent to participate in the study in accordance with the Declaration of Helsinki. Since the study did not expose the subjects to any risk and in agreement with the Regione Emilia Romagna and the University of Bologna Ethical Committees, instead of a written agreement form, a verbal consent was obtained from all the recruited patients. It was highlighted to all subjects that the tissue used for the study represents the usual surgical discard and that the nature of their participation in the study was entirely voluntary (freedom from coercion or undue influence, real, or imagined). Patients had sufficient opportunity to ask questions and consider their choice. The University of Bologna ethical committee approved this study.

## Acknowledgments

The authors kindly thank M. Nudi, BSc, MSc for proof reading the manuscript.

## References


About, I., Camps, J., Mitsiadis, T. A., Bottero, M. J., Butler, W., and Franquin, J. C. (2002). Influence of resinous monomers on the differentiation *in vitro* of human pulp cells into odontoblasts. *Biomed. Mater. Res.* 63, 418–423. doi: 10.1002/jbm.10253

Bakopoulou, A., Papadopoulos, T., and Garefis, P. (2009). Molecular toxicology of substances released from resin-based dental restorative materials. *Int. J. Mol. Sci.* 10, 3861. doi: 10.3390/ijms10093861

Botsali, M. S., Kuşgöz, A., Altintaş, S. H., Ülker, H. E., Tanriver, M., Kiliç, S., et al. (2014). Residual HEMA and TEGDMA release and cytotoxicity evaluation of resin-modified glass ionomer cement and compomers cured with different light sources. *Sci. World J.* 2014:218295. doi: 10.1155/2014/218295

Braga, R. R., Ballester, R. Y., and Ferracane, J. L. (2005). Factors involved in the development of polymerization shrinkage stress in resin-composites: a systematic review. *Dent. Mater.* 21, 962–970. doi: 10.1016/j.dental.2005.04.018

Burattini, S., Battistelli, M., and Falcieri, E. (2010). Morpho-functional features of *in vitro* cell death induced by physical agents. *Curr. Pharm. Des.* 16, 1376–1386. doi: 10.2174/138161210791033941

Chang, H. H., Guo, M. K., Kasten, F. H., Chang, M. C., Huang, G. F., Wang, Y. L., et al. (2005). Stimulation of glutathione depletion, ROS production and cell cycle arrest of dental pulp cells and gingival epithelial cells by HEMA. *Biomaterials* 26, 745–753. doi: 10.1016/j.biomaterials.2004.03.021

Edinger, A. L., and Thompson, C. B. (2004). Death by design: apoptosis, necrosis and autophagy. *Curr. Opin. Cell Biol.* 16, 663–669. doi: 10.1016/j.ceb.2004.09.011

Falconi, M., Ortolani, M., Teti, G., Zago, M., Orsini, G., Selan, L., et al. (2010). Suppression of procollagen {alpha}1 type 1 by long-term low-dose exposure to 2-hydroxyethylmethacrylate in human gingival fibroblasts *in vitro*. *Int. J. Toxicol.* 29, 523. doi: 10.1177/1091581810375003

Falconi, M., Teti, G., Zago, M., Pelotti, S., Breschi, L., and Mazzotti, G. (2007). Effects of HEMA on type I collagen protein in human gingival fibroblasts. *Cell Biol. Toxicol.* 23, 313–322. doi: 10.1007/s10565-006-0148-3

Filomeni, G., De Zio, D., and Cecconi, F. (2015). Oxidative stress and autophagy: the clash between damage and metabolic needs. *Cell Death Differ.* 22, 377. doi: 10.1038/cdd.2014.150

Galler, K. M., Schweikl, H., Hiller, K. A., Cavender, A. C., Bolay, C., D'Souza, R. N., et al. (2011). TEGDMA reduces mineralization in dental pulp cells. *J. Dent. Res.* 90, 257. doi: 10.1177/0022034510384618

Huang, J., Lam, G. Y., and Brumell, J. H. (2011). Autophagy signaling through reactive oxygen species. *Antioxid. Redox Signal* 14, 2215. doi: 10.1089/ars.2010.3554

Ilie, N., and Hickel, R. (2011). Resin composite restorative materials. *Aust. Dent. J.* 56, 59. doi: 10.1111/j.1834-7819.2010.01296.x

Krifka, S., Spagnuolo, G., Schmalz, G., and Schweikl, H. (2013). A review of adaptive mechanisms in cell responses towards oxidative stress caused by dental resin monomers. *Biomaterials* 34, 4555. doi: 10.1016/j.biomaterials.2013.03.019

Krysko, D. V., Vanden Berghe, T., D'Herde, K., and Vandenabeele, P. (2008). Apoptosis and necrosis: detection, discrimination and phagocytosis. *Methods* 44, 205. doi: 10.1016/j.ymeth.2007.12.001

Michelsen, V. B., Kopperud, H. B., Lygre, G. B., Björkman, L., Jensen, E., Kleven, I. S., et al. (2012). Detection and quantification of monomers in unstimulated whole saliva after treatment with resin-based composite fillings *in vivo*. *Eur. J. Oral. Sci.*120, 89. doi: 10.1111/j.1600-0722.2011.00897.x

Modena, K. C., Casas-Apayco, L. C., Atta, M. T., Costa, C. A., Hebling, J., Sipert, C. R., et al. (2009). Cytotoxicity and biocompatibility of direct and indirect pulp capping materials. *J. Appl. Oral. Sci.* 17, 544–554.

Nocca, G., Ragno, R., Carbone, V., Martorana, G. E., Rossetti, D. V., Gambarini, G., et al. (2011). Identification of glutathione-methacrylates adducts in gingival fibroblasts and erythrocytes by HPLC-MS and capillary electrophoresis. *Dent. Mater.* 27, 87–98. doi: 10.1016/j.dental.2011.01.002

Parzych, K. R., and Klionsky, D. J. (2014). An overview of autophagy: morphology, mechanism, and regulation. *Antioxid. Redox Signal* 20, 460. doi: 10.1089/ars.2013.5371

Peutzfeldt, A. (1997). Resin components in dentistry: the monomer systems. *Eur. J. Oral Sci.* 105, 97–116. doi: 10.1111/j.1600-0722.1997.tb00188.x

Reichl, F. X., Löhle, J., Seiss, M., Furche, S., Shehata, M. M., Hickel, R., et al. (2012). Elution of TEGDMA and HEMA from polymerized resin-based bonding systems. *Dent. Mater.* 28, 1120. doi: 10.1016/j.dental.2012.06.010

Saraste, A., and Pulkki, K. (2000). Morphologic and biochemical hallmarks of apoptosis. *Cardiovasc. Res.* 45, 528–537. doi: 10.1016/S0008-6363(99)00384-3

Schmalz, G., Krifka, S., and Schweikl, H. (2011). Toll-like receptors, LPS, and dental monomers. *Adv. Dent. Res.* 23, 302–306. doi: 10.1177/0022034511405391

Schweikl, H., Hartmann, A., Hiller, K. A., Spagnuolo, G., Bolay, C., Brockhoff, G., et al. (2007). Inhibition of TEGDMA and HEMA-induced genotoxicity and cell cycle arrest by N-acetylcysteine. *Dent. Mater.* 23, 688–695. doi: 10.1016/j.dental.2006.06.021

Schweikl, H., Spagnuolo, G., and Schmalz, G. (2006). Genetic and cellular toxicology of dental resin monomers. *J. Dent. Res.* 85, 870–877. doi: 10.1177/154405910608501001

Stanislawski, L., Lefeuvre, M., Bourd, K., Soheili-Majd, E., Goldberg, M., and Périanin, A. (2003). TEGDMA-induced toxicity in human fibroblasts is associated with early and drastic glutathione depletion with subsequent production of oxygen reactive species. *J. Biomed. Mater. Res. A* 66, 476–482. doi: 10.1002/jbm.a.10600

Teti, G., Mazzotti, G., Zago, M., Ortolani, M., Breschi, L., Pelotti, S., et al. (2009). HEMA down-regulates procollagen alpha1 type I in human gingival fibroblasts. *J. Biomed. Mater. Res. A* 90, 256. doi: 10.1002/jbm.a.32082

Van Landuyt, K. L., Nawrot, T., Geebelen, B., De Munck, J., Snauwaert, J., Yoshihara, K., et al. (2011). How much do resin-based dental materials release? A meta-analytical approach. *Dent. Mater.* 27, 723. doi: 10.1016/j.dental.2011.05.001

Zago, M., Teti, G., Mazzotti, G., Ruggeri, A., Breschi, L., Pelotti, S., et al. (2008). Expression of procollagen alpha1 type I and tenascin proteins induced by HEMA in human pulp fibroblasts. *Toxicol. In vitro* 22, 1153. doi: 10.1016/j.tiv.2008.03.008

19

# Biomimetically enhanced demineralized bone matrix for bone regenerative applications

**Edited by:**
*Thimios Mitsiadis,*
*University of Zurich, Switzerland*

***Correspondence:**
*Sriram Ravindran*
*sravin1@uic.edu*

*Sriram Ravindran [1]*, Chun-Chieh Huang [1], Praveen Gajendrareddy [2] and Raghuvaran Narayanan [1]*

*[1] Departments of Oral Biology, University of Illinois at Chicago, Chicago, IL, USA, [2] Departments of Periodontics, University of Illinois at Chicago, Chicago, IL, USA*

Demineralized bone matrix (DBM) is one of the most widely used bone graft materials in dentistry. However, the ability of DBM to reliably and predictably induce bone regeneration has always been a cause for concern. The quality of DBM varies greatly depending on several donor dependent factors and also manufacturing techniques. In order to standardize the quality and to enable reliable and predictable bone regeneration, we have generated a biomimetically-enhanced version of DBM (BE-DBM) using clinical grade commercial DBM as a control. We have generated the BE-DBM by incorporating a cell-derived pro-osteogenic extracellular matrix (ECM) within clinical grade DBM. In the present study, we have characterized the BE-DBM and evaluated its ability to induce osteogenic differentiation of human marrow derived stromal cells (HMSCs) with respect to clinical grade commercial DBM. Our results indicate that the BE-DBM contains significantly more pro-osteogenic factors than DBM and enhances HMSC differentiation and mineralized matrix formation *in vitro* and *in vivo.* Based on our results, we envision that the BE-DBM has the potential to replace DBM as the bone graft material of choice.

**Keywords: demineralized bone matrix, biomimetic materials, mesenchymal stem cells, bone regeneration and repair, extracellular matrix**

## INTRODUCTION

Bone is the second most transplanted organ in the human body (Marino and Ziran, 2010). Bone grafting is used in several aspects of medicine ranging from placement of dental implants and spinal fusions to regenerating lost bone resulting from trauma or congenital anomalies. With respect to children, over 75% of birth defects are craniofacial anomalies (such as cleft palate) that require bone reconstruction procedures (Zuk, 2008). Finally, with the many wars around the globe, the incidence of injuries requiring bone reconstruction is at an all time high.

Over the past decade several natural and synthetic biomaterials have been developed to aid bone regeneration (George and Ravindran, 2010). However, they have not been able to replace currently used bone graft materials successfully. On the other hand, the focus of current research has shifted away from improving the performance of existing clinical materials. The most immediate clinical need lies in the generation of products that improve the performance of existing materials or modified versions of existing clinical materials with improved performance. The focus of this study is the generation of a modified bone graft material with superior osteoinductive properties.

The gold standard for bone regenerative procedures is autografts. In situations that require significant quantity of bone to be regenerated, donor site morbidity becomes an issue with autografts. Under these circumstances, bone graft materials such as allograft bone are used. DBM is a commonly used allograft bone material. It is most commonly used in appendicular, axial and craniofacial bone regenerative applications (Gruskin et al., 2012). However, The quality and effectiveness of commercial DBM varies with processing techniques and several donor dependent factors (Zhang et al., 1997; Schwartz et al., 1998; Lohmann et al., 2001; Traianedes et al., 2004). As a result, bone regeneration and augmentation procedures do not have predictable outcomes. Additionally, the osteoinductive and osteogenic capacity of allograft DBM is significantly lesser than autografts (Marino and Ziran, 2010).

Very few medical products have as much variability in composition and performance as commercially available clinical grade DBM. Several inconsistencies have been reported with respect to DBM: The presence of osteoinductive growth factors (such as BMPs) varies significantly between batches of DBM and even amongst samples from the same batch (Bae et al., 2006, 2010). DBM from female donors has been shown to contain higher quantities of BMPs (Pietrzak et al., 2006). DBM shows variability in performance depending on donor age (Schwartz et al., 1998) and finally revascularization of DBM and allograft bone is poor (Delloye et al., 2007). Recently, several approaches have been studied to enhance the effectiveness of DBM such as remineralization (Soicher et al., 2013; Horváthy et al., 2015)and use of platelet rich plasma (Han et al., 2009) with limited and varied results. DBM in combination with bone marrow aspirates has been used to treat bone cysts effectively (Park et al., 2008; Di Bella et al., 2010), but it is not as effective when used for fracture healing and large quantity bone regenerative applications (Drosos et al., 2015).

Clinically, in order to augment bone regeneration, recombinant BMP2 is used clinically. Although it is very potent, dosage issues and ectopic effects are major problems facing BMP2 usage. Many complications have been reported recently causing serious safety concerns among clinicians (Thibault et al., 2010; Zara et al., 2011).

We have attempted to solve the inherent problems associated with DBM by generating a biomimetically-modified version of clinical grade DBM. We have achieved this by incorporating the native extracellular matrix (ECM) of differentiating mesenchymal stem cells (MSCs) within it. We chose MSCs as the source cell for creating the ECM, as the resulting matrix would be a combination of MSC matrix and that of MSCs differentiating into osteoblasts. This can provide an ideal environment for patient specific MSCs. The other alternative would be osteoblasts. However, osteoblasts have limited proliferative ability and hence would not be able to populate the DBM as effectively as MSCs. We have published previously on the standardization of conditions and advantages of using biomimetic scaffolds for tissue regeneration (Ravindran et al., 2012, 2014b). We have used these techniques to develop a modified clinical product with enhanced performance. The aim of this study was to evaluate the ability of our biomimetically enhanced DBM (BE-DBM) in comparison with commercial DBM using *in vitro* and *in vivo* experimental models to analyze if the BE-DBM depicts improved stem cell attachment, proliferation and differentiation abilities.

## MATERIALS AND METHODS

### Cell Culture

Human marrow stromal cells were used in this study (HMSCs). These primary cells were obtained from NIH-funded center for research resources, Tulane Center for the preparation and distribution of adult stem cells. The cells are representative of marrow stromal cells from five donors between the age groups of 19 and 29 consisting of both male and female donors (Sekiya et al., 2002). We have published previously using these cells and they have been verified for multipotetncy (Ravindran et al., 2012, 2014a, 2015). The cells were cultured in αMEM basal media (Gibco) with 20% FBS (Gibco), 1% L-glutamine (Gibco) and 1% antibiotic-antimycotic solution (Gibco).

### Generation of BE-DBM

BE-DBM was generated using clinical grade commercial DBM. Two different types of DBM were used to generate BE-DBM. For the *in vitro* experiments, we used DBM granules alone. For the *in vivo* experiments, we used DBM granules containing cortical bone chips to serve as internal control for mineralized matrix. For each of the two types of DBM, we used three vials to generate the BE-DBM. Once the BE-DBM was prepared, they were stored as lyophilized samples until required for experimental use.

BMSCs were seeded on to the DBM at a concentration of 1 million cells per 250 mg of DBM granules and cultured in standard BMSC culture media for a period of 24 h. After this, the cells were cultured for 2 weeks in osteogenic culture media (growth media containing100 μg/ml ascorbic acid, 10 mM β-glycerophosphate and 10 mM dexamethasone). This was performed to induce osteogenic differentiation of the BMSCs and to facilitate the generation of a pro-osteogenic matrix. After 2 weeks, the DBM granules containing BMSCs were decellularized using our published protocol (Ravindran et al., 2012, 2014a,b). Briefly, the samples were incubated for 1 h at 37°C in TBS containing 0.5% triton x-100. After this, the cells were lysed using 25 mM ammonium hydroxide solution. They were then washed extensively in TBS followed by one wash in HBSS. Finally, DNAse digestion was performed and the samples were washed in double deionized water extensively, lyophilized and stored. Decellularization was verified by immunostaining for tubulin and DAPI nuclear staining.

### Proliferation Experiment

Twenty thousand HMSCs were seeded on to equal amounts of DBM and BE-DBM in quadruplicates. Eight hours post seeding, the unattached cells were removed by aspiration and the samples were washed using three exchanges of fresh media to ensure complete removal of all unattached cells. Twenty-four hours post seeding, the number of live cells was quantitatively measured using an MTT cell titer assay (Promega). The number of cells present at various time points up to 1 week was also measured to obtain the proliferation rate.

### Electron Microscopy

Electron microscopic evaluation was performed on DBM and BE-DBM in their natural state as well as when subjected to *in vitro* mineralization. To generate mineralized DBM and BE-DBM, *in vitro* mineralization experiment was performed as per previously published protocols (Ravindran et al., 2014b). Electron microscopic evaluation of the samples was performed after coating the samples with platinum and palladium using Hitachi S3000 electron microscope. Energy dispersive X-ray (EDX) analysis in variable pressure mode was performed to obtain elemental information on the mineralized samples and also to obtain ratios of calcium to phosphorus in the samples. For all EDX analyses, the samples were not coated.

## *In Vitro* Differentiation of HMSCs

500,000 HMSCs were seeded on to 50 mg of DBM or BE-DBM and cultured in standard growth media for 2 weeks in quadruplicates. After 2 weeks, the RNA was isolated from both sets of samples. After first strand synthesis (BioRad first strand synthesis kit), quantitative real time PCR (qPCR) was performed using gene specific primers. **Table 1** lists the primer sequences used in this study. All expression data were normalized to housekeeping genes GAPDH and B2M.

## *In Vivo* Implantation

All experiments were performed in accordance with approved animal care protocols (Assurance No: A3460-01). 500,000 HMSCs were seeded on to 50 mg of DBM or BE-DBM encapsulated in collagen sponges (Zimmer collagen tape) and implanted subcutaneously on the back of 2-month-old athymic male nude mice for a period of 2 weeks. Experiments were performed in triplicate. We had two groups one with commercial DBM and the other with BE-DBM. Two implants were placed on the back of each mouse. On one side, we placed the DBM implant and the other side contained the BE-DBM implant. Therefore, a total of three mice were used for this study. After 2 weeks, the samples were extracted, fixed in 4% neutral buffered formalin, paraffin embedded and sectioned.

## Histology and Immunohistochemistry

Hematoxylin and eosin (H&E) staining and alizarin red staining was performed as per previously published protocols (Ravindran et al., 2014a). Expression of proteins in the explant sections as well as DBM and BE-DBM sections were performed either using peroxidase conjugated secondary antibodies (Vector Laboratories DAB kit) or using secondary antibodies conjugated to fluorescent probes. The following primary antibodies were used: rabbit polyclonal anti fibronectin antibody (1/250, abcam), mouse monoclonal anti tubulin antibody (1/1000, Sigma), mouse monoclonal anti bone morphogenetic protein 2 (BMP2) antibody (1/100, abcam), rabbit polyclonal anti transforming growth factor β1 (TGFβ) antibody (1/100, abcam), mouse monoclonal anti phosphorylated serine (pSer) antibody (1/100, Santa Cruz biotechnology), mouse monoclonal anti DMP-1 antibody (1/1000, a gift from Dr. Chunlin Qin, Baylor College of Dentistry), mouse monoclonal anti osteocalcin antibody (1/100, abcam), mouse monoclonal anti runt-related transcription factor x2 (RUNX2) antibody (1/100, abcam), mouse monoclonal anti von Willebrand factor antibody (1/100, Santa Cruz biotechnology), rabbit polyclonal anti VEGF antibody (1/100, abcam).

Fluorescent microscopy was performed using a Zeiss LSM 710 laser scanning confocal microscope or a BioRad Zoe fluorescent microscope. For all comparative samples, the imaging parameters were maintained constant. For peroxidase stained sections, microscopy was performed using a Zeiss Axio Observer D1 microscope or an EVOS XL Core microscope (Life Technologies).

## Quantitation of Proteins in DBM and BE-DBM

ELISA was used to quantitate the amount of a few important pro-osteogenic proteins in the DBM and BE-DBM. Equal amounts of both materials (10 mg) were placed in 96 well plates in quadruplicates. The material was blocked with 5% BSA for 1 h and incubated with the appropriate primary antibody overnight at 4°C. The samples were then washed four times in PBS and incubated with a biotinylated secondary antibody (1/250, Vector Laboratories) and then subsequently washed four times with PBS and incubated with peroxidase conjugated avidin (Vector Laboratories) for 1 h at room temperature. Finally, the samples were incubated with an ELISA substrate (Turbo TMB ELISA substrate, Thermo Scientific) for 5 min at room temperature. The reaction was stopped by the addition of 1 M sulfuric acid. The solution was then transferred to empty 96 well plate wells and absorbance at 490 nm was recorded. The following primary

**TABLE 1 | qPCR primer sequences.**

| Gene | Forward | Reverse |
|---|---|---|
| FGF2 | 5′-AGA AGA GCG ACC CTC ACA TCA-3′ | 5′-CGG TTA GCA CAC ACT CCT TTG-3′ |
| GDF10 | 5′-AGA TCG TTC GTC CAT CCA ACC-3′ | 5′-GGG AGT TCA TCT TAT CGG GAA CA-3′ |
| PHEX | 5′-GAG GCA CTC GAA TTG CCC T-3′ | 5′-ACT CCT GTT TAG CTT GGA GAC TT-3′ |
| OCN | 5′-AGC CCA TTA GTG CTT GTA AAG G-3′ | 5′-CCC TCC TGC TTG GAC ACA AAG-3′ |
| VEGFA | 5′-AGG GCA GAA TCA TCA CGA AGT-3′ | 5′-AGG GTC TCG ATT GGA TGG CA-3′ |
| GAPDH | 5′-CAG GGC TGC TTT TAA CTC TGG-3′ | 5′-TGG GTG GAA TCA TAT TGG AAC A-3′ |
| B2M | 5′-GAG GCT ATC CAG CGT ACT CCA-3′ | 5′-CGG CAG GCA TAC TCA TCT TTT-3′ |
| DMP1 | 5′-CTC CGA GTT GGA CGA TGA GG-3′ | 5′-TCA TGC CTG CAC TGT TCA TTC-3′ |

*Table showing the forward and reverse primer sequences for the genes used in the real time PCR analyses.*

antibodies were used: rabbit polyclonal anti fibronectin antibody (1/500), mouse monoclonal anti BMP2 antibody (1/250), rabbit polyclonal anti VEGF antibody (1/250), mouse monoclonal anti phosphorylated serine, threonine, and tyrosine antibody (1/1000, abcam).

## Statistical Analysis

Student's $t$-test was performed for the indicated experiments to verify statistical significance. A $P < 0.05$ (95% confidence interval) was considered as statistically significant.

# RESULTS

## Characterization of BE-DBM for Enhanced Presence of Pro-osteogenic Proteins

DBM and BE-DBM sections were immunostained for the presence of several ECM proteins and growth factors that play an important role in osteogenesis and osteogenic differentiation of MSCs. **Figure 1** shows representative images of 3D confocal microscopy. Results presented in **Figure 1** show that the BE-DBM contains more pro-osteogenic proteins when compared to the commercially available DBM. The BE-DBM was generated using the DBM from the same container and hence, the results are directly comparable. In the results presented in **Figure 1**, tubulin was used as a negative control to show the absence of intracellular proteins (**Figures 1B,B1**). DAPI staining was performed to show the absence of cellular DNA (**Figures 1C,C1**). Rabbit and mouse secondary antibody controls were performed to show absence of non-specific staining (**Figures 1D,D1**).

The results presented in **Figure 1** show that the BE-DBM contains more structural proteins such as fibronectin (**Figure 1A** vs. **Figure 1A1**), growth factors (**Figures 1F,G** vs. **Figures 1F2,G1**), pro-angiogenic factors such as VEGF (**Figure 1E** vs. **Figure 1E1**), phosphorylated proteins (**Figure 1H** vs. **Figure 1H1**) proteases (**Figure 1I** vs. **Figure 1I1**), and nucleating proteins (**Figure 1J** vs. **Figure 1J1**).

ELISA was used to quantify the increased presence of fibronectin, BMP2, VEGF, and phosphorylated proteins. The graph presented in **Figure 1K** shows a statistically significant increase in the presence of these proteins within the BE-DBM when compared to DBM.

## Electron Microscopic Evaluation of DBM and BE-DBM

The microstructure of DBM and BE-DBM was evaluated using electron microscopy. **Figure 2** represents results from

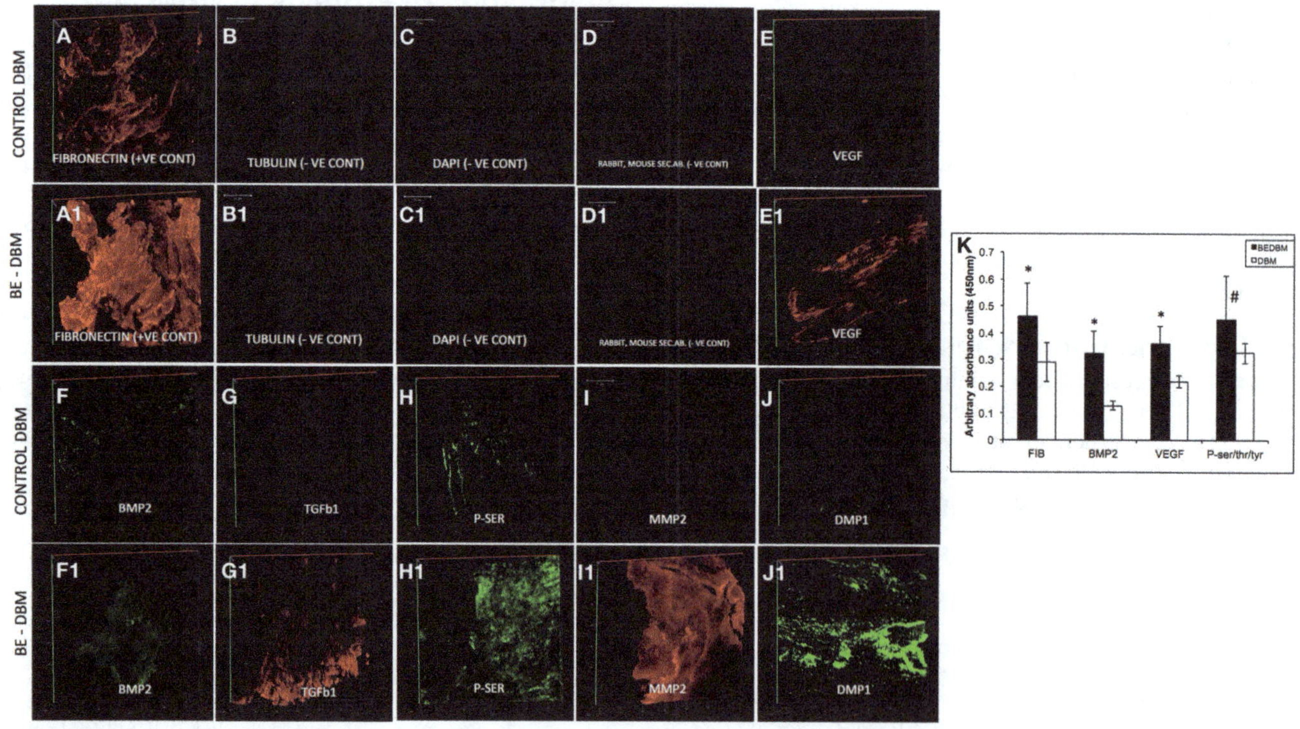


**FIGURE 1 | ECM proteins in DBM and BE-DBM.** Images compare the expression of representative ECM proteins in DBM **(A–J)** and BE-DBM **(A1–J1)**. All images except **B,B1,C,C1,D,D1** (scale bar represents 20 μm for these images) are 3D renderings of z-stack confocal images. Tubulin **(B,B1)** was used as a negative control for absence of intracellular proteins and DAPI **(C,C1)** nuclear staining was used as negative control for absence of cellular DNA. Immunostaining was performed for Fibronectin **(A,A1)**, VEGF **(E,E1)**, BMP2 **(F,F1)**, TGFβ1 **(G,G1)**, proteins containing phosphorylated serines **(H,H1)** matrix metalloproteinase 2 (MMP2, **I,I1**) and DMP1 **(J,J1)**. Panel **(K)** is a graphical representation of the relative amounts of select ECM proteins in both DBM and BE-DBM ($n = 4$). The quantified proteins were: Fibronectin (FIB), BMP2, VEGF, and phosphorylated proteins (P-ser/thr/tyr). Statistical significance was measured using student's $t$-test. *Represents statistical significance with $P < 0.05$ and #represents statistical significance with $P < 0.1$. Phosphorylated proteins were quantified using an antibody that recognizes phosphorylated serine, threonine and tyrosine residues.

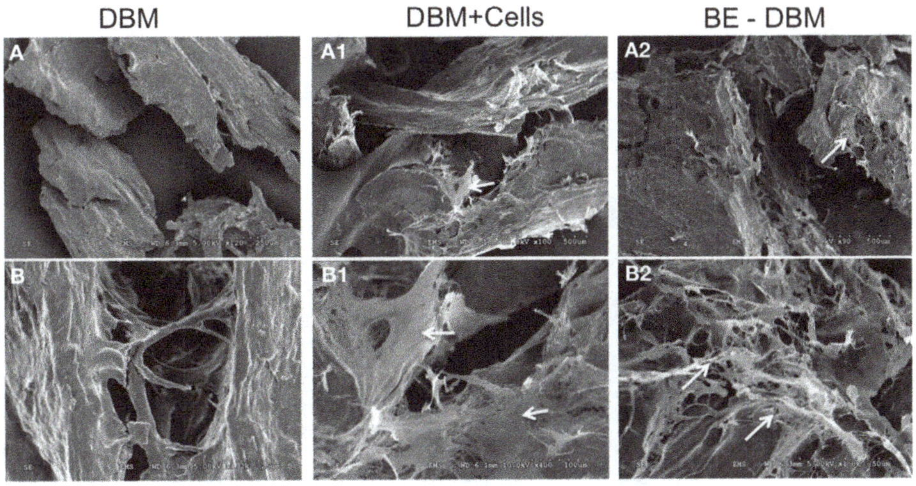


**FIGURE 2 | Electron microscopic evaluation of DBM and BE-DBM.** Images are representative electron micrographs of DBM **(A,B)**, DBM with HMSCs **(A1,B1)** and BE-DBM **(A2,B2)**. Panels **(A,A1,A2)** are low magnification images. Panels **(B–B2)** are higher magnification images showing the microstructure. The white arrows in **(A1,B1)** point to the cells. White arrows in **(A2,B2)** point to ECM deposition in the BE-DBM samples. Note the absence of such structures in images **(A,B)**.

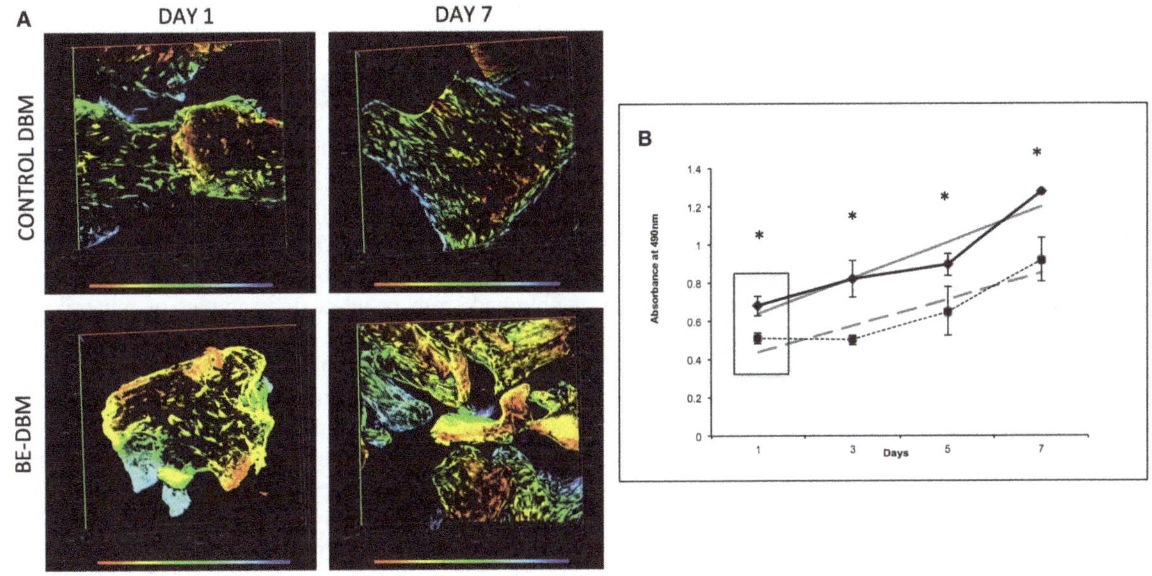


**FIGURE 3 | Attachment and proliferation of HMSCs in DBM and BE-DBM. (A)** Represents 3D renderings of z-stack confocal images of HMSCs within DBM and BE-DBM after 1 day and 1 week. These images provide qualitative proof that the BE-DBM promotes enhanced stem cell attachment and proliferation. The color-coding in the renderings represents depth as indicated by the depth scale below. **(B)** Represents proliferation of HMSCs in the DBM (dotted lines) and BE-DBM (solid lines) over 1 week. The data points represent mean of quadruplicates with standard deviation as error. The slope of the linear lines (dotted lines for DBM and solid lines for BE-DBM) provides the rate of proliferation. HMSCs in the BE-DBM showed a 34.52% increase in proliferation rate. The boxed region in the graph represents data obtained at day 1. A 34.07% ($P < 0.01$ by student's *t*-test) increase in initial cell attachment was seen in BE-DBM with respect to DBM. The data at all time points was statistically significant with $P < 0.05$. *above each point represents statistical significance.

this experiment. **Figures 2A,B** are images of commercial DBM. **Figures 2A1,B1** show the presence of HMSCs on the DBM before decellularization is performed. **Figures 2A2,B2** show images of BE-DBM containing the cell-secreted ECM. Upon comparing **Figures 2A,B** pertaining to DBM with **Figure 2A2** and **Figure 2B2** pertaining to BE-DBM it is possible to observe increased presence of fibrillar structures within the BE-DBM samples. The white arrows in **Figure 2A2** and **Figure 2B2** point to these structures. These structures represent the ECM deposition within the DBM.

## The BE-DBM Promotes Improved Stem Cell Attachment and Proliferation

An MTT assay was used to quantitate proliferation of HMSCs on DBM and BE-DBM. Results presented in **Figure 3B** show that the BE-DBM promotes improved stem cell attachment (boxed

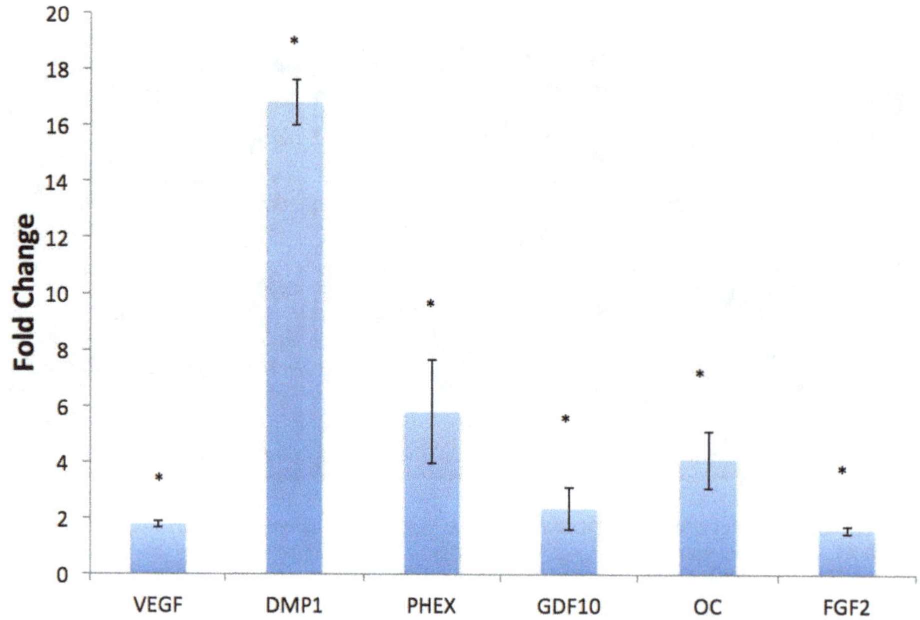


**FIGURE 4 | *In vitro* regulation of osteogenic genes.** The graph represents fold change in gene regulation of key pro-osteogenic genes and growth factors in BE-DBM with respect to control DBM. Data are represented as mean fold change obtained from quadruplicate experiments with standard deviation as error. Student's *t*-test used to obtain statistical significance with respect to control. *Represents significance of $P < 0.05$.

area representing the 1 day time point). A 34.07% ($P < 0.01$ by student's *t*-test) increase in cellular attachment was observed in the BE-DBM compared to DBM. Rate of proliferation was obtained by calculating the slope of the lines representing proliferation of the cells over a period of 1 week. The results showed that the BE-DBM enhanced the rate of proliferation of HMSCs by 34.52%.

**Figure 3A** shows representative images of HMSCs in DBM and BE-DBM after 1 day and 7 days. The images show qualitatively the increased presence of cells in the BE-DBM at these time points.

## The BE-DBM Promotes Improved Osteogenic Differentiation of HMSCs *in Vitro*

HMSCs were cultured under normal growth conditions in both DBM and BE-DBM for 2 weeks. qPCR results presented in **Figure 4** show a statistically significant change in the expression of several key pro-osteogenic proteins such as DMP1, phosphate regulating endopeptidase homolog X (PHEX) and osteocalcin. We also observed significant increase in the expression of osteogenic growth factors such as growth and differentiation factor 10 (GDF10) and FGF2 and pro angiogenic factor VEGF.

## The BE-DBM Promotes Improved Matrix Mineralization *in Vitro*

The ability of DBM and BE-DBM to promote nucleation of calcium phosphate crystals was evaluated using an *in vitro* nucleation experiment. Under these conditions, the DBM did not nucleate a large amount of calcium phosphate crystals. Results presented in **Figures 5A,B** show similar microstructure to DBM that was not subjected to *in vitro* nucleation experiment (**Figures 2A,B**). On the other hand, results presented in **Figures 5A1,B1** show the presence several structures resembling nucleated calcium phosphate crystals. These images were obtained from pt/pd-coated samples of mineralized DBM and BE-DBM. In addition, imaging of mineralized DBM and BE-DBM was performed on uncoated samples in variable pressure mode. Results presented in **Figure 5C** show the presence of a few calcium phosphate crystals in the DBM samples. The bright areas in the image (white arrows) are calcium phosphate deposits. The presence of calcium and phosphorus was verified by EDX elemental analysis (**Figure 5D**). The ratio of calcium to phosphorus in these deposits was 1.485 ($S.D = 0.175$, $n = 8$).

On the other hand, results presented in **Figure 5C1** show a very robust deposition of calcium phosphate throughout the BE-DBM sample (white arrows). Presence of calcium and phosphorus was verified using EDX analysis (**Figure 5D1**) and the ratio of calcium to phosphorus was 1.645 ($S.D = 0.106$, $n = 8$). The difference in the Calcium to phosphorus ratio between the two samples was statistically significant with a *P*-value of 0.033 using student's *t*-test.

## The BE-DBM Promotes Improved Osteogenic Differentiation *in Vivo*

Gene expression data is not valuable if protein expression does not follow *in vivo*. HMSCs were seeded on to DBM and BE-DBM, wrapped in clinical grade collagen sponges and implanted subcutaneously for 2 weeks in immunocompromised mice. Results presented in **Figure 6** show that the HMSCs in BE-DBM

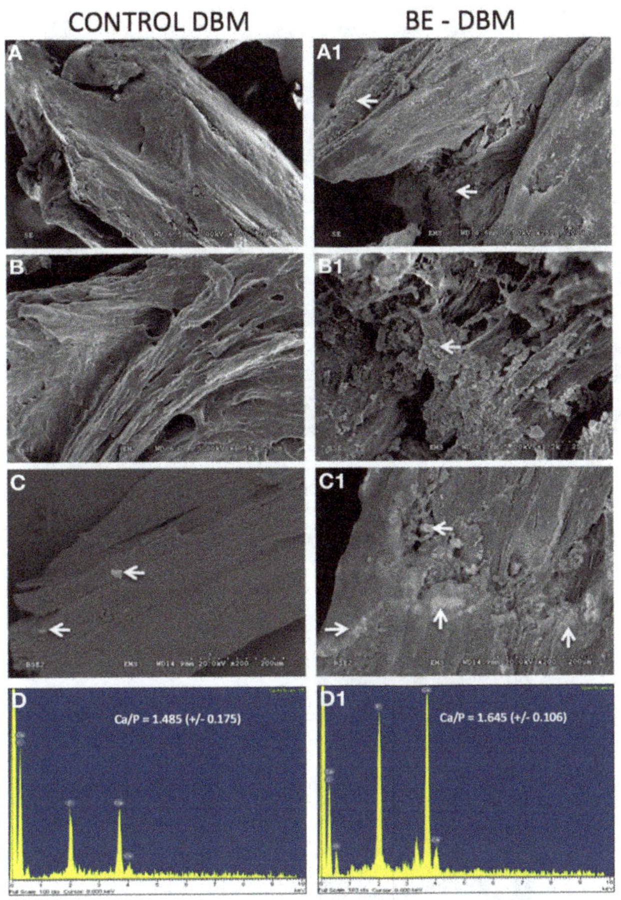


**FIGURE 5 | *In vitro* calcium phosphate nucleation.** Panels **(A–C)** are representative electron micrographs of DBM samples subjected to *in vitro* calcium phosphate nucleation. Panels **(A1–C1)** are electron micrographs of BE-DBM samples subjected to *in vitro* nucleation. Note the increased deposition on the BE-DBM samples. Panels **(C,C1)** were acquired using samples that were not coated with pt/pd. White arrows in **(C,C1)** indicate areas of calcium phosphate deposition. Panels **(D,D1)** are representative EDX spectrums of DBM and BE-DBM samples respectively showing the presence of calcium and phosphorus.

expressed higher amounts of osteocalcin, DMP1, BMP2, TGFβ1, and RUNX2 when compared to those in commercial DBM.

## The BE-DBM Promotes Enhanced Mineralization and Vascularization *in Vivo*

The key to successful bone regeneration is collagen deposition and matrix mineralization. The 2-week explant sections were stained with H&E to observe general tissue architecture. Results presented in **Figures 7A,A1** show more robust eosin staining in the BE-DBM sections compared to DBM sections indicating a higher presence of collagen. Alizarin red staining was performed to look for calcium deposition. Results presented in **Figures 7B,B1** show that the BE-DBM containing sections showed more robust staining with alizarin red indicating a higher calcium deposition in the matrix.

The DBM that was used for generating the BE-DBM and control DBM samples for *in vivo* experiments contained cortical bone chips. The cortical bone chips served as an internal control for collagen presence and calcium presence in natural bone. The black arrows in **Figures 7A,A1,B,B1** point to cortical bone chips.

Angiogenesis is vital for bone regeneration. Our results indicate that the BE-DBM contains more VEGF compared to commercially available DBM (**Figures 1E,E1**). We analyzed if this translated to improved vascularization *in vivo*. The BE-DBM sections showed a higher amount of von Willebrand factor positive endothelial cells than the DBM sections (**Figures 7C,C1**) indicating that the BE-DBM promoted migration of host endothelial cells better than DBM. We quantified the von Willebrand factor staining. Six images spanning three samples for each group were used for this purpose. In the BE-DBM samples, on an average 10.53% of the area in the images stained positive for von Willebrand factor as opposed to 2.15% in the DBM samples. Student's $t$-test on the data showed a $P$-value of 0.0196 indicating that the data was statistically significant.

Additionally, the DBM samples did not show any endothelial cells within the samples. In certain areas, we were able to observe endothelial cells in the periphery of the sample. However, these may include some mouse connective tissue as well. We included these areas as well in our calculation. The * in **Figures 7C,C1** indicate cortical bone chips. When the H&E stained sections were imaged using a confocal microscope, RBCs were observed only in the BE-DBM sections indicating active blood flow (**Figures 7D,D1**). This data corroborates well with the von Willebrand factor staining of the samples that indicated that there were no endothelial cells within the DBM samples. The presence of RBCs were not scattered, but concentrated in the shape of vessels (yellow arrows in **Figure 7D**) indicating that they were not from random bleeding. Finally, no secondary antibody non-specific staining was observed in our experiments (**Figures 7E,E1**).

## DISCUSSION

The ECM is a dynamic environment that dictates cellular behavior and tissue functionality. We have published several articles on the use of decellularized ECM as a biomimetic biomaterial for tissue regeneration (Ravindran et al., 2012, 2014a,b). Decellularized biomimetic matrices have gained prominence recently and have been evaluated for several tissue engineering applications such as heart (Moroni and Mirabella, 2014), lung (Petersen et al., 2012; Calle et al., 2015), and cartilage (Schwarz et al., 2012). The advantage of these matrices over other biomaterials is that they can provide a tissue specific environment. Several studies have shown the effectiveness and safety of this process (Crapo et al., 2011). The limitation however, is the maintenance of tissue integrity (Moroni and Mirabella, 2014). In the case of DBM this is not an issue as the starting material itself is demineralized and decellularized bone particles.

In this study, we have characterized a biomimetically-enhanced version of clinical DBM that has the potential to significantly improve the quality of bone regenerative procedures. Our results show that the BE-DBM contains significantly more pro-osteogenic factors. One of the significant observations was the increased presence of fibronectin.

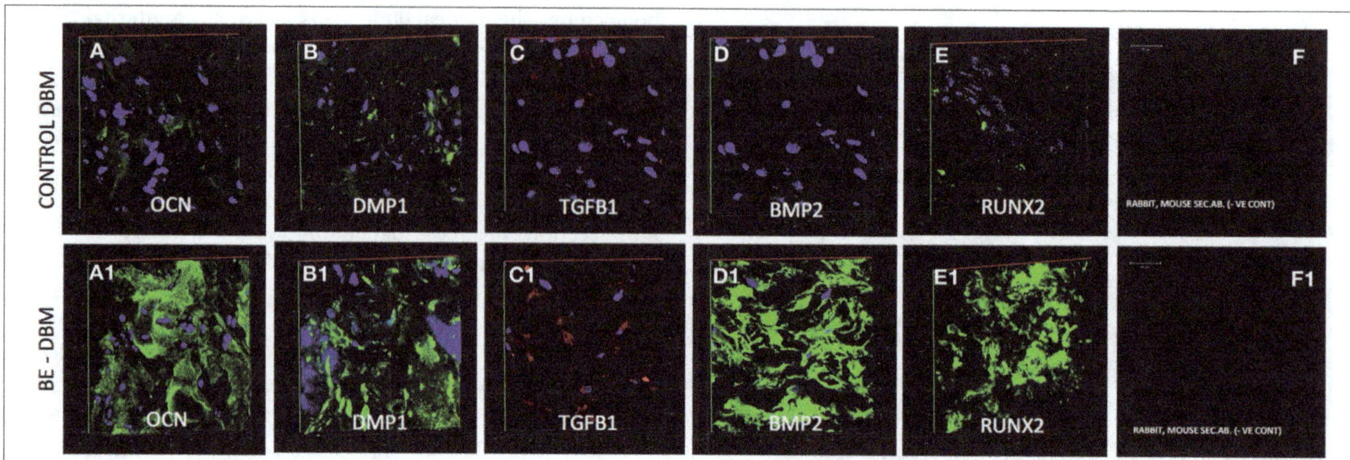


**FIGURE 6 | Immunohistochemistry of DBM and BE-DBM *in vivo* explants.** All images except secondary antibody controls **(F,F1)** are 3D renderings of z-stack confocal images. Scale bar in **(F,F1)** represents 20 μm. The 3D images represent expression of osteocalcin (OCN, **A,A1**), DMP1 **(B,B1)**, TGFβ1 **(C,C1)**, BMP2 **(D,D1)**, and RUNX2 **(E,E1)** in DBM **(A–E)** and BE-DBM **(A1–E1)** samples after 2 weeks of subcutaneous implantation with HMSCs in immunocompromised mice. Note the marked increase in the expression levels of all the proteins in the BE-DBM.

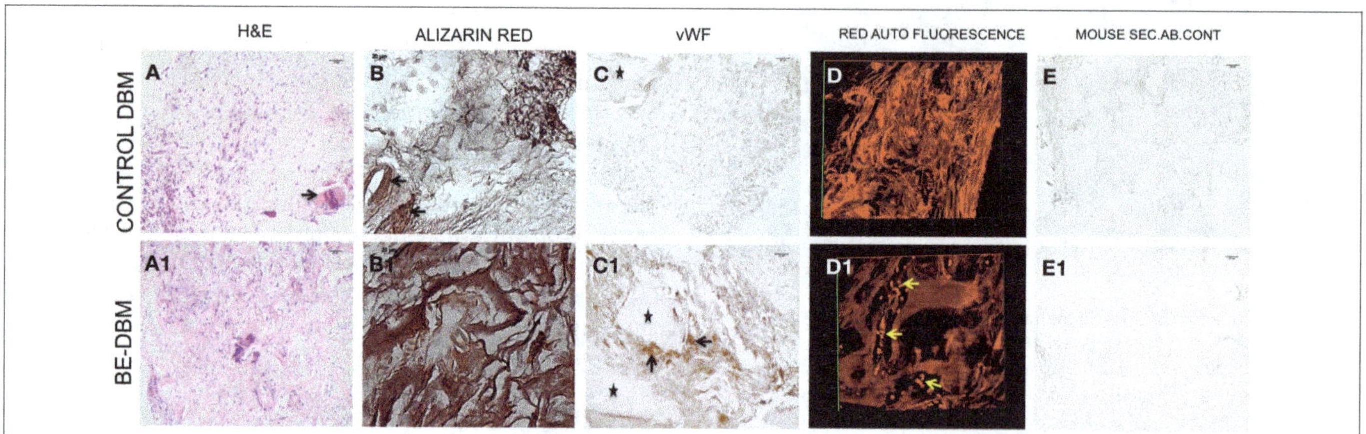


**FIGURE 7 | Histology of DBM and BE-DBM *in vivo* explants. (A,A1)** Represent H&E stained sections of DBM and BE-DBM explants, respectively. The arrow in **(A)** points to a cortical bone chip. **(B,B1)** Represent alizarin red stained sections from DBM and BE-DBM explants. **(C,C1)** Represent DBM and BE-DBM sections immunohistochemically stained for von Willebrand factor. The arrows in **(C1)** point to positively stained endothelial cells in the BE-DBM section. *Symbols in **(C,C1)** represent cortical bone chips. **(D,D1)** Represent 3D confocal images of red channel auto fluorescence from H&E stained DBM and BE-DBM sections. The yellow arrows in **(D1)** point to RBCs. **(E,E1)** Represent mouse secondary antibody controls for the DBM and BE-DBM sections. Scale bar in all other images represents 20 μm.

Fibronectin binds several growth factors (Goerges and Nugent, 2004; Zhu and Clark, 2014). Therefore, an increase in fibronectin can result in increased sequestration of growth factors *in vivo*. Apart from fibronectin, growth factors such as VEGF, BMP2, and TGFβ1 were also observed in increased amounts in the BE-DBM compared to DBM. The BE-DBM also contained significantly higher amounts of phosphorylated proteins. Phosphorylated proteins serve as the source for inorganic phosphorus during hydroxyapatite nucleation. Therefore, the increased presence of these proteins was an encouraging sign that the BE-DBM may promote faster and better nucleation. Although the qualitative and quantitative data provided in this study is not an exhaustive list of proteins present in the matrix, they provide a good overview to summarize that the BE-DBM that we have generated contains significantly more pro-osteogenic proteins.

During bone regeneration, recruitment of MSCs to the site is critical for new bone formation. Therefore, a bone regenerative material should possess the ability to promote stem cell attachment and proliferation. The BE-DBM promoted improved stem cell attachment and proliferation compared to DBM indicating its enhanced potential to recruit stem cells. Additionally, the BE-DBM also promotes better osteogenic differentiation of MSCs compared to DBM.

Our results indicated statistically significant regulation of key pro-osteogenic genes. Our results indicated a significant increase in the expression levels of PHEX, DMP1 and OC. PHEX and

DMP1 are extremely important for mineralized matrix formation and regulate FGF23 expression (Martin et al., 2011). PHEX is an endopeptidase that acts upon the mineralization inhibitor osteopontin to positively regulate mineralized matrix formation (Zhu and Clark, 2014). DMP1 is a multi-functional pro-osteogenic protein that possesses several intra and extracellular roles ranging from control of MSC differentiation to serving as a collagen binding protein that actively nucleates hydroxyapatite (He et al., 2003; He and George, 2004; Ravindran et al., 2008; Eapen et al., 2010). OC is one of the most abundant non-collagenous proteins in bone. OC acts as an endocrine hormone and plays a pivotal role in bone formation and increase in bone mineral density (Lee et al., 2007). Apart from these key regulators of bone formation, the BE-DBM also stimulated an increase in the expression levels of the pro-angiogenic growth factor VEGF and pro-osteogenic growth factors GDF10 (Kaihara et al., 2003; Marsell and Einhorn, 2009) and FGF2 (Hong et al., 2010; Kigami et al., 2013). These results indicated the enhanced potential of the BE-DBM to induce MSC differentiation.

When subjected to *in vitro* nucleation experiments to explore the calcium phosphate nucleating ability of the BE-DBM compared to DBM, the BE-DBM showed a more robust nucleating ability with calcium to phosphorus ratio similar to that of hydroxyapatite found in bone. Collectively, our *in vitro* experiments indicated that the BE-DBM is better than DBM in promoting stem cell attachment, proliferation, differentiation and hydroxyapatite nucleation.

When BE-DBM and DBM were compared *in vivo* in a subcutaneous implantation model with HMSCs, the BE-DBM promoted better collagen synthesis and formation of a better-calcified matrix as evidenced by our histological data. These observations are in line with our *in vitro* data that indicated the ability of the BE-DBM to promote these events better than DBM. Additionally, in line with the positive regulation of pro-angiogenic factors *in vitro,* the BE-DBM also promoted better migration of host endothelial cells and vascularization when compared to commercial DBM. Finally, fluorescence immunohistochemistry of the explant sections revealed that the BE-DBM was able to promote better osteogenic differentiation of MSCs by inducing higher levels of expression of pro-osteogenic non-collagenous proteins such as OC and DMP1, growth factors such as BMP2 and TGFβ1 (Yamamoto et al., 2000; Ozkan et al., 2007) and important pro-osteogenic transcription factors such as RUNX2 (Komori, 2008; Zhang et al., 2009). These results indicated that the BE-DBM accelerated osteogenic differentiation and matrix mineralization *in vivo.*

Overall, the data presented in this manuscript shows that the BE-DBM promotes better differentiation of HMSCs *in vitro* and *in vivo.* However, further investigation using large animal critical-size bone defect models is required to verify the improved osteoinductive properties of BE-DBM. Our efforts at present are focused on these models and if successful, this product can bring about standardization to the quality and performance of DBM that is critically lacking at present. DBM is widely used in craniofacial bone regeneration, spinal fusion and in non-union fracture healing in conjunction with autologous bone (Gruskin et al., 2012). Based on our results, we predict that the BE-DBM will enable faster regeneration of higher quality bone in these applications.

This is the first report that shows that it is possible to generate a biomimetic ECM incorporated DBM that has the potential replace the existing material. The amount of ECM incorporated within DBM to generate BE-DBM can be standardized by the use of cell lines and by controlling the cell number, density and culture conditions using a bioreactor. If these conditions are standardized, it is feasible to scale up the production of BE-DBM for commercial use.

## ACKNOWLEDGMENTS

This work was supported by NIH grant DE023806, UIC Chancellor's Discovery fund award and UIC Proof of Concept award to SR.

## REFERENCES

Bae, H., Zhao, L., Zhu, D., Kanim, L. E., Wang, J. C., and Delamarter, R. B. (2010). Variability across ten production lots of a single demineralized bone matrix product. *J. Bone Joint Surg. Am.* 92, 427–435. doi: 10.2106/JBJS.H.01400

Bae, H. W., Zhao, L., Kanim, L. E., Wong, P., Delamarter, R. B., and Dawson, E. G. (2006). Intervariability and intravariability of bone morphogenetic proteins in commercially available demineralized bone matrix products. *Spine (Phila Pa 1976)* 31, 1299–1306. discussion 1307–1298. doi: 10.1097/01.brs.0000218581.92992.b7

Calle, E. A., Mendez, J. J., Ghaedi, M., Leiby, K. L., Bove, P. F., Herzog, E. L., et al. (2015). Fate of distal lung epithelium cultured in a decellularized lung extracellular matrix. *Tissue Eng. Part A* 21, 1916–1928. doi: 10.1089/ten.TEA.2014.0511

Crapo, P. M., Gilbert, T. W., and Badylak, S. F. (2011). An overview of tissue and whole organ decellularization processes. *Biomaterials* 32, 3233–3243. doi: 10.1016/j.biomaterials.2011.01.057

Delloye, C., Cornu, O., Druez, V., and Barbier, O. (2007). Bone allografts: what they can offer and what they cannot. *J. Bone Joint Surg. Br.* 89, 574–579. doi: 10.1302/0301-620X.89B5.19039

Di Bella, C., Dozza, B., Frisoni, T., Cevolani, L., and Donati, D. (2010). Injection of demineralized bone matrix with bone marrow concentrate improves healing in unicameral bone cyst. *Clin. Orthop. Relat. Res.* 468, 3047–3055. doi: 10.1007/s11999-010-1430-5

Drosos, G. I., Touzopoulos, P., Ververidis, A., Tilkeridis, K., and Kazakos, K. (2015). Use of demineralized bone matrix in the extremities. *World J. Orthop.* 6, 269–277. doi: 10.5312/wjo.v6.i2.269

Eapen, A., Sundivakkam, P., Song, Y., Ravindran, S., Ramachandran, A., Tiruppathi, C., et al. (2010). Calcium-mediated stress kinase activation by DMP1 promotes osteoblast differentiation. *J. Biol. Chem.* 285, 36339–36351. doi: 10.1074/jbc.M110.145607

George, A., and Ravindran, S. (2010). Protein templates in hard tissue engineering. *Nano Today* 5, 254–266. doi: 10.1016/j.nantod.2010.05.005

Goerges, A. L., and Nugent, M. A. (2004). pH regulates vascular endothelial growth factor binding to fibronectin: a mechanism for control of extracellular matrix storage and release. *J. Biol. Chem.* 279, 2307–2315. doi: 10.1074/jbc.M308482200

Gruskin, E., Doll, B. A., Futrell, F. W., Schmitz, J. P., and Hollinger, J. O. (2012). Demineralized bone matrix in bone repair: history and use. *Adv. Drug Deliv. Rev.* 64, 1063–1077. doi: 10.1016/j.addr.2012.06.008

Han, B., Woodell-May, J., Ponticiello, M., Yang, Z., and Nimni, M. (2009). The effect of thrombin activation of platelet-rich plasma on demineralized bone matrix osteoinductivity. *J. Bone Joint Surg. Am.* 91, 1459–1470. doi: 10.2106/JBJS.H.00246

He, G., Dahl, T., Veis, A., and George, A. (2003). Nucleation of apatite crystals *in vitro* by self-assembled dentin matrix protein 1. *Nat. Mater.* 2, 552–558. doi: 10.1038/nmat945

He, G., and George, A. (2004). Dentin matrix protein 1 immobilized on type I collagen fibrils facilitates apatite deposition *in vitro*. *J. Biol. Chem.* 279, 11649–11656. doi: 10.1074/jbc.M309296200

Hong, K. S., Kim, E. C., Bang, S. H., Chung, C. H., Lee, Y. I., Hyun, J. K., et al. (2010). Bone regeneration by bioactive hybrid membrane containing FGF2 within rat calvarium. *J. Biomed. Mater. Res. A* 94, 1187–1194. doi: 10.1002/jbm.a.32799

Horváthy, D. B., Vácz, G., Toró, I., Szabó, T., May, Z., Duarte, M., et al. (2015). Remineralization of demineralized bone matrix in critical size cranial defects in rats: a 6-month follow-up study. *J. Biomed. Mater. Res. B Appl. Biomater.* doi: 10.1002/jbm.b.33446. [Epub ahead of print].

Kaihara, S., Bessho, K., Okubo, Y., Sonobe, J., Komatsu, Y., Miura, M., et al. (2003). Over expression of bone morphogenetic protein-3b (BMP-3b) using an adenoviral vector promote the osteoblastic differentiation in C2C12 cells and augment the bone formation induced by bone morphogenetic protein-2 (BMP-2) in rats. *Life Sci.* 72, 1683–1693. doi: 10.1016/S0024-3205(02)02477-3

Kigami, R., Sato, S., Tsuchiya, N., Yoshimakai, T., Arai, Y., and Ito, K. (2013). FGF-2 angiogenesis in bone regeneration within critical-sized bone defects in rat calvaria. *Implant Dent.* 22, 422–427. doi: 10.1097/ID.0b013e31829d19f0

Komori, T. (2008). Regulation of bone development and maintenance by Runx2. *Front. Biosci.* 13, 898–903. doi: 10.2741/2730

Lee, N. K., Sowa, H., Hinoi, E., Ferron, M., Ahn, J. D., Confavreux, C., et al. (2007). Endocrine regulation of energy metabolism by the skeleton. *Cell* 130, 456–469. doi: 10.1016/j.cell.2007.05.047

Lohmann, C. H., Andreacchio, D., Köster, G., Carnes, D. L. Jr., Cochran, D. L., Dean, D. D., et al. (2001). Tissue response and osteoinduction of human bone grafts *in vivo*. *Arch. Orthop. Trauma Surg.* 121, 583–590. doi: 10.1007/s004020100291

Marsell, R., and Einhorn, T. A. (2009). The role of endogenous bone morphogenetic proteins in normal skeletal repair. *Injury* 40(Suppl. 3), S4–S7. doi: 10.1016/S0020-1383(09)70003-8

Martin, A., Liu, S., David, V., Li, H., Karydis, A., Feng, J. Q., et al. (2011). Bone proteins PHEX and DMP1 regulate fibroblastic growth factor Fgf23 expression in osteocytes through a common pathway involving FGF receptor (FGFR) signaling. *FASEB J.* 25, 2551–2562. doi: 10.1096/fj.10-177816

Moroni, F., and Mirabella, T. (2014). Decellularized matrices for cardiovascular tissue engineering. *Am. J. Stem Cells* 3, 1–20.

Ozkan, K., Eralp, L., Kocaoglu, M., Ahishali, B., Bilgic, B., Mutlu, Z., et al. (2007). The effect of transforming growth factor beta1 (TGF-beta1) on the regenerate bone in distraction osteogenesis. *Growth Factors* 25, 101–107. doi: 10.1080/08977190701352594

Park, I. H., Micic, I. D., and Jeon, I. H. (2008). A study of 23 unicameral bone cysts of the calcaneus: open chip allogeneic bone graft versus percutaneous injection of bone powder with autogenous bone marrow. *Foot Ankle Int.* 29, 164–170. doi: 10.3113/FAI.2008.0164

Petersen, T. H., Calle, E. A., Colehour, M. B., and Niklason, L. E. (2012). Matrix composition and mechanics of decellularized lung scaffolds. *Cells Tissues Organs* 195, 222–231. doi: 10.1159/000324896

Pietrzak, W. S., Woodell-May, J., and McDonald, N. (2006). Assay of bone morphogenetic protein-2, -4, and -7 in human demineralized bone matrix. *J. Craniofac. Surg.* 17, 84–90. doi: 10.1097/01.scs.0000179745.91165.73

Ravindran, S., Gao, Q., Kotecha, M., Magin, R. L., Karol, S., Bedran-Russo, A., et al. (2012). Biomimetic extracellular matrix-incorporated scaffold induces osteogenic gene expression in human marrow stromal cells. *Tissue Eng. Part A* 18, 295–309. doi: 10.1089/ten.TEA.2011.0136

Ravindran, S., Huang, C. C., and George, A. (2014a). Extracellular matrix of dental pulp stem cells: applications in pulp tissue engineering using somatic MSCs. *Front. Physiol.* 4:395. doi: 10.3389/fphys.2013.00395

Ravindran, S., Kotecha, M., Huang, C. C., Ye, A., Pothirajan, P., Yin, Z., et al. (2015). Biological and MRI characterization of biomimetic ECM scaffolds for cartilage tissue regeneration. *Biomaterials* 71, 58–70. doi: 10.1016/j.biomaterials.2015.08.030

Ravindran, S., Narayanan, K., Eapen, A. S., Hao, J., Ramachandran, A., Blond, S., et al. (2008). Endoplasmic reticulum chaperone protein GRP-78 mediates endocytosis of dentin matrix protein 1. *J. Biol. Chem.* 283, 29658–29670. doi: 10.1074/jbc.M800786200

Ravindran, S., Zhang, Y., Huang, C. C., and George, A. (2014b). Odontogenic induction of dental stem cells by extracellular matrix-inspired three-dimensional scaffold. *Tissue Eng. Part A* 20, 92–102. doi: 10.1089/ten.TEA.2013.0192

Schwartz, Z., Somers, A., Mellonig, J. T., Carnes, D. L. Jr., Dean, D. D., Cochran, D. L., et al. (1998). Ability of commercial demineralized freeze-dried bone allograft to induce new bone formation is dependent on donor age but not gender. *J. Periodontol.* 69, 470–478. doi: 10.1902/jop.1998.69.4.470

Schwarz, S., Koerber, L., Elsaesser, A. F., Goldberg-Bockhorn, E., Seitz, A. M., Dürselen, L., et al. (2012). Decellularized cartilage matrix as a novel biomatrix for cartilage tissue-engineering applications. *Tissue Eng. Part A* 18, 2195–2209. doi: 10.1089/ten.TEA.2011.0705

Sekiya, I., Larson, B. L., Smith, J. R., Pochampally, R., Cui, J. G., and Prockop, D. J. (2002). Expansion of human adult stem cells from bone marrow stroma: conditions that maximize the yields of early progenitors and evaluate their quality. *Stem Cells* 20, 530–541. doi: 10.1634/stemcells.20-6-530

Soicher, M. A., Christiansen, B. A., Stover, S. M., Leach, J. K., and Fyhrie, D. P. (2013). Remineralization of demineralized bone matrix (DBM) via alternating solution immersion (ASI). *J. Mech. Behav. Biomed. Mater.* 26, 109–118. doi: 10.1016/j.jmbbm.2013.05.007

Thibault, R. A., Scott Baggett, L., Mikos, A. G., and Kasper, F. K. (2010). Osteogenic differentiation of mesenchymal stem cells on pregenerated extracellular matrix scaffolds in the absence of osteogenic cell culture supplements. *Tissue Eng. Part A* 16, 431–440. doi: 10.1089/ten.TEA.2009.0583

Traianedes, K., Russell, J. L., Edwards, J. T., Stubbs, H. A., Shanahan, I. R., and Knaack, D. (2004). Donor age and gender effects on osteoinductivity of demineralized bone matrix. *J. Biomed. Mater. Res. B Appl. Biomater.* 70, 21–29. doi: 10.1002/jbm.b.30015

Yamamoto, M., Tabata, Y., Hong, L., Miyamoto, S., Hashimoto, N., and Ikada, Y. (2000). Bone regeneration by transforming growth factor beta1 released from a biodegradable hydrogel. *J. Control. Release* 64, 133–142. doi: 10.1016/S0168-3659(99)00129-7

Zara, J. N., Siu, R. K., Zhang, X., Shen, J., Ngo, R., Lee, M., et al. (2011). High doses of bone morphogenetic protein 2 induce structurally abnormal bone and inflammation *in vivo*. *Tissue Eng. Part A* 17, 1389–1399. doi: 10.1089/ten.TEA.2010.0555

Zhang, M., Powers, R. M. Jr., and Wolfinbarger, L. Jr. (1997). Effect(s) of the demineralization process on the osteoinductivity of demineralized bone matrix. *J. Periodontol.* 68, 1085–1092. doi: 10.1902/jop.1997.68.11.1085

Zhang, S., Xiao, Z., Luo, J., He, N., Mahlios, J., and Quarles, L. D. (2009). Dose-dependent effects of Runx2 on bone development. *J. Bone Miner. Res.* 24, 1889–1904. doi: 10.1359/jbmr.090502

Zhu, J., and Clark, R. A. (2014). Fibronectin at select sites binds multiple growth factors and enhances their activity: expansion of the collaborative ECM-GF paradigm. *J. Invest. Dermatol.* 134, 895–901. doi: 10.1038/jid.2013.484

Zuk, P. A. (2008). Tissue engineering craniofacial defects with adult stem cells? Are we ready yet? *Pediatr. Res.* 63, 478–486. doi: 10.1203/PDR.0b013e31816bdf36

# 20

# Bone resorption: an actor of dental and periodontal development?

*Andrea Gama*[1,2†], *Benjamin Navet*[3,4†], *Jorge William Vargas*[3,4,5], *Beatriz Castaneda*[1,5] *and Frédéric Lézot*[3,4*]

[1] Institut National de la Santé et de la Recherche Médicale, UMR-1138, Equipe 5, Centre de Recherche des Cordeliers, Paris, France, [2] Odontologic Center of District Federal Military Police, Brasilia, Brazil, [3] Institut National de la Santé et de la Recherche Médicale, UMR-957, Equipe Ligue Nationale Contre le Cancer, Nantes, France, [4] Laboratoire de Physiopathologie de la Résorption Osseuse et Thérapie des Tumeurs Osseuses Primitives, Faculté de Médecine, Université de Nantes, Nantes, France, [5] Department of Basic Studies, Faculty of Odontology, University of Antioquia, Medellin, Colombia

**Edited by:**
Thimios Mitsiadis,
University of Zurich, Switzerland

***Correspondence:**
Frédéric Lézot
frederic.lezot@univ-nantes.fr

† These authors have contributed equally to this work.

Dental and periodontal tissue development is a complex process involving various cell-types. A finely orchestrated network of communications between these cells is implicated. During early development, communications between cells from the oral epithelium and the underlying mesenchyme govern the dental morphogenesis with successive bud, cap and bell stages. Later, interactions between epithelial and mesenchymal cells occur during dental root elongation. Root elongation and tooth eruption require resorption of surrounding alveolar bone to occur. For years, it was postulated that signaling molecules secreted by dental and periodontal cells control bone resorbing osteoclast precursor recruitment and differentiation. Reverse signaling originating from bone cells (osteoclasts and osteoblasts) toward dental cells was not suspected. Dental defects reported in osteopetrosis were associated with mechanical stress secondary to defective bone resorption. In the last decade, consequences of bone resorption over-activation on dental and periodontal tissue formation have been analyzed with transgenic animals (*RANK*$^{Tg}$ and *Opg*$^{-/-}$ mice). Results suggest the existence of signals originating from osteoclasts toward dental and periodontal cells. Meanwhile, experiments consisting in transitory inhibition of bone resorption during root elongation, achieved with bone resorption inhibitors having different mechanisms of action (bisphosphonates and RANKL blocking antibodies), have evidenced dental and periodontal defects that support the presence of signals originating bone cells toward dental cells. The aim of the present manuscript is to present the data we have collected in the last years that support the hypothesis of a role of bone resorption in dental and periodontal development.

**Keywords: bone resorption, RANKL, Zoledronic acid, tooth**

## INTRODUCTION

Early tooth development, more precisely initiation and morphogenesis, has been extensively studied in the last decades. Factors implicated in the cross-talk between epithelial and mesenchymal cells have been identified (for review Mitsiadis and Graf, 2009). Regarding later stages of tooth development, more precisely dental and periodontal histogenesis, the differentiation processes of mineralized tissue forming cells (namely amelogenesis, dentinogenesis and cementogenesis) have also been widely studied (Foster et al., 2007; Babajko et al., 2014; Bleicher, 2014). Pathologies associated with dysfunctions of these processes are nowadays well characterized as amelogenesis imperfecta and dentinogenesis imperfecta (Cobourne and Sharpe, 2013). Dental and periodontal histogenesis corresponds to an important volumetric growth of these tissues, more precisely regarding root formation. Consequently, the surrounding alveolar bone has to be remodeled simultaneously to enable normal tooth development and a dental functional achievement through the eruption process.Bone remodeling requires differentiation and activity of bone resorbing cells from hematopoietic origin called osteoclasts. Osteoclastogenesis is a well-characterized process with three consecutive steps corresponding to precursors recruitment, their fusion into mature polynucleated osteoclasts and finally the activation of these mature osteoclasts (Lézot et al., 2010). The two major signaling factors implicated in these differentiation steps are presented in **Figure 1**.

Signals coming from dental and periodontal tissues were shown to stimulate the alveolar bone remodeling (Wise, 2009). Indeed, these tissues secrete factors stimulating osteoclastogenesis (Wise, 2009). The absence of alveolar bone formation in the case of dental agenesis (**Figure 2A**) supported the assertion that dental and periodontal tissues are central coordinator elements in the development of the dento-alveolar bone complex. Moreover, the apparently normal development of the crown region observed in osteopetrotic mouse models (**Figure 2B**), despite the altered bone resorption, suggests that crown mineralized tissue formation is independent of bone resorption.

In this context it was not surprising that potential reverse signals from bone cells toward dental and periodontal tissues have been rarely considered. Recently, the analysis of dental and periodontal development in mouse models of hyper-resorption ($RANK^{Tg}$ and $Opg^{-/-}$) has changed the vision of the dento-alveolar bone complex development (Castaneda et al., 2011, 2013). Bone resorption was for the first time shown to be an active element of the dental and periodontal tissues development. This active implication was supported by results of studies comprising transitory inhibition of bone resorption during dental and periodontal tissue histogenesis, achieved with bisphosphonate or RANKL blocking antibody (Lézot et al., 2014, 2015). In these studies dental and periodontal tissue defects were associated and proportional to the induced delay of tooth eruption.

Here we present a hypothetical model of tooth root and periodontal development based on our own results as well as on previously reported by other findings.

## CURRENT STATUS CONCERNING TOOTH ROOT AND PERIODONTAL FORMATION: FACTS AND HYPOTHESES

### Consequences of RANK Over-expression in the Monocyte-macrophage Lineage (*RANK*$^{Tg}$ Mouse) on Dental and Periodontal Development

In order to analyze the consequences of RANK over-expression on dental and periodontal tissue growth, a transgenic mouse-line overexpressing *RANK* in the osteoclast precursors ($RANK^{Tg}$; Duheron et al., 2011) was used. The dental and periodontal phenotype of $RANK^{Tg}$ mouse was analyzed comparatively to

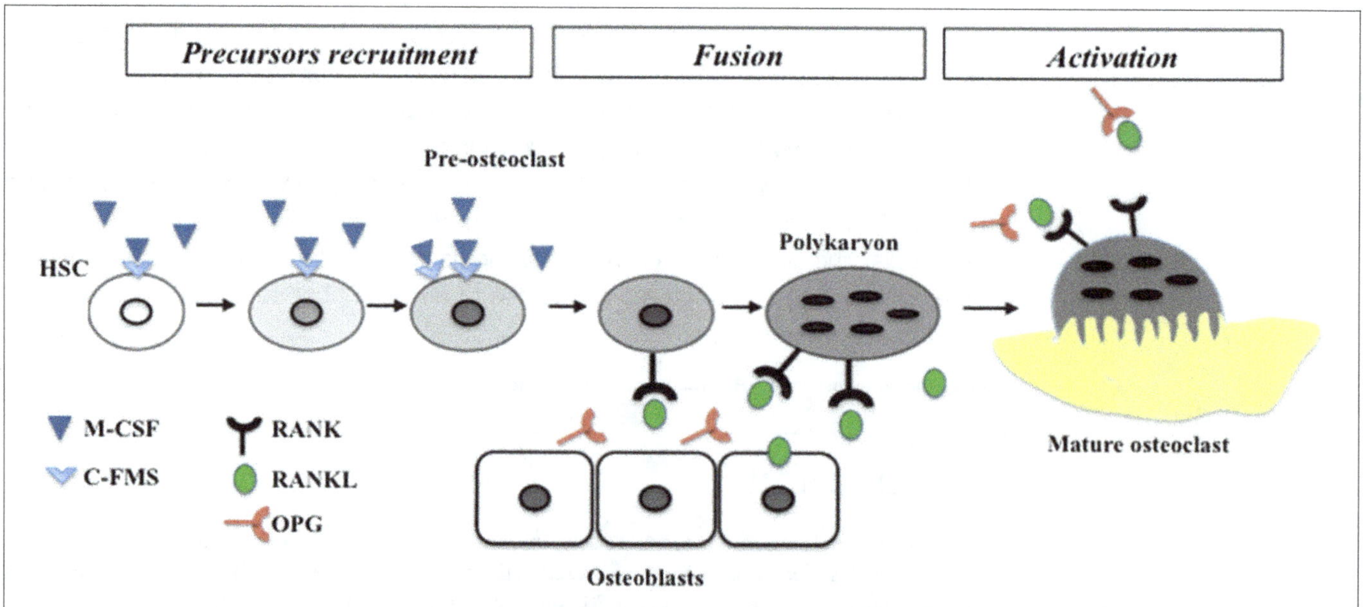


**FIGURE 1 | Schematic representation of different steps of osteoclastogenesis.** The two mains factors controlling the differentiation called M-CSF and RANKL are represented with their receptors. M-CSF is necessary to recruitment and expression of RANK at the surface of pre-osteoclasts. RANKL enable the fusion of pre-osteoclasts in polykaryon and the final differentiation in mature osteoclasts. HSC, hematopoietic stem cell.

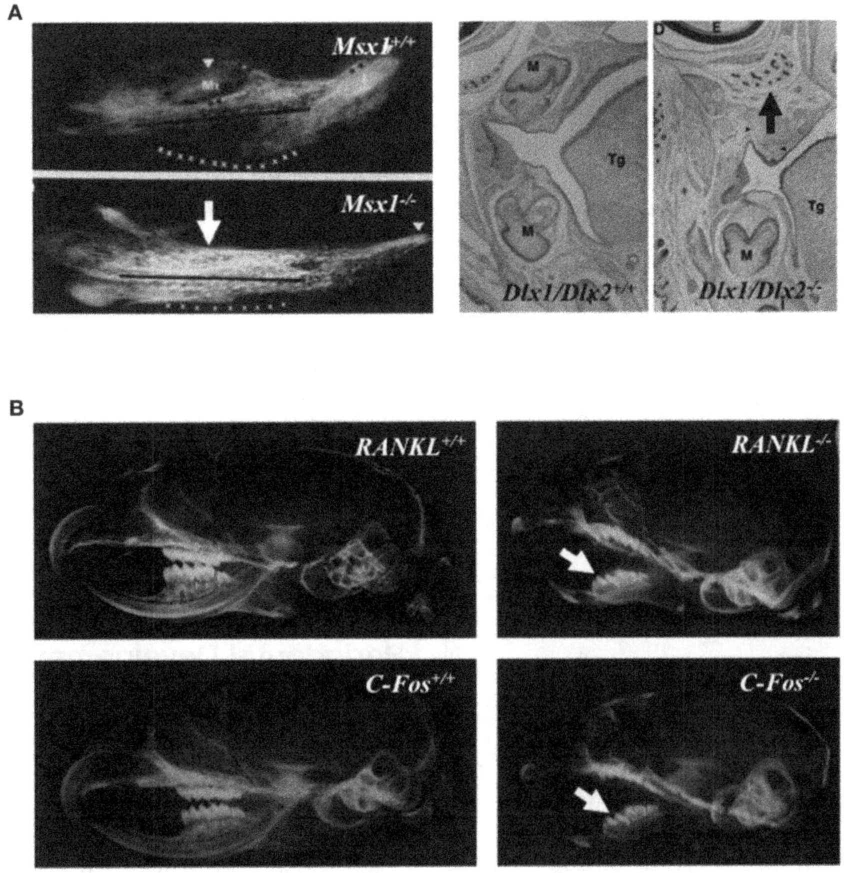


**FIGURE 2 | Tooth agenesis consequence on alveolar bone formation (A) and close to normal crown morphology in osteopetrotic animals (B).** Mandible micro-radiographies and head frontal sections of newborn *Msx1* and *Dlx1/Dlx2* null mutants **(A)**; *Msx1* null mutant mouse image taken form Orestes-Cardoso et al. (2002). Absence of alveolar bone formation in area of tooth agenesis (arrows). Micro-radiographies of wild type, *C-Fos*$^{-/-}$ and *RANKl*$^{-/-}$ 21 day-old mouse heads **(B)** the formation of dental crowns (arrows) in osteopetrotic mutant mice with morphologies close to those of control littermate mice. M, molar; Tg, tongue.

littermate from birth to 1 month (Castaneda et al., 2011). Results show a significant increase in the osteoclast number around the tooth at all ages. This led to an earlier tooth eruption and an accelerated tooth root elongation (**Figure 3**). The final root length is not affected (**Figure 4**) but an important reduction of the root diameter is observed no matter what the genetic background (wild-type or *Msx2* null mutant) considered (Castaneda et al., 2011, 2013).

Interestingly, the complex phenotype of *Msx2*$^{-/-}$ mouse combining amelogenesis imperfecta, root dysmorphia (defects in Hertwig epithelial root sheaths (HERS) and epithelial rests of Malassez), mild-osteopetrosis (with *RANKl* expression severely decreased in the dental epithelium and alveolar bone), and dentinogenesis imperfecta (Aïoub et al., 2007; Molla et al., 2010; Berdal et al., 2011) was partly rescued by RANK over-expression (Castaneda et al., 2013). Indeed, RANK over-expression resulted in significant recovery of all molar eruption and root elongation processes (**Figure 4**). However, the roots remained shorter than in wild-type mice and no improvement of the crown morphology was observed (**Figure 4**).

These results show that root length is genetically determined while root thickness is environmentally controlled, specifically by the bone resorption ability.

The complete analysis of the *RANK*$^{Tg}$ mouse dento-alveolar bone complex phenotype has so enabled to demonstrate that bone resorption is an important element of dental and periodontal tissue development (Castaneda et al., 2011, 2013). RANK over-expression induces an early tooth eruption and root elongation with, as a final consequence, a reduction of the root diameter. This accelerated tooth root elongation corresponds to an increase of HERS cells and adjacent follicular sac mesenchyme cells proliferation (Castaneda et al., 2011). The final root lengths of the RANK transgenic and wild type mice are similar suggesting that the interactions between epithelial and mesenchyme cells are correct but accelerated (Castaneda et al., 2011). The *Msx2*$^{-/-}$ mouse present many defects of the root formation (Aïoub et al., 2007) including an important reduction of the length as shown in **Figure 5**. The fact that, in the *Msx2*$^{-/-}$ mouse the RANK over-activation has no repercussion on the final root length validates that root length is genetically determined. Meanwhile, the root diameter appears to be micro-environmentally controlled, more specifically by the bone resorption capability (Castaneda et al., 2011, 2013). Finally the reverse relationship between bone resorption level and the root diameter established by these studies (Castaneda et al., 2011) could explain part of the root defects seen in diseases with perturbations of the osteoclast function. Concerning the root resorption observed in these diseases, the question of a relationship between root thinness and the prevalence of root resorption is raised. Interestingly, such thin root resorptions are observed in the $Opg^{-/-}$ mouse (Koide et al., 2013) in the context of a progressive loss of the alveolar bone.

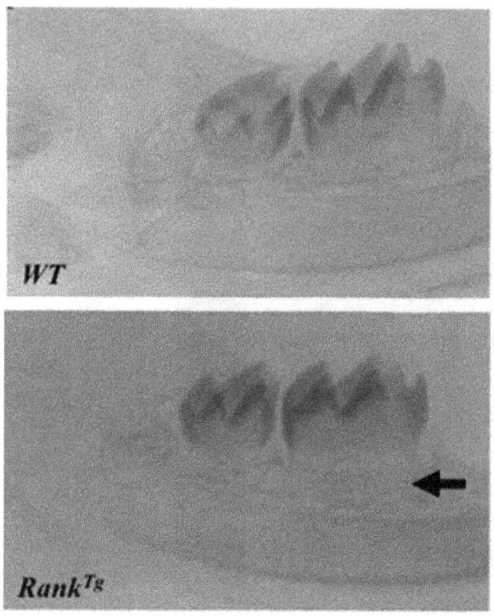


**FIGURE 3 | Accelerated root elongation in *RANK*$^{Tg}$ mouse.** Micro-CT section in the mandible main axis show in 11 day-old *RANK*$^{Tg}$ mouse a more advanced root elongation (arrow) compared to wild type mouse.

In humans, *RANK* gene gains of function mutations have been found in three seemingly distinctive disorders (the Familial Expansile Osteolysis, the Expansile Skeletal Hyperphosphatasia and the Early-onset Paget Disease of Bone). These mutations increase the RANK signal peptide length and alter its normal cleavage, what is believed to cause a NF-κB pathway over-activation (Whyte and Hughes, 2002; Nakatsuka et al., 2003). Such over-activation of the RANK-signaling pathway causes a hyper-osteoclastic activity that increases the bone turnover. A notable observation in these patients is an early tooth loss associated in some case with an idiopathic external resorption localized at either apical or cervical levels (Mitchell et al., 1990; Hughes et al., 1994; Whyte, 2006). This convergence of phenotype between human patients and *RANK*$^{Tg}$ mice qualified the *RANK*$^{Tg}$ mouse as a model of these three different pathologies and confirmed the importance of bone resorption for dental and periodontal tissue development.

## Consequences of Transitory Inhibition of Bone Resorption Using Zoledronic Acid or a RANKL Blocking Antibody on Dental and Periodontal Development

In order to analyze the consequences of transitory inhibitions of bone resorption on dental and periodontal tissue growth, a powerful pharmacologic inhibitor of bone resorption from the bisphosphonate family was injected (four injections in total every 2 days) in newborn or 1 week-old mice. The impact on dental and periodontal tissues was analyzed at the end of treatment, 1 and 3 months after the last injection. Zoledronic acid (ZOL), a third generation bisphosphonate, was chosen for experiments and C57BL/6J and CD1 mice used.

The different molars were not similarly affected by the treatment. A relationship appears between severity of dental and periodontal defects and each molar developmental period

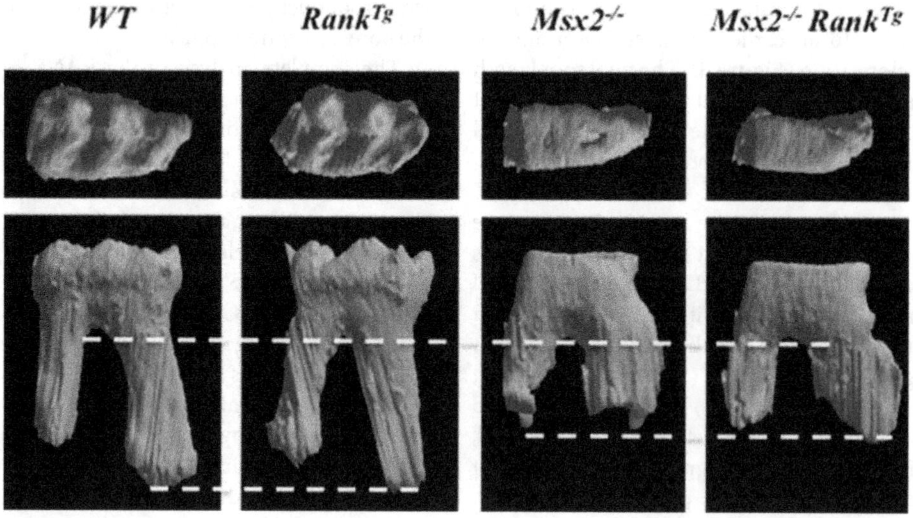


**FIGURE 4 | Roots and crown morphologies of the mandible first molars of adult wild-type, *RANK*$^{Tg}$, *Msx2*$^{-/-}$,and *Msx2*$^{-/-}$ *RANK*$^{Tg}$mice.** Roots of *RANK*$^{Tg}$ mouse molars are thinner and roots of *Msx2*$^{-/-}$ mouse molars are shorter as evidenced by dash lines. Crown of *Msx2*$^{-/--/-}$ mouse are flat with no cuspide independently of RANK over-expression.

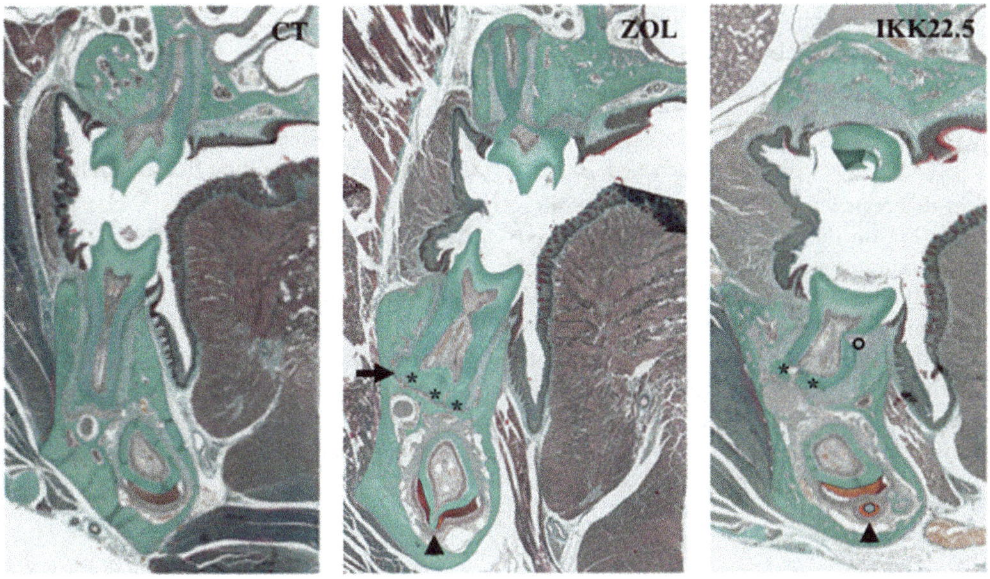


**FIGURE 5 | Dental and periodontal consequences of four injections of ZOL or IKK22.5 in newborn mice, 3 months after the last injection.** Head frontal sections in the plane of the first molars show the presence of ankylosis (arrow), hyper-cementosis (stars), enamel organ disorganization (arrow-heads), and root resorption (circle) in treated animals.

encompassed by the treatment. Indeed, when injections were performed in newborn pups, the first molar was the most affected and the third molar the least affected (Lézot et al., 2014, 2015). The C57BL/6J mice appear to be more sensitive to ZOL than the CD1 mice who need more elevated doses to obtain similar effects (Lézot et al., 2015). In addition to delayed eruption, the main observed defects of dental and periodontal tissues were abnormal amelogenesis with disorganized ameloblasts, root ankylosis, hypercementosis and with time presence of root resorption (**Figure 5**; Lézot et al., 2014). These results evidence that transitory inhibition of bone resorption with ZOL irreversibly impact the histogenesis of dental and periodontal tissues with long-term consequences that remain to be evaluated.

Similar experiments were performed with another powerful inhibitor of bone resorption, a RANKL blocking antibody named IKK22.5.

Experimental results evidenced that while C57BL/6J mice had several teeth included, CD1 mouse had only the upper first molars included confirming the difference of sensitivity to bone resorption inhibitors between these two mouse strains (Lézot et al., 2015). Regarding the dental and periodontal phenotype of non-included molars of CD1 mouse, similar defects to those induced by ZOL injections were observed (**Figure 5**). Interestingly, after the end of treatment with the IK22.5 antibody, a shorter period is necessary to observe neo-osteoclasts presence on the alveolar bone surface than observed after ZOL treatment (Lézot et al., 2015) signaling a more stable inhibition with ZOL than with IKK22.5.

These results demonstrate that transitory use of two different pharmacological bone resorption inhibitors during root elongation induces dental and periodontal defects. This supports our hypothesis of the existence of signaling from bone cells toward dental cells. These powerful pharmacological inhibitors were developed for the treatment of pathologies characterized by excessive bone resorption such as juvenile Paget's disease, osteoporosis, primary or metastatic bone tumors and familial expansile osteolysis (Silverman, 2011; Zwolak and Dudek, 2013; Tella and Gallagher, 2014). In pediatric patients, a RANKL-blocking antibody (Denosumab) is currently under clinical evaluation for osteogenesis imperfecta (phase 2 clinical trial NCT01799798) and for Giant Cell Tumor of Bone (phase 2 clinical trial NCT00680992) with promising preliminary reports in both cases (Semler et al., 2012; Chawla et al., 2013; Karras et al., 2013; Demirsoy et al., 2014; Federman et al., 2014). Bisphosphonates are currently used for the treatment of osteogenesis imperfecta (Barros et al., 2012; Bishop et al., 2013; Ward and Rauch, 2013; Sousa et al., 2014) and juvenile Paget's disease (Demir et al., 2000; Cundy et al., 2004; Polyzos et al., 2010; Saki et al., 2013). In addition, they are under evaluation for treatment of primary bone tumors (Goldsby et al., 2013; phase 3 Clinical trials NCT00987636, NCT00742924, and NCT004470223) and Fibrous Dysplasia of Bone (phase 2 clinical trial NCT00445575). Concerning all these young patients, dental and periodontal tissue developmental defects may occur as a consequence of the bone resorption inhibition. Preclinical studies and clinical observations have already demonstrated that bisphosphonates, in particular alendronate and ZOL, delay or inhibit tooth eruption causing several dental abnormalities (Grier and Wise, 1998; Bradaschia-Correa et al., 2007; Kamoun-Goldrat et al., 2008; Hiraga et al., 2010) and may, as in the juvenile Paget's disease of bone, exert an inhibitory effect on bone mineralization

(Polyzos et al., 2011). Such inhibition of mineralization has been observed for various bisphosphonate in *in vitro* tests using calvaria osteoblast culture (Widler et al., 2002).

## CONCLUSION

The data presented in this review are unambiguous concerning the role of bone resorption on the development of dental and periodontal tissues and supports the hypothesis of a direct implication of osteoclasts in dental and periodontal tissue formation. Further studies will be necessary to decipher, at the molecular level, signals originating from bone cells (presumably osteoclasts) toward dental and periodontal cells. These signals could be directly secreted by bone cells or released from the bone matrix during the resorption.

## FUNDING

The presented projects have received the financial support of the French Association for Cancer Research (ARC, Project # ECL;2010R00778), the "ligue contre le cancer" Association, the Liddy Shriver Sarcoma Initiative (grant) and the French National Cancer Institute (Funding INCa-6001).

## ACKNOWLEDGMENTS

The authors wish to thank G. Hamery and P. Monmousseau from the Therapeutic Experimental Unit (Nantes, France) for their technical assistance. We thank Aguamemnon Gregoriadis, Yongwon Choi and Christopher Mueller for sharing their *C-Fos*, *RANKl*, and *RANK* mouse models, respectively. Meadhbh Brennan is thanked for kindly editing the manuscript.

## REFERENCES

Aïoub, M., Lézot, F., Molla, M., Castaneda, B., Robert, B., Goubin, G., et al. (2007). Msx2 -/- transgenic mice develop compound amelogenesis imperfecta, dentinogenesis imperfecta and periodental osteopetrosis. *Bone* 41, 851–859. doi: 10.1016/j.bone.2007.07.023

Babajko, S., de La Dure-Molla, M., Jedeon, K., and Berdal, A. (2014). MSX2 in ameloblast cell fate and activity. *Front. Physiol.* 5:510. doi: 10.3389/fphys.2014.00510

Barros, E. R., Saraiva, G. L., de Oliveira, T. P., and Lazaretti-Castro, M. (2012). Safety and efficacy of a 1-year treatment with zoledronic acid compared with pamidronate in children with osteogenesis imperfecta. *J. Pediatr. Endocrinol. Metab.* 25, 485–491. doi: 10.1515/jpem-2012-0016

Berdal, A., Castaneda, B., Aïoub, M., Néfussi, J. R., Mueller, C., Descroix, V., et al. (2011). Osteoclasts in the dental microenvironment: a delicate balance controls dental histogenesis. *Cells Tissues Organs* 194, 238–243. doi: 10.1159/000324787

Bishop, N., Adami, S., Ahmed, S. F., Antón, J., Arundel, P., Burren, C. P., et al. (2013). Risedronate in children with osteogenesis imperfecta: a randomised, double-blind, placebo-controlled trial. *Lancet* 382, 1424–1432. doi: 10.1016/S0140-6736(13)61091-0

Bleicher, F. (2014). Odontoblast physiology. *Exp. Cell Res.* 325, 65–71. doi: 10.1016/j.yexcr.2013.12.012

Bradaschia-Correa, V., Massa, L. F., and Arana-Chavez, V. E. (2007). Effects of alendronate on tooth eruption and molar root formation in young growing rats. *Cell Tissue Res.* 330, 475–485. doi: 10.1007/s00441-007-0499-y

Castaneda, B., Simon, Y., Ferbus, D., Robert, B., Chesneau, J., Mueller, C., et al. (2013). Role of RANKL (TNFSF11)-dependent osteopetrosis in the dental phenotype of Msx2 null mutant mice. *PLoS ONE* 8:e80054. doi: 10.1371/journal.pone.0080054

Castaneda, B., Simon, Y., Jacques, J., Hess, E., Choi, Y.-W., Blin-Wakkach, C., et al. (2011). Bone resorption control of tooth eruption and root morphogenesis: involvement of the receptor activator of NF-$\kappa$B (RANK). *J. Cell. Physiol.* 226, 74–85. doi: 10.1002/jcp.22305

Chawla, S., Henshaw, R., Seeger, L., Choy, E., Blay, J.-Y., Ferrari, S., et al. (2013). Safety and efficacy of denosumab for adults and skeletally mature adolescents with giant cell tumour of bone: interim analysis of an open-label, parallel-group, phase 2 study. *Lancet Oncol.* 14, 901–908. doi: 10.1016/S1470-2045(13)70277-8

Cobourne, M. T., and Sharpe, P. T. (2013). Diseases of the tooth: the genetic and molecular basis of inherited anomalies affecting the dentition. *Wiley Interdiscip. Rev. Dev. Biol.* 2, 183–212. doi: 10.1002/wdev.66

Cundy, T., Wheadon, L., and King, A. (2004). Treatment of idiopathic hyperphosphatasia with intensive bisphosphonate therapy. *J. Bone Miner. Res.* 19, 703–711. doi: 10.1359/jbmr.040127

Demir, E., Bereket, A., Ozkan, B., and Topçu, M. (2000). Effect of alendronate treatment on the clinical picture and bone turnover markers in chronic idiopathic hyperphosphatasia. *J. Pediatr. Endocrinol. Metab.* 13, 217–221. doi: 10.1515/JPEM.2000.13.2.217

Demirsoy, U., Karadogan, M., Selek, O., Anik, Y., Aksu, G., Müezzinoglu, B., et al. (2014). Golden bullet-denosumab: early rapid response of metastatic giant cell tumor of the bone. *J. Pediatr. Hematol. Oncol.* 36, 156–158. doi: 10.1097/MPH.0000000000000034

Duheron, V., Hess, E., Duval, M., Decossas, M., Castaneda, B., Klöpper, J. E., et al. (2011). Receptor activator of NF-kappaB (RANK) stimulates the proliferation of epithelial cells of the epidermo-pilosebaceous unit. *Proc. Natl. Acad. Sci. U.S.A.* 108, 5342–5347. doi: 10.1073/pnas.1013054108

Federman, N., Brien, E. W., Narasimhan, V., Dry, S. M., Sodhi, M., and Chawla, S. P. (2014). Giant cell tumor of bone in childhood: clinical aspects and novel therapeutic targets. *Paediatr. Drugs* 16, 21–28. doi: 10.1007/s40272-013-0051-3

Foster, B. L., Popowics, T. E., Fong, H. K., and Somerman, M. J. (2007). Advances in defining regulators of cementum development and periodontal regeneration. *Curr. Top. Dev. Biol.* 78, 47–126. doi: 10.1016/S0070-2153(06)78003-6

Goldsby, R. E., Fan, T. M., Villaluna, D., Wagner, L. M., Isakoff, M. S., Meyer, J., et al. (2013). Feasibility and dose discovery analysis of zoledronic acid with concurrent chemotherapy in the treatment of newly diagnosed metastatic osteosarcoma: a report from the Children's Oncology Group. *Eur. J. Cancer* 49, 2384–2391. doi: 10.1016/j.ejca.2013.03.018

Grier, R. L., and Wise, G. E. (1998). Inhibition of tooth eruption in the rat by a bisphosphonate. *J. Dent. Res.* 77, 8–15. doi: 10.1177/00220345980770011201

Hiraga, T., Ninomiya, T., Hosoya, A., and Nakamura, H. (2010). Administration of the bisphosphonate zoledronic acid during tooth development inhibits tooth eruption and formation and induces dental abnormalities in rats. *Calcif. Tissue Int.* 86, 502–510. doi: 10.1007/s00223-010-9366-z

Hughes, A. E., Shearman, A. M., Weber, J. L., Barr, R. J., Wallace, R. G., Osterberg, P. H., et al. (1994). Genetic linkage of familial expansile osteolysis to chromosome 18q. *Hum. Mol. Genet.* 3, 359–361. doi: 10.1093/hmg/3.2.359

Kamoun-Goldrat, A., Ginisty, D., and Le Merrer, M. (2008). Effects of bisphosphonates on tooth eruption in children with osteogenesis imperfecta. *Eur. J. Oral Sci.* 116, 195–198. doi: 10.1111/j.1600-0722.2008.00529.x

Karras, N. A., Polgreen, L. E., Ogilvie, C., Manivel, J. C., Skubitz, K. M., and Lipsitz, E. (2013). Denosumab treatment of metastatic giant-cell tumor of bone in a 10-year-old girl. *J. Clin. Oncol.* 31, e200–e202. doi: 10.1200/jco.2012.46.4255

Koide, M., Kobayashi, Y., Ninomiya, T., Nakamura, M., Yasuda, H., Arai, Y., et al. (2013). Osteoprotegerin-deficient male mice as a model for severe alveolar bone loss: comparison with RANKL-overexpressing transgenic male mice. *Endocrinology* 154, 773–782. doi: 10.1210/en.2012-1928

Lézot, F., Chesneau, J., Battaglia, S., Brion, R., Castaneda, B., Farges, J.-C., et al. (2014). Preclinical evidence of potential craniofacial adverse effect of zoledronic acid in pediatric patients with bone malignancies. *Bone* 68, 146–152. doi: 10.1016/j.bone.2014.08.018

Lézot, F., Chesneau, J., Navet, B., Gobin, B., Amiaud, J., Choi, Y., et al. (2015). Skeletal consequences of RANKL-blocking antibody (IK22-5) injections during growth: mouse strain disparities and synergic effect with zoledronic acid. *Bone* 73, 51–59. doi: 10.1016/j.bone.2014.12.011

Lézot, F., Thomas, B. L., Blin-Wakkach, C., Castaneda, B., Bolanos, A., Hotton, D., et al. (2010). Dlx homeobox gene family expression in osteoclasts. *J. Cell. Physiol.* 223, 779–787. doi: 10.1002/jcp.22095

Mitchell, C. A., Kennedy, J. G., and Wallace, R. G. (1990). Dental abnormalities associated with familial expansile osteolysis: a clinical and radiographic study. *Oral Surg. Oral Med. Oral Pathol.* 70, 301–307. doi: 10.1016/0030-4220(90)90145-I

Mitsiadis, T. A., and Graf, D. (2009). Cell fate determination during tooth development and regeneration. *Birth Defects Res. C Embryo Today* 87, 199–211. doi: 10.1002/bdrc.20160

Molla, M., Descroix, V., Aïoub, M., Simon, S., Castañeda, B., Hotton, D., et al. (2010). Enamel protein regulation and dental and periodontal physiopathology in MSX2 mutant mice. *Am. J. Pathol.* 177, 2516–2526. doi: 10.2353/ajpath.2010.091224

Nakatsuka, K., Nishizawa, Y., and Ralston, S. H. (2003). Phenotypic characterization of early onset Paget's disease of bone caused by a 27-bp duplication in the TNFRSF11A gene. *J. Bone Miner. Res.* 18, 1381–1385. doi: 10.1359/jbmr.2003.18.8.1381

Orestes-Cardoso, S., Nefussi, J. R., Lezot, F., Oboeuf, M., Pereira, M., Mesbah, M., et al. (2002). Msx1 is a regulator of bone formation during development and postnatal growth: *in vivo* investigations in a transgenic mouse model. *Connect. Tissue Res.* 43, 153–160. doi: 10.1080/03008200290000547

Polyzos, S. A., Anastasilakis, A. D., Litsas, I., Efstathiadou, Z., Kita, M., Arsos, G., et al. (2010). Profound hypocalcemia following effective response to zoledronic acid treatment in a patient with juvenile Paget's disease. *J. Bone Miner. Metab.* 28, 706–712. doi: 10.1007/s00774-010-0198-8

Polyzos, S. A., Anastasilakis, A. D., Makras, P., and Terpos, E. (2011). Paget's disease of bone and calcium homeostasis: focus on bisphosphonate treatment. *Exp. Clin. Endocrinol. Diabetes* 119, 519–524. doi: 10.1055/s-0031-1284365

Saki, F., Karamizadeh, Z., Nasirabadi, S., Mumm, S., McAlister, W. H., and Whyte, M. P. (2013). Juvenile paget's disease in an Iranian kindred with vitamin D deficiency and novel homozygous TNFRSF11B mutation. *J. Bone Miner. Res.* 28, 1501–1508. doi: 10.1002/jbmr.1868

Semler, O., Netzer, C., Hoyer-Kuhn, H., Becker, J., Eysel, P., and Schoenau, E. (2012). First use of the RANKL antibody denosumab in osteogenesis imperfecta type VI. *J. Musculoskelet. Neuronal Interact.* 12, 183–188.

Silverman, S. L. (2011). Bisphosphonate use in conditions other than osteoporosis. *Ann. N.Y. Acad. Sci.* 1218, 33–37. doi: 10.1111/j.1749-6632.2010. 05769.x

Sousa, T., Bompadre, V., and White, K. K. (2014). Musculoskeletal functional outcomes in children with osteogenesis imperfecta: associations with disease severity and pamidronate therapy. *J. Pediatr. Orthop.* 34, 118–122. doi: 10.1097/BPO.0b013e3182a006a0

Tella, S. H., and Gallagher, J. C. (2014). Prevention and treatment of postmenopausal osteoporosis. *J. Steroid Biochem. Mol. Biol.* 142, 155–170. doi: 10.1016/j.jsbmb.2013.09.008

Ward, L. M., and Rauch, F. (2013). Oral bisphosphonates for paediatric osteogenesis imperfecta? *Lancet* 382, 1388–1389. doi: 10.1016/S0140-6736(13)61531-7

Whyte, M. P. (2006). Paget's disease of bone and genetic disorders of RANKL/OPG/RANK/NF-kappaB signaling. *Ann. N.Y. Acad. Sci.* 1068, 143–164. doi: 10.1196/annals.1346.016

Whyte, M. P., and Hughes, A. E. (2002). Expansile skeletal hyperphosphatasia is caused by a 15-base pair tandem duplication in TNFRSF11A encoding RANK and is allelic to familial expansile osteolysis. *J. Bone Miner. Res.* 17, 26–29. doi: 10.1359/jbmr.2002.17.1.26

Widler, L., Jaeggi, K. A., Glatt, M., Müller, K., Bachmann, R., Bisping, M., et al. (2002). Highly potent geminal bisphosphonates. From pamidronate disodium (Aredia) to zoledronic acid (Zometa). *J. Med. Chem.* 45, 3721–3738. doi: 10.1021/jm020819i

Wise, G. E. (2009). Cellular and molecular basis of tooth eruption. *Orthod. Craniofac. Res.* 12, 67–73. doi: 10.1111/j.1601-6343.2009. 01439.x

Zwolak, P., and Dudek, A. Z. (2013). Antineoplastic activity of zoledronic acid and denosumab. *Anticancer Res.* 33, 2981–2988.

# 21

# Stem cell origin differently affects bone tissue engineering strategies

**Edited by:**
*Thimios Mitsiadis,*
*University of Zurich, Switzerland*

***Correspondence:**
*Monica Mattioli-Belmonte,*
*Department of Clinical and Molecular Sciences, Università Politecnica delle Marche, Via Tronto 10/a, 60126 Ancona, Italy*
*m.mattioli@univpm.it*

***Monica Mattioli-Belmonte [1]*, Gabriella Teti [2], Viviana Salvatore [2], Stefano Focaroli [2], Monia Orciani [1], Manuela Dicarlo [1], Milena Fini [3], Giovanna Orsini [4], Roberto Di Primio [1] and Mirella Falconi [2]***

*[1] Department of Clinical and Molecular Sciences, Università Politecnica delle Marche, Ancona, Italy, [2] Department of Biomedical and Neuromotor Sciences, University of Bologna, Bologna, Italy, [3] Laboratory of Preclinical and Surgical Studies, Rizzoli Orthopaedic Institute, Bologna, Italy, [4] Department of Clinical Sciences and Stomatology, Università Politecnica delle Marche, Ancona, Italy*

Bone tissue engineering approaches are encouraging for the improvement of conventional bone grafting technique drawbacks. Thanks to their self-renewal and multi-lineage differentiation ability, stem cells are one of the major actors in tissue engineering approaches, and among these adult mesenchymal stem cells (MSCs) hold a great promise for regenerative medicine strategies. Bone marrow MSCs (BM-MSCs) are the first- identified and well-recognized stem cell population used in bone tissue engineering. Nevertheless, several factors hamper BM-MSC clinical application and subsequently, new stem cell sources have been investigated for these purposes. The fruitful selection and combination of tissue engineered scaffold, progenitor cells, and physiologic signaling molecules allowed the surgeon to reconstruct the missing natural tissue. On the basis of these considerations, we analyzed the capability of two different scaffolds, planned for osteochondral tissue regeneration, to modulate differentiation of adult stem cells of dissimilar local sources (i.e., periodontal ligament, maxillary periosteum) as well as adipose-derived stem cells (ASCs), in view of possible craniofacial tissue engineering strategies. We demonstrated that cells are differently committed toward the osteoblastic phenotype and therefore, taking into account their specific features, they could be intriguing cell sources in different stem cell-based bone/periodontal tissue regeneration approaches.

**Keywords: PDPCs, ASCs, PDL-SCs, tissue engineering, q-RT-PCR, SEM, TEM**

## Introduction

Reconstruction of large bone and/or complex craniofacial defects is a clinical challenge in situations of injury, congenital defects or disease. The use of cell-based therapies represents one of the most advanced methods to enhance the regenerative response for bone wound healing. As suggested by Giannoudis et al. (2007), in addition to 3D dimensional structures, mechanical, and/or physical signals, cell type as well as environmental bioactive factors are critical to direct tissue repair and regeneration. Both somatic and stem cells have been adopted in the treatment of complex osseous defects and, among these, mesenchymal stem cells (MSCs) held the greatest promise for regenerative therapies in the skeletal system. MSCs are multipotent and self-renewing cells owning endogenous functions for tissue renewal and repair within their individual local tissues (van der Kooy and Weiss, 2000). The term MSCs was originally generated considering a theoretical common progenitor of a wide range of "mesenchymal" tissues (Caplan, 1991) and these cells are commonly identified because of their surface phenotype and *in vitro* ability to differentiate into specific lineages (Dominici et al., 2006). Even though it has been widely accepted that MSCs reside ubiquitously throughout a variety of post-natal tissues and organs (Crisan et al., 2008), this concept undergoes to strong criticism for the missing of an essential *in vivo* experimental support (Bianco et al., 2013). Moreover, recent literature suggests that not all MSCs are certainly created equal in their differential and proliferative capacities, or in their capability to respond to external influences (i.e., microenvironment). Cells harvested from different sources may in fact show phenotypic heterogeneity and dissimilar *in vivo* results after transplantation (Rebelatto et al., 2008). For researchers investigating stem cell-based tissue engineering, it is essential to select the most appropriate type of MSCs source naturally suited to obtain a more efficient treatment for the regeneration of injured skeletal tissues of different anatomical districts.

To this aim, we tested the cross-talk between 3D porous scaffolds and MSCs derived from different adult human tissues. The choice of the different MSCs population harvesting sites (i.e., periosteum, periodontal ligament and adipose tissue) was based on their possible regenerative medicine applications in complex craniofacial lesions.

Periosteum derived precursor cells (PDPCs) reside in the inner "cambium layer" of periosteum which is a connective structure comprised of 2 layers that covers the external surface of bone (Roberts et al., 2015). Specifically, besides osteoblasts and bone lining cells, the inner layer has adult mesenchymal skeletal progenitor cells, smaller and more isodiametric fibroblasts, and sympathetic nerves that make periosteum a structure with regenerative capacity (Ferretti and Mattioli-Belmonte, 2014a; Lin et al., 2014). Periodontal ligament stem cells (PDL-SCs) that reside at the perivascular regions possess characteristics of MSCs and are a promising tool for periodontal regeneration (Zhu and Liang, 2015). At last, Adipose-derived Stem Cells (ASCs) were found to be more suitable in clinical application in comparison with those derived by bone marrow for higher stem cells harvest from lipoaspirates, faster cell proliferation and less discomfort and morbidities during collecting procedure. However, conflicting results on their osteogenic capacity is now still debated (Liao and Chien, 2014).

In this study, PDPCs, PDL-SCs, and ASCs were seeded on two kinds of gelatin/genipin scaffolds for 14 and 21 days and cultured in appropriate differentiating media in order to mimic a chondrogenic or osteogenic microenvironment. Cell proliferation assay, light microscopy, transmission (TEM) and scanning (SEM) electron microscopies and qRT-PCR were carried out to evaluate cell viability, morphological and functional changes induced by cell/scaffold interaction.

# Materials and Methods

## Cell Culture

### Periosteal Derived Progenitor Cells (PDPCs)

PDPCs were obtained from maxillary periosteal tissue of four subjects undergoing routine oral surgery (mean age 34 years), after the obtainment of their informed consent. As previously described (Ferretti et al., 2012, 2014b), tissue was washed in Dulbecco's Phosphate-Buffered Saline (D-PBS) lacking in $Ca^{2+}$ and $Mg^{2+}$, minced into small pieces (4–9 $mm^2$) and then placed in a 100 mm Petri dish in Dulbecco's Modified Eagle Medium: Nutrient Mixture F-12 (DMEM/F-12, Sigma-Aldrich, Milan, Italy) supplemented with 10% Fetal Bovine Serum (FBS) and 1% penicillin-streptomycin (100 U/ml), all from GIBCO® (Life Technologies Corporation, USA). DMEM-F12 provides optimal and appropriate culture conditions for MSCs isolation and *ex vivo* expansion, preserving the correct morphology, population doubling time and immunophenotype (Pal et al., 2009). Periosteum explants were positioned with their cambium side placed against the dishes to allow cell adhesion. Petri dishes were incubated at 37°C in a humidified, $CO_2$-controlled (5%) incubator. Medium was changed twice a week. As soon as cells migrating from the explants reached 50% of confluence, they were collected by treatment with 0.25% trypsin/1 mM EDTA (Sigma-Aldrich, Milan, Italy) and subcultured at 1:3 dilutions under the same culture condition. Cells were used at the 3rd passage to assess their MSC phenotype and their ability to differentiate into mesenchymal lineages.

### Periodontal Ligament Stem Cells (PDL-SCs)

Periodontal ligaments tissues were obtained from extracted human molars, of 10 healthy volunteers aged 16–30 years. Written informed consent was obtained from all donors. As previously described (Orciani et al., 2012), periodontal ligaments tissues were cut in small pieces and cultured in Petri dishes in Dulbecco's Modified Eagle Medium: Nutrient Mixture F-12 (DMEM/F-12) (Gibco, Life Technologies, Milan, Italy) containing 10% FBS, penicillin (100 U/mL) and streptomycin (100 μg/mL) (Gibco, Life Technologies, Milan, Italy). Cells were grown until 50% confluence was reached, then they were harvested by treatment with 0.25% trypsin/1 mM EDTA (Gibco, Life Technologies, Milan, Italy) and re-plated at 1:2 dilutions under the same culture condition. Cells were used at the 3rd passage for phenotypic characterization and differentiation.

### Adipose Derived Stem Cells (ASCs)

StemPro® Human ASCs were purchased from Life Technologies Corporation (Monza, Italy). Cells were grown in MesenPRO RS™ Basal Medium (Life Technologies, Monza, Italy) supplemented with MesenPRO RS™ Growth Supplement (Life Technologies, Milan, Italy) according to the manufacture's suggestions. ASCs were expanded to 4–5 passages before they lost the capacity to grow or differentiate into all potential phenotypes.

## Cell Characterization

According to The International Society for Cellular Therapy for identification of human MSCs (Dominici et al., 2006), PDPCs, PDL-SCs, and ASCs were analyzed by flow cytometry and subjected to differentiation into mesenchymal lineages.

For immunophenotyping, $2.5 \times 10^5$ cells were washed with D-PBS and then stained for 45 min with the following antibodies: fluorescein isothiocyanate-(FITC)-labeled mouse anti-human CD90 (Stem Cell Technologies—Milan, Italy), CD105, CD14, CD19 (Diaclone, France), and R-phycoerythrin-(PE)-labeled mouse anti-human CD34, CD45 (Diaclone, France), CD73 (Becton Dickinson) and anti HLA-DR purchased from Diaclone. Control for FITC or PE coupled antibodies was an isotypic mouse IgG1.

Flow cytometric analysis was performed on a FACSCalibur system (Becton Dickinson, CA, USA) using CellQuest software (Becton Dickinson). To evaluate fibroblastic contamination, we tested FITC-labeled mouse anti-human CD9 monoclonal antibody (ImmunoTools GmbH, Germany) (Halfon et al., 2011).

Cell differentiation into osteoblasts, adipocytes and chondrocytes was evaluated using STEMPRO® Osteogenesis, Adipogenesis and Chondrogenesis Kits (Life Technologies Corporation, USA) respectively. Cells cultured in DMEM/F-12 with 10%FBS were used as negative controls.

For osteoblastic differentiation, cells were plated at a density of $4.5 \times 10^4$ cells with appropriate medium for 10 days, refreshing the medium every 2 days. In order to assess the osteoblastic differentiation von Kossa and Alkaline phosphatise (ALP) stainings were performed. For von Kossa stain, cells were fixed with 4% Paraformaldehyde (PFA) for 15 min at room temperature (RT) and incubated with 1% silver nitrate solution under UV light for 20 min at RT. Unreacted silver was removed with 5% sodium thiosulfate for 5 min. For ALP staining, cells were fixed with 4% PFA for 15 min RT and washed in 100 mM Tris-HCl pH 9.5, 100 mM NaCl and 10 mM MgCl2 buffer for 10 min RT. Cells were then stained with fast 5-bromo-4-chloro-3-indolyl phosphate and nitroblue tetrazolium alkaline phosphate substrate (Sigma-Aldrich, Milan, Italy) for 10 min and rinsed in $dH_2O$. Reaction was observed with a light microscope (Nikon Eclipse 600, Nikon, Milan, Italy).

For adipogenic differentiation $9 \times 10^4$ cells were seeded and treated with the appropriate medium for 15 days, changing the media twice a week. Differentiation was assessed by Oil Red staining and CD36 immunoreaction. Briefly, cells fixed in 4% PFA were exposed to Oil Red O solution (0.5% in 100% isopropyl alcohol) for 20 min RT, cleared with isopropanol 60% and finally washed in $dH_2O$. For the detection of CD36 positivity, PDPCs were incubated with monoclonal anti-CD36 (ImmunoTools GmbH, Friesoythe, Germany) diluted 1:100. The reaction was visualized using the streptavidin-biotin-peroxidase technique (DAKO LSAB+/HRP peroxidase kit; Dako SpA, Milano, Italy). Cells were incubated with 3,3-diaminobenzidine-DAB (10 mg diaminobenzidine in 15 ml 0.05 M Tris buffer, pH 7.6 and 12 μl hydrogen peroxide 30%) and counterstained with Mayer's haematoxylin (Bio-Optica SpA, Milan, Italy). Reaction was examined with a light microscope (Nikon Eclipse 600).

For chondrogenic differentiation, cells were cultured in pellet culture system. For the preparation of each pellet, aliquots of $1 \times 10^6$ cells in 1 ml of appropriate medium were spun down at 1200 rpm for 5 min. Pellets were cultured for 20 days changing the medium twice a week. Pellets were then fixed in 4% PFA, paraffin embedded and sectioned. Sections were exposed to a solutions of Alcian Blue pH 1 (Bio-Optica) for 20 min RT or Safranin-O (0.1 g in EtOH 100%, working dilution 1: 2 $dH_2O$) for 5 min RT and observed with a light microscope (Nikon Eclipse 600).

## Scaffold Preparation

3D Gelatin (G) scaffolds (GEL) were obtained using type A gelatin from pig skin cross-linked with genipin as previously described (Panzavolta et al., 2013). Briefly, following the addition of genipin, the foam assumed a blue color due to the binding with primary amino-groups of the gelatin. For the preparation of scaffolds containing hydroxyapatite (HA), 10 wt% powders was added to 140 ml of a gelatin solution in order to obtain a suspension (G/HA). The suspension was maintained under constant mechanical stirring and subsequently cross-linked with genipin. The samples were then allowed to jellify in an oven, washed in a glycine aqueous and finally frozen in liquid $N_2$ and freeze-dried (GEL/HA scaffold).

Before seeding the scaffolds were sterilized in 70% ethyl alcohol solution (ETOH; Sigma-Aldrich, Milan, Italy) for 2 h, washed two times in PBS (GIBCO) for 30 min and placed under UV 15 min for each side. In order to improve cell adhesion, scaffolds were then conditioned overnight in suitable media at 5% CO2, 37°C. The media were then discarded and scaffolds considered ready for seeding. Cells were detached using 0.25% trypsin in 1 mM ethylene-diamine- tetracetic -acid (EDTA, Sigma-Aldrich, Milan; Italy) and seeded at a density of $1 \times 10^4$ cell/cm$^3$ by applying 50 μL of cell suspension on the samples placed at 37°C for 30 min in a humified chamber, in order to avoid the slip down of cells. After 1.5 ml of STEMPRO® Osteogenesis or STEMPRO® Chondrogenesis medium was added to cover G/HA or G scaffolds placed in Corning® ultra-low attachment multiwell plates, respectively. Cells were cultured for 7, 14, and 21 days.

## MTT (3-dimethylthiazol-2,5-diphenyltetrazolium Bromide) Viability Assay

Cell viability was assessed in PDPCs, ASCs, and PDL-SCs after 7, 14, and 21 days of culture in basal and differentiating osteogenic or chondrogenic media. Cell viability was also evaluated in cells cultured on GEL and GEL/HA scaffolds. Briefly, after removing the culture media, 200 μL of MTT (3-dimethylthiazol-2,5-diiphenyltetrazolium bromide, 135038 Sigma-Aldrich) solution (5 mg/mL in phenol red-free DMEM) and 1.8 mL DMEM were added to the multi-well plates and incubated at 37°C for 3 h. After discarding the supernatants, 2 mL of solvent (4%HCl 1N in isopropanol absolute) were added to dissolve the dark blue formazan crystals and quantify them spectrophotometrically measuring the absorbance at 570 nm (Secoman, Anthelie light, version 3.8, Contardi, Italy). Data were expressed as percentage over the respective control culture (see **Figure 1** legend).

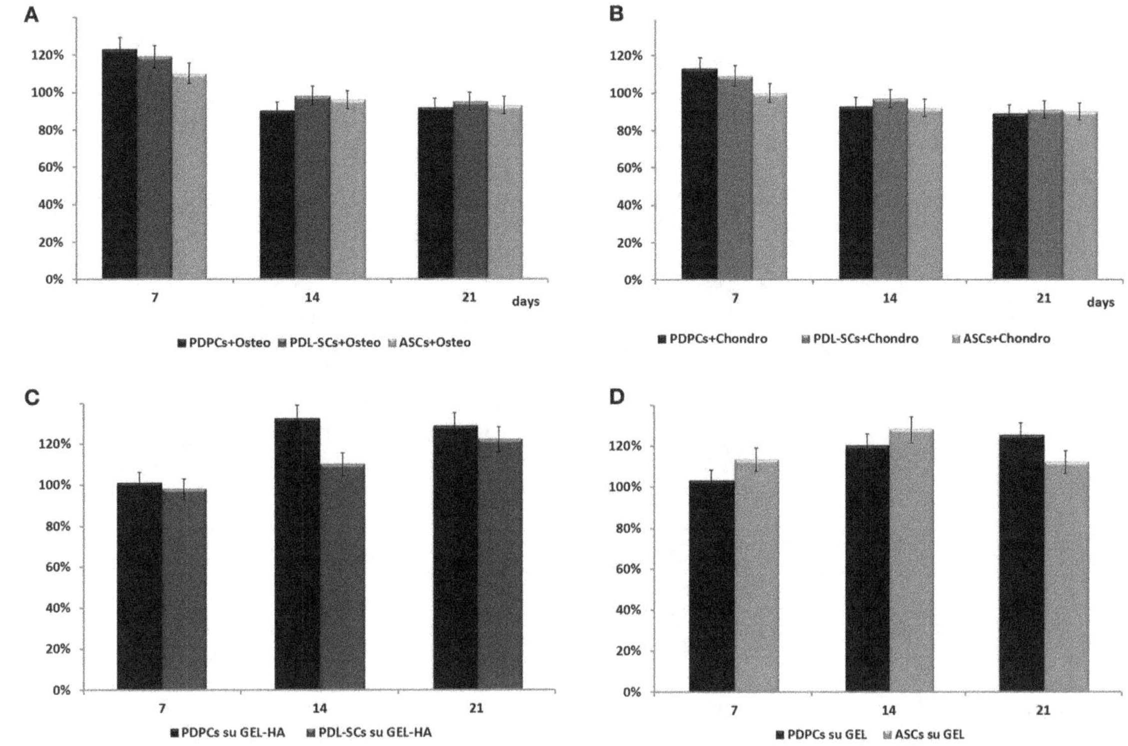


**FIGURE 1 | Histograms depict MTT viability test performed in PDPCs, PDL-SCs, and ASCs cultured in tissue culture plates for 7, 14, and 21 days in osteogenic (A) or chondrogenic (B) medium.** Data are expressed respectively as percentage over PDPCs, PDL-SCs, and ASCs cultured for 7, 14, and 21 days in undifferentiating medium; **(C)** PDPCs and PDL-SCs cultured on GEL/HA scaffolds for 7, 14, and 21 days in osteogenic medium. Data are expressed respectively as percentage over PDPCs and PDL-SCs cultured in osteogenic media in tissue culture plates in osteogenic media. **(D)** PDPCs and ASCs cultured on GEL scaffolds for 7, 14, and 21 days in chondrogenic medium. Mean values ± SD are reported.

**TABLE 1 | Analysed genes description.**

| Gene | Detected transcript | Primer forward (5′->3′) | Primer reverse (5′->3′) | Annealing T (°C) |
|---|---|---|---|---|
| RUNX2 | NM_004348.3 | CTCGTCCGCACCGACAGCC | TACCTCTCCGAGGGCTACCACC | 60 |
| BMP2 | NM_001200.2 | CCAGCCGAGCCAACACTGTGC | TCTCCGGGTTGTTTTCCCACTCG | 60 |
| SPARC | NM_003118.3 | CCTGAGGCTGTAACTGAGAGAAAG | GTGGGAGGGGAAACAAGAAGATAA | 65 |
| BGLAP | NM_199173 | GACTGTGACGAGTTGGCTGA | GCCCACAGATTCCTCTTCTG | 64 |
| SOX9 | NM_000346 | GAGGAAGTCGGTGAAGAACG | ATCGAAGGTCTCGATGTTGG | 65 |
| Type II Collagen | NM_001248899 | GGCAATAGCAGGTTCACGTACA | CGATAACAGTCTTGCCCCACTT | 60 |
| GAPDH * | NM_002046.3 | AGCCACATCGCTCAGACAC | GCCCAATACGACCAAATCC | 60 |
| GUSB* | NM_000181.2 | AAACGATTGCAGGGTTTCAC | TCTCGTCGGTGACTGTTCA | 81 |

*Runx2, runt-related transcription factor 2; Bmp2, bone morphogenetic protein 2; Sparc, Osteonectin; Bglap, osteocalcin; Sox9, SRY (sex determining region Y)-box 9; Gusb, beta glucuronidase; Gapdh, glyceraldehyde-3-phosphate dehydrogenase. *Reference genes.*

## Scanning Electron Microscopy (SEM)

Samples from cell culture tests were fixed in 2% glutaraldehyde (Sigma-Aldrich) in 0.1 M cacodylate buffer (pH 7.4, Sigma-Aldrich), post-fixed in 1% osmium tetroxide (Sigma, Milan, Italy), dehydrated in increasing ethanol (Sigma-Aldrich) concentrations (25, 50, 70, 80, and 100%), CPD-dried, mounted on aluminum stubs, gold-sputtered by the Edwards Sputter Coater B150S equipment and observed with a Philips XL 20 SEM (FEI Italia SRL, Milan, Italy) microscope.

## Transmission Electron Microscopy (TEM)

Cells cultured on scaffolds were fixed in 2.5% glutaraldehyde in 0.1 M cacodylate buffer for 2 h at 4°C and post-fixed in 1% Osmium tetroxide in 0.1 M cacodylate buffer for 30 min at room temperature. Samples were dehydrated in graded ethanol and finally infiltrated and embedded in RL London White (Fluka, Sigma Aldrich, St. Louis, Missouri, USA). 100 nm ultra-thin sections were cut using a Diatome (Diatome, Hatfield, PA, USA) diamond knife on a NOVA LKB Ultratome. Sections were

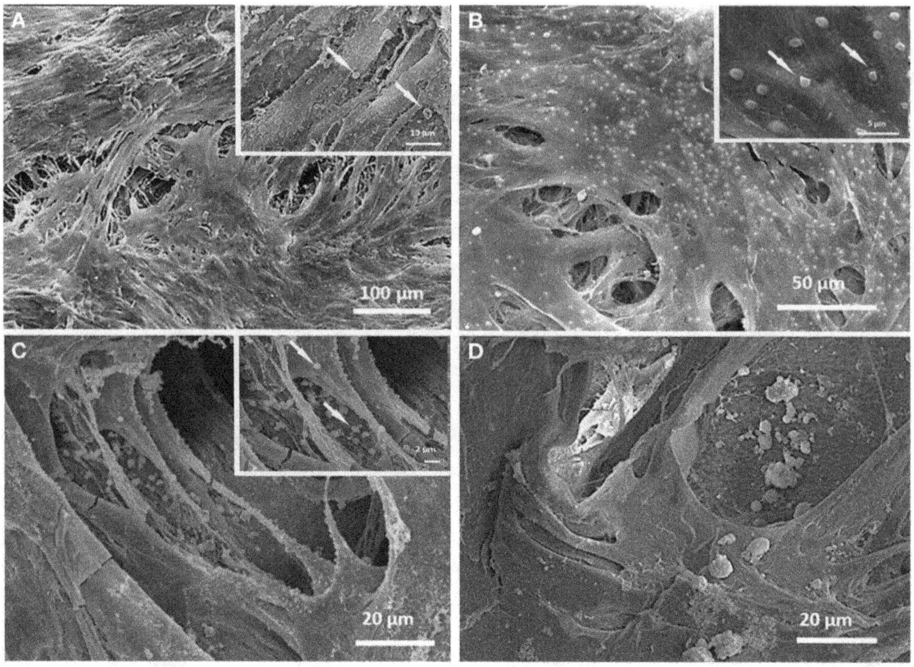


**FIGURE 2 | SEM micrographs of cells cultured on GEL/HA (A,B) and GEL (C,D) displaying a good colonization of the 3D scaffolds.** At 21 days (insets), spherical structures (arrows) were present in PDPCs cultured on both tested scaffolds. Similar features were evidenced also in PDL-SCs seeded on GEL/HA (inset **Figure 1C**).

picked up on nickel grids and stained with alcoholic uranyl acetate and Reynold's lead citrate. Ultrastructural examination was performed using the Philips CM10 Transmission Microscope (FEI Company, Eindhoven, The Netherlands). Images were recorded by Megaview III digital camera (FEI Company, Eindhoven, The Netherlands).

## Quantitative Real-time Polymerase Chain Reaction (qRT-PCR)

### RNA Extraction, Quantitation and Reverse Transcription

Total RNA was extracted from cells with TRIzol® Reagent (Life Technologies, Milan, Italy) according to the manufacturer's protocol. RNA samples were quantified by measuring their absorbance at 260 nm (bioPhotometer plus, Eppendorf GmbH, Germany). The Go Script™ RT System (Promega Corporation—Italy) was used to reverse transcribe 1 μg of total RNA in a 20-μL reaction volume. cDNA neo-synthesized was stored at −20°C.

### qRT- PCR

Real-time PCR was carried out in white plastic-ware with a Mastercycler Realplex2 thermocycler (Eppendorf GmbH, Germany) using the SsoFast™ EvaGreen® Supermix 1X. All PCR assays contained 1 μL of cDNA (corresponding to 50 ng of total RNA template) in a 10-μL reaction volume.

The following program was used for amplification: enzyme activation for 30 s at 95°C, followed by 40 cycles of denaturation for 5 s at 95°C, annealing and extension at 60°C for 20 s. Each primer was used at a 200 nM final concentration. Primer sequences were designed by Primer 3 (v. 0.4.0) software and their specificity was tested by BLAST Assembled RefSeq Genomes in order to avoid any appreciable homology to pseudo-genes or other unexpected targets (**Table 1**). In each assay, the mRNA of both reference genes and each gene of interest were measured simultaneously under equal conditions. Primers showed the same amplification efficiency. Melting curve analysis furthermore confirmed the specificity of qRT-PCR reactions.

### Quantification of mRNA Expression

Real-time PCR reactions were performed in triplicate and Ct values of reference genes were used to normalize cellular mRNA data. In this instance, normalization involved the ratio of mRNA concentrations of specific genes of interest (as mentioned above) to that corresponding to Ct medium values for glyceraldehyde-3-phosphate dehydrogenase (GAPDH) and beta glucuronidase (GUSB) (Ragni et al., 2013). Data were expressed as gene relative expression ($2^{-\Delta Ct}$). Furthermore, in order to highlight the effect of mechanical stimuli on cells, the $\Delta\Delta$Ct method for the evaluation of Fold-Change was employed and cells seeded on plastic were used as an internal control. The relative amount of each mRNA was calculated using the comparative threshold (Ct) method with $\Delta Ct = Ct(mRNA) - Ct(GAPDH)$ and relative quantification of mRNA expression was calculated with the $2^{-\Delta\Delta Ct}$ method (Livak and Schmittgen, 2001). The qPCR efficiency in all our experiments was more than 90%, as the difference between the actual and theoretical (100%) efficiencies would result in an

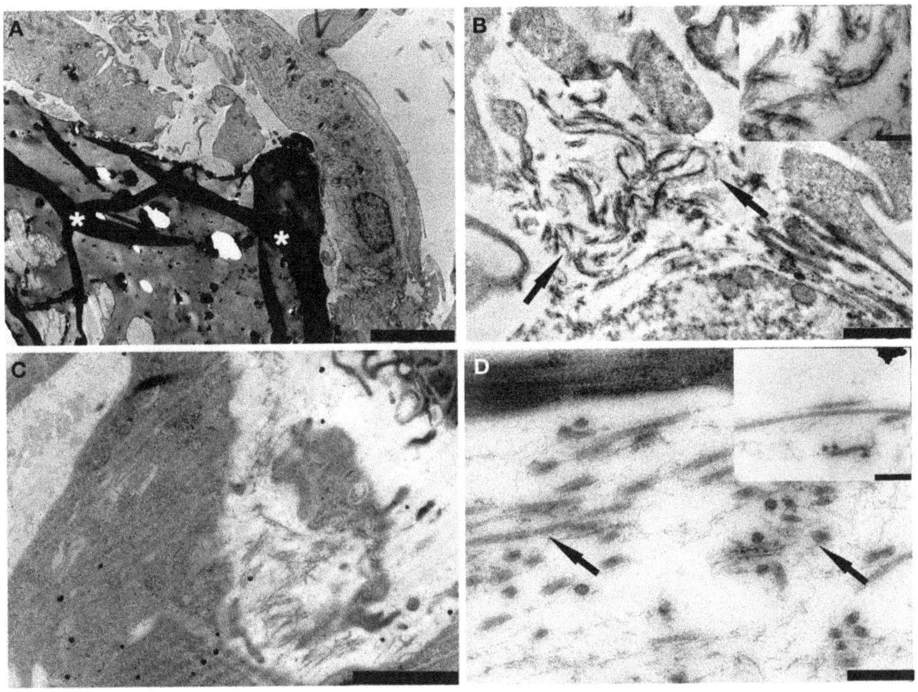


**FIGURE 3 | TEM micrographs of (A) PDL-SCs cultured on gelatin/hydroxyapatite (white asterisks) for 14 days (bar: 5 μm); (B) Fibrils (arrows) resembling the early deposition of extracellular matrix components were detected (bar: 1000 nm).** The inset shows a detail on collagen type I fibers (bar: 200 nm); **(C)** PDL-MSCs cultured on gelatin/hydroxyapatite for 21 days (bar: 2000 nm); **(D)** A high synthesis of extracellular matrix components (arrows) was observed (bar: 200 nm). The inset shows details on collagen type I fibers detected in the extracellular matrix (bar: 200 nm).

underestimation of the mRNA concentration of all analyzed samples.

Data in histograms were expressed as fold-regulation that represents fold-change results in a biologically meaningful way. In particular, the fold-regulation is equal to the fold-change ($2^{-\Delta\Delta Ct}$) for fold-change values greater than one, which indicate an up-regulation. Fold-change values less than one indicate a down-regulation: in this case the fold-regulation is the negative inverse of the fold-change ($-1/2^{-\Delta\Delta Ct}$).

## Statistical Analysis

Mean and standard deviation of three different experiments are reported. Data were analyzed by One-Way ANOVA, Student-Newman-Keuls's and Student's T tests. Statistical significance was tested at $p < 0.05$

# Results

## Cell Characterization

PDPCs, PDL-SCs, and ASCs were all plastic-adherent under standard culture conditions with a fibroblastic, spindle-shape appearance. All cell populations expressed stromal surface markers CD73, CD90, and CD105 and were negative for hematopoietic lineage markers CD45, HLA-DR, CD14, CD19, and CD34 in agreement with the criteria of the International Society for Cell Therapy (Dominici et al., 2006). Moreover they were able to differentiate into all the mesenchymal lineages (data not shown).

## MTT Viability Test

A significant decrease in cell viability was observed in all tested cells after 14 days of culture in osteogenic or chondrogenic medium. No changes were detected between 14 and 21 days of culture (**Figures 1A,B**). These results well-matched with cell differentiation.

PDPCs cultured on GEL/HA scaffolds showed a significant increase of cell viability up to 21 days. A similar behavior was detected also for PDL-SCs even though at a lower extent (**Figure 1C**).

As far as cell seeded on GEL scaffold, PDPCs showed a trend similar to that observed on GEL/HA, whilst ASCs exhibited an increase in cell viability after 14 days of culture and then a decrease at 21 days (**Figure 1D**).

## SEM

Morphological analyses showed the ability of cells to colonize the porosity of both tested scaffolds (**Figure 2**). After 21 days (**Figure 2** insets) cells covered the entire surface of the scaffolds, and on PDL-SCs features indicative of induction of mineralization were detected.

## TEM

ASCs cultured for 14 days on gelatin scaffold showed a good cell adhesion on the surface of the material (**Figure 3A**).

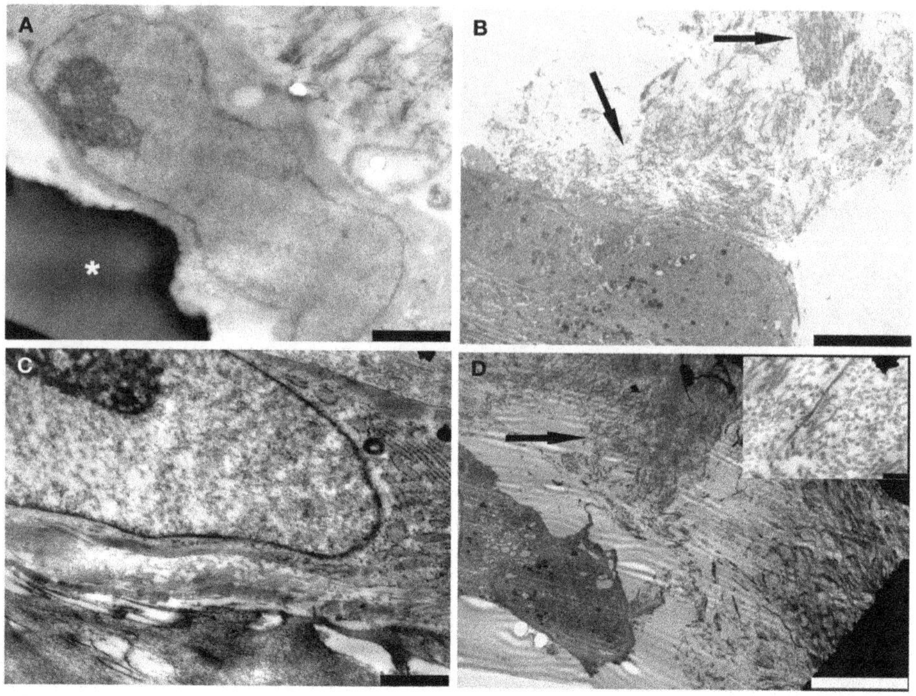


**FIGURE 4 | TEM micrographs of (A) ASCs observed after 14 days of cultured on gelatin scaffold (white asterisks) (bar: 2000 nm); (B) components (arrows) of the extracellular matrix were detected in ASCs cultured for 14 days on scaffold (bar: 10 μm); (C) ASCs cultured on gelatin scaffold for 21 days.** Cells showed a well preserved nucleus and rough endoplasmic reticulum (bar: 1000 nm); **(D)** Several fibrillary structures (arrow) resembling collagen fibers were easily observed in the extracellular matrix (bar: 10 μm). The inset shows a detail on collagen fibers (bar: 200 nm).

Nucleus and nucleolus were well-evident (**Figure 3A**) and a good production of extracellular matrix (ECM) components was observed (**Figure 3B**).

After 21 days of culture on gelatin scaffolds, cells showed a well-developed rough endoplasmic reticulum (RER) suggesting a high protein synthesis (**Figure 3C**). ECM matrix was well-noticed (**Figure 3D**) and fibrillar structures connected to collagen fibers were easily observed (**Figure 3D** inset).

TEM images regarding PDL-SCs cultured on gelatin/hydroxyapatite for 14 days demonstrated well-adhered cells on the scaffold surface (**Figure 4A**). Nucleus and cytoplasmic organelles, such as RER, were well-detected (**Figure 4A**). Small fibrils resembling the early deposition of collagen type I were observed (**Figure 4B**). After 21 days of scaffold culture PDL-SCs showed a high synthesis of ECM components with ultrastructurally identified collagen type I fibrils (**Figures 4C,D**) inset.

## qRT-PCR

Comparison of gene expression results in cells seeded onto GEL/HA with control culture in plastic are shown in **Figure 5A**. Both PDPCs and PDL-SCs showed a reduction in the expression of runx2 after 14 days of culture on GEL/HA, that was detected also after 21 days of culture, being significantly marked in PDPCs. The same trend was observed in PDPCs for osteonectin (sparc) mRNA expression. In PDL-SCs we observed a reduction of mRNA for osteonectin (Fold regulation = $-1.5 \pm 0.1$) after 14 days of culture and its increase (Fold regulation = $2.8 \pm 0.6$) after 21 days. As far as osteocalcin (bglap) mRNA expression is concerned, PDPCs showed its moderate up regulation after 14 days of culture, that became significantly marked after 21 days (Fold regulation = $6.6 \pm 1.2$). On the contrary, in PDL-SCs bglap mRNAexpression was down regulated at both time point analyzed with a significant decrease after 21 days of culture.

The assessment of changes in gene expression between 21 and 14 days in cells seeded onto GEL/HA scaffolds compared to those cultured in tissue control plates suggested a different "commitment" of the diverse MSCs populations studied (**Figure 5B**). In PDPCs we observed a significant up-regulation of bglap on cells seeded on the scaffolds respect to controls. This up-regulation was concomitant with the down regulation of sparc mRNA expression and with a reduced activation of runx2. On the contrary in PDL-SCs seeded on the GEL/HA scaffolds there were slight changes in runx2 and sparc mRNA expression in comparison with controls, whilst we observed a reduction in bglap mRNA expression.

Overall, these results suggested that PDPCs are more committed toward an osteoblastic phenotype compared to PDL-SCs and concomitantly we observed that the scaffold architecture/composition affect osteoblastic differentiation.

As far as cells seeded on GEL scaffold and induced toward a chondrogenic differentiation Bmp2 resulted significantly down regulated in PDPCs, while it remained unchanged in ASCs.

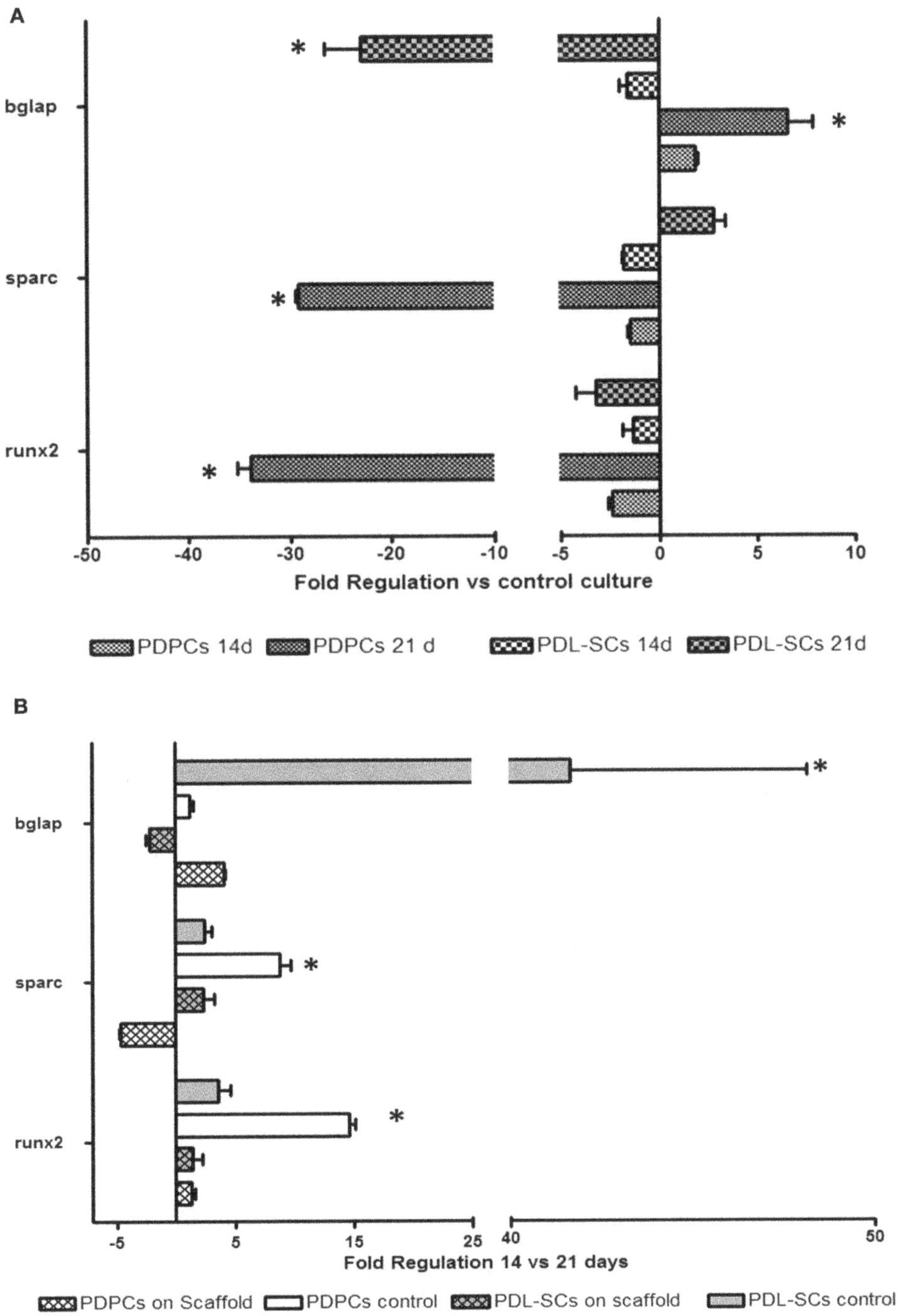


**FIGURE 5 | Histograms depict changes between PDPCs and PDL-SCs mRNA expression of runx2, osteonectin (sparc) and osteocalcin (bglap) observed after culturing cells for 14 and 21 days on GEL/HA with osteogenic differentiating medium. (A)** Fold-changes of PDPCs and PDL-SCs seeded on scaffold with respect to PDPCs and PDL-SCs control cultures (i.e., PDPCs and PDL-SCs in tissue culture plates with osteogenic differentiating medium); **(B)** Fold changes of PDPCs and PDL-SCs seeded on GEL/HA (scaffold) or in tissue control plates (control) at 14 vs. 21 days. Data are expressed as fold-regulation which represents fold-change results in a biologically expressive manner (see Materials and Method section). Statistical differences with relative controls are denoted with an asterisk (*$p < 0.05$).

Sox9 expression was down regulated in both cell cytotypes at 14 days of culture, whilst it appeared unmodified at 21 days of culture. Results of the comparison of Type II collagen mRNA expression in cells seeded onto the scaffolds with control culture in plastic showed a down regulation of this gene at 14 days that was more marked in ASCs. On the contrary, after 21 days the production of Type II collagen increased for both tested cytotypes (**Figure 6A**).

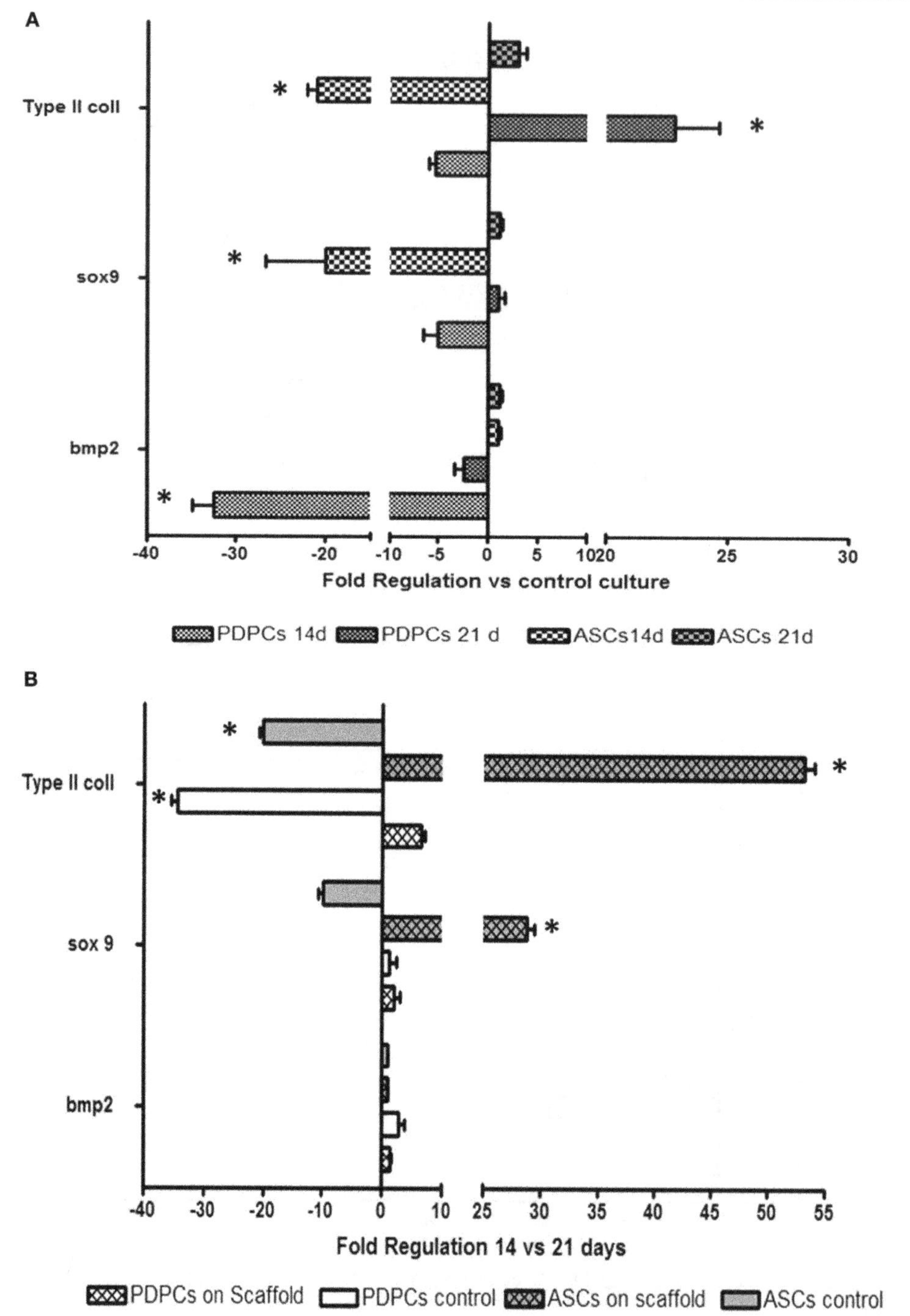


**FIGURE 6 | Histograms depict changes between PDPCs and ASCs mRNA expression of bmp2, Sox 9 and Collagen Type II observed after culturing cells for 14 and 21 days on GEL with chondrogenic differentiating medium. (A)** Fold-changes of PDPCs and ASCs seeded on scaffolds with respect to control cultures (i.e., PDPCs and ASCs in tissue culture plates with chondrogenic differentiating medium); **(B)** Fold changes of PDPCs and ASCs seeded on GEL (scaffold) or in tissue control plates (control) at 14 vs. 21 days. Data are expressed as fold-regulation which represents fold-change results in a biologically expressive manner (see Materials and Method section). Statistical differences with relative controls are denoted with an asterisk ($^{*}p < 0.05$).

The role of a 3D structure in the production of Sox9 and Type II collagen (i.e., chondrogenic commitment) was confirmed by changes in gene expression between 21 and 14 days in cells seeded onto GEL (**Figure 6B**), in which the increase of mRNA for both genes was observed only in cells seeded on scaffolds.

## Discussion

To restore extensive or complex fracture and/or maxillofacial defects, autograft has been widely used and it is still considered as a gold standard (Dimitriou et al., 2011). Autogenous tissue is endowed of all the basic elements essential for an effective tissue regeneration: it provides cells, extracellular matrix and cytokines (Khan et al., 2005; Pape et al., 2010). Nevertheless, the use of autograft possesses drawbacks in terms of costs, procedure time, patient discomfort and possible complications. Moreover, given the limited availability of autogenous tissues, harvested volume could be insufficient to fill or cover a defect (Zouhary, 2010). To overcome these limitations, a variety of exogenous substitutes has been introduced in clinical practice over the last decades (De Long et al., 2007). Indeed, the presence of cells, which orchestrate the release of growth factors and the maintenance of a stable scaffold is key factor for a positive tissue regeneration as cells play a pivotal role in the healing process (Taba et al., 2005). Both somatic and stem cells can be used: the former can be harvested, cultured and implanted to engineer new tissues. Restrictions in the application of somatic cells are related to the lack of self-renewal capability and limited potency, which are exclusive characteristics of stem cells (Garcia-Godoy and Murray, 2006). Among the latter, MSCs has held a great promise. After their initial detection in bone marrow, several other sources of MSCs were identified, including embryonic tissues (umbilical cord, amnion or placenta), as well as different adult tissues (skin, dental pulp, periosteum and adipose tissue, among others) (Salvolini et al., 2010; Ferretti and Mattioli-Belmonte, 2014a; Lazzarini et al., 2014). Indeed, MSCs of different origin may vary in their ability to proliferate and/or respond to external influences (i.e., microenvironment), this behavior could entail different *in vivo* results after transplantation. In this respect, it is crucial to select the most appropriate MSC type for the healing of different anatomical district injured skeletal tissues. Moreover, to improve bone healing, researchers must develop and/or select a scaffold able to maintain, induce and restore biological functions. Therefore, scaffolds must be evaluated not only for their capability to preserve MSC survival, but also to promote their proliferation and differentiation.

In the present study we compared the functional behavior of MSCs of different origin on two kind of 3D porous scaffolds intended for bone (GEL/HA) or cartilage (GEL) regeneration. In order to mimic microenvironment cell cultures were performed in osteogenic or chondrogenic differentiating medium. MSC harvesting site (periosteum, periodontal ligament or adipose tissue) was selected on the basis of experimental evidences of their possible use in clinical practice.

Periosteum has an inner cambium layer with skeletal progenitor cells that constantly give rise to osteoblasts for appositional bone growth and for cortical bone modeling and remodeling in concert with osteoclasts. The outstanding periosteum property has produced widespread research on the use of periosteum-derived cells (PDPCs) for regenerative approaches. Preclinical studies showing the potential of PDPCs in the treatment of non-healing bone fractures and large bone defects are currently available (Ferretti and Mattioli-Belmonte, 2014a). Upon bone injury, PDPCs tend to initiate endochondral bone formation. This feature seems to be a unique periosteal characteristic, as endosteal or bone marrow lesions heal by intramembranous ossification (Colnot, 2009). This dissimilarity in preferred bone formation is maintained even when cells have been expanded *ex vivo* (van Gastel et al., 2014). Indeed, during post-natal bone repair periosteum is the tissue mainly involved in the generation of tissue-forming progenitors. However, multiple adult stem cell populations can be induced into the osteogenic and/or chondrogenic lineages *in vitro*, and as a consequence used for skeletal regeneration.

Periodontal ligament (PDL) contains cell populations that can differentiate into either cementum-forming cells (cementoblasts) or bone-forming cells (osteoblasts) (Huang et al., 2009). This suggests that PDL contains progenitor cells that maintain periodontal tissue homeostasis and regeneration (Huang et al., 2009). Indeed, PDL-SCs are able to form both soft and hard periodontal tissues *in vivo* and are able to stimulate alveolar bone formation (Seo et al., 2004).

At last, ASCs are easily achievable by lipoaspirates from human adipose tissue (Kim and Heo, 2014). In current literature, confident results of tissue engineering strategies for the reconstruction of large osseous defects in orthopedic and craniofacial surgery are available (Griffin et al., 2014; Marmotti et al., 2014). At present, significant efforts have been made for their application in cartilage regeneration (Griffin et al., 2014; Marmotti et al., 2014).

For these reasons we decided to test PDPCs on both type of scaffolds (with or without HA), using them to check PDL-SCs osteogenic differentiation and ASCs chondrogenic differentiation capability, respectively.

Our results evidenced that PDL-SCs are less osteoblastic committed in comparison with PDPCs and the latter seems to be affected by scaffold structure/composition that accelerates cell differentiation toward osteoblasts. This finding is in agreement with our previous results in which we demonstrated the importance of mechanical properties in the expression of PDPC osteogenic genes and of HA in fastening this event (Mattei et al., 2015). Studies comparing the osteogenic capacity of PDL-SCs with other MSCs sources report conflicting data and this contradiction may be at least in part explained by technical differences between these researches, including cell passage number and osteogenic conditions used. Therefore, as reported by Liu et al. (2008) in an experimental animal model PDL-SCs could be an ideal cellular source for periodontal ligament regeneration and this PDL-SC mediated treatment could in turn recover the heights of alveolar bone. As far as chondrogenic differentiation is concerned, scaffold geometry seemed essential to favor cells chondroblast differentiation, confirming recent observation of other researchers (Chen et al., 2015; Dinescu et al., 2015; Roberts et al., 2015).

In conclusion, the proposed 3D porous scaffolds differing in chemical composition are confirmed as promising candidates for osteochondral tissue regeneration applications. However, in order to achieve a successful cell-based skeletal therapy of different anatomical regions a correct stem cell source selection is mandatory.

## Author Contributions

Each author substantially contributed to experimental procedure. In particular MMB planned the whole research and performed

SEM analysis; GT performed TEM observation; GO and MF supplied tissue samples for the different cytotypes, VS, SF, and MD executed cell cultures and qRT-PCR, MO was responsible for qRT-PCR analysis. MFa and RD oversaw the whole research. All authors equally and competently contributed to the draft.

## Ethical Statement

All patients provided their informed consent to participate in the study in accordance with the Declaration of Helsinki. Since the study did not expose the subjects to any risk and in agreement with the Regione Marche Ethical Committee, instead of a written agreement form, a verbal consent was obtained from all the recruited patients. It was highlighted to all subjects that the tissue used for the study represents the usual surgical discard and that the nature of their participation in the study was entirely voluntary (freedom from coercion or undue influence, real or imagined). Patients had sufficient opportunity to ask questions and consider their choice.

## Funding

This work was supported by FIRB (RBAP10MLK7) and PRIN (2010J8RYS7) grants.

## Acknowledgments

The Author would like to thank PhD Concetta Ferretti for her scientific contribution and the Prof. Adriana Bigi and Roberto Giardino of the University of Bologna for the supply of the porous 3D scaffolds and for the useful suggestions during the realization of the whole FIRB research project.

## References

Bianco, P., Barker, R., Brüstle, O., Cattaneo, E., Clevers, H., Daley, G. Q., et al. (2013). Regulation of stem cell therapies under attack in Europe: for whom the bell tolls. *EMBO J.* 32, 1489–1495. doi: 10.1038/emboj.2013.114

Caplan, A. I. (1991). Mesenchymal stem cells. *J. Orthop. Res.* 9, 641–650. doi: 10.1002/jor.1100090504

Chen, X., Li, J., Wang, E., Zhao, Q., Kong, Z., and Yuan, X. (2015). Dynamic compression combined with SOX-9 overexpression in rabbit adipose-derived mesenchymal stem cells cultured in a three-dimensional gradual porous PLGA composite scaffold upregulates HIF-1α expression. *J. Biomed. Mater. Res. A.* doi: 10.1002/jbm.a.35530. [Epub ahead of print].

Colnot, C. (2009). Skeletal cell fate decisions within periosteum and bone marrow during bone regeneration. *J. Bone Miner. Res.* 24, 274–282. doi: 10.1359/jbmr.081003

Crisan, M., Yap, S., Casteilla, L., Chen, C. W., Corselli, M., Park, T. S., et al. (2008). A perivascular origin for mesenchymal stem cells in multiple human organs. *Cell Stem Cell* 3, 301–313. doi: 10.1016/j.stem.2008.07.003

De Long, W. G. Jr., Einhorn, T. A., Koval, K., McKee, M., Smith, W., Sanders, R., et al. (2007). Bone grafts and bone graft substitutes in orthopaedic trauma surgery. A critical analysis. *J. Bone Joint Surg. Am.* 89, 649–658. doi: 10.2106/JBJS.F.00465

Dimitriou, R., Jones, E., McGonagle, D., and Giannoudis, P. V. (2011). Bone regeneration: current concepts and future directions. *BMC Med.* 9:66. doi: 10.1186/1741-7015-9-66

Dinescu, S., Galateanu, B., Radu, E., Hermenean, A., Lungu, A., Stancu, I. C., et al. (2015). A 3D porous gelatin-alginate-based-IPN acts as an efficient promoter of chondrogenesis from human adipose-derived stem cells. *Stem Cells Int.* 2015:252909. doi: 10.1155/2015/252909

Dominici, M., Le Blanc, K., Mueller, I., Slaper-Cortenbach, I., Marini, F., Krause, D., et al. (2006). Minimal Criteria for deifying multipotent mesenchymal stem cells. The International Society for Cellular Therapy position statement. *Cytotherapy* 8, 315–317. doi: 10.1080/14653240600855905

Ferretti, C., Borsari, V., Falconi, M., Gigante, A., Lazzarini, R., Fini, M., et al. (2012). Human periosteum-derived stem cells for tissue engineering applications: the role of VEGF. *Stem Cell Rev.* 8, 882–890. doi: 10.1007/s12015-012-9374-7

Ferretti, C., and Mattioli-Belmonte, M. (2014a). Periosteum derived stem cells for regenerative medicine proposals: boosting current knowledge. *World J. Stem Cells* 6, 266–277. doi: 10.4252/wjsc.v6.i3.266

Ferretti, C., Vozzi, G., Falconi, M., Orciani, M., Gesi, M., Di Primio, R., et al. (2014b). Role of IGF1 and IGF1/VEGF on human mesenchymal stromal cells in bone healing: two sources and two fates. *Tissue Eng. Part A* 20, 2473–2482. doi: 10.1089/ten.tea.2013.0453

Garcia-Godoy, F., and Murray, P. E. (2006). Status and potential commercial impact of stem cell-based treatments on dental and craniofacial regeneration. *Stem Cells Dev.* 15, 881–887. doi: 10.1089/scd.2006.15.881

Giannoudis, P. V., Einhorn, T. A., and Marsh, D. (2007). Fracture healing: the diamond concept. *Injury* 38, S3–S6. doi: 10.1016/S0020-1383(08)70003-2

Griffin, M., Kalaskar, D. M., Butler, P. E., and Seifalian, A. M. (2014). The use of adipose stem cells in cranial facial surgery. *Stem Cell Rev.* 10, 671–685. doi: 10.1007/s12015-014-9522-3

Halfon, S., Abramov, N., Grinblat, B., and Ginis, I. (2011). Markers distinguishing mesenchymal stem cells from fibroblasts are downregulated with passaging. *Stem Cells Dev.* 20, 53–66. doi: 10.1089/scd.2010.0040

Liao, H. T., and Chen, C. T. (2014). Osteogenic potential: comparison between bone marrow and adipose-derived mesenchymal stem cells. *World J. Stem Cells* 6, 288–295. doi: 10.4252/wjsc.v6.i3.288

Huang, G. T., Gronthos, S., and Shi, S. (2009). Mesenchymal stem cells derived from dental tissues vs. those from other sources: their biology and role in regenerative medicine. *J. Dent. Res.* 88, 792–806. doi: 10.1177/0022034509340867

Khan, S. N., Cammisa, F. P. Jr., Sandhu, H. S., Diwan, A. D., Girardi, F. P., and Lane, J. M. (2005). The biology of bone grafting. *J. Am. Acad. Orthop. Surg.* 13, 77–86.

Kim, E. H., and Heo, C. Y. (2014). Current applications of adipose-derived stem cells and their future perspectives. *World J. Stem Cells* 6, 65–68. doi: 10.4252/wjsc.v6.i1.65

Lazzarini, R., Olivieri, F., Ferretti, C., Mattioli-Belmonte, M., Di Primio, R., and Orciani, M. (2014). mRNAs and miRNAs profiling of mesenchymal stem cells derived from amniotic fluid and skin: the double face of the coin. *Cell Tissue Res.* 355, 121–130. doi: 10.1007/s00441-013-1725-4

Lin, Z., Fateh, A., Salem, D. M., and Intini, G. (2014). Periosteum: biology and applications in craniofacial bone regeneration. *J. Dent. Res.* 93, 109–116. doi: 10.1177/0022034513506445

Liu, Y., Zheng, Y., Ding, G., Fang, D., Zhang, C., Bartold, P. M., et al. (2008). Periodontal ligament stem cell-mediated treatment for periodontitis in miniature swine. *Stem Cells* 26, 1065–1073. doi: 10.1634/stemcells.2007-0734

Livak, K. J., and Schmittgen, T. D. (2001). Analysis of relative gene expression data using real-time quantitative PCR and the 2(-Delta Delta C(T)) Method. *Methods* 25, 402–408. doi: 10.1006/meth.2001.1262

Marmotti, A., de Girolamo, L., Bonasia, D. E., Bruzzone, M., Mattia, S., Rossi, R., et al. (2014). Bone marrow derived stem cells in joint and bone diseases: a concise review. *Int. Orthop.* 38, 1787–1801. doi: 10.1007/s00264-014-2445-4

Mattei, G., Ferretti, C., Tirella, A., Ahluwalia, A., and Mattioli-Belmonte, M. (2015). Decoupling the role of stiffness from other hydroxyapatite signalling cues in periosteal derived stem cell differentiation. *Sci. Rep.* 5:10778. doi: 10.1038/srep10778

Orciani, M., Di Primio, R., Ferretti, C., Orsini, G., Salvolini, E., Lazzarini, R., et al. (2012). *In vitro* evaluation of Mesenchymal stem cell isolation possibility from different intra-oral tissues. *J. Biol. Regul. Homeost. Agents* 26, 57S–63S.

Pal, R., Hanwate, M., Jan, M., and Totey, S. (2009). Phenotypic and functional comparison of optimum culture conditions for upscaling of bone marrow-derived mesenchymal stem cells. *J. Tissue Eng. Regen. Med.* 3, 163–174. doi: 10.1002/term.143

Panzavolta, S., Torricelli, P., Amadori, S., Parrilli, A., Rubini, K., della Bella, E., et al. (2013). 3D interconnected porous biomimetic scaffolds: *in vitro* cell response. *J. Biomed. Mater. Res. A* 101, 3560–3570. doi: 10.1002/jbm.a.34662

Pape, H. C., Evans, A., and Kobbe, P. (2010). Autologous bone graft: properties and techniques. *J. Orthop. Trauma* 24, S36–S40. doi: 10.1097/bot.0b013e3181tcec4a1

Ragni, E., Viganò, M., Rebulla, P., Giordano, R., and Lazzari, L. (2013). What is beyond a qRT-PCR study on mesenchymal stem cell differentiation properties: how to choose the most reliable housekeeping genes. *J. Cell. Mol. Med.* 17, 168–180. doi: 10.1111/j.1582-4934.2012.01660.x

Rebelatto, C. K., Aguiar, A. M., Moretão, M. P., Senegaglia, A. C., Hansen, P., Barchiki, F., et al. (2008). Dissimilar differentiation of mesenchymal stem cells from bone marrow, umbilical cord blood, and adipose tissue. *Exp. Biol. Med. (Maywood).* 233, 901–913. doi: 10.3181/0712-RM-356

Roberts, S. J., van Gastel, N., Carmeliet, G., and Luyten, F. P. (2015). Uncovering the periosteum for skeletal regeneration: the stem cell that lies beneath. *Bone* 70, 10–18. doi: 10.1016/j.bone.2014.08.007

Salvolini, E., Orciani, M., Vignini, A., Mattioli-Belmonte, M., Mazzanti, L., and Di Primio, R. (2010). Skin-derived mesenchymal stem cells (S-MSCs) induce endothelial cell activation by paracrine mechanisms. *Exp. Dermatol.* 19, 848–850. doi: 10.1111/j.1600-0625.2010.01104.x

Seo, B. M., Miura, M., Gronthos, S., Bartold, P. M., Batouli, S., Brahim, J., et al. (2004). Investigation of multipotent postnatal stem cells from human periodontal ligament. *Lancet* 364, 149–155. doi: 10.1016/S0140-6736(04)16627-0

Taba, M. Jr., Jin, Q., Sugai, J. V., and Giannobile, W. V. (2005). Current concepts in periodontal bioengineering. *Orthod. Craniofac. Res.* 8, 292–302. doi: 10.1111/j.1601-6343.2005.00352.x

van der Kooy, D., and Weiss, S. (2000). Why stem cells? *Science* 287, 1439–1441. doi: 10.1126/science.287.5457.1439

van Gastel, N., Stegen, S., Stockmans, I., Moermans, K., Schrooten, J., Graf, D., et al. (2014). Expansion of murine periosteal progenitor cells with fibroblast growth factor 2 reveals an intrinsic endochondral ossification program mediated by bone morphogenetic protein 2. *Stem Cells* 32, 2407–2418. doi: 10.1002/stem.1783

Zhu, W., and Liang, M. (2015). Periodontal ligament stem cells: current status, concerns, and future prospects. *Stem Cells Int.* 2015:972313. doi: 10.1155/2015/972313

Zouhary, K. J. (2010). Bone graft harvesting from distant sites: concepts and techniques. *Oral Maxillofac. Surg. Clin. North Am.* 22, 301–316. doi: 10.1016/j.coms.2010.04.007

# 22

# NZ-GMP Approved Serum Improve hDPSC Osteogenic Commitment and Increase Angiogenic Factor Expression

**Edited by:**
*Giovanna Orsini,*
*Marche Polytechnic University, Italy*

***Correspondence:**
*Marcella La Noce*
*marcella.lanoce@unina2.it*

***Anna Spina [1], Roberta Montella [1], Davide Liccardo [1], Alfredo De Rosa [2], Luigi Laino [3], Thimios A. Mitsiadis [4] and Marcella La Noce [1]****

*[1] Sezione di Biotecnologie, Dipartimento di Medicina Sperimentale, Istologia Medica e Biologia Molecolare, Seconda Università degli Studi di Napoli, Napoli, Italy, [2] Sezione di Odontostomatologia, Dipartimento Multidisciplinare Medico-chirurgico, Seconda Università degli Studi di Napoli, Napoli, Italy, [3] Dipartimento di Medicina Clinica e Sperimentale, Università degli Studi di Foggia, Foggia, Italy, [4] Orofacial Development and Regeneration, ZZM, Institute of Oral Biology, University of Zurich, Zurich, Switzerland*

Human dental pulp stem cells (hDPSCs), selected from the stromal-vascular fraction of dental pulp, are ecto-mesenchymal stem cells deriving from neural crests, successfully used in human bone tissue engineering. For their use in human therapy GMP procedures are required. For instance, the use of fetal bovine serum (FBS) is strongly discouraged in clinical practice due to its high risk of prions and other infections for human health. Alternatively, clinical grade sera have been suggested, including the New Zealand FBS (NZ-FBS). Therefore, the aim of this study was to evaluate the behavior of hDPSCs expanded in culture medium containing NZ-FBS. Since it was widely demonstrated hDPSCs display relevant capabilities to differentiate into osteogenic and angiogenic lineages, we performed a comparative study to assess if these features are also retained by cultivating the cells with a safer serum never tested on this cell line. hDPSCs were grown using NZ-FBS and conventional (C-FBS) for 7, 14, and 21 days, in both 2D and 3D cultures. Growth curves, expression of bone-related markers, calcification and angiogenesis were evaluated. NZ-FBS induced significant cell growth with respect to C-FBS and promoted an earlier increase expression of osteogenic markers, in particular of those involved in the formation of mineralized matrix (BSP and OPN) within 14 days. In addition, hDPSCs cultured in presence of NZ-FBS were found to produce higher mRNA levels of the angiogenic factors, such as VEGF and PDGFA. Taken together, our results highlight that hDPSCs proliferate, enhance their osteogenic commitment and increase angiogenic factors in NZ-FBS containing medium. These features have also been found when hDPSC were seeded on the clinical-grade collagen I scaffold (Bio-Gide®), leading to the conclusion that for human therapy some procedures and above all the use of GMP-approved materials have no negative impact.

**Keywords: hDPSCs, osteogenesis, angiogenesis, bone differentiation, bioscaffold**

## INTRODUCTION

There is an increasing interest in the regeneration of organs and tissues damaged by diseases, trauma or aging. In human regeneration, the use of autologous and allogeneic stem cells isolated from various tissues of adult individuals has fewer ethical problems than the use of embryonic stem cells (Caplan, 2007; Ferro et al., 2012). An easily accessible source of mesenchymal stem cells is the dental pulp, which is a stromal, fibrous, highly vascularized structure located in the inner part of the tooth (d'Aquino et al., 2007). Stem cells from dental follicles and human dental pulp stem cells (hDPSCs) express several transcription factors that are involved in the maintenance of self-renewal and pluripotency such as Sox2 and Nanog (d'Aquino et al., 2011), and specific mesenchymal stem cell markers such as CD90 (Ponnaiyan et al., 2012) and CD34, used for the first time by Laino et al. to isolate a population of stromal stem cells of neural crest origin (Laino et al., 2005). Under definite culture conditions, hDPSCs differentiate into numerous cell types, including osteogenic, adipogenic, neurogenic, and neural crest-derived cells (Almushayt et al., 2006; Zhang et al., 2006; Arthur et al., 2008; Paino et al., 2010). Several studies have shown that hDPSCs can be successfully used in clinical practice as a new therapeutic tool for healing bone defects (d'Aquino et al., 2009; Mitsiadis et al., 2011; Giuliani et al., 2013) since it was demonstrate that DPSCs are self-committed to osteogenic and angiogenic differentiation (d'Aquino et al., 2007).

However, various important issues have been addressed concerning the clinical use of hDPSCs, namely the generation of an adequate number of cells in a short period of time; the characterization of cells at all stages of culture before their use in clinic (Tirino et al., 2012); and the development of safe-for-human-use materials for the isolation and maintenance of cells selected for therapy (Desiderio et al., 2014). For these reasons, it is necessary to standardize procedures and good manufacturing practice (GMP) protocols for the culture of the stem cells for clinical use (La Noce et al., 2014). To this end, the development of international standards for the production of hDPSCs, in accordance with GMP, holds a paramount importance.

In this context, physical and chemical factors play a pivotal role since they can influence the cell culture conditions and, therefore, the cells' fate. Stem cells display different behaviors and answers in culture and it is extremely complex to obtain similar stem cell stocks following a standard protocol. Moreover, the serum added to basic medium may contain growth factors and nutrients that mimic the extracellular environment, which may be crucial for cell proliferation and differentiation. Usually, cells are cultured in media containing animal-origin sera which are not recommended for clinical practice because of concerns about human safety. In fact, viruses, prions, mycoplasma or any other animal pathogen could contaminate the sera. Bovine sera are the most commonly used and, in particular, fetal bovine serum (C-FBS) has become the standard supplement for cell culture media. It is a cocktail of most of the factors required for cell proliferation and maintenance, and thus is an almost universal growth supplement. FBS sourced from New Zealand (NZ-FBS) is a valid bovine serum as it offers greater safety due to the fact that New Zealand has the fewest reported bovine diseases in the world for its geographically isolation. Indeed, one of the benefits of this isolation is that New Zealand has been determined to be free from BSE and FMD.

Additionally, the use of DPSCs in clinical applications requires a support system. The choice of scaffolds for tissue engineering is rather critical due to the large amount of existing variables and the GMP procedures require that these scaffolds are clinical-grade, ready for human use (Naddeo et al., 2015; Mele et al., 2016).

In this study, two different sera have been assayed and compared, namely the commonly used C-FBS, and a more controlled FBS, originating from New Zealand (NZ-FBS), that is GMP-approved. In addition, the influence of two different sera on a three-dimensional (3D) culture of hDPSC *in vitro*, using a commercially available clinical-grade collagen I bioscaffold, the Bio-Gide® (Geistlich, Wolhusen, CH), has been assessed.

## MATERIALS AND METHODS

### Human Dental Pulp Extraction and Cell Culture

Human dental pulps were extracted from teeth of healthy adults (21–38 years of age). Prior to the extraction, each subject ($n$ = 40) was checked for systemic and oral infections or diseases. Only patients undergoing a third molar or supernumerary tooth extraction were interviewed and enlisted. All subjects signed the Ethical Committee (Second University Internal Ethical Committee) consent brochure before being enrolled. Every subject was pretreated for a week with professional dental hygiene. The dental crown was covered with 0.3% chlorhexidine gel (Forhans, New York, USA) for 2 min prior to the extraction. Dental pulp was obtained with a dentinal excavator or a Gracey curette. The pulp was delicately removed and immersed for 1 h at 37°C in a digestive solution composed of 3 mg/ml type I collagenase and 4 mg/ml dispase in phosphate buffered saline (PBS) containing 40 mg/ml gentamicin. Once digested, the solution was filtered through 70 μm Falcon strainers (Becton & Dickinson, Franklin Lakes, NJ, USA). Cells were cultured in basal growth medium consisting of Dulbecco's modified Eagle's medium (DMEM) with 100 U/mL penicillin, 100 mg/mL streptomycin and 200 mM L-glutamine (all from GIBCO, Monza, Italy), supplemented with the two sera to get the different culture conditions: (a) 10% fetal bovine serum (C-FBS; GIBCO, Monza, Italy), and (b) 10% New Zealand origin FBS (NZ-FBS; SAFC Biosciences). Cultures were maintained in a humidified atmosphere under 5% $CO_2$ at 37°C. Media were changed twice a week. The analyses were conducted at 7, 14, and 21 days of culture.

### Growth Analysis

Cells in the two different culture media were plated at a density of 50,000 cells/well in 6-well plates and at a density of 100,000 cells in T25 flasks. The cells were harvested and re-suspended in PBS. An aliquot of cell suspension was diluted with 0.4% trypan blue (Sigma-Aldrich, Milan, Italy), pipetted onto a hemocytometer and counted under a microscope. The number of viable cells for each experimental condition was counted and represented on a linear graph. The doubling time (DT) was determined from the growth curves or by using the formula.

$$DT = (t - t_0) \log 2/(\log N - \log N_0)$$

where t and $t_0$ were the times at which the cells were counted, and N and $N_0$ were the cell numbers at times t and $t_0$, respectively.

## FACs Analysis

Flow cytometry analyses were performed on hDPSCs cultured in medium supplemented with C-FBS or NZ-FBS at first passage of culture. Cells were incubated with FITC-conjugated anti-CD90, PerCP-Cy5.5-conjugated anti-CD105, APC-Cy7-conjugated anti-CD45 (all purchased from BD Pharmingen, San Diego, CA), and PE-conjugated anti-CD34 (Miltenyi Biotech, Calderara di Reno, Bologna, Italy) for phenotypic characterization; and anti-Bone sialoprotein (BSP) (Abcam, Cambridge, UK), anti-CFS-conjugated anti-Osteopontin (OPN), PE-conjugated anti-Osteocalcin (OC) (both from R&D Systems, Minneapolis, MN) and PerCP-Cy 5.5-conjugated anti-Nanog (BD Pharmingen, Milan, Italy) to evaluate osteogenic differentiation and mesenchymal stemness. hDPSCs were sorted by CD34 expression. The purity of sorting was 90%. As negative controls, cells were stained with an isotype control antibody. After incubation with the antibody, cells were resuspended in PBS and analyzed with a FACS ARIA III (BD Biosciences, San Jose, CA). For intracellular staining of Osteocalcin, Osteopontin and Nanog, cells were processed using Fix & Perm Kit (Invitrogen, Milan, Italy) following the manufacturer's guidelines. All data were analyzed using FCS express version 3 (De Novo Software, Glendale, CA).

## RNA Isolation and qRT-PCR

Total RNA was extracted from hDPSCs after 7, 14, and 21 days of culture in DMEM supplemented with 10% C-FBS or 10% FBS New Zealand, using an AMBION kit (Life Technologies Italia, Monza, Italy) following the manufacturer's instructions. RNA was treated with DNase (Promega, Milan, italy) to exclude DNA contamination and stored at −80°C. cDNA synthesis was carried out from total RNA (1 µg) using VILO SUPERSCRIPT (Invitrogen, Monza, Italia,). Samples were analyzed using real-time quantitative PCR. PCR reactions were performed using StepOne Thermocycler (Applied Biosystems, Monza, Italy) and the amplifications were done using the SYBR Green PCR Master Mix (Applied Biosystems, Monza, Italy). The thermal cycling conditions were: 50°C for 2 min followed by an initial denaturation step at 95°C for 2 min, 40 cycles at 95°C for 30 s, 60°C for 30 s and 72°C for 30 s. Real-time PCR was performed using the primer sequences shown in **Table 1**. The experiments were carried out in triplicate for each data point. Gene expression was normalized to *GAPDH* considered as internal control.

**TABLE 1 | Primers for real time RT-PCR.**

| Gene | Primer sequence | Ta (°C) |
|---|---|---|
| *GAPDH* | Fw: GGAGTCAACGGATTTGGTCG<br>Rev: CTTCCCGTTCTCAGCCTTGA | 57 |
| *CD90* | Fw: CCCAGTGAAGATGCAGGTTT<br>Rev: GACAGCCTGAGAGGGTCTTG | 60 |
| *RUNX2* | Fw: CACTCACTACCACACCTACC<br>Rev: TTCCATCAGCGTCAACACC | 52 |
| *CD34* | Fw: TCAAATGTTCAGGCATCAGAG<br>Rev: TCAGGTCAGATTGGTGCTT | 56 |
| *NANOG* | Fw: TTCAGTCTGGACACTGGCTG<br>Rev: CTCGGTGATTAGGGTCCAAC | 58 |
| *BGLAP (OSTEOCALCIN)* | Fw: CTCACACTCCTCGCCCTATTG<br>Rev: CTTGGACACAAAGGCTGCAC | 57 |
| *SPP1 (OSTEOPONTIN)* | Fw: GCCGAGGTGATAGTGTGGTT<br>Rev: TGAGGTGATGTCCTCGTCTG | 58 |
| *IBSP* | Fw: GGGCAGTAGTGACTCATCCG<br>Rev: TTCTCAGCCTCAGAGTCTTCA | 58 |
| *SP7 (OSTERIX)* | Fw: TCCTCCCTGCTTGAGGAGGA<br>Rev: AGTCCCGCAGAGGGCTAGAG | 60 |
| *CXCR4* | Fw: CCTATGCAAGGCAGTCCATGT<br>Rev: GGTAGCGGTCCAGACTGATGA | 57 |
| *ITGB1 (INTEGRIN-BETA1)* | Fw: CATCTGCGAGTGTGGTGTCT<br>Rev: GGGGTAATTTGTCCCGACTT | 57 |
| *VEGF* | Fw: TGACAGGGAAGAGGAGGAGA<br>Rev: CGTCTGACCTGGGGTAGAGA | 59 |
| *PDGFA* | Fw: ACACGAGCAGTGTCAAGTGC<br>Rev: GGCTCATCCTCACCTCACAT | 60 |

## Alizarin Red Staining and Quantification

After 21 days of culture in the different sera, osteogenic differentiation was evaluated by Alizarin Red staining to visualize calcium-rich deposits produced by the cells. The samples were washed twice in PBS, fixed with 4% paraformaldehyde (PFA) in PBS for 30 min at 4°C, and stained with Alizarin Red solution (2%, pH 4.2; Sigma Aldrich, Milan, Italy) for 20 min at room temperature. Stained cells were extensively washed with deionized water to remove any nonspecific precipitation. Micrographs were taken with a microscope Eclipse TE2000-S (Nikon, Firenze, Italy) and a Nikon camera (Nikon, Firenze, Italy).

For the quantification of Alizarin Red S staining, 4 ml 10% (vol/vol) acetic acid was added to each well and the plate was incubated at room temperature for 30 min under gentle agitation. The monolayer was scraped off the plate and transferred to a 1.5 ml microcentrifuge tube after adding 1 ml of 10% (vol/vol) acetic acid. After vortexing for 30 s, the slurry was overlaid with 1.25 ml mineral oil (Sigma-Aldrich, St. Louis, MO), heated to 85°C for 10 min, and transferred to ice for 5 min. The slurry was then centrifuged at 20,000 g for 15 min, and 500 µl of the supernatant then removed to a new 1.5 ml microcentrifuge tube. 200 µl of 10% (vol/vol) ammonium hydroxide was added to neutralize the acid. Absorbance of aliquots (150 µl) of the supernatant was measured in triplicate at 405 nm in a 96-well format.

## Quantification of Osteocalcin in Supernatant

Osteocalcin levels were evaluated in the culture supernatants of hDPSCs at different time and tested sera by a solid phase Enzyme Amplified Sensitivity Immunoassay (EASIA) kit (Invitrogen, Monza, Italy). Standards and samples were analyzed in duplicate. The assay was performed according to the manufacturer's protocols. The absorbance of each well was read at 450 nm and the concentration of Osteocalcin was determined by interpolation from the standard curve.

## Cell Seeding on Bio-Gide® Collagen Scaffolds

In order to both better analyze the hDPSCs performances in presence of the two sera, and understand the DPSCs's potential differentiation capabilities, we challenged these stem cells in a 3D culture system, in order to determine to what extent these cells were capable of differentiating toward bone and vessel progenitors, in presence of GMP-approved or FBS serum. For this purpose, hDPSCs were seeded onto BioGide® (Geistlich Pharma AG, Switzerland), a clinical-grade collagen I reabsorbable bilayer membrane composed of a superior thick and an inferior smooth surface. The scaffold's membrane is made of a natural collagen I without further cross-linking: the superior thick and porous surface allows the adhesion of osteoblasts on the surface, whereas the dense and smooth surface hinders cells to both adhere and penetrate inside it.

This scaffold, commercially used in dentistry, has a low antigenicity and excellent biocompatibility.

The membranes were cut under sterile conditions into pieces of equal size (5 × 5 mm). Scaffolds were placed in 6-well-plates and a cell suspension of $1 \times 10^6$ cells/ 200 µl of medium was pipetted onto the top (thick and porous surface) of each piece. Cells were allowed to adhere under a humidified atmosphere at 37°C and 5% $CO_2$ for 4 h. The seeded scaffolds were then placed in tubes containing DMEM supplemented with the two different sera (C-FBS and NZ-FBS) for 30 days in an incubator at 37°C and 5% $CO_2$. Media were changed twice a week.

## Cryostat Sectioning

After 3D culture, samples were fixed in 4% paraformaldehyde (PFA) and cryoprotected overnight at 4°C by immersion in a 30% (wt/vol) sucrose solution before being embedded in Tissue-Tek® O.C.T. Compound (Tissue-Tek; Sakura Finetek, Torrance,

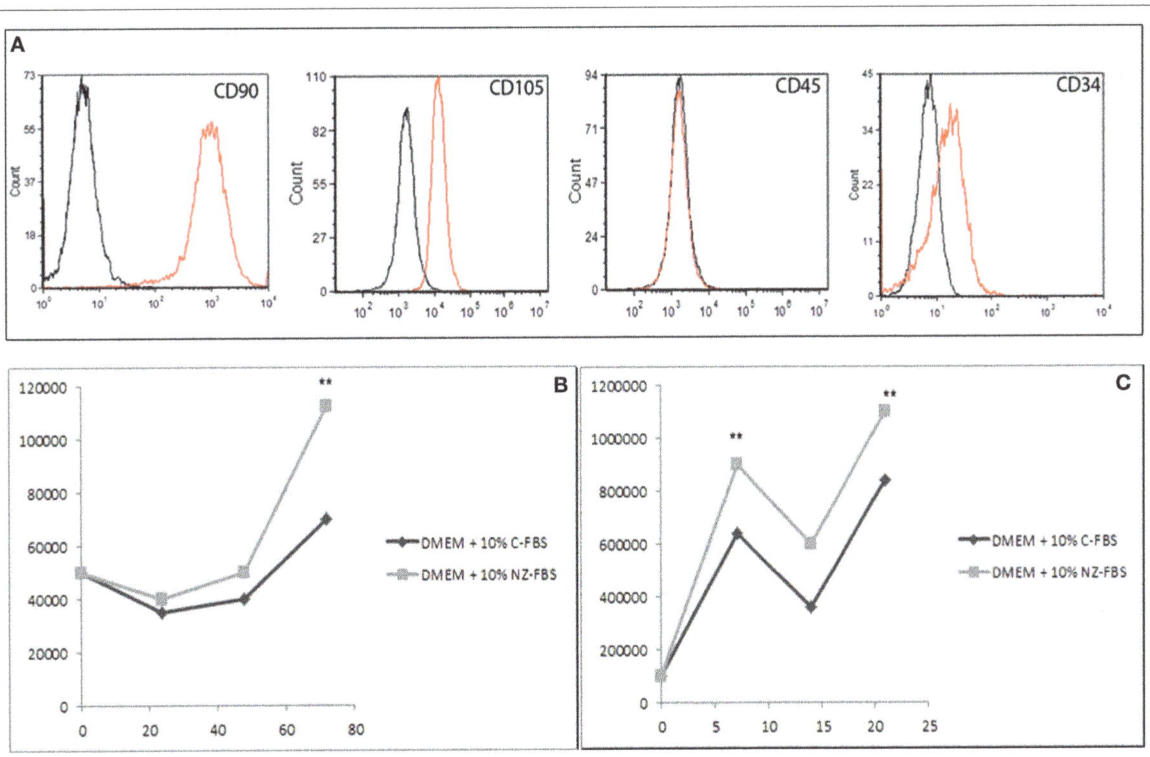


**FIGURE 1 | (A)** Characterization of DPSCs at the first passage of culture: cytometric analysis of CD90, CD105, CD45, and CD34 markers in DPSCs. Histograms represent the number of cells (y axis) and the fluorescence intensity (x axis) relative to unstained control cells (dot line) and cells marked with specific antibodies against surface proteins (solid line). **(B)** Growth curve of DPSCs cultured in DMEM + 10% of standard FBS and in DMEM + 10% of New Zealand FBS up to 72 h. **(C)** Growth performance was studied up to 21 days. **$p < 0.001$.

CA,) and frozen. Sections were cut 5-μm thick with a cryostat at −20°C and then processed for immunostaining.

## Immunohistochemistry/ Immunofluorescence Analysis

hDPSCs cultured in 24-well plates were fixed with 4% PFA in PBS for 20 min at room temperature. After washing in PBS, samples were permeabilized with 0.1% Triton X-100 for 5 min and blocked with 1% BSA in PBS. Incubation with primary anti-OC antibody (sc-30044 Santa Cruz) was performed overnight at 4°C. Primary antibody was revealed using a FITC-conjugated anti-rabbit IgG secondary antibody. Nuclei were stained with Hoechst.

Frozen sections were stained by Hematoxylin and Eosin or permeabilized with 0.1% Triton X-100 for 15 min. Incubation with primary antibodies anti-OPN (ab8448 Abcam, Cambridge, UK), anti-OC (sc-30044 Santa Cruz), and anti-VEGF (ab39250 Abcam Cambridge, UK) was performed overnight at 4°C. FITC conjugated secondary antibody to rabbit IgG was used to reveal primary antibodies. Micrographs were taken with a microscope EVOS FL Cell Imaging System (Life Technologies).

## Statistical Analysis

Values are shown as the mean ± S.E.M. of measurements of at least three independently performed experiments to avoid possible variation of cell cultures. Student's $t$-test was employed, and $p < 0.05$ was considered to be statistically significant.

**TABLE 2 | Doubling time of DPSCs under different culture conditions.**

| Culture conditions | Doubling Time (hours) | *P*-value |
|---|---|---|
| DMEM + 10% C-FBS | 126 ± 12 | $P < 0.001$ |
| DMEM + 10% NZ-FBS | 94 ± 7 | $P < 0.005$ |

# RESULTS

## Characterization of hDPSCs by Flow Cytometric Analysis

At the first culture passage, cells were characterized by evaluating the expression of CD90, CD105, CD45, and CD34 using cytometric analysis. Cells were all positive for the mesenchymal markers CD90 and CD105, and negative for CD45. Approximately 20% of cells were positive for CD34 (**Figure 1A**). Then cells were sorted by CD34.

## Evaluation of Cell Proliferation after Sera Treatment

Cell proliferation under the different conditions was evaluated at 24, 48, and 72 h (**Figure 1B**) and at 7, 14, and 21 days (**Figure 1C**) of culture. To this purpose, equal numbers of cells were initially plated and the relative time of duplication was assessed. Either C-FBS and NZ-FBS promoted hDPSC proliferation. However, there were lower numbers of cells in bovine-origin sera compared with NZ-FBS, a difference already detectable at 48 h (**Figure 1B**). NZ-FBS stimulated earlier cell duplication with a reduction in the doubling time to less than a half of that of NZ-FBS (**Table 2**).

## Phenotypic Characterization of DPSCs during Cell Culture

In order to evaluate the effect of different sera on the expression of stemness and osteogenic markers, a flow cytometric assay at different days of culture for CD34, NANOG, CD90, BSP, and

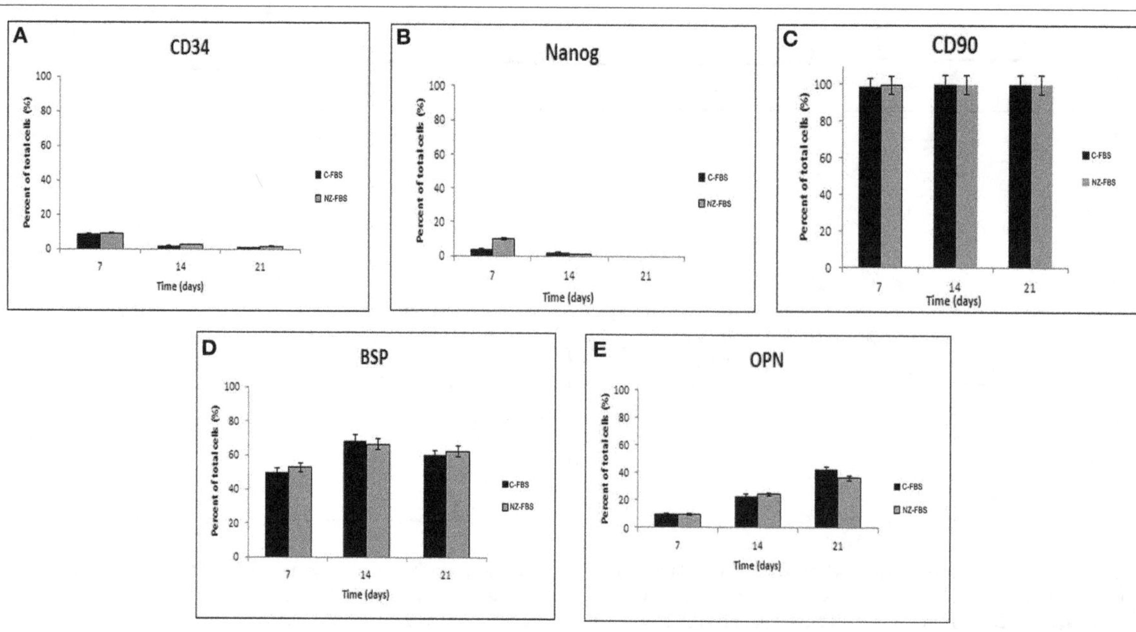


**FIGURE 2 | Cytometric analysis for stemness markers (A–C), and osteogenic markers (D,E) in DPSCs.**

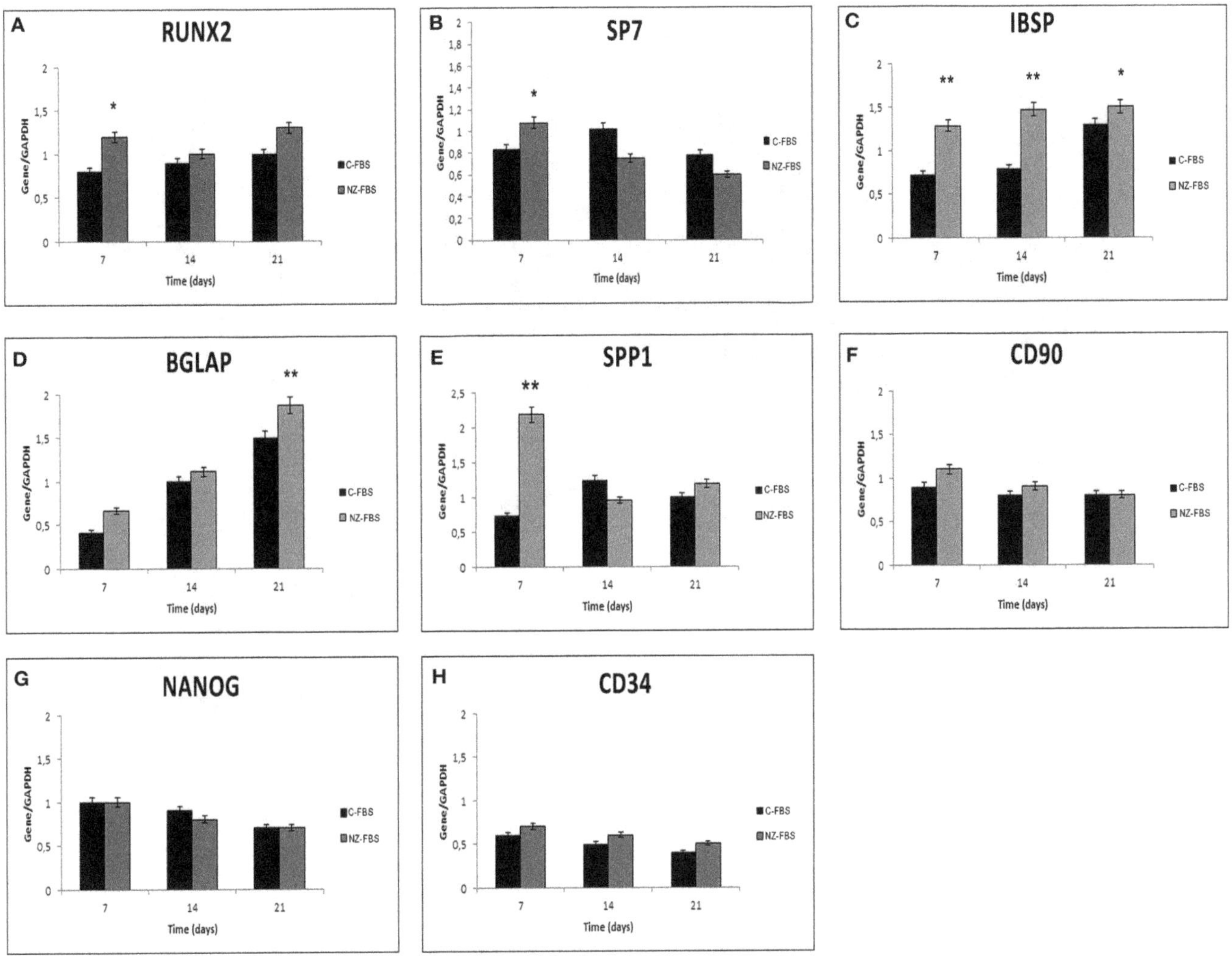


**FIGURE 3 | Gene expression analysis for osteogenic markers (A–E), and stemness markers (F–H) in DPSCs.** *$p < 0.05$; **$p < 0.001$.

OPN, was performed (**Figures 2A–E**). Levels of the stromal-vascular antigen CD34 decreased up to day 21 (**Figure 2A**) in both sera. Expression of the stemness marker NANOG also decreased, although its protein level was higher at 7 days of culture in NZ-FBS (**Figure 2B**). All hDPSCs expanded with C-FBS and NZ-FBS, showed positivity (>98%) for the mesenchymal marker CD90 (**Figure 2C**).

The expression of osteogenic markers BSP and OPN did not show substantial differences during culture time using both sera (**Figures 2D,E**).

Further investigations on osteogenic features and the maintenance of stemness were also performed using a quantitative RT-PCR for *RUNX2, SP7 (OSTERIX), IBSP, BGLAP(OSTEOCALCIN), SPP1 (OSTEOPONTIN), CD90, NANOG,* and *CD34* at 7, 14, and 21 days of culture (**Figures 3A–H**). The expression of *RUNX2*, the master transcription factor of osteogenic differentiation, was higher in FBS-NZ at 7 days of culture and then decreased at 14 and 21 days in both sera without significant differences (**Figure 3A**). *SP7* mRNA, another transcription factor involved in osteogenic differentiation, showed an increase only at 7 days of culture (**Figure 3B**).

mRNA levels of *IBSP*, *BGLAP* and *SPP1* increased in cells cultured with FBS-NZ starting from 7 days (**Figures 3C–E**).

The mRNA levels of *CD90* were comparable in all the experimental conditions (**Figure 3F**). *NANOG* was always expressed but decreased during culture time as well as *CD34* mRNA (**Figures 3G,H**).

## Intracellular Localization of Osteocalcin, Evaluation of Mineralization, and Osteocalcin Secretion

Immunoreactivity for OC was strongest and distributed throughout the cell in hDPSCs cultured with NZ-FBS at 21 days of culture (**Figure 4B**). hDPSCs cultured with C-FBS were only weakly positive for OC that was mostly localized in the perinuclear region (**Figure 4A**).

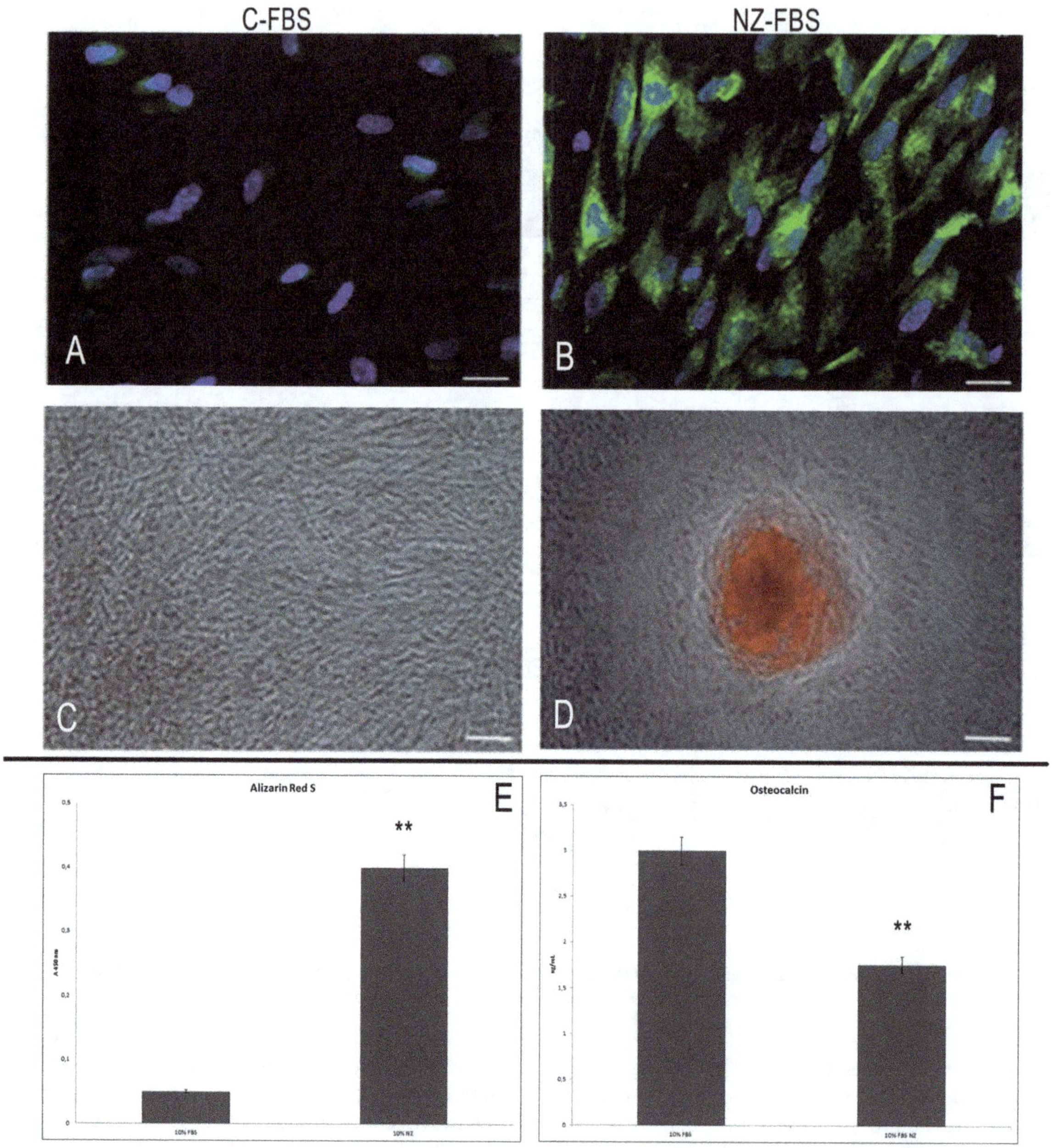


**FIGURE 4 | Immunofluorescence analysis for osteocalcin in DPSCs cultured with C-FBS (A) and NZ-FBS (B).** Scale bar = 10 μm. Alizarin red analysis of DPSCs cultured with C-FBS **(C)** and NZ-FBS **(D)**. Scale bar = 100 μm. **(E)** Alizarin Red Quantification. **(F)** Osteocalcin concentration with C-FBS and NZ-FBS. $^{**}p < 0.001$.

Alizarin red staining was used to evaluate calcium-rich deposits after 21 days of culture (**Figures 4C,D**). Calcified nodules were absent in cultures with C-FBS (**Figure 4C**) but small areas of staining were evident, whereas mineral deposition was observed in cultures with NZ-FBS (**Figure 4D**). This observation was confirmed by Alizarin red quantification (**Figure 4E**).

Moreover, we determined the concentration of OC in the culture supernatants after 21 days. A significant difference was observed between the two tested sera (**Figure 4F**). In FBS-NZ the amount of osteocalcin in the medium was very low.

## Homing, Chemotaxis and Evaluation of Angiogenesis

In order to evaluate a possible effect of FBS-NZ on DPSCs homing and chemotaxis, we assessed the expression of *ITGB1* (*INTEGRIN-β1*) and *CXCR4*. *ITGB1* mRNA showed a slight increase at 7 days of culture with NZ-FBS, but then remained almost unchanged in the two different tested sera (**Figure 5A**).

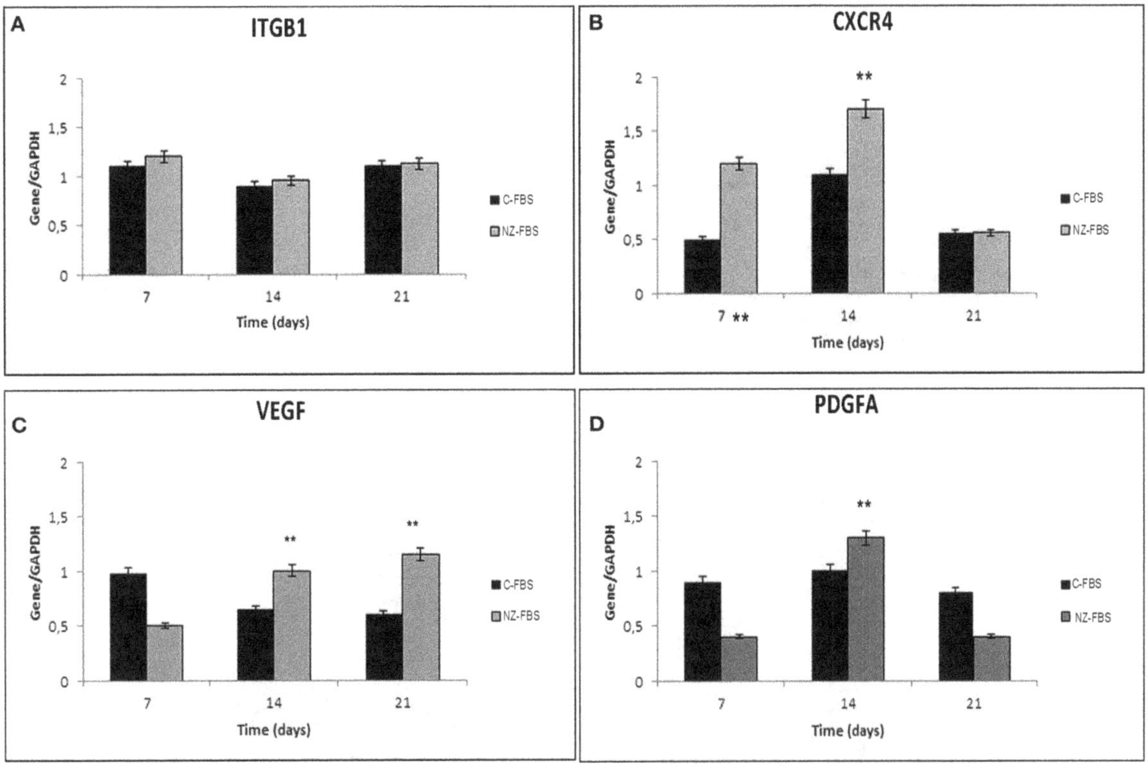


**FIGURE 5 | Real time PCR for genes involved in chemotaxis and cell adhesion.** In **(A,B)** are respectively shown expression of Integrin beta 1 (Intβ1) and chemokine receptor 4 (CXCR4) mRNA in DPSCs. Real time PCR for genes involved in angiogenesis: VEGF **(C)** and PDGFA **(D)** mRNA levels in DPSCs. All results were normalized to GAPDH expression. $^{**}p < 0.001$.

The expression of *CXCR4* was more induced by NZ-FBS at 7 and 14 days of culture, and drastically decreased at 21 days (**Figure 5B**).

The expression of *VEGF* and Platelet-derived growth factor A (*PDGFA*) mRNAs in hDPSCs was also evaluated after numerous days of culture (**Figures 5C,D**). The *VEGF* expression was significantly promoted by NZ-FBS at 14 and 21 days of culture (**Figure 5C**); the expression of *PDGFA* gene was higher in NZ-FBS samples only at 14 days of culture, then decreased (**Figure 5D**). hDPSCs were negative for *PDGFB* mRNA in all the experimental conditions (data not shown).

## 3D Culture Experiments

The results of 3D cultures are shown in **Figure 6**. In this figure, the cross section of the scaffold is depicted in IA: it is made of collagen I fibers surrounded on the two sides by a membrane (one thick and porous and another smooth).

Challenging hDPSCs with this scaffold, in presence of the two sera, hDPSCs displayed on the scaffold's surface constituting a cell monolayer as shown in **Figure 6IB**. Specifically, through the use of specific antibodies for osteo-angiogenesis, we found that cells expressed all the markers, including OPN, OC, VEGF (**Figures 6IIA–F**), through the whole cell layer.

In particular, using NZ-FBS in cultures, DPSCs were found to be noticeably positive for the said markers of bone and vessels (**Figures 6IIB,D,F**).

# DISCUSSION

The use of animal sera for stem cell cultures may be unsafe for human cell-based therapies as they may contain factors or pathogens that could be transferred to patients or cause immune rejection during cell transplantations (Mackensen et al., 2000; Sundin et al., 2007).

In the present study, a GMP-approved serum was compared with a commercial fetal bovine serum during isolation and expansion of hDPSCs *in vitro*.

Freshly isolated hDPSCs, were characterized and found to be positive for common mesenchymal stem cells markers. Later, hDPSCs phenotype was characterized during culture and the differences in cell proliferation, stemness, and osteogenic features were assessed.

In this study it has been shown that NZ-FBS induced significant cell growth with respect to C-FBS. The expression of CD90 marker remained unchanged throughout all experimental conditions, indicating that these cells maintained the mesenchymal lineage, whereas the expression of stemness markers CD34 and NANOG decreased with time, as expected.

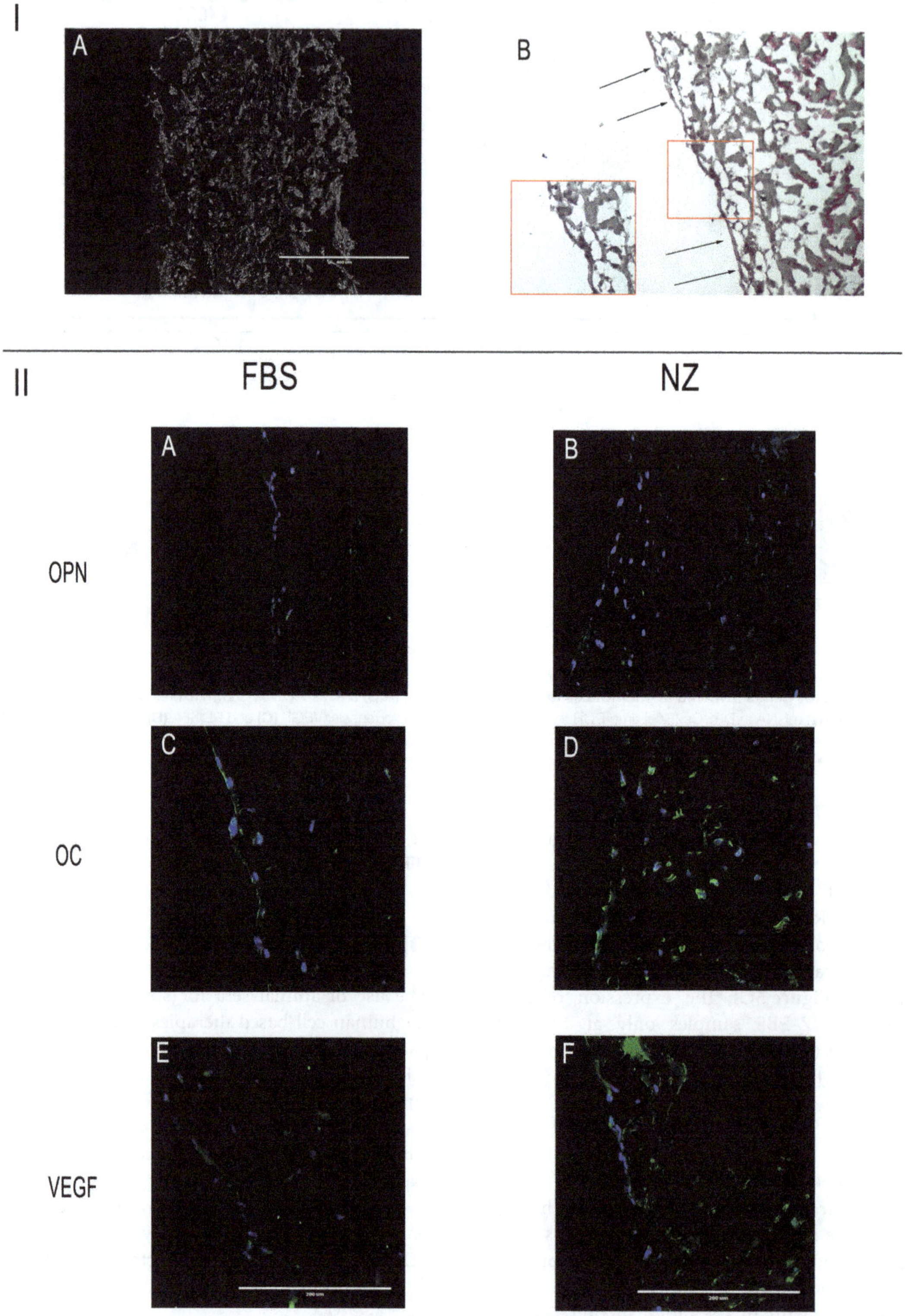


**FIGURE 6 | I: (A)** Cross section of the scaffold; **(B)** hDPSCs on the scaffold's surface constitute a cell monolayer. Scale bar = 400 μm. **II:** Immunofluorescence analysis of specific antibodies for osteo-angiogenesis, (OPN, OC, VEGF) in cells seeded on scaffolds and cultured with C-FBS **(A,C,E)** and NZ-FBS **(B,D,F)**. Scale bar = 200 μm.

This suggested that DPSCs progressively lose their stem cell property during *in vitro* expansion. In addition, we observed that the use of NZ-FBS promoted an earlier increase expression of osteogenic markers, in particular of those involved in the formation of mineralized matrix (BSP and OPN) within 14 days as well as evidenced by Alizarin Red staining. Moreover, the osteocalcin expression in 2D culture, during time, showed a significant increase: *BGLAP* mRNA was higher with NZ-FBS compared with C-FBS cultures, and its protein detected by immunofluorescence, was more evident and distributed throughout the cytoplasm. In addition, we noted that the lowest amount of osteocalcin was found in medium recovered from cells cultured with NZ-FBS. This suggested that released osteocalcin can bind to the extracellular matrix and guide hydroxyapatite to form mineralized nodules (Neve et al., 2013).

*RUNX2* and *SP7* are the key transcription factors initiating and regulating the osteogenesis, respectively (Zhou et al., 2010; Bruderer et al., 2014). NZ-FBS induced a slight increase in *RUNX2* and *SP7* at 7 days of culture. In summary, NZ-FBS induced a positive effect on DPSCs culture allowing an earlier commitment to differentiation toward osteogenic fates, when compared with C-FBS. The differences in osteogenic potential were detectable already at 7 days of culture, when NZ-FBS enhanced the expression of bone-related markers.

When a tissue or organ is damaged, several mechanisms may contribute to the success of wound repair, both under physiological conditions and after administration of stem cells. Angiogenesis, chemotaxis, homing, and engraftment are crucial in equal measure to allow the repair of an injured tissue by stem cells. Chemotactic stimuli recruit various cell types to the injury site. The interaction between the chemokine SDF1 and its receptor CXCR4 expressed on the hDPSCs' surface is a key factor in the recruitment of these cells to the damaged area (Jiang et al., 2008; Kim et al., 2013). The use of both sera induced an increase in *CXCR4* expression on hDPSCs within 14 days of culture but this was more evident in cells expanded with NZ-FBS. In addition to cell migration, cell-matrix, and cell-cell interactions play essential roles in tissue reparation. The expression of surface molecules such as integrins may influence the maintenance of stemness, cell proliferation and changes during the differentiation process. Our findings show that there are no substantial differences in the effects of integrins between the various sera, suggesting that culture conditions did not interfere with cell adhesion.

When an injury, such as a fracture occurs, the vasculature is compromised and hinders the supply of nutrients and oxygen to the site of the lesion. Angiogenesis is a crucial process for bone healing. During tissue reparation, the migration and organization of endothelial cells into capillary tubes is regulated by a paracrine and autocrine action of VEGF (Lamalice et al., 2007). When the damaged tissue involves bone, the cells located in its inner part have a limited blood and oxygen supply. This major issue must necessarily be overtaken in order to obtain good results in clinical practice. At this purpose, we considered the expression of *VEGF* and *PDGFA*. hDPSCs cultured in presence of NZ-FBS were found to produce higher mRNA levels of the said angiogenic factors.

In addition, hDPSC's capabilities in culture were examined by evaluating a 3D environment. To this aim, we seeded hDPSCs on the Bio-Gide scaffold.

This scaffold was chosen because of the following features: it is made of collagen I, the physiological collagen of bone; it is clinically approved and commonly used mainly in order to constitute a biological barrier between bone and soft tissues. In fact, during surgical procedures such as craniofacial and orthopedic surgeries, the correct growth of both bone and the surrounding connective tissue must be ensured. For this purpose, the aforementioned scaffold has been manufactured as a biological barrier to cell penetration on one of the two surfaces: one thick and porous (upper) and another smooth (lower), generally facing the soft tissues. The thick surface allows the ingrowth of bone-forming cells, whereas the latter prevents the ingrowth of fibrous tissue into the bone defect. Therefore, cells are not allowed to penetrate it and they cannot invade the re-absorbable scaffold. Thereby, the cells remain on the surface and our aim, devoted to observe the level of differentiation under the different sera, was better evidenced by observing them at the surface of the scaffold, without other possible interferences. Finally, based on the clinical observations, this scaffold is fully biocompatible. As evidenced by the results, hDPSCs on the scaffold's surface strongly expressed OC, OPN and VEGF in all the cases above all in presence of NZ-FBS. Taken together, our results strongly indicate that NZ-FBS (clinical grade) has a positive effect on replicative potentials and self-commitment of hDPSCs. Therefore, NZ-FBS can be considered a reliable tool for cell-based treatments in autologous grafts and GMP conditions for bone repair and regeneration. Under these conditions, hDPSCs retain their features directing toward osteo-angiogenesis lineage, which represents the gold standard in order to obtain a well-vascularized bone.

In addition, the use of sera belonging to controlled animals could overcome the problems related to GMP standards, that require developing well-defined culture conditions, guaranteeing the maintenance of stem cell multipotency and/or differentiation.

## AUTHOR CONTRIBUTIONS

MN: Designed the study, performed the experiments, wrote the manuscript and approved it. AS, RM, DL, LL, AR: Performed experiments, collected data. TM: Designed the experiment, approved the manuscript.

## ACKNOWLEDGMENTS

This study was supported by MIUR-EU funds (PON 01_02834 and PRIN 2011/13).

## REFERENCES

Almushayt, A., Narayanan, K., Zaki, A. E., and George, A. (2006). Dentin matrix protein 1 induces cytodifferentiation of dental pulp stem cells into odontoblasts. *Gene Ther.* 13, 611. doi: 10.1038/sj.gt.3302687

Arthur, A., Rychkov, G., Shi, S., Koblar, S. A., and Gronthos, S. (2008). Adult human dental pulp stem cells differentiate toward functionally active neurons under appropriate environmental cues. *Stem Cells.* 26, 1787. doi: 10.1634/stemcells.2007-0979

Bruderer, M., Richards, R. G., Alini, M., and Stoddart, M. J. (2014). Role and regulation of RUNX2 in osteogenesis. *Eur. Cell. Mater.* 28, 269–286.

Caplan, A. I. (2007). Adult mesenchymal stem cells for tissue engineering versus regenerative medicine. *J. Cell. Physiol.* 213, 341–347. doi: 10.1002/jcp.21200

d'Aquino, R., De Rosa, A., Lanza, V., Tirino, V., Laino, L., Graziano, A., et al. (2009). Human mandible bone defect repair by the grafting of dental pulp stem/progenitor cells and collagen sponge biocomplexes. *Eur. Cell. Mater.* 18, 75–83.

d'Aquino, R., Graziano, A., Sampaolesi, M., Laino, G., Pirozzi, G., De Rosa, A., et al. (2007). Human postnatal dental pulp cells codifferentiate into osteoblasts and endotheliocytes: a pivotal synergy leading to adult bone tissue formation. *Cell Death Differ.* 14, 1162. doi: 10.1038/sj.cdd.4402121

d'Aquino, R., Tirino, V., Desiderio, V., Studer, M., De Angelis, G. C., Laino, L., et al. (2011). Human neural crest-derived postnatal cells exhibit remarkable embryonic attributes either *in vitro* or *in vivo*. *Eur. Cell. Mater.* 21, 304–316.

Desiderio, V., Tirino, V., Papaccio, G., and Paino, F. (2014). Bone defects: molecular and cellular therapeutic targets. *Int. J. Biochem. Cell Biol.* 51, 75. doi: 10.1016/j.biocel.2014.03.025

Ferro, F., Spelat, R., Beltrami, A. P., Cesselli, D., and Curcio, F. (2012). Isolation and characterization of human dental pulp derived stem cells by using media containing low human serum percentage as clinical grade substitutes for bovine serum. *PLoS ONE.* 7:e48945. doi: 10.1371/journal.pone.0048945

Giuliani, A., Manescu, A., Langer, M., Rustichelli, F., Desiderio, V., Paino, F., et al. (2013). Three years after transplants in human mandibles, histological and in-line holotomography revealed that stem cells regenerated a compact rather than a spongy bone: biological and clinical implications. *Stem Cells Transl. Med.* 2, 316. doi: 10.5966/sctm.2012-0136

Jiang, L., Zhu, Y. Q., Du, R., Gu, Y. X., Xia, L., Qin, F., et al. (2008). The expression and role of stromal cell-derived factor-1alpha-CXCR4 axis in human dental pulp. *J. Endod.* 34, 939. doi: 10.1016/j.joen.2008.05.015

Kim, D. S., Kim, Y. S., Bae, W. J., Lee, H. J., Chang, S. W., Kim, W. S., et al. (2013). The role of SDF-1 and CXCR4 on odontoblastic differentiation in human dental pulp cells. *Int. Endod. J.* 47, 534. doi: 10.1111/iej.12182

Lamalice, L., Le Boeuf, F., and Huot, J. (2007). Endothelial cell migration during angiogenesis. *Circ. Res.* 100, 782. doi: 10.1002/dvdy.22389

La Noce, M., Paino, F., Spina, A., Naddeo, P., Montella, R., Desiderio, V., et al. (2014). Dental pulp stem cells: state of the art and suggestions for a true translation of research into therapy. *J. Dent.* 42, 761. doi: 10.1016/j.jdent.2014.02.018

Mackensen, A., Dräger, R., Schlesier, M., Mertelsmann, R., and Lindemann, A. (2000). Presence of IgE antibodies to bovine serum albumin in a patient developing anaphylaxis after vaccination with human peptide-pulsed dendritic cells. *Cancer Immunol. Immunother.* 49, 152. doi: 10.1007/s002620050614

Mele, L., Vitiello, P. P., Tirino, V., Paino, F., De Rosa, A., Liccardo, D., et al. (2016). Changing paradigms in cranio-facial regeneration: current and new strategies for the activation of endogenous stem cells. *Front. Physiol.* 7:62. doi: 10.3389/fphys.2016.00062

Mitsiadis, T. A., Feki, A., Papaccio, G., and Catón, J. (2011). Dental pulp stem cells, niches, and notch signaling in tooth injury. *Adv. Dent. Res.* 23:275. doi: 10.1177/0022034511405386

Naddeo, P., Laino, L., La Noce, M., Piattelli, A., De Rosa, A., Iezzi, G., et al. (2015). Surface biocompatibility of differently textured titanium implants with mesenchymal stem cells. *Dent. Mater.* 31, 235–243. doi: 10.1016/j.dental.2014.12.015

Neve, A., Corrado, A., and Cantatore, F. P. (2013). Osteocalcin: skeletal and extra-skeletal effects. *J. Cell. Physiol.* 228, 1149. doi: 10.1002/jcp.24278

Paino, F., Ricci, G., De Rosa, A., D'Aquino, R., Laino, L., Pirozzi, G., et al. (2010). Ecto-mesenchymal stem cells from dental pulp are committed to differentiate into active melanocytes. *Eur. Cell. Mater.* 20, 295–305.

Ponnaiyan, D., Bhat, K. M., and Bhat, G. S. (2012). Comparison of immuno-phenotypes of stem cells from human dental pulp and periodontal ligament. *Int. J. Immunopathol. Pharmacol.* 25, 127–134.

Sundin, M., Ringdén, O., Sundberg, B., Nava, S., Götherström, C., and Le Blanc, K. (2007). No alloantibodies against mesenchymal stromal cells, but presence of anti-fetal calf serum antibodies, after transplantation in allogeneic hematopoietic stem cell recipients. *Haematologica* 92, 1208–1215. doi: 10.3324/haematol.11446

Tirino, V., Paino, F., De Rosa, A., and Papaccio, G. (2012). Identification, isolation, characterization, and banking of human dental pulp stem cells. *Methods Mol. Biol.* 879, 443–463. doi: 10.1007/978-1-61779-815-3_26

Zhang, W., Walboomers, X. F., Shi, S., Fan, M., and Jansen, J. A. (2006). Multilineage differentiation potential of stem cells derived from human dental pulp after cryopreservation. *Tissue Eng.* 12, 2813. doi: 10.1089/ten.2006.12.2813

Zhou, X., Zhang, Z., Feng, J. Q., Dusevich, V. M., Sinha, K., Zhang, H., et al. (2010). Multiple functions of Osterix are required for bone growth and homeostasis in postnatal mice. *Proc. Natl. Acad. Sci. U.S.A.* 107, 12919. doi: 10.1073/pnas.0912855107

# 23

# *In vivo* administration of dental epithelial stem cells at the apical end of the mouse incisor

**Edited by:**
Gianpaolo Papaccio,
Second University of Naples, Italy

***Correspondence:**
Thimios A. Mitsiadis,
Orofacial Development and Regeneration Division, Faculty of Medicine, Center for Dental Medicine, Institute of Oral Biology, University of Zürich, Plattenstrasse 11, 8032 Zürich, Switzerland
thimios.mitsiadis@zzm.uzh.ch

*Giovanna Orsini[1], Lucia Jimenez-Rojo[2], Despoina Natsiou[2], Angelo Putignano[1] and Thimios A. Mitsiadis[2]**

[1] *Orofacial Development and Regeneration, Centre for Dental Medicine, Institute of Oral Biology, University of Zürich, Zürich, Switzerland,* [2] *Department of Clinical Sciences and Stomatology, Marche Polytechnic University, Ancona, Italy*

Cell-based tissue regeneration is an attractive approach that complements traditional surgical techniques for replacement of injured and lost tissues. The continuously growing rodent incisor provides an excellent model system for investigating cellular and molecular mechanisms that underlie tooth renewal and regeneration. An active population of dental epithelial progenitor/stem cells located at the posterior part of the incisor, commonly called cervical loop area, ensures the continuous supply of cells that are responsible for the secretion of enamel matrix. To explore the potential of these epithelial cells in therapeutic approaches dealing with enamel defects, we have developed a new method for their *in vivo* administration in the posterior part of the incisor. Here, we provide the step-by-step protocol for the isolation of dental epithelial stem cells and their delivery at targeted areas of the jaw. This simple and yet powerful protocol, consisting in drilling a hole in the mandibular bone, in close proximity to the cervical loop area of the incisor, followed up by injection of stem cells, is feasible, reliable, and effective. This *in vivo* approach opens new horizons and possibilities for cellular therapies involving pathological and injured dental tissues.

**Keywords: mouse incisor, enamel, tooth, dental injury, dental pathology, regeneration, stem cells, cervical loop**

## Introduction

The continuously erupting rodent incisor represents a suitable model system for studying cell proliferation, migration, differentiation, and mineral matrix deposition during development, homeostasis and regeneration of organs. Two of the hardest tissues of the body, the enamel and dentin, form as the outcome of interactions between oral epithelium cells and the cranial neural crest-derived mesenchyme during odontogenesis (Mitsiadis and Graf, 2009; Mitsiadis and Luder, 2011). The mineralized dental tissues are vulnerable to various external harmful agents, and to traumatic injuries that jeopardize tooth integrity. Loss of dental hard tissues in rodents caused by the frequent chewing and gnawing is balanced by constant cell divisions at the apical end of the incisor, allowing thus *de novo* enamel and dentin matrix formation by newly differentiated cells. Indeed, *in vivo* and *in vitro* cell tracing studies have shown that the cervical loops, which are located at the posterior part of the incisor, are niches for dental epithelial stem cells (DESCs) (Harada et al., 1999; Mitsiadis et al., 2007; Mitsiadis and Graf, 2009; Li et al., 2012). It has been demonstrated that DESCs are able to give rise to all epithelial cell layers of the incisor, including the enamel-forming layer of ameloblasts (Juuri et al., 2012; Biehs et al., 2013). Despite the obvious differences between rodent incisors and human teeth that include morphological, physiological and functional criteria there are fundamental similarities in dental hard tissue formation and structure in most of the species (Warshawsky et al., 1981; Jheon et al., 2013). However, damaged enamel cannot be repaired naturally in human teeth since ameloblasts are not present anymore after tooth eruption. Therefore, dental stem cells combined with tissue engineering products could be useful for the development of innovative strategies for cell-based dental tissue regeneration in the clinics (Mitsiadis et al., 2012).

To investigate the potential of DESCs in dental tissue regeneration and repair, we have applied an experimental model consisting of drilling a "window" in the alveolar bone of the mouse mandible, which overlies the apical part of the incisor. The creation of this bone window allows the injection of the DESCs at precise areas of the jaw, without affecting the overall physiology and masticatory attitudes of the animal. Here we demonstrate that this technique is successful and can be efficiently used to *in vivo* administer DESCs that could eventually be used for the repair of damaged or pathological dental tissues.

## Materials and Methods

### Isolation of Dental Epithelial Stems Cells

I. Dissect incisors from postnatal day 7 (PN7) ROSA26-EGFP mice. Incubate the incisors for 20 min at RT in Dispase (2 mg/ml) and DNAse (20 U/ml) solution in HBSS. Separate mechanically the epithelium from mesenchyme and dissect the cervical loop area.
II. Add the tissues in 15 ml Falcon tubes with 14 ml of PBS/10% CS.
III. Centrifuge at 300 g for 5 min.
IV. Remove supernatant.
V. Add 1 ml of PBS.
VI. Centrifuge at 300 g for 5 min.
VII. Remove supernatant.
VIII. Add 200 μl of 0.25% Trypsin (in PBS) and incubate 30 min at 37°C.
IX. Mix gently and pipet up and down vigorously.
X. Add DNase I (2 U/ml) and incubate 5 min at 37°C.
XI. Add 700 μl of PBS/10% CS.
XII. Centrifuge at 300 g for 5 min.
XIII. Remove supernatant.
XIV. Add 1 ml of PBS.
XV. Centrifuge at 300 g for 5 min.
XVI. Remove supernatant and resuspend DESCs in DMEM/F12 medium (1 ml).
XVII. Filter the cells through 40 μm cell strainer.
XVIII. Count the cells.
XIX. Pellet the cells at 300 g for 5 min.
XX. Resuspend DESCs in a solution of Growth Factor Reduced (GFR) Matrigel:PBS (1:8) at a concentration of 500000 cells/ml and keep them on ice.

### Animal Surgery Procedure

I. Use immunocompromised RAG1 -/- mice at 8–12 weeks of age.
II. Before the surgery, inject intraperitoneally the anesthesia solution consisting of Ketamine (65 mg/kg body weight) and Xylacine (13 mg/kg body weight).
III. Place the mice in the warming pad.
IV. Apply Vitamin A ointment (Bausch & Lomb) to the mice, in order to prevent eye dryness.
V. Start the surgery when loss of response to reflex stimulation is observed.
VI. Make an incision about 4 mm long through the skin of the animal to expose the vestibular surface of the hemimandible, along an imaginary line joining the auditory meatus and the lip commissure, to access the muscle layer (**Figure 1A**).
VII. Separate the masseter fibers along their longitudinal axis using a scalpel blade, following an imaginary line parallel to the posterior border of the mouse eye (**Figure 1A**).
VIII. Pay attention not to damage to the blood vessels and keep the muscle retracted using surgical tweezers.
IX. Use a periosteal separator to elevate the periosteum and expose the underlying bone surface.
X. Drill the bone window approximately 2 mm from the posterior border of the ramus, estimating its position using a 1.8 mm dental Woodson condenser (Brassler, Montreal, QC, Canada).
XI. Use a slow-speed dental drill mounting a carbide round burr (Brassler) size 008 to make the bone window (**Figure 1B**).
XII. Irrigate using physiological saline solution during drilling.
XIII. Use a Hamilton syringe Model 702N (with a 22-gauze needle) to inject 10 μl of the prepared solution of DESCs (5000 cells/injection).
XIV. Seal the bone hole using dental canal sealer (AH Plus, Root Canal Sealing Material).
XV. Suture the masseter muscle using absorbable suture 6.0 (Ethicon Inc., Somerville, NJ).
XVI. Suture the skin using non-absorbable silk suture 6.0 (Sherwood Davis & Geck, Wayne, NJ).
XVII. Clean and disinfect the surgical site.
XVIII. Put mice onto a warming pad and observe until they reach consciousness.
XIX. Follow pain management after surgery, by injecting Buprenorphine (0.1 mg/kg bodyweight) subcutaneously, every 6–8 h during the working day and orally administering it overnight, via the drinking water (buprenorphine 0.3 mg/ml are dissolved in 160 ml of water).
XX. Apply Buprenorphine treatment until day three after the surgery.

All mice were maintained and handled according to the Swiss Animal Welfare Law and in compliance with the regulations of the Cantonal Veterinary office, Zurich.

### Tissue Processing

I. At the desired time point of analysis, perfuse the mice with freshly prepared 4% Paraformaldehyde (PFA).
II. Dissect the heads and postfix them in 4% PFA overnight at 4°C.

III. Divide the heads in two equal halves along the longitudinal axis.
IV. Dissect the hemimandibles.
V. Decalcify the samples during 6 ± 2 weeks using 10% EDTA at 4°C. Change the EDTA solution every 2–3 days.
VI. Process the samples for paraffin embedding.
VII. Section paraffin blocks at 5 μm and perform immunofluorescence against GFP antibody.
VIII. Analyse the slides with Leica DM6000 FS microscope and take pictures with the Leica DFC350FX camera for the fluorescence imaging and the Leica DFC420C camera for bright-field imaging.

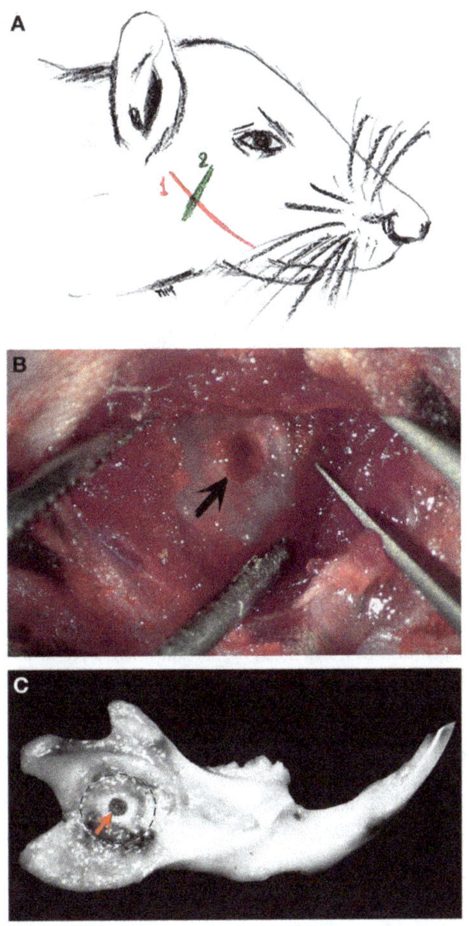


**FIGURE 1 | The various steps of the bone "window" technique. (A)** Schematic representation of a mouse head showing the incision areas (in red and green colors) in order to expose the alveolar bone of the mouse mandible. The first incision line (in red color, 1) follows an imaginary line that joins the auditory meatus and the lip commissure. The incision is performed through the skin of the animal to expose the masseter muscle. The second incision line (in green color, 2) follows an imaginary line parallel to the posterior border of the mouse eye. This incision serves to separate the masseter muscle fibers in order to expose the alveolar bone in the proximity of the apical end of the incisor. **(B)** After incisions, the drilled bone "window" (arrow) is visible in the exposed mandibular alveolar bone. **(C)** Mouse dissected hemimandible, showing the drilled "window" approximately 2 mm from the incisure of the posterior mandibular border (red arrow).

## Results

We have used immunocompromised (RAG1-/-) mice as recipients of DESCs in order to prevent the rejection of the transplanted cells. Thus, all mice recovered well and no complications were observed during the healing period.

The appropriate position of the bone window was confirmed at time of hemimandibles dissection (**Figure 1C**). In all cases the bone windows performed at the labial mandibular bone were drilled very close to the apical part of the incisor. Histologically, there was no alteration of the enamel organ: the drilling did not disrupt the dental tissues and more precisely the external epithelial layer of the incisor (**Figure 2A**). Green fluorescence protein (GFP) positive DESCs were observed in the hole (**Figure 2B**), showing that the GFP-expressing DESCs were successfully delivered to the vicinity of the apical part of the mouse incisor.

## Discussion

Cell-based regenerative therapies consist of the *in vivo* administration of stem cells to patients (Mitsiadis et al., 2012). Stem cell transplantation has already been shown to be successful

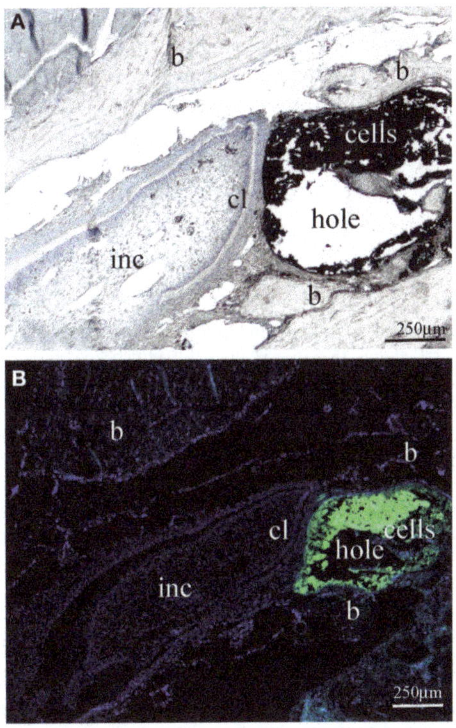


**FIGURE 2 | Longitudinal sections through the mouse mandible after the creation of the bone "window" and the injection of GFP-positive dental epithelial stem cells. (A)** Light micrograph showing the area of the alveolar bone "window" in close proximity to the posterior end of the mouse incisor. **(B)** Fluorescence micrograph showing the GFP positive dental epithelial stem cells in the drilled hole of the alveolar bone. Abbreviations: b, bone; cl, cervical loop area; inc, incisor. Bars: 250 μm.

for the treatment of several damaged or pathological tissues. For instance, cultured human keratinocyte stem cells have been largely used for the treatment of patients with third-degree burns (Pellegrini et al., 2009). Similarly, human corneal regeneration has been achieved after transplantation of diverse sources of cells such as limbal stem cells (Rama et al., 2010) and oral mucosal epithelial cells (Burillon et al., 2012). Therefore, specific stem cell populations derived from different organs and tissues are extremely interesting for clinical tissue engineering applications. The present step-by-step protocol provides a comprehensive view of a novel experimental procedure for the isolation and local delivery of DESCs in precise areas of the mouse mandible. Isolation of DESCs was based on previous protocols for dental (Chavez et al., 2013, 2014) or other non-dental tissues (Smalley, 2010; De Marval et al., 2014).

Several earlier reports have demonstrated that the formation of a bone window in the rat mandible, where osmotic minipumps can be adapted, constitutes an efficient method for the local and continuous delivery of various substances (Orsini et al., 2001; Nanci et al., 2004), as well as for gene transfer purposes (Wazen et al., 2006). Here we have adapted these techniques in order to develop a new method for *in vivo* stem cells delivery into precise areas of the mouse incisor such as its apical part. This newly described approach would be useful to trace the *in vivo* fate of the DESCs after their injection, and further analyse their integration capacity within the dental tissues.

The bone window technique allows the administration of a relatively high number of stem cells *in situ* that will be necessary for tissue repair and regeneration. However, some caveats cannot be exclused when realizing this technique. For example, because of the confined and narrow space separating the alveolar bone and the underlying dental epithelium, inappropriate position of the hole can either damage the apical end of the incisor or perforate the thin alveolar bone. Another parameter that has to be taken into consideration is time. It is necessary to obtain an efficient strategy for controlling the time period that will eventually vary according to the quantity of injected DESCs. Future developments of this technique are the tracing of injected GFP-positive DESCs and their fate when will incorporate the dental tissues.

To date, this method can be considered a useful *in vivo* approach for delivering DESCs in the mouse incisor. This could lead to greater biologic responsiveness, since the administered cells can endogenously synthesize proteins that may continue to exert its effect *in situ*. Thus, this technique could be easily adapted for the needs of the practitioners in the future. For instance, a potential applications of this technique in humans could be the repair of alveolar bone defects or bone loss during periodontal disease. However, it is still a great challenge to find appropriate sources of cells that ideally could be *in vitro* expanded without losing their regenerative capacity and, in addition, do not cause rejection by the recipient's immune system once transplantated into the target tissue.

## Acknowledgments

This work was supported by the Swiss National Foundation (SNSF) grant 31003A_135633 (TM), by institutional funds from the University of Zürich (TM, LJ, DN), and by funds from the Marche Polytechnic University (GO, AP). GO has realized a short-term mission (STSM-MP1005-271013-033583) to the Institut of Oral Biology (University of Zürich, Switzerland), funded by the COST Action NAMABIO MP1005.

## References

Biehs, B., Hu, J. K., Strauli, N. B., Sangiorgi, E., Jung, H., Heber, R. P., et al. (2013). BMI1 represses Ink4a/Arf and Hox genes to regulate stem cells in the rodent incisor. *Nat. Cell Biol.* 15, 846–852. doi: 10.1038/ncb2766

Burillon, C., Huot, L., Justin, V., Nataf, S., Chapuis, F., Decullier, E., et al. (2012). Cultured autologous oral mucosal epithelial cell sheet (CAOMECS) transplantation for the treatment of corneal limbal epithelial stem cell deficiency. *Invest. Ophthalmol. Vis. Sci.* 53, 1325–1331. doi: 10.1167/iovs.11-7744

Chavez, M. G., Hu, J., Seidel, K., Li, C., Jheon, A., Naveau, A., et al. (2014). Isolation and culture of dental epithelial stem cells from the adult mouse incisor. *J. Vis. Exp.* doi: 10.3791/51266

Chavez, M. G., Yu, W., Biehs, B., Harada, H., Snead, M. L., Lee, J. S., et al. (2013). Characterization of dental epithelial stem cells from the mouse incisor with two-dimensional and three-dimensional platforms. *Tissue Eng. Part C Methods* 19, 15–24. doi: 10.1089/ten.tec.2012.0232

De Marval, P. L., Kim, S. H., and Rodriguez-Puebla, M. L. (2014). Isolation and characterization of a stem cell side-population from mouse hair follicles. *Methods Mol. Biol.* 1195, 259–268. doi: 10.1007/7651_2013_61

Harada, H., Kettunen, P., Jung, H. S., Mustonen, T., Wang, Y. A., and Thesleff, I. (1999). Localization of putative stem cells in dental epithelium and their association with Notch and FGF signaling. *J. Cell Biol.* 147, 105–120. doi: 10.1083/jcb.147.1.105

Jheon, A. H., Seidel, K., Biehs, B., and Klein, O. D. (2013). From molecules to mastication: the development and evolution of teeth. *Wiley Interdiscip. Rev. Dev. Biol.* 2, 165–182. doi: 10.1002/wdev.63

Juuri, E., Saito, K., Ahtiainen, L., Seidel, K., Tummers, M., Hochedlinger, K., et al. (2012). Sox2+ stem cells contribute to all epithelial lineages of the tooth via Sfrp5+ progenitors. *Dev. Cell* 23, 317–328. doi: 10.1016/j.devcel.2012.05.012

Li, C. Y., Cha, W., Luder, H. U., Charles, R. P., McMahon, M., Mitsiadis, T. A., et al. (2012). E-cadherin regulates the behavior and fate of epithelial stem cells and their progeny in the mouse incisor. *Dev. Biol.* 366, 357–366. doi: 10.1016/j.ydbio.2012.03.012

Mitsiadis, T. A., Barrandon, O., Rochat, A., Barrandon, Y., and De Bari, C. (2007). Stem cell niches in mammals. *Exp. Cell Res.* 313, 3377–3385. doi: 10.1016/j.yexcr.2007.07.027

Mitsiadis, T. A., and Graf, D. (2009). Cell fate determination during tooth development and regeneration. *Birth Defects Res. C Embryo Today* 87, 199–211. doi: 10.1002/bdrc.20160

Mitsiadis, T. A., and Luder, H. U. (2011). Genetic basis for tooth malformations: from mice to men and back again. *Clin. Genet.* 80, 319–329. doi: 10.1111/j.1399-0004.2011.01762.x

Mitsiadis, T. A., Woloszyk, A., and Jimenez-Rojo, L. (2012). Nanodentistry: combining nanostructured materials and stem cells for dental tissue regeneration. *Nanomedicine (Lond.)* 7, 1743–1753. doi: 10.2217/nnm.12.146

Nanci, A., Wazen, R. M., Zalzal, S. F., Fortin, M., Goldberg, H. A., Hunter, G. K., et al. (2004). A tracer study with systemically and locally administered dinitrophenylated osteopontin. *J. Histochem. Cytochem.* 52, 1591–1600. doi: 10.1369/jhc.4A6452.2004

Orsini, G., Zalzal, S., and Nanci, A. (2001). Localized infusion of tunicamycin in rat hemimandibles: alteration of the basal lamina associated with maturation stage ameloblasts. *J. Histochem. Cytochem.* 49, 165–176. doi: 10.1177/002215540104900204

# 24

# *In vitro* osteogenic and odontogenic differentiation of human dental pulp stem cells seeded on carboxymethyl cellulose-hydroxyapatite hybrid hydrogel

**Edited by:**
Gianpaolo Papaccio,
Second University of Naples, Italy

***Correspondence:**
Giovanna Orsini
giovorsini@yahoo.com

*Gabriella Teti[1], Viviana Salvatore[1], Stefano Focaroli[1], Sandra Durante[1], Antonio Mazzotti[2], Manuela Dicarlo[3], Monica Mattioli-Belmonte[3] and Giovanna Orsini[4]**

*[1] Department of Biomedical and Neuromotor Sciences, University of Bologna, Bologna, Italy, [2] 1st Orthopaedic and Traumatologic Clinic, Rizzoli Orthopedic Institute, Bologna, Italy, [3] Department of Clinical and Molecular Sciences, Polytechnic University of Marche, Ancona, Italy, [4] Department of Clinical Sciences and Stomatology, Polytechnic University of Marche, Ancona, Italy*

Stem cells from human dental pulp have been considered as an alternative source of adult stem cells in tissue engineering because of their potential to differentiate into multiple cell lineages. Recently, polysaccharide based hydrogels have become especially attractive as matrices for the repair and regeneration of a wide variety of tissues and organs. The incorporation of inorganic minerals as hydroxyapatite nanoparticles can modulate the performance of the scaffolds with potential applications in tissue engineering. The aim of this study was to verify the osteogenic and odontogenic differentiation of dental pulp stem cells (DPSCs) cultured on a carboxymethyl cellulose—hydroxyapatite hybrid hydrogel. Human DPSCs were seeded on carboxymethyl cellulose—hydroxyapatite hybrid hydrogel and on carboxymethyl cellulose hydrogel for 1, 3, 5, 7, 14, and 21 days. Cell viability assay and ultramorphological analysis were carried out to evaluate biocompatibility and cell adhesion. Real Time PCR was carried out to demonstrate the expression of osteogenic and odontogenic markers. Results showed a good adhesion and viability in cells cultured on carboxymethyl cellulose—hydroxyapatite hybrid hydrogel, while a low adhesion and viability was observed in cells cultured on carboxymethyl cellulose hydrogel. Real Time PCR data demonstrated a temporal up-regulation of osteogenic and odontogenic markers in dental pulp stem cells cultured on carboxymethyl cellulose—hydroxyapatite hybrid hydrogel. In conclusion, our *in vitro* data confirms the ability of DPSCs to differentiate toward osteogenic and odontogenic lineages in presence of a carboxymethyl cellulose—hydroxyapatite hybrid hydrogel. Taken together, our results provide evidence that DPSCs and carboxymethyl cellulose—hydroxyapatite hybrid hydrogel could be considered promising candidates for dental pulp complex and periodontal tissue engineering.

**Keywords: osteogenic differentiation, odontogenic differentiation, dental pulp stem cells, hydrogel, tissue engineering**

## INTRODUCTION

The goal of tissue engineering and regenerative medicine is to improve or restore the functions of diseased tissues and organs. Tissue engineering strategies require main elements such as stem cells, scaffold or matrix, and growth factors (Kabir et al., 2014).

Adult mesenchymal stem cells (MSCs) have the potential to renew themselves for long periods through cell division and, under certain physiological or experimental conditions, they can be induced to become specialized cells (Verma et al., 2014; Potdar and Jethmalani, 2015).

Five types of MSCs have been isolated from dental tissues and demonstrated to have high proliferative and multilineage differentiation properties: dental pulp stem cells (DPSCs; Gronthos et al., 2000; Tirino et al., 2011; Pisciotta et al., 2012, 2015; La Noce et al., 2014), stem cells from human exfoliated deciduous teeth (SHEDs; Miura et al., 2003), periodontal ligament stem cells (PDLSCs; Seo et al., 2004), dental follicle progenitor stem cells (DFPCs; Morsczeck et al., 2005) and stem cells from apical papilla (SCAPs; Sonoyama et al., 2008).

Dental pulp is considered a rich source of DPSCs, suitable for tissue engineering applications (La Noce et al., 2014). It has been shown that DPSCs can be differentiated by modulation with growth factors, transcriptional factors, extracellular matrix proteins, and receptor molecules into different cell types including odontoblasts, osteoblasts, chondrocytes, cardiomyocytes, neuron cells, adipocytes, corneal epithelial cells, melanoma cells, and insulin secreting Beta cells (Pisciotta et al., 2012; La Noce et al., 2014; Paino et al., 2014; Potdar and Jethmalani, 2015).

DPSCs isolated from dental pulp co-express typical MSCs markers such as CD44, CD73, CD90, CD105, CD271, and STRO-1, while negative markers are CD34, CD45, and HLA-DR (La Noce et al., 2014; Verma et al., 2014; Potdar and Jethmalani, 2015). Pisciotta et al. (2015) recently demonstrated the co-existence of two subpopulations of adult stem cells derived from human DPSCs, one of mesodermal origin and a second of neural crest derivation, increasing the potential application of DPSCs in regenerative medicine. However, there is no specific or strict marker characterizing DPSCs, which are considered a heterogeneous population.

Recent attention has been focused on the utilization of DPSCs in tissue engineering (d'Aquino et al., 2009a; Verma et al., 2014). Several scaffolds have been used to promote 3-D tissue formation and studies have demonstrated that DPSCs show good adherence and bone tissue formation on microconcavity surface textures (Graziano et al., 2008; Naddeo et al., 2015). In oro-maxillo-facial bone repair DPSCs have been seeded on collagen sponge scaffolds, producing an optimal biocomplex for regeneration of DSPCs for bone repair (d'Aquino et al., 2009b). A 3-year follow-up demonstrated the synthesis of adult bone tissue with good vascularization (Giuliani et al., 2013), showing the powerful application of DPSCs in periodontal and dental pulp tissue engineering.

In tissues engineering strategies, the choice of an appropriate scaffold is a crucial step (Galler et al., 2011). Hydrogels have been employed as an emerging and promising tool in regenerative medicine but also as an injectable filler material (Varma et al., 2014; Vashist and Ahmad, 2015). A variety of natural and synthetic polymers have been used to fabricate hydrogels. Collagen, hyaluronic acid, chondroitin sulfate, fibrin, fibronectin, alginate, agarose, chitosan, and silk have been the most commonly used natural polymers (Geckil et al., 2010). Cellulose is one of the most ubiquitous and abundant of biopolymers produced in the biosphere. Tissue engineering and regenerative medicine researchers have shown an interest in cellulose because it has a low density and an excellent biodegradability associated with low ecotoxicological risks (Domingues et al., 2014). One of the main drawbacks of cellulose-based hydrogels is the lack of good mechanical proprieties (Pasqui et al., 2012).

Recently, a semisynthetic natural polymer obtained from the carboxymethylation of natural cellulose, named carboxymethyl cellulose (CMC) was developed with hydroxyapatite (HA) crystals to generate a new hybrid hydrogel for bone tissue engineering (Pasqui et al., 2014). Although the chemical and mechanical proprieties were well described (Pasqui et al., 2014), data on the biological performance of CMC-HA hydrogels on stem cells differentiation is lacking.

The aim of this study was to investigate the *in vitro* osteogenic and odontogenic differentiation of DPSCs seeded on a CMC-HA hydrogel. DPSCs were seeded on a CMC-HA hydrogel in presence of osteogenic factors for a period of up to 21 days. Biocompatibility was measured by MTT assay, while electron microscopy analyses were carried out to demonstrate cell adhesion on the scaffold surface.

The markers alkaline phosphatase (ALP), Runt-related transcription factor 2 (RUNX2), type I collagen and osteonectin (SPARC) were chosen for the examination of osteogenic differentiation, while the markers dentin matrix protein I (DMP1), and dentin sialophospho protein (DSPP) were chosen for the examination of odontogenic differentiation. Gene expression was tested by Real Time PCR. Results were compared to DPSCs seeded on CMC-based hydrogels and to DPSCs seeded on 2D system.

## MATERIALS AND METHODS

### Scaffold Synthesis and Characterization

CMC-based hydrogels without and with hydroxyapatite (HA) were synthesized and characterized as already described in Pasqui et al. (2014). Briefly, the crosslinking agent 1,3-diaminopropane (DAP) was added to the mixture at a molar ratio of 0.5 with respect to the moles of carboxylic acid of the polymers and to the activating agents 1-ethyl-3-[3-(dimethyl-amino)propyl)carbodiimide hydrochloride (EDC) and N-hydroxysuccinimide (NHS) moles. The molar ratio of EDC and NHS mole is 1 to 1. The pH of the mixture was adjusted to 4.75 by the addition of HCl 1M solution and the reaction was allowed to go on under stirring overnight at room temperature. Once formed, the hydrogel was purified by dipping it in water for 4–5 days until no traces of free EDC or NHS were revealed by UV spectrophotometry and finally freeze-dried. To load HA inside CMC hydrogel, an exactly weighted amount of freeze-dried hydrogel was dipped in a five solutions containing increasing amounts of HA in a range from 0.5 to 2.5 mg mL. Above this concentration, HA crystals form aggregates which precipitate. The hydrogel was let to swell under moderate stirring for 48 h that is a sufficient time to allow it to reach the maximum swelling degree. Finally, the hydrogel was removed from the solution washed with deionized water until no trace of HA was revealed in the washing solution and freeze-dried again.

## Human Dental Pulp Stem Cells (DPSCs) Isolation

DPSCs were obtained from healthy permanent premolars extracted during orthodontic treatment, under informed consent. Cells were isolated from dental pulp as described in a previous study (Teti et al., 2013). Briefly, the dental pulp was harvested from the teeth, carefully minced and collected in 60 × 15 mm cell-cultured dishes in Dulbecco's Modified Eagle Medium/F12 (DMEM, Gibco, Life Technologies, Monza, Italy) supplemented with 10% Fetal Bovine Serum (FBS, Gibco, Life Technologies, Monza, Italy) and 1% penicillin/streptomycin and then incubated at 37°C in a humidified atmosphere of 5% $CO_2$. At day 7–10 of culture, cells obtained from the minced dental pulp were subsequently trypsinized, resuspended, and plated in T25 tissue flasks in DMEM /F12 medium supplemented with 10% FBS and 1% penicillin/streptomycin. The cells were subcultured once a week using 1% trypsin (Gibco, Life Technologies, Monza, Italy), expanded in new T25 flasks and maintained at 37°C in a humidified atmosphere at 5% $CO_2$. Cells from passages 3–5th were utilized for the experiments described.

## FACS Analysis

The cells obtained were checked for their staminal profile by FACSCalibur flow cytometry system (Becton Dickinson, CA, USA). In agreement with minimal criteria for the identification of human MSCs (Dominici et al., 2006), $2.5 \times 10^5$ cells were removed with Dulbecco Phosphate buffer saline (D-PBS) and were then stained for 45 min with the following antibodies: fluorescein isothiocyanate-(FITC)-labeled mouse anti-human CD90 (StemCell Technologies, Milan, Italy), CD105, CD14, CD19, (Diaclone, France), R-phycoerythrin-(PE)-labeled mouse anti human CD34, CD45 (Diaclone, France), CD73 (Becton Dickinson, CA, USA), and anti HLA-DR (Diaclone, France). The control for FITC- or PE-coupled antibodies was isotypic mouse IgG1. The data were evaluated using CellQuest software (Becton Dickinson, CA, USA).

## Osteogenic Differentiation

$2 \times 10^5$ cells/ 100 μl of medium were seeded on CMC and CMC-HA scaffolds and incubated with the osteogenic medium for 1, 3, 5, 7, 14, and 21 days. The osteogenic medium consisted in alpha MEM medium (Life Technologies, Milan, Italy) supplemented with 10% FBS and 1% penicillin/streptomycin, 250 μmol/L ascorbic acid phosphate, 10 mmol/L beta glycerophosphate, and 10 nmol/L dexamethasone. DPSCs were incubated at 37°C with 5% $CO_2$. DPSCs between the 3rd and 5th passages were used throughout the study.

## MTT Assay

After each incubation time, the medium was changed to a fresh one containing 0.5 mg/ml of 3-(4,5-dimethylthiazol-2-yl)-2,5-diphenyltetrazolium bromide (MTT) and left for 2 h at 37°C. The formazan produced was dissolved by solvent solution (0.1 N HCl in isopropanol) and the optical density was read at 570 nm by Microplate Reader (Model 680, Biorad Lab Inc., CA, USA).

## High Resolution Scanning Electron Microscopy (HR-SEM)

At each experimental point, DPSCs seeded on CMC and CMC-HA scaffolds were washed in 0.15 M sodium cacodylate buffer, fixed with a solution of 2.5% glutaraldehyde in 0.1 M cacodylate buffer (Sigma Aldrich, St. Louis, Missouri, USA) for 2 h at 4°C and subsequently fixed with 1% $OsO_4$ in 0.1 M cacodylate buffer (Societa' Italiana Chimici, Roma, Italy) for 1 h at RT (room temperature). After washes in 0.15 M cacodylate buffer, the samples were dehydrated in an ascending alcohol series and CPD (critical point dried 030, Bal-Tec, Leica Microsystems GmbH, Wetzlar, Germany). The samples were then metal coated with a thin layer of carbon/platinum (Bal-Tec, Leica Microsystems GmbH, Wetzlar, Germany) and observed under HR-SEM (JSM 890, Jeol Company, Tokio, Japan) with 10 kV accelerate voltage and $1 \times 10^{-11}$ mA.

## Transmission Electron Microscopy (TEM)

At each experimental point, DPSCs seeded on CMC and CMC-HA scaffolds were fixed with 2.5% glutaraldehyde in 0.1 M cacodylate buffer for 2 h at 4°C and subsequently post-fixed with 1% $OsO_4$ in 0.1 M cacodylate buffer for 1 h at RT. After several washes, the samples were dehydrated in an acetone series (70, 90, 100%) and embedded in LR London white resin (Fluka, Sigma-Aldrich, St. Louis, Missouri, USA). Sections of 100 nm were collected on nickel grids, stained with uranyl acetate and lead citrate, and observed by Philips CM10 (FEI Company, Eindhoven, The Netherlands). Images were recorded by Megaview III digital camera (FEI Company, Eindhoven, The Netherlands). Some sections were stained with toluidine blue staining solution and observed under a light microscopy Nikon Eclipse E800 (Nikon Corporation, Tokyo, Japan).

## RNA Extraction and Quantitative Real Time Polymerase Chain Reaction (qRTPCR)

Total RNA was extracted in DPSCs seeded on CMC and CMC-HA scaffolds for 1, 3, 5, 7, 14, and 21 days, by NucleoSpin RNA I kit (Machery-Nagel, Duren, Germany), quantified using a NanoDrop® ND-1000 UV-Vis Spectrophotometer (Thermo Scientific, Wilmington, DE, USA), and cDNA was transcribed with reverse transcriptase SUPIII (Invitrogen, Carlsbad, CA, USA). The expression of mRNA was analyzed by quantitative Real Time PCR using 7500 Real Time PCR (Applied Biosystem, Life Technologies, Monza, Italy). For the analysis, the following TaqMan assays (Applied Biosystems, Life Technologies, Monza, Italy) were used: phosphatase alkaline (ALP Hs01029144_m1), runt-related transcription factor2 (RUNX2 Hs00231692_m1), osteonectin (SPARC Hs00234160_m1), collagen type I alpha 1 (COL1A1 Hs00164004_m1), dentin matrix protein 1 (DMP1 Hs01009390_m1), dentin sialophospho protein (DSPP Hs00171962_m1).

The relative gene expressions were normalized to glyceraldehyde 3-phosphate dehydrogenase (GAPDH Hs99999905_m1), and the data were presented as the fold change using the formula $2^{-\Delta\Delta CT}$ as recommended by the manufacturer (User Bulletin No.2 P/N 4303859, Applied Biosystems). The gene expression of DPSCs cultured on CMC-HA samples was relative to DPSCs cultured on tissue flasks for 21 days (2D system) in absence of osteogenic medium. Total RNA was extracted as previously described.

Data showed the average of triplicates ± SD and were representative from three independent experiments.

## Statistical Analysis

For cell viability data, the statistical differences were assessed by One-way ANOVA ($P < 0.05$) and Dunnet's Multiple Comparison Test ($P < 0.05$). For Real Time data the statistical differences were assessed by Two-way ANOVA ($P < 0.05$) and Bonferroni Multiple Comparison Test ($P < 0.05$).

The statistical analysis was performed with GraphPad Prism 5.0 software (San Diego, CA, USA).

# RESULTS

## Flow Cytometry (FACS) Analysis of Human Dental Pulp Stem Cells (DPSCs)

The MSCs utilized for all additional experiments were characterized for CD105, CD14, CD19, CD34, CD45, CD73, CD90, and HLADR using flow cytometric analysis. It was found that these cells were highly positive for CD105, CD73, and CD90, and negative for CD34, CD19, CD45, CD14, and HLA-DR (**Figure 1**).

## MTT Assay

In order to evaluate the biocompatibility of CMC and CMC-HA scaffolds cultured with DPSCs for 3, 5, and 7 days, an MTT assay was carried out. Cell viability results showed a high biocompatibility for CMC-HA material, while a lower cell viability is observed in CMC sample (**Figure 2**).

## High Resolution Scanning Electron Microscopy (HR-SEM)

To demonstrate the cell adhesion on both scaffold surfaces, high resolution scanning electron microscopic analysis was carried out.

CMC scaffold showed a smooth surface where just a few cells were weakly fixed on it after 1 day of culture (**Figure 3A**).

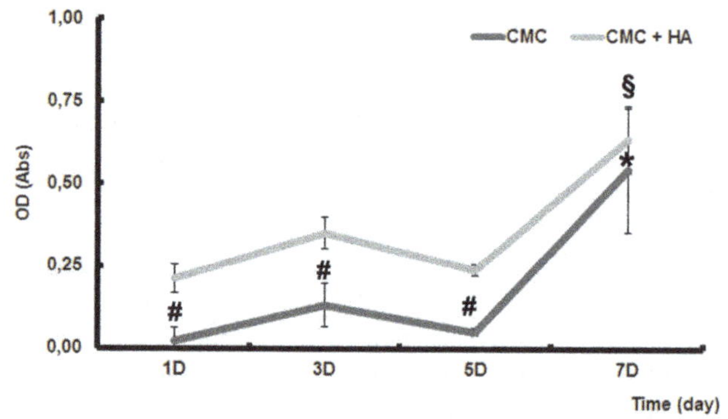


**FIGURE 2 | MTT assay of DPSCs seeded on CMC and CMC-HA scaffold for 1, 3, 5, and 7 days.** Data were expressed as mean of percentage ± SD. *represents a significant difference compared to DPSCs cultured for 1 day on CMC scaffold, $P < 0.05$. §represents a significant difference compared to DPSCs cultured for 1 day on CMC-HA scaffold, $P < 0.05$. # represents a significant difference of DPSCs cultured on CMC scaffold to DPSCs cultured on CMC-HA scaffold, $P < 0.05$.

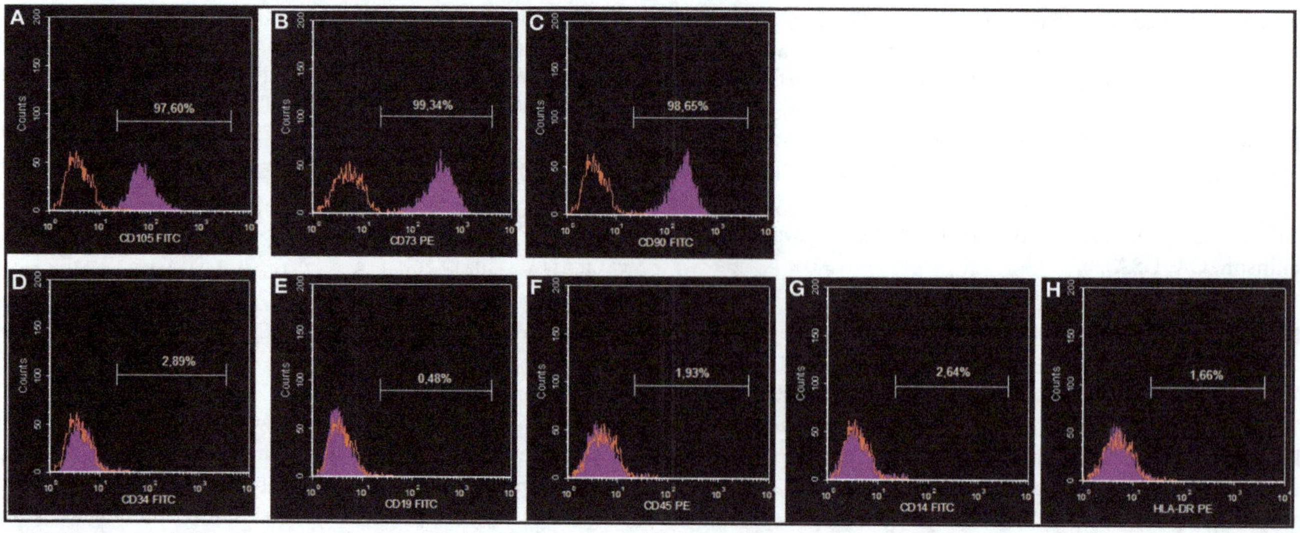


**FIGURE 1 | DPSC phenotypic profile.** Cells showing a positive reaction for CD105 **(A)**, CD73 **(B)** and CD90 **(C)**, and a negative reaction for CD34 **(D)**, CD19 **(E)**, CD45 **(F)**, CD14 **(G)** and HLA-DR **(H)**.

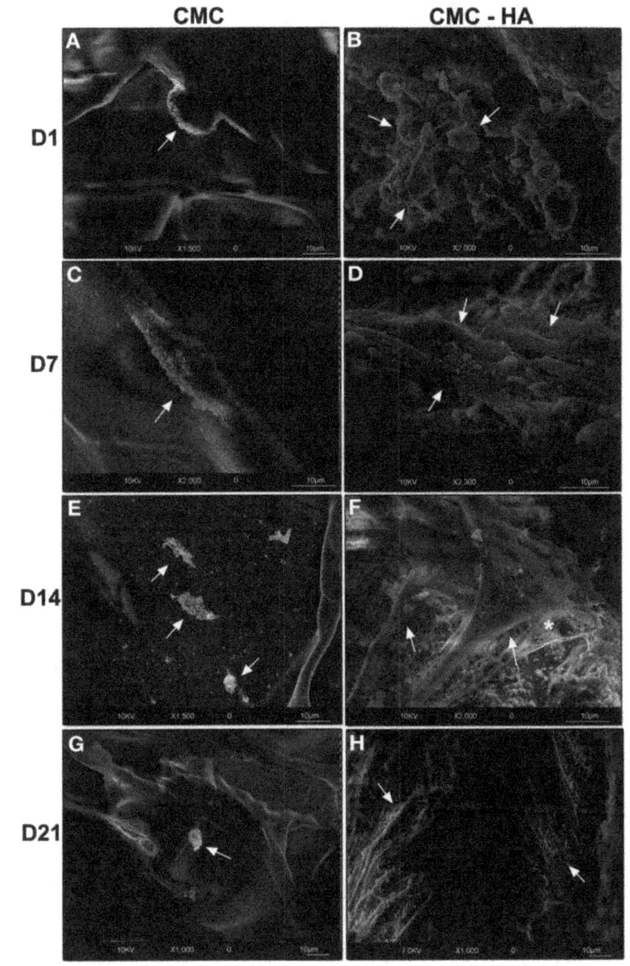


**FIGURE 3 | HRSEM showing DPSCs on scaffold surface. (A)** Cells (arrow) on CMC scaffold surface after 1 day of culture (bar: 10 um); **(C)** DPSCs (arrow) on CMC surface after 7 days (bar: 10 um); **(E)** cell debris (arrows) at day 14 on CMC surface (bar: 10 um); **(G)** cell debris (arrow) after 21 days on CMC surface (bar: 10 um); **(B)** DPSCs (arrows) after 1 day of differentiation on CMC-HA material (bar: 10um); **(D)** CMC-HA scaffold showing DPSCs with a fibroblast shape (arrows) morphology after 7 days of culture (bar: 10 um); **(F)** DPSCs (arrows) on CMC—HA scaffold after 14 days of culture. Some extracellular matrix components (*) are detected (bar: 10 um); **(H)** CMC-HA hydrogel surface is completely covered by DPSCs (arrows) (bar: 10um).

They appeared with a round shape morphology (**Figure 3A**). After 7 days of differentiation, a few cells with fibroblast like morphology were detected (**Figure 3C**). Only cell debris were observed after 14 (**Figure 3E**) and 21 (**Figure 3G**) days of differentiation.

On the contrary, CMC-HA scaffold showed a rough surface due to HA crystals. After 1 day of incubation, several cells appeared with a round-shaped morphology (**Figure 3B**). After 7 and 14 days of differentiation, cells with a fibroblast like morphology were observed (**Figures 3D,F**). CMC-HA surface was completely covered by DPSCs at day 21 (**Figures 3H, 4A**). Several secretory vesicles were observed on the cell surface (**Figure 4B**).

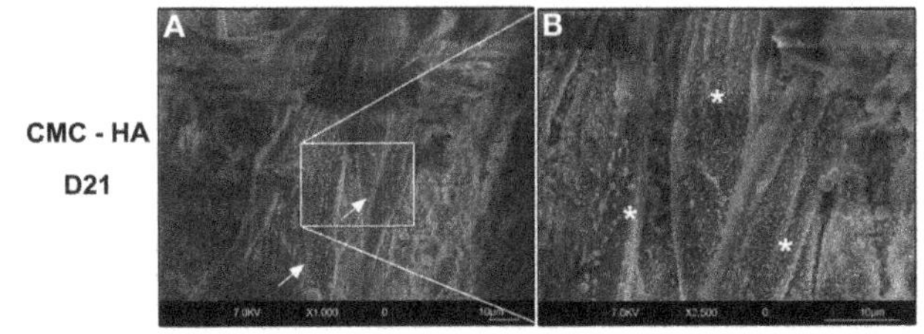


**FIGURE 4 | (A)** DPSCs (arrows) completely covered the surface of CMC—HA hydrogel after 21 days of differentiation (bar: 10 um). **(B)** Higher magnification of the surface of cells characterized by several secretory vesicles (*) (bar:10um).

## Light Microscopy of DPSCs Differentiated on CMC and CMC-HA Hydrogels

After 1 day of culture, sections of CMC samples showed small clusters of DPSCs on the surface of the material (**Figure 5A**). After 7, 14, and 21 days of culture, just a few cells were detected on the scaffold surface (**Figures 5C,E,G**).

Sections of CMC-HA hydrogels, showed small clusters of DPSCs on the material after 1 day of culture (**Figure 5B**). After 7 days of differentiation, several cells with a fibroblast-shaped morphology were detected on the scaffold (**Figure 5D**). By the end of Day 14 (**Figure 5F**) and 21 (**Figure 5H**), the hydrogel surface was completely covered by DPSCs.

Due to the low adhesion of cells on CMC based hydrogels, confirmed also by HRSEM analysis, we decided to perform the next experiments only on CMC-HA based hydrogels.

## TEM Analysis of DPSCs Differentiated on CMC-HA Scaffold

To better visualize the ultrastructure of DPSCs cultured on CMC-HA hydrogel, a TEM analysis was carried out.

**Figure 6A** shows DPSCs cultured for 1 day on CMC-HA scaffolds. Cells appeared organized in clusters, showing a well-preserved morphology (**Figure 6A**). CMC-HA hydrogel fibers with small crystals of HA were also detected (**Figure 6A**). By the end of the first week of differentiation, DPSCs were spread out on scaffold surface and they showed a fibroblast like morphology (**Figure 6B**). The nucleus and cytoplasmic organelles were well-preserved. No sign of extracellular matrix deposition was observed. After 14 days of differentiation, DPSCs showed several, fibrillary components in the extracellular space related to extracellular matrix (**Figures 6C,D**). By the end of the third week of differentiation, DPSCs completely covered the surface of the hydrogel (**Figure 6E**). In the extracellular matrix several fibrillary structure, with a banding organization, were observed (**Figure 6F**).

## Real Time PCR Analysis

To confirm osteogenic and odontogenic differentiation, the expression of some osteogenic markers such as ALP, RUNX2, COL1A1, SPARC, and odontogenic markers such as DMP1 and DSPP were analyzed in DPSCs cultured on CMC-HA samples for 1, 3, 5, 7, 14, and 21 days.

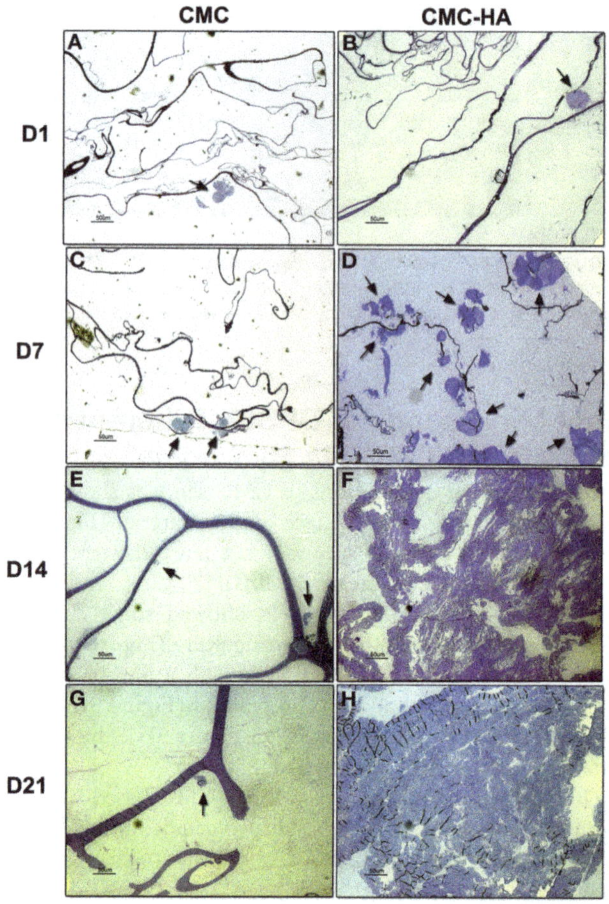


**FIGURE 5 | Resin embedded sections of (A) DPSCs cultured on CMC hydrogel for 1 day.** Cells organized in small clusters (arrow) on scaffold surface (bar: 50 um); **(B)** DPSCs cultured on CMC-HA hydrogel for 1 day. Cells organized in small clusters (arrow) (bar: 50 um); **(C)** DPSCs cultured for 7 days on CMC hydrogel. Just a few cell (arrows) were detected (bar: 50 um); **(D)** DPSCs cultured on CMC-HA hydrogel for 7 days. Cells proliferated and spread out on scaffold surface (arrows) (bar: 50 um); **(E)** DPSCs grown on CMC scaffold for 14 days. Cellular debris were observed (arrows) (bar: 50 um); **(F)** After 14 days of culture DPSCs covered completely the surface of CMC-HA material (Bar: 50 um); **(G)** DPSCs grown on CMC hydrogel for 21 days. Cellular debris were detected (arrow) (bar: 50 um); **(H)** CMC—HA scaffold with DPSCs cultured for 21 days. Cells still covered surface of the material (bar: 50 um).

The transcription factor RUNX2 showed an increase of expression just after 7 days of culture, according to the first steps of osteogenesis (**Figure 7A**). A significant up-regulation of COL1A1 expression was detected at day 14 and 21 of differentiation, according to TEM images in which fibrillary structures resembling type I collagen protein were detected in the extracellular matrix. Transcript of ALP and SPARC were also significant higher after 14 and 21 days of differentiation (**Figure 7A**).

Regarding odontogenic differentiation, the expression of DMP-1 and DSPP showed a gradually up-regulation during the time of differentiation with the highest level at D21 compared to control samples (**Figure 7B**).

## DISCUSSION

Highly proliferative and multi-lineage subpopulations of mesenchymal stem cells isolated from dental tissues are capable of differentiating toward odontoblast and osteoblast phenotypes (Gronthos et al., 2000; Miura et al., 2003; Tirino et al., 2011; La Noce et al., 2014; Pisciotta et al., 2015). These stem cells are readily available and easily accessible, making them promising tools for regenerative medicine.

Beside the well-known ability of DPSCs to be *in vitro* differentiated into functional osteoblasts producing extracellular and mineralized matrix in abundance (Riccio et al., 2010; Pisciotta et al., 2012), there are *in vivo* studies reporting the capacity of human DPSCs to reconstruct bone structures (d'Aquino et al., 2009b; Giuliani et al., 2013). These results suggest that DPSCs can be successfully utilized for dental pulp complex and periodontal tissue engineering.

In such strategies, the interaction between stem cells and the material applied as scaffold plays a critical role in the generation of a cell-friendly microenvironment, which must be conducive to the regeneration of dental structures (Conde et al., 2015).

The two categories of materials that are most commonly used in tissue engineering are synthetic polymers such as poly(lactic) acid (PLA) and poly(glycolic) acid (PGA) (Galler et al., 2011) and matrices derived from biological sources such as reconstituted collagen (Falconi et al., 2013; Focaroli et al., 2014; Ivanovski et al., 2014). In the last years, hydrogel systems were proposed as new biomaterials for minimally invasive surgery, repair of bone defects with irregular shape, such as periodontal defects, filling materials and *in vivo* delivery of bioactive signals or cells (Barbucci et al., 2010; Pasqui et al., 2012). Cellulose based hydrogels are well-known for their low toxicity, high biocompatibility, and low degradation rates. The main drawback is the lack of good mechanical proprieties. The presence of HA crystals in the scaffold offers suitable mechanical proprieties, and roughness which can increase cell adhesion (Geckil et al., 2010; Pasqui et al., 2012). The aim of this study was to evaluate the osteogenic and odontogenic differentiation of DPSCs cultured on a CMC-HA hydrogel and to verify the biological proprieties of this biomaterial which can subsequently be utilized in tissue regeneration. To our knowledge, the present experimental study is the first report demonstrating a favorable biological performance of CMC-HA hydrogels toward stem cell osteogenic and odontogenic differentiation.

Our cell viability assay of DPSCs seeded on CMC-HA showed a good biocompatibility of the material in agreement with previous studies on cellulose-based scaffolds (Pasqui et al., 2014). The MTT assay in particular demonstrated a slight increase in cell proliferation the first day of culture and a peak of proliferation at day 7, suggesting a period of adaption for the cells on scaffold surface prior to the proliferation phase. This behavior was already demonstrated for mesenchymal stem cells separated by bone marrow (Teti et al., 2012) and cultured on collagen-based scaffold (Focaroli et al., 2014). On the other end, cells seeded on CMC based hydrogel, although showing an increased metabolic activity up to day 7, had values of cell viability always lower than CMC-HA samples. Considering that the number of cells

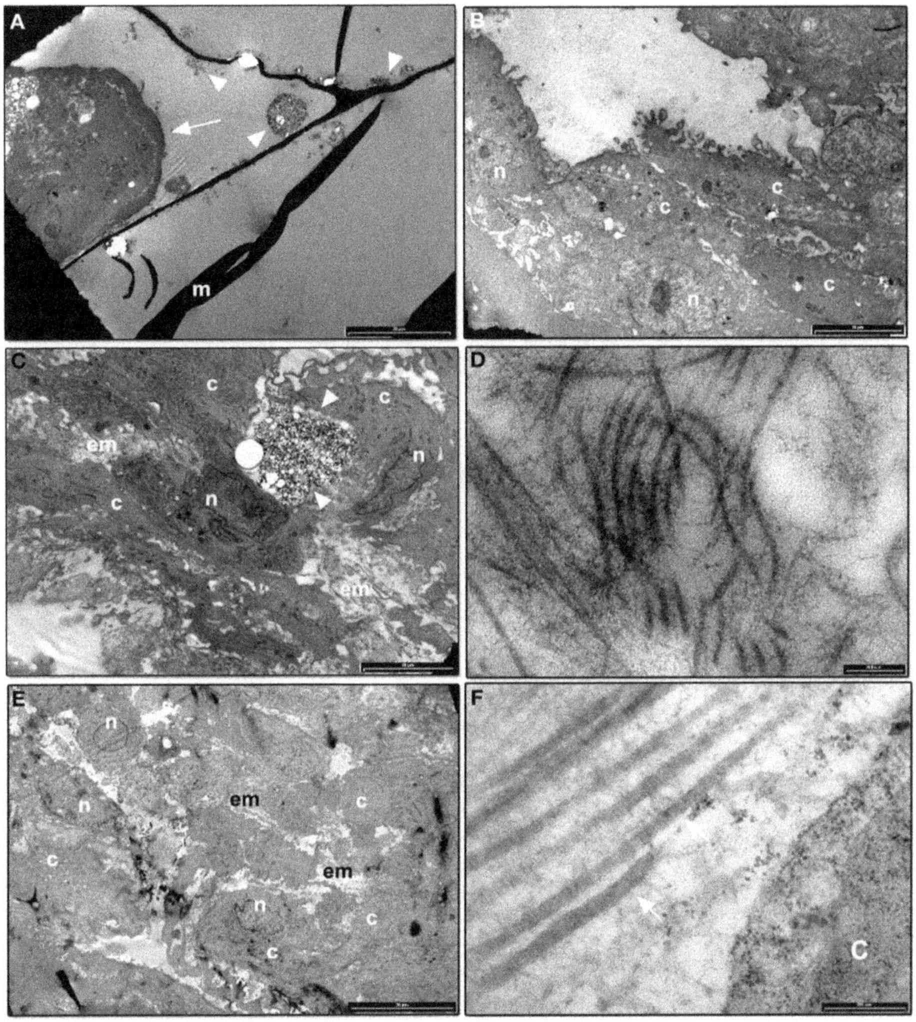


**FIGURE 6 | (A)** TEM image of CMC-HA scaffold with DPSCs organized in cluster (arrow) after 1 day of culture (m: hydrogel material; arrowheads: HA crystals; bar: 20 um); **(B)** TEM image of DPSCs cultured on CMC-HA hydrogel for 7 days. Cells appear well-preserved (n, nucleus; c, cytoplasm; bar: 10 um); **(C)** TEM analysis of DPSCs cultured for 14 days. An initial deposition of the extracellular matrix (em) was observed (n, nucleus; c, cytoplasm; arrowhead, HA crystals; bar: 10 um); **(D)** High magnification of the fibrillary structures observed in the extracellular matrix of DPSCs cultured on CMC—HA for 14 days (bar: 200 nm); **(E)** TEM image of DPSCs grown for 21 days on CMC—HA hydrogel. Cells completely covered hydrogel surface (n, nucleus; c, cytoplasm; em, extracellular matrix; bar: 20 um). **(F)** High magnification of fibrillary structures observed in the extracellular matrix of cells culture on CMC—HA hydrogel for 21 days. A banding structure connected with type I collagen fibers is observed (arrow) (c, cytoplasm; bar: 200 nm).

seeded on both materials was initially the same, we concluded that in CMC samples there was a weaker adhesion of cells to the scaffold surface and less proliferation during the time of incubation. These findings reflect one of the common problems associated with non-human polysaccharide based hydrogels (carboxymethylcellulose, chitosan, alginates, etc.) utilized for tissue engineering applications, characterized by a lack of bioactivity, which usually limits cell adhesion to biomaterials and further tissue integration (Shin et al., 2004; Jing et al., 2015). One approach to promote polysaccharide biomaterials interactions with surrounding tissue has been to tether cell-binding peptides to the biomaterial, through physical or chemical modification methods, to provide biological cues to mimic cell–extracellular matrix protein interactions (Jing et al., 2015).

Polysaccharide based hydrogels, designed for bone tissue engineering, need stronger mechanical proprieties to regenerate hard tissues (Pasqui et al., 2014; Mattei et al., 2015; Michel et al., 2015). To this aim, it has been demonstrated that the combination of hydroxyapatite with natural or synthetic hydrogels improves bioactivity, osteoinductivity, and osteoconductivity (Michel et al., 2015).

A previous investigation reports that the CMC-HA hybrid hydrogel showed the presence of HA crystal homogenously distributed inside and on the hydrogel surface, improving inherent mechanical and adhesive proprieties (Pasqui et al., 2012, 2014).

HR-SEM analysis confirmed a poor adhesion of DPSCs on the CMC surface. At the end of day 21, no cells were detected on

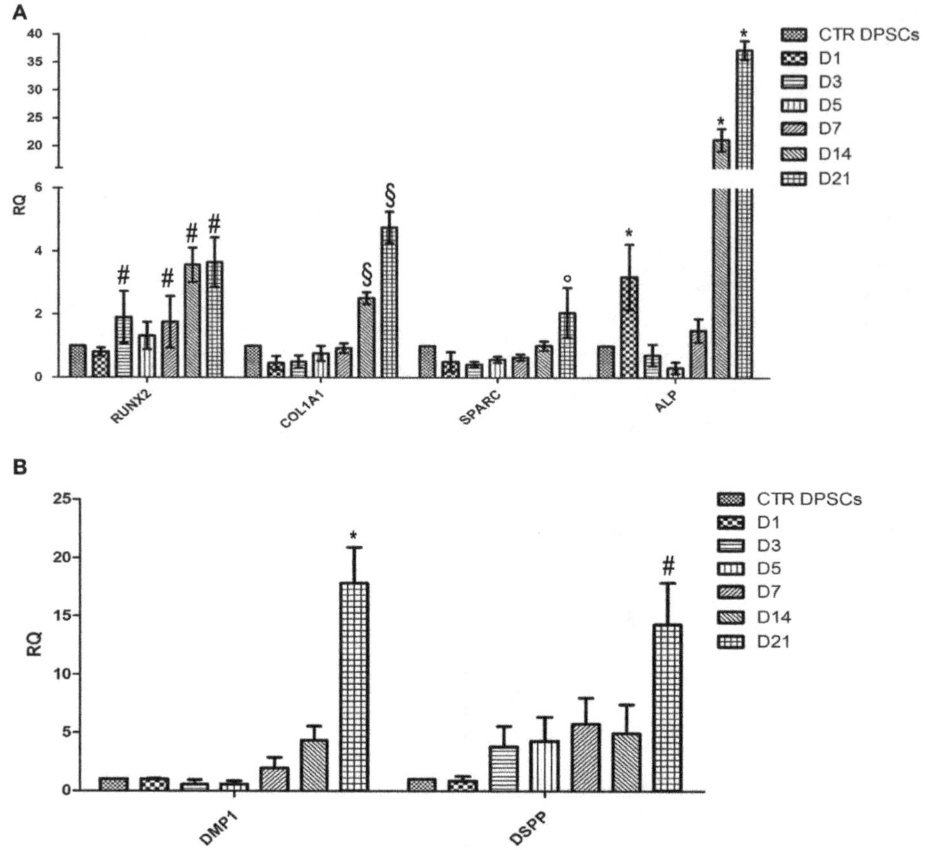


**FIGURE 7 | (A)** Quantitative Real Time PCR analysis of mRNA of RUNX-2, COL1A1, SPARC, and ALP of DPSCs cultured on CMC-HA scaffold for 1, 3, 5, 7, 14, and 21 days. Each individual assay was performed in triplicates and expressed as mean ± SD; # represents a significant difference of RUNX-2 expression relative to control DPSCs (CTR DPSCs), $P < 0.05$; §represents a significant difference of COL1A1 expression relative to control DPSCs (CTR DPSCs), $P < 0.05$; ° represents a significant difference of SPARC expression relative to control DPSCs (CTR DPSCs), $P < 0.05$; *represents a significant difference of ALP expression relative to control DPSCs (CTR DPSCs), $P < 0.05$; **(B)** Quantitative Real Time PCR analysis of mRNA of DMP-1and DSPP of DPSCs cultured on CMC-HA scaffold for 1, 3, 5, 7, 14, and 21 days. Each individual assay was performed in triplicates and expressed as mean ± SD; *represents a significant difference of DMP1 expression relative to control DPSCs (CTR DPSCs), $P < 0.05$; # represents a significant difference of DSPP expression relative to control DPSCs (CTR DPSCs).

the hydrogel surface. This result is apparently in contrast with cell viability data, where at day 7 a peak of cell viability was observed. We speculate that during the preparation of the sample for electron microscopy analysis, cells were lost due to a weak adhesion on the CMC scaffold.

HR-SEM images of the CMC-HA scaffold showed a good adhesion of cells after 1 day of culture. By the end of day 21, the cells covered the scaffold surface, showing a fibroblast-like morphology and several secretory vesicles on the cellular membrane, suggesting intense protein synthesis mainly connected with the differentiation process (Venugopal et al., 2010; Teti et al., 2012). TEM images demonstrated the presence of extracellular matrix fibrils resembling type I collagen protein at day 14 and 21, in agreement with the commitment of MSCs toward the osteogenic and odontogenic lineage (Riccio et al., 2010; Teti et al., 2012).

To fully confirm the osteogenic differentiation of DPSCs cultured on CMC-HA hydrogel, a Real Time PCR analysis was carried out to test mRNA expression of osteogenic markers such as ALP, RUNX2, COL1A1, and SPARC. RUNX2 is a transcription factor involved in osteoblastic differentiation and skeletal morphogenesis. It has been shown to affect the expression of type I collagen and SPARC by binding to the promoters of these genes. RUNX2 and COL1A1 are known to be early markers of osteoblastic differentiation while SPARC is involved in initiating mineralization and promoting mineral crystal formation during bone formation. ALP appears to be intimately related to pre-osseous cellular metabolism and to the elaboration of a calcifying bone matrix (Siffert, 1951).

The data obtained showed the expected expression profiles of the osteoblast phenotype. Results showed an up-regulation of all osteogenic markers after day 14 and 21, compared to control DPSCs. These data are in agreement with the temporal gene expression demonstrated during osteogenesis (Kulterer et al., 2007; Raggatt and Partridge, 2010; Fakhry et al., 2013). An up-regulation of RUNX2 was evident during the whole period of differentiation. COL1A1 reached a maximum of expression on day 21 in agreement with TEM images that showed the presence of extracellular fibrillary structures, resembling type I collagen protein. Also SPARC showed a nearly constant, up-regulated expression level with a peak on day 21 of differentiation.

To demonstrate odontogenic differentiation, the mRNA expression of DMP1 and DSPP genes was investigated by Real Time PCR. DMP1 plays crucial roles in the formation of dentin mineralized tissues (Ye et al., 2004). DSPP is a large protein which subsequently undergoes cleavage to generate two products: dentin sialoprotein (DSP) and dentin phosphoprotein (DPP) (Yamakoshi et al., 2006). DPP is thought to play a role during the nucleation of calcium phosphate while DSP has little or no effect on mineralization; its real function remains unclear (Yamakoshi et al., 2006). Our data demonstrated an upregulation of both odontogenic markers during the process of differentiation reaching peak levels at D14 and D21, corresponding to the phase of deposition of extracellular matrix and mineralization (Kulterer et al., 2007).

In conclusion, our *in vitro* data demonstrated that the CMC-HA hybrid hydrogel has suitable proprieties in supporting DPSCs adhesion, proliferation and osteogenic and odontogenic differentiation. This novel biomaterial could be a promising candidate for periodontal and dental pulp tissue engineering.

## AUTHOR CONTRIBUTIONS

Each author substantially contributed to experimental procedures. In particular, Dr. Teti and Prof. Orsini planned the research and experiments. Dr. Mazzotti, Dr. Dicarlo, and Dr. Durante were responsible for cell culture, differentiation treatment and hydrogel synthesis. Dott. Salvatore performed Real Time PCR data. Dott. Focaroli performed TEM analysis; Dr. Monica Mattioli Belmonte performed SEM observation. Prof. Orsini oversaw the whole research. All authors equally and competently contributed to the draft.

## FUNDING

This work was supported by Fondazione del Monte di Bologna e Ravenna.

## ACKNOWLEDGMENTS

The authors kindly thank M. Nudi, BSc, MSc for proof reading the manuscript.

## ETHICAL STATEMENT

Human dental pulp cells, utilized in this study, were obtained from healthy patients subjected to the molar extraction for orthodontic reasons. This study did not expose the donors to any risk. In lieu of a written consent form, a verbal authorization was obtained from all the recruited patients, in accordance with the Ethical Committee guidelines of the Polytechnic University of Marche.

## REFERENCES

Barbucci, R., Giardino, R., De Cagna, M., Golinia, L., and Pasqui, D. (2010). Inter-penetrating hydrogels (IPHs) as a new class of injectable polysaccharide hydrogels with thixotropic nature and interesting mechanical and biological properties. *Soft Matter.* 6, 3524. doi: 10.1039/c001949f

Conde, M. C., Chisini, L. A., Demarco, F. F., Nör, J. E., Casagrande, L., and Tarquinio, S. B. (2015). Stem Cell-Based Pulp Tissue Engineering: variables enrolled in translation from the bench to the bedside, a systematic review of literature. *Int. Endod. J.* doi: 10.1111/iej.12489. [Epub ahead of print].

d'Aquino, R., De Rosa, A., Laino, G., Caruso, F., Guida, L., Rullo, R., et al. (2009a). Human dental pulp stem cells: from biology to clinical applications. *J. Exp. Zool. B. Mol. Dev. Evol.* 312B, 408. doi: 10.1002/jez.b.21263

d'Aquino, R., De Rosa, A., Lanza, V., Tirino, V., Laino, L., Graziano, A., et al. (2009b). Human mandible bone defect repair by the grafting of dental pulp stem/progenitor cells and collagen sponge biocomplexes. *Eur. Cell Mater.* 18, 75–83.

Domingues, R. M., Gomes, M. E., and Reis, R. L. (2014). The potential of cellulose nanocrystals in tissue engineering strategies. *Biomacromolecules* 15, 2327. doi: 10.1021/bm500524s

Dominici, M., Le Blanc, K., Mueller, I., Slaper-Cortenbach, I., Marini, F., et al. (2006). Minimal criteria for defining multipotent mesenchymal stromal cells The Inter. Society for Cellular Therapy position statement. *Cytotherapy* 8, 315–317. doi: 10.1080/14653240600855905

Fakhry, M., Hamade, E., Badran, B., Buchet, R., and Magne, D. (2013). Molecular mechanisms of mesenchymal stem cell differentiation towards osteoblasts. *World J. Stem. Cells.* 5:136. doi: 10.4252/wjsc.v5.i4.136

Falconi, M., Salvatore, V., Teti, G., Focaroli, S., Durante, S., Nicolini, B., et al. (2013). Gelatin crosslinked with dehydroascorbic acid as a novel scaffold for tissue regeneration with simultaneous antitumor activity. *Biomed. Mater.* 8:035011. doi: 10.1088/1748-6041/8/3/035011

Focaroli, S., Teti, G., Salvatore, V., Durante, S., Belmonte, M. M., Giardino, R., et al. (2014). Chondrogenic differentiation of human adipose mesenchimal stem cells: influence of a biomimetic gelatin genipin crosslinked porous scaffold. *Microsc. Res. Tech.* 77, 928. doi: 10.1002/jemt.22417

Galler, K. M., D'Souza, R. N., Hartgerink, J. D., and Schmalz, G. (2011). Scaffolds for dental pulp tissue engineering. *Adv. Dent. Res.* 3, 333. doi: 10.1177/0022034511405326

Geckil, H., Xu, F., Zhang, X., Moon, S., and Demirci, U. (2010). Engineering hydrogels as extracellular matrix mimics. *Nanomedicine* 5, 469. doi: 10.2217/nnm.10.12

Giuliani, A., Manescu, A., Langer, M., Rustichelli, F., Desiderio, V., Paino, F., et al. (2013). Three years after transplants in human mandibles, histological and in-line holotomography revealed that stem cells regenerated a compact rather than a spongy bone: biological and clinical implications. *Stem. Cells Transl. Med.* 2:316. doi: 10.5966/sctm.2012-0136

Graziano, A., d'Aquino, R., Cusella-De Angelis, M. G., De Francesco, F., Giordano, A., Laino, G., et al. (2008). Scaffold's surface geometry significantly affects human stem cell bone tissue engineering. *J. Cell Physiol.* 214, 166–172. doi: 10.1002/jcp.21175

Gronthos, S., Mankani, M., Brahim, J., Robey, P. G., and Shi, S. (2000). Postnatal human dental pulp stem cells (DPSCs) *in vitro* and *in vivo*. *Proc. Natl. Acad. Sci. U.S.A.* 97, 13625–13630. doi: 10.1073/pnas.240309797

Ivanovski, S., Vaquette, C., Gronthos, S., Hutmacher, D. W., and Bartold, P. M. (2014). Multiphasic scaffolds for periodontal tissue engineering. *J. Dent. Res.* 93, 1212. doi: 10.1177/0022034514544301

Jing, J., Fournier, A., Szarpak-Jankowska, A., Block, M. R., and Auzély-Velty, R. (2015). Type, density, and presentation of grafted adhesion peptides on polysaccharide-based hydrogels control preosteoblast behavior and differentiation. *Biomacromolecules* 16:715. doi: 10.1021/bm501613u

Kabir, R., Gupta, M., Aggarwal, A., Sharma, D., Sarin, A., and Kola, M. Z. (2014). Imperative role of dental pulp stem cells in regenerative therapies: a systematic review. *Niger. J. Surg.* 20, 1. doi: 10.4103/1117-6806.127092

Kulterer, B., Friedl, G., Jandrositz, A., Sanchez-Cabo, F., Prokesch, A., Paar, C., et al. (2007). Gene expression profiling of human mesenchymal stem cells derived from bone marrow during expansion and osteoblast differentiation. *BMC Genomics* 8:70. doi: 10.1186/1471-2164-8-70

La Noce, M., Paino, F., Spina, A., Naddeo, P., Montella, R., Desiderio, V., et al. (2014). Dental pulp stem cells: state of the art and suggestions for a true translation of research into therapy. *J. Dent.* 42, 761. doi: 10.1016/j.jdent.2014.02.018

Mattei, G., Ferretti, C., Tirella, A., Ahluwalia, A., and Mattioli-Belmonte, M. (2015). Decoupling the role of stiffness from other hydroxyapatite signalling cues in periosteal derived stem cell differentiation. *Sci Rep.* 5:10778. doi: 10.1038/srep10778

Michel, J., Penna, M., Kochen, J., and Cheung, H. (2015). Recent advances in hydroxyapatite scaffolds containing mesenchymal stem cells. *Stem Cells Int.* 2015:305217. doi: 10.1155/2015/305217

Miura, M., Gronthos, S., Zhao, M., Lu, B., Fisher, L. W., Robey, P. G., et al. (2003). SHED: Stem cells from human exfoliated deciduous teeth. *Proc. Natl. Acad. Sci. U.S.A.* 100, 5807–5812. doi: 10.1073/pnas.0937635100

Morsczeck, C., Gotz, W., Schierholz, J., Zeilhofer, F., Kühn, U., Möhl, C., et al. (2005). Isolation of precursor cells (PCs) from human dental follicle of wisdom teeth. *Matrix Biol.* 24, 155–165. doi: 10.1016/j.matbio.2004.12.004

Naddeo, P., Laino, L., La Noce, M., Piattelli, A., De Rosa, A., Iezzi, G., et al. (2015). Surface biocompatibility of differently textured titanium implants with mesenchymal stem cells. *Dent. Mater.* 31, 235. doi: 10.1016/j.dental.2014.12.015

Paino, F., La Noce, M., Tirino, V., Naddeo, P., Desiderio, V., Pirozzi, G., et al. (2014). Histone deacetylase inhibition with valproic acid downregulates osteocalcin gene expression in human dental pulp stem cells and osteoblasts: evidence for HDAC2 involvement. *Stem Cells* 32, 279. doi: 10.1002/stem.1544

Pasqui, D., De Cagna, M., and Barbucci, R. (2012). Polysaccharide-based hydrogels: the key role of water in affecting mechanical properties. *Polymers* 3:1517. doi: 10.3390/polym4031517

Pasqui, D., Torricelli, P., De Cagna, M., Fini, M., and Barbucci, R. (2014). Carboxymethyl cellulose-hydroxyapatite hybrid hydrogel as a composite material for bone tissue engineering applications. *J. Biomed. Mater. Res. A.* 102, 1568–1579. doi: 10.1002/jbm.a.34810

Pisciotta, A., Carnevale, G., Meloni, S., Riccio, M., De Biasi, S., and Gibellini, L. (2015). Human dental pulp stem cells (hDPSCs): isolation, enrichment and comparative differentiation of two sub-populations. *BMC Dev. Biol.* 15:14. doi: 10.1186/s12861-015-0065-x

Pisciotta, A., Riccio, M., Carnevale, G., Beretti, F., Gibellini, L., Maraldi, T., et al. (2012). Human serum promotes osteogenic differentiation of human dental pulp stem cells *in vitro* and *in vivo*. *PLoS ONE* 7:e50542. doi: 10.1371/journal.pone.0050542

Potdar, P. D., and Jethmalani, Y. D. (2015). Human dental pulp stem cells: applications in future regenerative medicine. *World J. Stem Cells* 7:839. doi: 10.4252/wjsc.v7.i5.839

Raggatt, L. J., and Partridge, N. C. (2010). Cellular and molecular mechanisms of bone remodeling. *J. Biol. Chem.* 285, 25103. doi: 10.1074/jbc.R109.041087

Riccio, M., Resca, E., Maraldi, T., Pisciotta, A., Ferrari, A., and Bruzzesi, G. (2010). Human dental pulp stem cells produce mineralized matrix in 2D and 3D cultures. *Eur. J. Histochem.* 54:e46. doi: 10.4081/ejh.2010.e46

Seo, B. M., Miura, M., Gronthos, S., Bartold, P. M., Batouli, S., and Brahim, J. (2004). Investigation of multipotent postnatal stem cells from human periodontal ligament. *Lancet* 364, 149–155. doi: 10.1016/S0140-6736(04)16627-0

Shin, H., Zygourakis, K., Farach-Carson, M. C., Yaszemski, M. J., and Mikos, A. G. (2004). Modulation of differentiation and mineralization of marrow stromal cells cultured on biomimetic hydrogels modified with Arg-Gly-Asp containing peptides. *J. Biomed. Mater. Res. A.* 69, 535–543. doi: 10.1002/jbm.a.30027

Siffert, R. S. (1951). The role of alkaline phosphatase in osteogenesis. *J. Exp. Med.* 93, 415–426. doi: 10.1084/jem.93.5.415

Sonoyama, W., Liu, Y., Yamaza, T., Tuan, R. S., Wang, S., Shi, S., et al. (2008). Characterization of the apical papilla and its residing stem cells from human immature permanent teeth: a pilot study. *J. Endodon.* 34, 166–171. doi: 10.1016/j.joen.2007.11.021

Teti, G., Cavallo, C., Grigolo, B., Giannini, S., Facchini, A., Mazzotti, A., et al. (2012). Ultrastructural analysis of human bone marrow mesenchymal stem cells during *in vitro* osteogenesis and chondrogenesis. *Microsc. Res. Tech.* 75, 596. doi: 10.1002/jemt.21096

Teti, G., Salvatore, V., Ruggeri, A., Manzoli, L., Gesi, M., and Orsini, G. (2013). *In vitro* reparative dentin: a biochemical and morphological study. *Eur. J. Histochem.* 57:e23. doi: 10.4081/ejh.2013.e23

Tirino, V., Paino, F., d'Aquino, R., Desiderio, V., De Rosa, A., and Papaccio, G. (2011). Methods for the identification, characterization and banking of human DPSCs: current strategies and perspectives. *Stem Cell Rev.* 7, 608. doi: 10.1007/s12015-011-9235-9

Varma, D. M., Gold, G. T., Taub, P. J., and Nicoll, S. B. (2014). Injectable carboxymethylcellulose hydrogels for soft tissue filler applications. *Acta Biomater.* 10, 4996. doi: 10.1016/j.actbio.2014.08.013

Vashist, A., Ahmad, S. (2015). Hydrogels in tissue engineering: scope and applications. *Curr. Pharm. Biotechnol.* 16, 606–620. doi: 10.2174/1389201016607150427111651

Venugopal, J., Prabhakaran, M. P., Zhang, Y., Low, S., Choon, A. T., and Ramakrishna, S. (2010). Biomimetic hydroxyapatite-containing composite nanofibrous substrates for bone tissue engineering. *Philos. Trans. A. Math. Phys. Eng. Sci.* 368, 2065–2081. doi: 10.1098/rsta.2010.0012

Verma, K., Bains, R., Bains, V. K., Rawtiya, M., Loomba, K., and Srivastava, S. C. (2014). Therapeutic potential of dental pulp stem cells in regenerative medicine: an overview. *Dent. Res. J.* 11, 302–308.

Yamakoshi, Y., Hu, J. C., Iwata, T., Kobayashi, K., Fukae, M., and Simmer, J. P. (2006). Dentin sialophosphoprotein is processed by MMP2 and MMP20 *in vitro* and *in vivo*. *J. Biol. Chem.* 281, 38235–38243. doi: 10.1074/jbc.M607767200

Ye, L., MacDougall, M., Zhang, S., Xie, Y., Zhang, J., Li, Z., et al. (2004). Deletion of dentin matrix protein-1 leads to a partial failure of maturation of predentin into dentin, hypomineralization, and expanded cavities of pulp and root canal during postnatal tooth development. *J. Biol. Chem.* 279, 19141–19148. doi: 10.1074/jbc.m400490200

# Permissions

All chapters in this book were first published in DPTFRCAFC, by Frontiers Media SA; hereby published with permission under the Creative Commons Attribution License or equivalent. Every chapter published in this book has been scrutinized by our experts. Their significance has been extensively debated. The topics covered herein carry significant findings which will fuel the growth of the discipline. They may even be implemented as practical applications or may be referred to as a beginning point for another development.

The contributors of this book come from diverse backgrounds, making this book a truly international effort. This book will bring forth new frontiers with its revolutionizing research information and detailed analysis of the nascent developments around the world.

We would like to thank all the contributing authors for lending their expertise to make the book truly unique. They have played a crucial role in the development of this book. Without their invaluable contributions this book wouldn't have been possible. They have made vital efforts to compile up to date information on the varied aspects of this subject to make this book a valuable addition to the collection of many professionals and students.

This book was conceptualized with the vision of imparting up-to-date information and advanced data in this field. To ensure the same, a matchless editorial board was set up. Every individual on the board went through rigorous rounds of assessment to prove their worth. After which they invested a large part of their time researching and compiling the most relevant data for our readers.

The editorial board has been involved in producing this book since its inception. They have spent rigorous hours researching and exploring the diverse topics which have resulted in the successful publishing of this book. They have passed on their knowledge of decades through this book. To expedite this challenging task, the publisher supported the team at every step. A small team of assistant editors was also appointed to further simplify the editing procedure and attain best results for the readers.

Apart from the editorial board, the designing team has also invested a significant amount of their time in understanding the subject and creating the most relevant covers. They scrutinized every image to scout for the most suitable representation of the subject and create an appropriate cover for the book.

The publishing team has been an ardent support to the editorial, designing and production team. Their endless efforts to recruit the best for this project, has resulted in the accomplishment of this book. They are a veteran in the field of academics and their pool of knowledge is as vast as their experience in printing. Their expertise and guidance has proved useful at every step. Their uncompromising quality standards have made this book an exceptional effort. Their encouragement from time to time has been an inspiration for everyone.

The publisher and the editorial board hope that this book will prove to be a valuable piece of knowledge for researchers, students, practitioners and scholars across the globe.

# List of Contributors


**Maitane Aurrekoetxea, Patricia Garcia-Gallastegui, Igor Irastorza, Jon Luzuriaga, Verónica Uribe-Etxebarria, Fernando Unda and Gaskon Ibarretxe**
Department of Cell Biology and Histology, Faculty of Medicine and Dentistry, University of the Basque Country, Leioa, Spain

**Daisuke Akita, Naoki Tsukimura and Tomohiko Ishigami**
Department of Partial Denture Prosthodontics, School of Dentistry, Nihon University, Tokyo, Japan

**Koichiro Kano**
Laboratory of Cell and Tissue Biology, College of Bioresource Science, Nihon University, Fujisawa, Japan

**Yoko Saito-Tamura and Niina Tsurumachi**
Department of Orthodontics, School of Dentistry, Nihon University, Tokyo, Japan

**Takayuki Mashimo**
Department of Oral and Maxillofacial Surgery, Faculty of Medicine, Juntendo University, Tokyo, Japan

**Momoko Sato-Shionome**
Department of Pediatric Dentistry, School of Dentistry, Nihon University, Tokyo, Japan

**Katsuyuki Yamanaka and Tadashi Kaneko**
GC Corp. R&D, Tokyo, Japan

**Taku Toriumi and Keitaro Isokawa**
Department of Anatomy, School of Dentistry, Nihon University, Tokyo, Japan

**Yoshinori Arai**
School of Dentistry, Nihon University, Tokyo, Japan

**Taro Matsumoto**
Division of Cell Regeneration and Transplantation, Department of Functional Morphology, School of Medicine, Nihon University, Tokyo, Japan

**Masaki Honda**
Department of Oral Anatomy, School of Dentistry, Aichi-Gakuin University, Nagoya, Japan

**Hugo Fabre, Frédéric Mallein-Gerin and Emeline Perrier-Groult**
Laboratoire de Biologie Tissulaire et Ingénierie thérapeutique, UMR5305 Centre National de la Recherche Scientifique/Université Claude Bernard Lyon 1, Lyon, France

**Giovanna Orsini**
Department of Clinical Sciences and Stomatology, Polytechnic University of Marche, Ancona, Italy

**Maria C. Mazzotti**
Department of Medical and Surgical Sciences, University of Bologna, Italy

**Olivier Degoul, Gianluigi Atzeni, Colin McGuckin and Nico Forraz**
CTI-BIOTECH, Cell Therapy Research Institute, Meyzieu, France

**Brigitte Alliot-Licht**
Faculté d'Odontologie, Institut National de la Santé et de la Recherche Médicale UMR1064, Centre de Recherche en Transplantation et Immunologie, Université de Nantes, Nantes, France

**Luigi Mele, Virginia Tirino, Francesca Paino, Davide Liccardo, Gianpaolo Papaccio and Vincenzo Desiderio**
Department of Experimental Medicine, Section of Biotechnology and Medical Histology and Embryology, Second University of Naples, Naples, Italy

**Pietro Paolo Vitiello**
Medical Oncology, Dipartimento Medico-Chirurgico di Internistica Clinica e Sperimentale "F. Magrassi e A. Lanzara," Second University of Naples, Naples, Italy

**Alfredo De Rosa**
Department of Odontology and Surgery, Second University of Naples, Naples, Italy

**Anna Woloszyk and Thimios A. Mitsiadis**
Orofacial Development and Regeneration, Center of Dental Medicine, Institute of Oral Biology, University of Zurich, Zurich, Switzerland

**Johanna Buschmann**
Plastic Surgery and Hand Surgery, University Hospital Zurich, Zurich, Switzerland

**Conny Waschkies**
Institute for Biomedical Engineering, ETH and University of Zurich, Zurich, Switzerland
Visceral and Transplant Surgery, University Hospital Zurich, Zurich, Switzerland

**Bernd Stadlinger**
Clinic of Cranio-Maxillofacial and Oral Surgery, University of Zurich, University Hospital Zurich, Zurich, Switzerland

**Davide Liccardo**
Section of Biotechnology and Medical Histology and Embryology, Department of Experimental Medicine, Second University of Naples, Naples, Italy

**Igor Adameyko**
Department of Physiology and Pharmacology, Karolinska Institutet, Stockholm, Sweden
Department of Molecular Neurosciences, Center of Brain Research, Medical University of Vienna, Vienna, Austria

**Kaj Fried**
Department of Neuroscience, Karolinska Institutet, Stockholm, Sweden

**Min Oh**
Department of Cariology, Restorative Sciences, Endodontics, University of Michigan School of Dentistry, Ann Arbor, MI, USA

**Jacques E. Nör**
Department of Cariology, Restorative Sciences, Endodontics, University of Michigan School of Dentistry, Ann Arbor, MI, USA
Department of Otolaryngology, University of Michigan School of Medicine, Ann Arbor, MI, USA
Department of Biomedical Engineering, University of Michigan College of Engineering, Ann Arbor, MI, USA

**Zhi Chen**
The State Key Laboratory Breeding Base of Basic Science of Stomatology (Hubei-MOST) and Key Laboratory of Oral Biomedicine Ministry of Education, School and Hospital of Stomatology, Wuhan University, Wuhan, China

**Jingwen Yang and Guohua Yuan**
The State Key Laboratory Breeding Base of Basic Science of Stomatology (Hubei-MOST) and Key Laboratory of Oral Biomedicine Ministry of Education, School and Hospital of Stomatology, Wuhan University, Wuhan, China
Department of Pediatric Dentistry, School and Hospital of Stomatology, Wuhan University, Wuhan, China

**Agathoklis D. Passos, Aikaterini A. Mouza and Spiros V. Paras**
Department of Chemical Engineering, Aristotle University of Thessaloniki, Thessaloniki, Greece

**Christos Gogos and Dimitrios Tziafas**
Department of Endodontology, School of Dentistry, Aristotle University of Thessaloniki, Thessaloniki, Greece

**Aurélie Bellanger and Françoise Bleicher**
Institut de Génomique Fonctionnelle de Lyon, UMR5242 Centre National de la Recherche Scientifique/ENS/ Université Lyon 1, Equipe Physiopathologie des Odontoblastes, Lyon, France

**Florence Carrouel**
Institut de Génomique Fonctionnelle de Lyon, UMR5242 Centre National de la Recherche Scientifique/ENS/ Université Lyon 1, Equipe Physiopathologie des Odontoblastes, Lyon, France
Faculté d'Odontologie, Université Lyon 1, Université de Lyon, Lyon, France

**Béatrice Richard**
Institut de Génomique Fonctionnelle de Lyon, UMR5242 Centre National de la Recherche Scientifique/ENS/ Université Lyon 1, Equipe Physiopathologie des Odontoblastes, Lyon, France
Faculté d'Odontologie, Université Lyon 1, Université de Lyon, Lyon, France
Hospices Civils de Lyon, Service de Consultations et Traitements Dentaires, Lyon, France

**Jean-Christophe Farges**
Institut de Génomique Fonctionnelle de Lyon, UMR5242 Centre National de la Recherche Scientifique/ENS/ Université Lyon 1, Equipe Physiopathologie des Odontoblastes, Lyon, France
Faculté d'Odontologie, Université Lyon 1, Université de Lyon, Lyon, France
Hospices Civils de Lyon, Service de Consultations et Traitements Dentaires, Lyon, France
Laboratoire de Biologie Tissulaire et Ingénierie Thérapeutique, Institut de Biologie et Chimie des Protéines, UMR5305 Centre National de la Recherche Scientifique/Université Lyon 1, Lyon, France

**Maxime Ducret**
Faculté d'Odontologie, Université Lyon 1, Université de Lyon, Lyon, France
Hospices Civils de Lyon, Service de Consultations et Traitements Dentaires, Lyon, France
Laboratoire de Biologie Tissulaire et Ingénierie Thérapeutique, Institut de Biologie et Chimie des Protéines, UMR5305 Centre National de la Recherche Scientifique/Université Lyon 1, Lyon, France

**Elisabeth Aubert-Foucher**
Laboratoire de Biologie Tissulaire et Ingénierie Thérapeutique, Institut de Biologie et Chimie des Protéines, UMR5305 Centre National de la Recherche Scientifique/Université Lyon 1, Lyon, France

**Masaki Sato, Maki Kimura, Yuki Kojima, Masakazu Tazaki and Yoshiyuki Shibukawa**
Department of Physiology, Tokyo Dental College, Tokyo, Japan

**Toru Sato**
Department of Crown and Bridge Prosthodontics, Tokyo Dental College, Tokyo, Japan

**Tadashi Furuya**
Department of Physiology, Tokyo Dental College, Tokyo, Japan
Department of Crown and Bridge Prosthodontics, Tokyo Dental College, Tokyo, Japan

**Asha Eapen and Anne George**
Brodie Tooth Development Genetics and Regenerative Medicine, Department of Oral Biology, University of Illinois at Chicago, Chicago, IL, USA

**Hans U. Luder**
Center of Dental Medicine, Institute of Oral Biology, University of Zurich, Zurich, Switzerland

**Christiaan M. Suttorp, Rui Xie, Ditte M. S. Lundvig, Anne Marie Kuijpers-Jagtman, Jasper Tom Uijttenboogaart, René Van Rheden, Jaap C. Maltha and Frank A. D. T. G. Wagener**
Department of Orthodontics and Craniofacial Biology, Radboud university medical centre, Radboud Institute for Molecular Life Sciences, Nijmegen, Netherlands

**Min Liu**
Department of Periodontology, Stomatological Hospital, Jilin University, Changchun, China

**David A. Reed, Xuanyu Lu and Xianghong Luan**
Department of Oral Biology, University of Illinois, Chicago, IL, USA

**Giancarlo M. Cecchini**
College of Dentistry, Midwestern University, Downers Grove, IL, USA

**Karan Ganjawalla**
School of Dental Medicine, Harvard University, Boston, MA, USA

**Carol S. Gonzales and Richard Monahan**
Department of Oral Diagnosis, University of Illinois College of Dentistry, Chicago, IL, USA

**Thomas G. H. Diekwisch**
Department of Oral Biology, University of Illinois, Chicago, IL, USA
Center for Craniofacial Research and Diagnosis and Department of Periodontics, Texas A&M University Baylor College of Dentistry, Dallas, TX, USA

**David W. Green and Han-Sung Jung**
Division in Anatomy and Developmental Biology, Department of Oral Biology, Oral Science Research Center, BK21 PLUS Project, Yonsei University College of Dentistry, Seoul, South Korea
Oral Biosciences, Faculty of Dentistry, the University of Hong Kong, Hong Kong, Hong Kong

**Jung-Seok Lee**
Department of Periodontology, Research Institute for Periodontal Regeneration, Yonsei University College of Dentistry, Seoul, South Korea

**Sriram Ravindran, Chun-Chieh Huang and Raghuvaran Narayanan**
Departments of Oral Biology, University of Illinois at Chicago, Chicago, IL, USA

**Praveen Gajendrareddy**
Departments of Periodontics, University of Illinois at Chicago, Chicago, IL, USA

**Andrea Gama**
Institut National de la Santé et de la Recherche Médicale, UMR-1138, Equipe 5, Centre de Recherche des Cordeliers, Paris France
Odontologic Center of District Federal Military Police, Brasilia, Brazil

**Benjamin Navet and Frédéric Lézot**
Institut National de la Santé et de la Recherche Médicale, UMR-957, Equipe Ligue Nationale Contre le Cancer, Nantes, France
Laboratoire de Physiopathologie de la Résorption Osseuse et Thérapie des Tumeurs Osseuses Primitives, Faculté de Médecine, Université de Nantes, Nantes, France

**Jorge William Vargas**
Institut National de la Santé et de la Recherche Médicale, UMR-957, Equipe Ligue Nationale Contre le Cancer, Nantes, France
Laboratoire de Physiopathologie de la Résorption Osseuse et Thérapie des Tumeurs Osseuses Primitives, Faculté de Médecine, Université de Nantes, Nantes, France
Department of Basic Studies, Faculty of Odontology, University of Antioquia, Medellin, Colombia

**Beatriz Castaneda**
Institut National de la Santé et de la Recherche Médicale, UMR-1138, Equipe 5, Centre de Recherche des Cordeliers, Paris France
Department of Basic Studies, Faculty of Odontology, University of Antioquia, Medellin, Colombia

**Milena Fini**
Laboratory of Preclinical and Surgical Studies, Rizzoli Orthopaedic Institute, Bologna, Italy

**Anna Spina, Roberta Montella, Davide Liccardo and Marcella La Noce**
Sezione di Biotecnologie, Dipartimento di Medicina Sperimentale, Istologia Medica e Biologia Molecolare, Seconda Università degli Studi di Napoli, Napoli, Italy

**Alfredo De Rosa**
Sezione di Odontostomatologia, Dipartimento Multidisciplinare Medico-chirurgico, Seconda Università degli Studi di Napoli, Napoli, Italy

**Luigi Laino**
Dipartimento di Medicina Clinica e Sperimentale, Università degli Studi di Foggia, Foggia, Italy

**Lucia Jimenez-Rojo and Despoina Natsiou**
Department of Clinical Sciences and Stomatology, Marche Polytechnic University, Ancona, Italy

**Gabriella Teti, Viviana Salvatore, Stefano Focaroli, Mirella Falconi, Alessandra Ruggeri and Sandra Durante**
Department of Biomedical and Neuromotor Sciences, University of Bologna, Bologna, Italy

**Antonio Mazzotti**
1st Orthopaedic and Traumatologic Clinic, Rizzoli Orthopedic Institute, Bologna, Italy

**Manuela Dicarlo, Monia Orciani, Roberto Di Primio and Monica Mattioli-Belmonte**
Department of Clinical and Molecular Sciences, Polytechnic University of Marche, Ancona, Italy